Lucia Raggetti

ʿĪsā ibn ʿAlī's Book on the Useful Properties of Animal Parts

Science, Technology, and Medicine in Ancient Cultures

Edited by
Markus Asper
Philip van der Eijk
Mark Geller
Heinrich von Staden
Liba Taub

Volume 6

Lucia Raggetti

ʿĪsā ibn ʿAlī's Book on the Useful Properties of Animal Parts

Edition, translation and study of a fluid tradition

DE GRUYTER

ISBN 978-3-11-054986-7
e-ISBN (PDF) 978-3-11-055036-8
e-ISBN (EPUB) 978-3-11-054994-2
ISSN 2194-976X

Library of Congress Control Number: 2018961123

Bibliographic information published by the Deutsche Nationalbibliothek
The Deutsche Nationalbibliothek lists this publication in the Deutsche Nationalbibliografie; detailed bibliographic data are available on the Internet at http://dnb.dnb.de.

Printing and binding: CPI books GmbH, Leck

www.degruyter.com

FSC www.fsc.org MIX Papier aus verantwortungsvollen Quellen FSC® C083411

Preface

This book is based on my PhD dissertation, defended in April 2012. Two lines of thought led me to select this topic: a desire to keep working on Arabo-Islamic animal literature—an important section of readings in my curriculum of study—and curiosity about working with manuscripts. Curiosity is fundamental for the scholar and, luckily, it is not fatal to all animals. The literature on properties and especially the textual criticism on fluid traditions in Arabic is mostly uncharted territory. I tried to develop linear and empirical ways to handle this large and complex tradition, and make it available in a reliable edition with an English translation. The publication has been designed as a research tool, not just for arabists, but also scholars of the history of ancient medicine and science in different cultural and linguistic traditions. Once it has been tamed, such an unruly tradition—in which 'everything is similar but nothing is the same'—opens large horizons and new perspectives on the 'science of properties', its transmission and its contents. Looking at any opening of the edition with its mirror translation, one is immediately struck by a *horror vacui* inspired by the blank space at the bottom of the odd pages. The annotation of the text, with the *loci similes* in Arabic literature as well as in other traditions, would have occupied several other volumes and years. It remains, however, a *desideratum* for the continuation of my research.

Acknowledgements

I would like to thank Giovanni Canova, who inspired my passion for Mediaeval Arabic literature. Remke Kruk deserves special thanks for all the support and time she generously gave during the years of the PhD, and the dear friendship that resulted from our cooperation. To Mark Geller—and his research group—my thanks for all the formative experiences, the unique scholarly opportunities and the enthusiastic support: the years in Berlin really made the difference. For his linguistic help and all the interesting discussions we had in our years together in Berlin, I am grateful to Pavel Pavlovic who shared with me his exquisite knowledge of the Arabic language and his unfailing sympathy. I would also like to thank Philip van der Eijk and his research group, who always welcomed me and gave me important feedback. In particular, my friend and colleague Matteo Martelli, who shared his vast knowledge and encouraged me in the final metres. I am grateful, too, for the friendly advice and constant support of Alessandro Bausi, Antonella Brita and Caroline Macé, from whom I learnt the philological trade.

Table of Contents

Edition and translation

Introduction

I. Authorship and Genre

I.1 ʿĪsā ibn ʿAlī and his fate

Arabic sources unanimously present ʿĪsā ibn ʿAlī as both one of Ḥunayn Ibn Isḥāq's most brilliant students and the author of a book on the properties of animals. ʿĪsā ibn ʿAlī served as court physician to the Abbasid Caliph al-Muʿtamid (256–279 H/870–892 AD), during an era noteworthy in Islamic culture for its extraordinary vitality and creativity. This portrait of ʿĪsā ibn ʿAlī emerges from a review of several bio-bibliographical sources. The first mention of him is in the *Fihrist*.[1]

> ʿĪsā ibn ʿAlī
> He was one of the pupils of Ḥunayn [Ibn Isḥāq] and an excellent man. Among his books there was *The Book of Useful Properties obtained from the parts of animals.*

In the later tradition, however, the fact that his name so closely resembles that of another physician has partially hidden the historical tracks left by our author. Indeed, he was soon mistaken for the famous oculist ʿAlī ibn ʿĪsā, even though the latter lived a century and half after ʿĪsā ibn ʿAlī.[2] ʿĪsā ibn ʿAlī appears in both the well-known reference works of medieval Islamic medicine, viz. in Ibn abī ʿUṣaybiʿa's *ʿUyūn al-anbāʾ fī-ṭabaqāt al-aṭibbāʾ* ('The Sources of information about the Generations of Physicians') and Ibn al-Qifṭī's *Taʾrīḫ al-ḥukamāʾ* ('Chronology of the Learned Men').

Ibn Abī ʿUṣaybiʿa mentions both physicians in two different entries. ʿĪsā ibn ʿAlī can be found in the eighth chapter, alongside several members of the Buḫtišūʿ's family, where they are referred to as 'Syriac physicians who lived in the early times of the Abbasid rule'.[3]

> He was a noteworthy physician who was also prominent in the field of philosophy and wrote various works on this subject. He studied the practice of medicine under the guidance of Ḥunayn ibn Isḥāq and was considered one of his more brilliant disciples. He served Aḥmad ibn al-Mutawakkil, that is al-Muʿtamid bi-Allāh. He was his personal physician for a long time and when [Aḥmad] obtained the dignity of the Caliphate, he favoured and honoured ʿĪsā ibn ʿAlī and lavishly bestowed precious gifts on him. Several books are ascribed to ʿĪsā ibn ʿAlī: *The Book of Useful Properties obtained from the Parts of Animals*, and a *Book of Poisons* [in two chapters].

The almost homonymous ʿAlī ibn ʿĪsā (d. 400 H/1010 AD) is mentioned in the tenth chapter as an outstanding ophtalmologist, who composed the famous *Taḏkirat al-Kaḥḥālīn* ('The Reference Work for the Ophtalmologist') in three books.[4] So in Ibn Abī ʿUṣaybiʿa's work at least the distinction between the two figures is clear. In Ibn al-Qifṭī's *Taʾrīḫ al-Ḥukamāʾ*, however, the two physicians are conflated and their entries merged.[5]

> ʿĪsā ibn ʿAlī, one of the disciples of Ḥunayn [ibn Isḥāq], an author famous for his book *Reference work for Oculists* (*Taḏkirat al-Kaḥḥālīn*), on which the doctors in this field subsequently based their work—*The Book of Useful Properties obtained from the Parts of Animals.*

1 See Ibn al-Nadīm 1970, II 699; for the Arabic text, see Ibn al-Nadīm 1872, I 297.

2 See Mittwoch, E., "ʿAlī b. ʿĪsā', in: *Encyclopaedia of Islam*, Second Edition, Edited by: P. Bearman, Th. Bianquis, C.E. Bosworth, E. van Donzel, W.P. Heinrichs. Consulted online on 13 February 2018 http://dx.doi.org/10.1163/1573-3912_islam_SIM_0513.

3 See Ibn abī ʿUṣaybiʿa 1884, 123 and 203.

4 Ibid., 247.

5 Ibn al-Qifṭī 1903, 237. This problematic passage misled Ibn al-Qifṭī's editor, who added a cross-reference to the passage on ʿĪsā ibn ʿAlī in Ibn Abī ʿUṣaybiʿa, see Ibn al-Qifṭī 1903, 247. Wüstenfeld and Leclerc instead followed Ibn al-Nadīm, so the two physicians remain entirely distinct. They blame the misunderstanding on the problematic manuscript tradition of the eighth chapter of Ibn Abī ʿUṣaybiʿa's work, see Wüstenfeld 1840,39, and Leclerc 1876, I 303–304). Both Ullmann and Eisenstein mention ʿĪsā ibn ʿAlī as a prominent figure in the earliest phase of medico-zoographical literature, see Ullmann 1972, 21–22 and Eisenstein 1991, 96).

The figure that emerges from the sources is that of a prestigious author who lived at a very early and golden moment of Arabo-Islamic civilization. However, as a result of the aforementioned confusion over his identity, ʿĪsā ibn ʿAlī partly disappeared from the biographical tradition. Inevitably, this biographical state of affairs affected the transmission of ʿĪsā ibn ʿAlī's text. On the one hand, an ancient and prestigious authorship prevented this collection of recipes from getting lost among the anonymous mass of similar compositions; on the other hand, the long time span of the transmission, and the uncertainty about the authorship created the conditions for a fluid transmission of the text.

This unfortunate homonymic case is not enough, however, to explain the oblivion into which ʿĪsā ibn ʿAlī sank. The extraordinary development of Arabic medicine probably played a role as well. There is no reason to doubt that, during his lifetime, and proably for at least a century after, ʿĪsā ibn ʿAlī enjoyed a reputation as a brillant and important physician. His appointment at the court is a tangible sign of his professional prestige. However, if one compares the collection of recipes edited here with the medical encyclopedias and treatises composed shortly thereafter—al-Tabārī's (3rd cent. H/9th cent. AD) *Firdaws al-ḥikma* ('The Paradise of Wisdom'),[6] al-Rāzī's (250–313 or 323 H/834–925 or 935 AD) *Kitāb al-ḥāwī* ('*Liber Continens*'), Ibn Sīnā's (370–428 H/980–1037 AD) *Qānūn fi-l-ṭibb* ('Canon of Medicine'), to name a few examples—the book by ʿĪsā ibn ʿAlī seems to correspond to a more archaic phase that preceded the unfolding of the golden age of Arabic medicine. The titles mentioned became reference works in the field of medicine, casting their shadow over other 'minor' works. It would be inappropriate, however, to see ʿĪsā ibn ʿAlī's *Manāfiʿ* as the petty result of a primitive age, in which Arabic medicine was clumsily taking its first steps. This was rather a moment when contacts and interactions with a large number of non-Arabic sources were particularly intense, no doubt thanks to the multicultural background of the author: his native language was probably Syriac, he wrote in Arabic, and it highly likely that he came into contact with the Greco-Arabic translation movement.

One may wonder, then, how, in spite of all these disadvantages, the text managed to survive. It is likely that, even as medical interest in this text was waning, a new kind of interest in its contents arose. The recipes started to be read as a collection of curious and wondrous tricks. This delineates two different readerships: one interested in medical knowledge, the other attracted by the more curious aspects of the recipes. However, it would be unwise to trace any kind of sharp division in terms of periods and readership, for the use of animal substances for healing purposes clearly survived alongside new models of medicine and pharmacology. Even after Arabic medicine had moved on, the text survived as a collection of curious and amusing tales, in Arabic *ʿaǧāʾib wa-ġarāʾib*, which maintained a literary interest in the materials.[7] In other words, the textual tradition did not die, but rather shifted in the direction of a 'Book of Secrets'.[8] This change also made the text prone to including all kinds of heterogeneous materials.

According to this scenario, the name of ʿĪsā ibn ʿAlī as the author of a collection of recipes based on animal ingredients remained an important element, conferring authority and reliability upon the text. He was either identified as the most outstanding ophtalmologist, or as a nebulous character, who nevertheless lived during the great and highly idealized phase of early Abbasid rule, an authorial presence that, in any case, would have strengthened the importance of the text.

I.2 Title and introduction

Even if Arabic sources did not always attribute the work to the correct physician, they are in agreement about the title of the work: *Kitāb al-manāfiʿ allatī tustafādu min aʿḍāʾ al-ḥayawān* ('The Book of Useful Properties That

6 The *Firdaws al-ḥikma* is the first medical encyclopedia in Arabic: for this and its early composition date, it is particularly relevant to compare it with ʿĪsā ibn ʿAlī's work, see Ṭabarī 1928; see also Ullmann 1978, 108..

7 Clues to this shift can be found in the manuscript tradition, where one often finds comments in the margins of the recipes. These marginalia often consist of a single word, either *ʿaǧīb* (wondrous) or *ġarīb* (strange). Moreover, the more technical and positive *muǧarrab* ('tried out') can also be found among the marginal comments, see Raggetti 2015.

8 See Eamon's description of this tradition in Mediaeval and Early Modern Europe (Eamon 1994).

Can Be Obtained From Parts of Animals'). The manuscript tradition reveals a number of different titles, but does not include the one recorded by Ibn al-Nadīm and the other sources.[9]

The passage in the text highlighting the authorship is the introduction to the book. It is not possible to ascertain whether this passage really does originate from the pen of the author;[10] nonetheless, there are some clear indications about the composition of the work, the use of the sources, the organization and the purpose of the book. These key elements of the composition cut across the whole manuscript tradition, in spite the general fluidity of its wording. The adherence of later compilers and copyists to the guidelines announced in the introduction should not be taken for granted.

The first point in the introduction describes the author's efforts to collect materials. The composition of the book began with the collection of relevant passages from a variety of ancient sources. The names of a number of authorities in the field of medicine and *physiologika* are mentioned here, whereas in the rest of the text the sources remain unattributed. All the manuscript witnesses mention Hermes Trismegistos and Democritus as sources, and they were almost certainly responsible for the transmission of large amounts of materials on the sympathetic properties of natural objects in the Greek tradition.[11] Other authorities are mentioned as well, for instance Euclides and Hippocrates. Such names, however, appear to have been added in order to give authority to the text of a specific copy, rather than as reference to actual sources. The actual number of sources may well have been much higher, but all of them remain implicit. In the branch (b) of the tradition, there is a further remark on the selection of materials. The author sieved through his sources, discarding any materials that were not relavant for his book, in particular any spells and charms that implied an opposition to the useful properties.[12] This awareness of the problematic relationship between these two entities is evidenced by the author's decision to select recipes on a qualitative base.

The originality of the book emerges on a formal level. While the materials were known and drawn from authoritative ancient sources—so well known or so easily recognized that they could remain implicit—the structure is presented as entirely innovative: the materials are organized in chapters and divided by animal.[13]

All these efforts to reorganize the materials, creating a new arrangement, were carried out for the benefit of the prospective reader: the author aims to facilitate the search for particular pieces of information within the book.[14]

The general impression is that the author is inscribing himself in a long tradition that goes back to antiquity and Hellenism. While the Greek component in the sources is predominant, it does not muffle the echo of other texts. The nature of ʿĪsā ibn ʿAlī's innovation was chiefly formal, and consisted of a radically new organization of the materials.

---

9 For the titles attested to in the manuscript tradition, see the description of the manuscript witnesses, ch. IV.

10 In theory, it may well be a fictional literary construction.

11 Only fragments of his works survive, transmitted in the form of short passages arranged on a thematic base with, as a consequence, a particularly fluid transmission. Still, there are enough fragments to state that the analogy between their works and the *manāfiʿ/ḫawāṣṣ* literature is real, see Wellmann 1928, 10 and Laurenti 1985, 91.

12 Nevertheless, a number of recipes mention magic, describing practices and suggesting how to protect oneself from it, see 'Thematic Index'.

13 If we are to believe what the introduction says about the ancient sources, properties and sympathies had to be listed simply without any particular criterion for their order. If the perception in the 9th century was such, then the organization in chapters by animal already represents a huge innovation. This lack of internal organization is mirrored more widely by the section on pharmacological preparations based on animal ingredients in the *Naturalis Historia* (XXVIII–XXXII), which ultimately results in an overwhelming entanglement: if we take the introduction at face value, we might have expected arbitrary lists of properties and sympathies. This is just an example, illustrating that, in the perception of the 9th-century audience, the organization of this material in chapters—with each chapter dedicated to ingredients deriving from a particular animal—might genuinely have been perceived as a huge innovation.

14 The introduction in (b) even mentions numbers assigned to the chapters.

I.3 Manāfiʿ vs. ḫawāṣṣ

In connection with ʿĪsā ibn ʿAlī, the Arabic sources only speak of *manāfiʿ* (useful properties), and not about *ḫawāṣṣ* (occult properties). In most of the texts dealing with the 'science of properties',[15] the two terms go side by side, and are used to label a diverse accumulation of recipes and a huge amount of animal lore. In the wider manuscript tradition, the expressions *manāfiʿ* (useful properties) and *ḫawāṣṣ* (occult properties) are used interchangeably.

The apparently inextricable entanglement can be overcome by focusing on the common traits shared by all the recipes and prescriptions: they are all based on the properties of natural objects and circulated under the aforementioned labels of *manāfiʿ*, and *ḫawāṣṣ*. The lexicographical significance of these two categories has turned out to be quite a productive approach to defining their distinct characteristics.

> *Manāfiʿ* (sing. *manfaʿa*): a cause, or means of advantage, profit, utility; or benefit: and simply, advantage; profit or profitableness; utility, use, usefulness; or benefit. Contrary of *maḍarra*.[16]
> *Ḫawāṣṣ* (sing. *ḫāṣṣa*): A property of a thing not found, or not existing, either wholly or partly in another thing.
> *Ḫawāṣṣ* (sing. *ḫāṣṣiyya*): a property, or particular or peculiar virtue which is an unknown cause of a known effect; as that by which a medicine operates: the former differs from the latter in being conventionally applied to an effect, or effective property, whether the cause of its existence be known or not. And *ḫawāṣṣ* is a quasi-plural noun, not a plural.[17]

The difference between *manāfiʿ* and *ḫawāṣṣ* seems to be in the transparency of the underlying causal correlations. When the relation between cause and effect is clear and, indeed, can be deduced and known, then it can be classified as *manafiʿ*; by contrast, in respect of *ḫawāṣṣ*, only the effect is known, while the causal process remains unintellegible.

The hidden causal process of the *ḫawāṣṣ* is presented as their signature, also in the theoretical statements formulated by al-Ṭabarī and al-Rāzī shortly after the composition of ʿĪsā ibn ʿAlī's book. The *Firdaws al-ḥikma* can be considered as the first medical encyclopedia in Arabic and, as well as having the features of a genre pioneer, it preserves a number of archaicizing traits,[18] among them a long section on the useful properties of animals. At a different place in the work, al-Ṭabarī defines the *ḫawāṣṣ* in contrast to the *quwwa* ('faculty', often used to translate the Greek term *dynamis*, especially in the context of the Galenic translations).[19] Al-Ṭabarī wrote that the senses can grasp the *quwwa*, whereas hidden properties can be comprehended only through experience.[20]

> **Occult properties of things**
> With the help of God, I have already written what I wanted to write about the faculty (*quwwa*) of the bodies, the diseases and their own peculiar moments, and also other things about the tests, the urine, and other similar issues that the physician should not neglect. Now I will mention the faculty of the natural objects (litt. *ašiyāʾ*, things), the signs of this faculty in the colours, in the flavours, and in the senses, with the permission and the help of God. Each natural object, in fact, has a faculty that can be perceived with the senses, but it has also an occult property (*ḫāṣṣa*) that is unknown, whose depth cannot be grasped but by trying it out several times (*taǧārib*, lit. 'experiences'), because the occult properties are a mystery hidden in the natural objects. Like the occult property of the magnet that attracts iron and the particles of chaff. Among the natural objects whose occult property is to make the bladder stones crumble, when they reach the bladder, there are things like burnt scorpions and wild celery seeds.

15 I borrowed this expression from Paul Kraus, who used it for a particular section of the *Corpus Gabirianum* dealing with the properties of natural objects. See Kraus 1942, 61–70, and Raggetti 2015.

16 Lane 1863, VIII 3036.

17 Ibid., II 747.

18 I discuss the commission of innovative and archaic elements in the *Firdaws al-ḥikma* in a forthcoming article 'The Paradise of Wisdom: Streams of Tradition in the First Medical Encyclopaedia in Arabic', in *Cultural Systems of Classification: Sickness, Health and Local Epistemologies*, in the Routledge Series 'Body and Medicine in Antiquity'

19 Ullmann 2002, 208–209.

20 See al-Ṭabarī 1928, 355.

Al-Rāzī composed a short essay on occult properties, the *Kitāb al-ḫawāṣṣ*, collecting quotations from Classical Greek authors and a few contemporary colleagues, the materials here are arranged alphabetically. Its sharply polemic introduction opposes those who refuse to take advantage of such properties because their underlying *ratio* is not transparent.[21]

***Kitāb al-Ḫawāṣṣ* — Introduction**

Muḥammad ibn Zakariyya al-Rāzī said: 'I do know that there are people whose occupation is the accusation, the opposition, and the hastiness for the derogation of what they ignore, they are quick in censuring us while [in this way they are] declaring themselves stupid. We have observed in the composition of this book that there is no need for us to omit the things—in which we believe there is some usefulness—for the sake of people who are ignorant, and therefore against it. This could have been avoided if only those had been people of reason, careful examination, and waiting before rushing into the refusal of something they have no proof against.

[...]

And then how is it that in every moment they see things that go against them, which change in front of them, like the condition of the things that they reject, in spite of the fact that these things that are found evident in front of them, and what situation they see with their own eyes but do not realize it. In fact, they constantly see that the magnet attracts iron, but if someone claims the existence of a stone that attracts copper, or a stone that attracts gold or glass they hastily deny it, and dismiss it as a silly construct'.

Considering the statements of the two physicians, it seems that a clear distinction between *manāfiʿ* and *ḫawāṣṣ* existed at an early phase of the use of these labels, but they soon became inextricably linked. A concrete example is given by the titles transmitted by the manuscript tradition of ʿĪsā ibn ʿAlī, in which the words *manāfiʿ* and *ḫawāṣṣ* are either interchangeable or used side by side.

Al-Ṭabarī's definition introduces a third lexical element to the discussion—the role of experience—already mentioned among the lexicographical remarks. The passive participle *muǧarrab*, 'tried out', can be found—isolated or in some periphrastic expression—not only in the margins, but also at the end of many recipes in the body of the text. The *Muǧarrabāt*, intended as a medical literary genre, comprises records of physicians' case histories, treatments, medical experiences and remedies presented as real cases.[22] Manfred Ullmann argues that these texts are recipes that have proven to be effective through the actual treatment of a patient, making them more *empirica* rather then *experimenta*.[23] Again, lexicography may help our understanding of some of the implications of this expression. The Arabic 'intensive', a verbal stem known to imply a notion of plurality, can be seen as an indication of a particular kind of successfully repeated operation or procedure. The *Muǧarrabāt* seem to depend upon the human experience of a certain recipe or procedure. Based on the curious mixtures and procedures described in these recipes, the addition of the expression 'tried out' readily gives the impression of an 'experimental' phase in its prehistory, thus bestowing its contents with a greater reliability. Any emphasis on the existence of a modern empirical procedure (a test or an experiment), however, would almost certainly turn out to be anachronistic.

The expression *muǧarrab* was also used in manuscripts outside its eponymous and rather limited textual genre: the word was simply added at the end of some recipes, as a comment on their alleged efficacy. In this way, it was possible for the expression to find its way into many different textual traditions: the personal point of view and comment of a single copyist or a particularly active reader—who, for some reason, felt confident enough to 'certify' a recipe's potency—could, potentially, be included anywhere in the text and at any moment of the transmission. Whether the *Manāfiʿ* and *Ḫawāṣṣ* absorbed this expression, extrapolating it from its genre

---

21 See al-Rāzī, *Kitāb al-ḫawāṣṣ*, MS Cairo DAK Ṭibb Taymūr 264, p. 2; see also Ullmann 1978, 109. The existence of a whole range of magnets capable of attacting a large assortment of substances (hair, cotton, wool, nails, gold, silver, etc.) is attested to in the tradition of the Ps. Aristotle *Book of Stones*, see Ruska 1912, 108–111 and 154–160. The same example was discussed by Ibn al-Ǧazzār in the introduction to his *Kitāb al-ḫawāṣṣ*, see Käs 2012, 31.

22 See Álvarez Millán 2010, 195–197 and Álvarez Millán 1994.

23 See Ullmann 1970, 311–13 and Ullmann 1978, 110.

context, or whether the *Muğarrabāt* genre originated from further reflection on the importance of medical observation, or even from some kind of need in the professional readership, remains an open question.[24]

Combining the lexicographical perspective with the different genres in which these properties appear might give the impression that the riddle is not as obscure as it seemed. The actual state of the texts, however, is much more complex and characterized by many inconsistencies in employing the words *manāfiʿ* and *ḫawāṣṣ*. Each textual tradition has its own peculiarities and a huge number of unedited texts still require study in order to test the validity of these categories.[25]

II. The Structure of ʿĪsā ibn ʿAlī's *Manāfiʿ*

A thorny and ambitious question looms over this and other similar texts. How and where should the line between magic and medicine be drawn?[26] If an ordinary liver complaint, for instance, is cured by a series of knots made on a thread of camel wool, should one focus on the healing properties of this item or on the procedure designed to restore health, which could easily be classified as a kind of ritual or a magical manipulation? Without wishing to deny the intrinsic value of these categories, one is forced to admit that this approach often results in a stalemate. Since the dichotomy and opposition between medicine and magic cannot not be applied consistently to the analysis of the considerable amount of materials transmitted under the name of ʿĪsā ibn ʿAlī, I suggest, here, the combination of a formal approach for the structure of the text with a thematic analysis of its contents.

---

24 Cristina Álvarez-Millán underlines a singular point: the word *muğarrab* never occurs in a proper collection of medical experiences, but only at the end of other kinds of recipes, see Álvarez-Millán 2010, 198. Moreover, the three main books identified as *Kutub al-Muğarrabāt* ('Book of the Tried Out Remedies', by al-Rāzī, al-Hāšimī, and Abū al-ʿAlā ibn Zuhr) were posthumous compilations of medical cases dealt with by a physician, usually collected by one of the pupils. On the whole, this does not support the hypothesis that the word *muğarrab* migrated from a formal, medical genre to a decontextualized use in popular medicine and magic. On later *Muğarrabāt* and their relationship with magic, see Dorpmüller 2005.

25 The *Nuʿūt* and *Ṭabāʾiʿ*—the 'characteristics' and the 'natures'—of animals are other categories that can be related to *manāfiʿ* and *ḫawāṣṣ*, not least because some of them entered collection of different properties. They deal with the habits and behaviours of animals in a more descriptive way. Although all these words are mixed up in titles, their contents are rather distinct. In the Ps. Aristotelian *Nuʿūt al-Ḥayawān*, the chapters include distinct paragraphs devoted either to useful properties or to the habits of an animal (see MS Tunis 16385, for which I would thank Prof. Remke Kruk, who let me work with her copy of this manuscript), whereas in Ibn Buḫtīšūʿ, this information about the innate habits of animals is concentrated in a specific section that opens the chapter (see MS Dublin Chester Beatty 5006, MS Istanbul Aya Sofya 2916, and MS Istanbul Aya Sofya 2943). These materials have their origin in the book on animals composed by Timotheus of Gaza, see Ullmann 1972,15, and Kruk 2001. Ullmann maintains that the difference between the *ṭabāʾiʿ* and *manāfiʿ* / *ḫawāṣṣ* lies in their main sources, which, for the latter, are to be found in the pseudo-Democritean and Hermetic writings, in Xenochrates of Aphrodisia, and Anassilaos of Larissa (Ullmann 1972, 10). An example of *Ṭabāʾiʿ* in the work of ʿĪsā ibn ʿAlī can be found at the end of the chapter on the lion (2.33 and 2.34). Since *nuʿūt* and *ṭabāʾiʿ* are invariably found at the beginning or at the end of a chapter, there is a concrete basis for the hypothesis that they are a later addition. Another difference can be observed in the textual form: *manāfiʿ* and *ḫawāṣṣ* are structured as prescriptive texts (recipes), whereas *nuʿūt* and *ṭabāʾiʿ* are, on the whole, descriptive ones or narratives. However, the fact that ʿĪsā ibn ʿAlī was counted among the sources of Ibn Buḫtīšūʿ, at least for the contents related to *manāfiʿ*, is attested to in the manuscript MS Escurial 893 (f. 140r), see Ruiz Bravo-Villasante 1980, 125.

26 The scientific literature on this distinction is vast. An attempt to apply a modern, Western distinction to shed some light on complex textual and human phenomena has been a distinctive feature of almost every attempt to write about the history of science. It would be far too ambitious to attempt an acceptable bibliography on the topic here. I will therefore limit the list to those readings that, in different ways, have provided me with a general background for my research questions, namely Frazer 1906–15, Thorndike 1923, Lloyd 1979 and Lloyd 1983, Ullmann 1972.

II.1 Macro level: the chapters and their organization

The work of ʿĪsā ibn ʿAlī is organized in chapters, whose number varies greatly from one manuscript witness to another. Each chapter deals with a single animal and contains a number of recipes.[27] Although the order of the entries is not uniform in the manuscript tradition, it is still possible to detect some trends in the arrangement of the contents. The list begins with man, as the most elevated living being at the peak of the creation. A small group of large carnivorous animals follows (lion, wolf, hyena, bear, chapters 2–5). The chapters 6 to 14 (jerboa, pig, dog, gazelle, mountain goat, deer, fox, and crocodile), present a quite heterogeneous ensemble, and its *ratio* is less clear. The next group includes cattle and beasts of burden, both domestic and wild (chapters 15–24). Chapters 25–44 mainly deal with small animals, such as cat, lynx, badger, weasel, jackal, monkey, etc. The presence among them of the exotic and huge rhinoceros, or the most famous of all lizards—the salamander—is peculiar. The groups of birds (chapters 45–78), creeping animals (chapters 79–100), and water creatures (chapters 101–110) delineate themselves with much less uncertainty. In this picture, one can recognize the different organizational criteria from ancient systems of classification, which were inherited by the Arabo-Islamic tradition: food and diet (carnivorous, herbivorous, onmivorous), relations with men (domestic and wild), method of locomotion (creep, fly, swim) and preferred environment (air, water).[28]

In ʿĪsā ibn ʿAlī's table of contents, all these different criteria are weighted equally and groups are defined on the basis of different overlapping and coexisting principles. The boundaries dividing the groups, however, are quite elastic. This makes the inclusion of additional chapters plausible and could explain some of the odd inclusions and configurations of the groups in the classification. In cases when the addition of an entire chapter entered the tradition and was somehow misplaced in the list, one can imagine that either there was no place considered appropriate for the animal, or that the author of the interpolation exercised his own ingenuity.

The manuscript tradition bears signs of this interest in classification, and the branch (b) is the most conspicuous in this regard. Here, there are additional headings marking the classification and labelling large groups of chapters. In this same branch of the tradition, the MSS T and W include a list of the chapters prior to the beginning of the text. In terms of the sub-groups within some chapters, four groups were singled out in the manuscript tradition: *insān* (human being),[29] *bahāʾim* (animals, possibly with four legs), *ṭuyūr* (birds) and, finally, *ḫišāš al-arḍ* (insects of the earth). Notably, there is no specific classification of water creatures.[30] In the MS Istanbul Saray Ahmet III, 2083, in particular, the headings are rubricated, and the final number of one hundred chapters is also given.[31] In the list of chapters that opens MS Wien 1481/2, there are three different labels: *sibāʿ* (beasts of prey), *ṭuyūr* (birds), and *ḥašarāt* (creeping animals).[32] The text is incomplete, so it is impossible to check whether the classification labels were consistently applied in the text. Although the interpretation of these clues of classification remains open, there is a clear intention to define clusters of animals in a consistent way, and to organize the table of contents as a multi-oriented classification system.

27 Focusing on a single animal is more a tendency for the chapters than a rule. Also, those chapters with a single protagonist tend to call the animal by different names when referring to the male or female specimen, to the young, etc. In the chapter dedicated to sheep for example, five different names are used: *ḍaʾn* and *šāʾ* as collective nouns, with the addition of the more general *ġanam* for small cattle, *ḫarūf* for the young, *naʿǧa* for the female and *kabš* for the ram. The chapter about the dog, in an associative way, includes a recipe based on the shark, literally called 'sea dog' (*kalb al-baḥr*). A similar approach is taken with the horse (*faras*) and the hippopotamus (*faras al-nahr*). By association, I suppose, the chapter devoted to the pearl oyster includes a mineral, meerschaum, as distinctive ingredient (106.15). In the case of chickens, there are two distinct chapters, one for the hen and one for the rooster. There appears to be some confusion, at least at the semantic level, for less common animals. The chameleon (*ḥirbāʾ*), for instance, is mentioned in three different chapters (83, 89 and 94).

28 For a summary of the different classifications in Arabic scientific literature, see Ullmann 1972, 50–54. See also Ibn Qutayba 1949.

29 This sections includes three distinct chapters for man, woman and child.

30 See MS Istanbul Saray Ahmet III 2055 (T), ff. 1v–3r and MS Wien 1482/2.

31 See Ibid., ff. 5v–7v. These quotations deal with: animals with a bony or non-bony penis, animals with a large tongue, fish bones, fish eggs, etc.

32 MS Wien 1481/2 (W), ff. 134r–134v.

II.2 Fortunes and misfortunes of the structure

If the case of homonymity can be seen as an unlucky and unpredictable setback, the problematic aspects of the structure affected its fortune more predictably. The text, as ʿĪsā ibn ʿAlī arranged it, can be searched only by animal, and the search is possible only at a chapter level. Within chapters, there is no systematic order to the recipes (*a capite ad calcem*, for instance, or, alternatively, distinctive ingredients presented in alphabetical order). If, however, the reader wants to search for a remedy for a specific disease, the whole book must be leafed through, or indeed, the contents learned by heart.

It is not surprising, then, that this structure was soon abandoned in favour of something more practical.[33] Nevertheless, in the first medical encyclopedia ever composed in Arabic, the *Firdaws al-ḥikma* by ʿAlī ibn Rabbān al-Ṭabarī,[34] the fourth *maqāla* deals with the useful properties of animals. Forty-two animals are listed, each of them in a dedicated chapter.[35] A single chapter in the *Firdaws* usually contains less recipes than in ʿĪsā ibn ʿAlī, but the recipes are basically given in the same order. The classification implied in the list of animals in al-Ṭabarī strenghtens the hypothesis about ʿĪsā ibn ʿAlī's composition. The main difference between the two texts lies in the position of the predatory and the domestic animals: in ʿĪsā ibn ʿAlī, man is followed first by predators and then by domestic animals, whereas al-Ṭabarī inverts their positions, placing domestic animals immediately after the chapter on man. The fact that portions of text could be moved within a larger textual frame confirms the presence of coherent blocks of chapters defined by an implicit classification.

This formal analogy between the structures of the two works, together with the cultural features shared by the two authors, offers another clue to the fact that we are dealing with a very early stage of this textual genre. In this early phase, the authors were still familiar with the ancient sources, also thanks to the multilingual dimension of their personal and professional lives. They experimented with new textual forms, new structures—not all of them meeting with the same success—to reshape materials inherited from the past.

While later authors radically changed the formal paradigm and adopted a completely different arrangement of the materials, the readership, too, had to cope with the problems posed by ʿĪsā ibn ʿAlī's text. Traces of different attempts to limit the discomfort caused by the textual structure are clear in the manuscript tradition. For instance, the copyist or another hand added marginal glosses, with the aim of indexing the text; another solution was that this text circulated together with others containing similar recipes arranged by illness, from head to toe.[36]

II.3 Micro level: the recipes

If the chapters and their arrangement represent the macro-level of this work, the micro-level is represented by its smallest structural component, i.e. the recipe. Recipes often coincide with a syntactic unit. Thus, the recipes' role is mirrored by some codicological features of the manuscript witnesses, where the coherence of the recipe as a unit of text is explicitly marked by various dividers. The composition of the basic textual unit (the recipe) can also be approached in a formal way. This allows recipes to be compared and helps us understand whether we are dealing with the same one, in spite of the huge number of variants. Each recipe has three constitutional elements: the animal ingredient, processing of the ingredient(s), and the purpose or aim of the recipe.[37]

---

33 For the stategies and tools devised in the Arabo-Islamic Middle Age by scholars, see Rosenthal 1947.

34 ʿAlī ibn Rabbān al-Ṭabarī was born near Marw at the beginning of the 9th century, to a Christian Persian family. He worked on the *Firdaws al-Ḥikma* for more than twenty years, completing it at the beginning of al-Mutawakkil's reign (850 ca.). See Meyerhof 1931 and Thomas, D., 'al-Ṭabarī', in: *Encyclopaedia of Islam*, Second Edition, Edited by: P. Bearman, Th. Bianquis, C.E. Bosworth, E. van Donzel, W.P. Heinrichs. Consulted online on 13 February 2018 <http://dx.doi.org/10.1163/1573-3912_islam_SIM_7248>.

35 Ṭabarī 1928, 420–444.

36 For a description of the manuscript witnesses, see ch. IV. For a specific description of their material features to be interpreted as clues of evolution and clues of transmission, see Raggetti 2015.

37 Anna Contadini has suggested the existence of a treatment syntagm composed by five elements (condition, choice of body part, manner of preparation, specification of dosage, result). She seems, however, quite pessimistic about the possibility of identifying

II.3.1 The distinctive animal ingredient

The distinctive element of every recipe in this collection is an ingredient of animal origin and this determines its inclusion within a specific chapter. These ingredients include organs (liver, testicle, brain, etc.), tissues (skin, horn, hoof, etc), fluids and secretions (blood, urine, sweat, etc.), and body parts (leg, wing, paw, etc). The origins of some ingredients, however, are more opaque. One recipe, for instance, is based on a worm that can be found inside the head of wild cattle: the presence of such a worm makes the animal restless; therefore, if this worm is placed on a man, he will not be able to sleep (29.1).[38] Bezoar stones are another peculiar ingredient. They are not actual stones or minerals, bur rather conglomerates of hair and other materials, usually found in the digestive tracts of animals. ʿĪsā ibn ʿAlī's work features a number of animals from which these 'stones' can be obtained: cow (15.58), rooster (61.10), goose (64.6), swallow (50.14), and chameleon (84.X). In the chapter on the dog (8.28), a pseudo-bezoar is mentioned. This is a stone that has been swallowed and which is subsequently regurgitated by the animal. Moreover, this text refers to a greater diversity of useful properties of bezoar stones than the purpose for which they became famous, that is as a powerful and universal antidote.

The inherent beneficial power of the animal ingredient—its 'vis' or faculty—can be more or less transparent. In many recipes, the effect depends on a sympathetic or antipathetic interaction. For instance, the ingredients provided by the mule—a notoriously sterile crossbreed—are meant either to act against sterility, or to provoke it. Similarly, the sparrow, believed to hold a record among animals for the frequency of its sexual intercourse, serves as a key source for ingredients that affect desire and sexual potency.[39] Sympathy is stated and interpreted in many different ways. An immediate association occurs when a particular organ cures the corresponding body part in a human patient. In many cases, however, the connection between the intrinsic power of a certain ingredient and its effect is less clear, and none of the solutions suggested until now is valid. By applying the lexicographical observations on the possible difference between *manāfiʿ* and *ḫawāṣṣ* to this collection of recipes, the properties that can somehow be reconnected to a sympathetic relationship—or that, generally, have a transparent causality—can be considered *manāfiʿ*; whereas those whose causal relation remains obscure are *ḫawāṣṣ*. Nevertheless, the issue of the difference between *manāfiʿ* and *ḫawāṣṣ* is so complex that this criterion is only the first tentative step, rather than a definitive solution. What cannot be excluded, however, is that a cause that today remains unintelligible, may well have been self-evident in the context of the composition and circulation of this work.

The fact that some effects are governed by sympathies suggests that the ingredients are literally meant as animal organs and substances; that is, they are the actual vehicle for the *vis animalium*.[40] The power preserved

common materials through formal analysis. See Contadini 2008, 146. Medical recipes, in different fields of study, have recently been the object of scholarly attention. See, for instance Totelin 2009 and Lehmhaus-Martelli 2017.

38 This parasite is mentioned in connection with two different animals, the wild cow in branch (b), and the buffalo in branch (a) and branch (c).

39 See al-Ǧāḥiẓ 1965, II 330.

40 Robert Muth suggested the name *Träger des Lebenskraft* for some of these substances, and offers a collection of examples from Greek and Latin on the use of saliva, urine, and excrement. He reiterates, however, a dichotomy between magic and medicine in the two groups of materials in his analysis: *Zaubermittel* and *Volksmedizin und Heilungswunder*, see Muth 1954. Pliny vehemently attacked the use of disgusting animal ingredients in Greek medicine, and, from the sources mentioned, it seems that this use was imported from the East: 'To examine human entrails is deemed an act of impiety; what then must it be to devour them? Say, Osthanes, who was it that first devised these practices; for it is thee that I accuse, thou uprooter of all human laws, thou inventor of these monstrosities; devised, no doubt, with the view that mankind might not forget thy name! Who was it that first thought of devouring each member of the human body? By what conjectural motives was he induced? What can possibly have been the origin of such a system of medicine as this? Who was it that thus made the very poisons less baneful than the antidotes prescribed for them? Granted that barbarous and outlandish tribes first devised such practices, must the men of Greece, too, adopt these as arts of their own? We read, for instance, in the memoirs of Democritus, still extant, that for some diseases, the skull of a malefactor is most efficacious, while for the treatment of others, that of one who has been a friend or guest is required. Apollonius, again, informs us in his writings, that the most effectual remedy for tooth-ache is to scarify the gums with the tooth of a man who has died a violent death; and, according to Miletus, human gall is a cure for cataract. For epilepsy, Artemon has prescribed water drawn from a spring in the night, and drunk from the skull of a man who has been slain, and whose body remains unburnt. From the skull, too, of a man who had been hanged, Antæus made pills that were to be an antidote to the bite of mad dog. Even more than this, man has resorted to similar remedies for the cure of four-footed beasts even—for tympanitis in oxen, for instance, the horns have been perforated, and in the animal body parts is activated by the processing, and then transferred to the patient. However, the phenomenon of zoological *Decknamen* to encode the names of mineral and vegetal ingredients is attested to in other Arabic sources, and in Ancient technical literature more generally.[41] A number of recipes raise the suspicion that the animal ingredient may, in fact, be a code name for other substances, for instance, the recipe stating that crows' eggs are able to negate the effects of lime (59.12), while bat droppings congeal it (52.25), swallow droppings are used to slake chalk (50.16), and horse hooves can be used to harden glass and make gold and silver look like copper (16.13). A recipe based on the abdomen of a black cat equates its effect to that of tar (30.2), and given the resemblance in colour this could be a clue to a *Deckname*. In general, however, the trend in the ʿĪsā ibn ʿAlī tradition seems to be towards a literal interpretation. Some recipes are based on a single animal ingredient, but it is common to find a longer list of ingredients that includes plants, oils, and mineral substances.

Any kind of ingredient needs to be quantified on order for a procedure to be repeated and to obtain a specific result. If an ingredient is quantifiable in units, then a precise number is given, for instance, seven lice taken from a dog (8.23). If, instead, the weight or the volume of the ingredients has to be quantified as a whole, there are three distinct approaches. The first adopts a precise unit of measurement (*raṭl*, *dirham*, *qīrāṭ*, *dāniq*, *miṯqāl*, etc.), the second uses empirical units of measurement, determined by common sense and daily life experience (a handful the quantity equivalent to a chickpea, etc.), while the third adopts a relative measurement based on the part against which the other ingredients can be proportionally measured. In the pre-modern world—and Arabo-Islamic society was no exception—the units of measure could vary not only from place to place, but also from one individual to the other.[42] This implies that, in the transmission of a text, relative measures represent a more reliable approach to preserving the intended proportion of ingredients in a recipe.

II.3.2 Processing the ingredients

The second structural element in the recipes can be considered from several perspectives. It may deal with the application or administration of the animal substance (salves, pills, compresses, fumigations, eyedrops, mixed with food or beverages, etc.), or with the preparation of an intermediary object to convey the effect of the animal ingredient (talismans, lanterns, phylacteria, etc.). Different operations may coexist in the formal space of the 'main ingredient's processing', and this component of the recipes can easily be enlarged by selecting and combining different procedures. Moreover, additional indications are easily introduced into this part of a recipe. They also consist of supplementary therapeutic indications: whether the medicament must be applied to the right or the left part of the body, taken in the bath or on an empty stomach, additional handling of the main ingredient (to be pulverized, ground, burnt, filed, liquefied, etc.), and the indication of different media for the administration of the medicament.

---

human bones inserted; and when swine have been found to be diseased, fine wheat has been given them which has lain for a night in the spot where a human being has been slain or burnt!' (*Nat. Hist.* XXVIII.2). For the nature of his work, Pliny as been chosen here as an example of a wide collection of many different traditions circulating in antiquity. Despite the many centuries and cultures in between, there still it a resemblance between the recipes mentioned by Pliny and ʿĪsā ibn ʿAlī. See Pliny 1963, 5–9.

41 In a manuscript witness to the astro-mineralogical work attributed to ʿUṭārid ibn Muḥammad, dealing with the stones associated with the seven planets and their engraved seals (MS Paris BnF Ar. 2775, f. 108v), there is one clear example of a *Deckname*. In the chapter describing the preparation of the seal of Mars, there is an explicit identification of a vegetal ingredient alongside a second name referring to a plant: 'the tongue of the black bird, which is a mollusc which lives in the ponds, and a medicinal plant called scorpion'. In the copy preserved in MS Istanbul Aya Sofya 3610, f. 156v, the indication of an equivalent name in Greek is missing. On the use of *Decknamen* in alchemy, see Siggel 1951.

42 For this complex technical topic, see the second edition of the *Encyclopaedia of Islam* s.v. *Makāyil*, (Ashtor, E. and Burton-Page, J., 'Makāyil (a.)', in: *Encyclopaedia of Islam, Second Edition*, Edited by: P. Bearman, Th. Bianquis, C.E. Bosworth, E. van Donzel, W.P. Heinrichs. Consulted online on 13 February 2018 <http://dx.doi.org/10.1163/1573-3912_islam_COM_0635>); see also Sauvaire 1884a, 1884b, and 1885. Armin Schopen borrows the values given by Oliver Kahl, see Schopen 2006, 236 and Kahl 2002, 225–228; see also Bos 2009. Sara Fani has formulated an admirable synthesis of the question in her PhD dissertation, summarizing in the glossary what is stated in primary sources, as well as the discussion in the secondary literature, see Fani 2013.

There are two distinct approaches to the processing of the main ingredient. The first points at those mechanical and technical processes that belong to the ordinary activities of an apothecary. The second, by contrast, refers to all those magical and ritual actions involved in the preparation.

The first group includes many different procedures aimed at reducing the main ingredient to the most suitable consistency, in order to mix it with other components. Hard materials are ground up and pulverized, while fluid or soft ones are diluted with decoctions of plants and oils. The different kinds of meats have to be cooked until they dissolve in a broth, alternatively they are baked in a clay oven or roasted. Different kinds of oven are mentioned, used in connection with specific activities: the kiln for lime (79.6), the oven in which the seller of sheep heads prepares his goodies (21.8), and an already warm oven used to bake bread (50.12). Some alchemical instruments are mentioned as well, like the alembic and the 'cucurbit' (16.13).

Some recipes prescribe that one or more ingredients are to be left to putrefy for a certain number of days, sometimes in a vessel buried in the ground or in manure. The creatures generated during the process of fermentation can be used as a source for medical ingredients. Fermentation and generation of peculiar creatures from the decayed matter are also used in other works as a metaphor for the description of alchemical operations.[43]

Some of the preparations are not meant for immediate use, but rather are to be preserved in small bottles or containers, so that they are at hand in moments of need.

As for the 'magical' and ritual processing, the most common procedure suggested by the recipes is the preparation of a phylactery, usually consisting of a part of an animal that is carried around in a small purse made of skin, either from the same or from a different animal. Significant attention is paid to the correspondence between left and right. In the case of paired limbs and organs, it is not uncommon to find a precise indication about the side from which the part has to be taken, or to which the medicament must be applied. There are less indications about colours, but they are still significant. They deal with the specific nuance of a thread or a piece of cloth to be used in the preparation of a protective talisman (15.58, 16.13 and 56.10). Other traces of magical procedure can be seen in a recipe to bind someone's tongue (where the mouth of a frog has to be sewn shut with a silk thread, 108.9), in the dismembered parts of a large rat arranged in a particular configuration in order to chase pests away from the fields (43.10), and with the cat, whose blood is used for a love potion (30.9). Only in one case, an animal, namely the turtle, is presented as a medical scapegoat, to be burnt once the disease has been transferred to it (104.15). Among the few examples of written amulets, there is a little scroll against fever (1.29)—the recipes suggest modifying the text in accordance with the kind of fever to be cured—and a tanned piece of weasel skin inscribed against epilepsy (33.5).

As for the administration of medicaments, some recipes contain more detailed indications: the dosage may be different for adults and children (1.35), some preparations have to be taken in the bath on an empty stomach or at certain intervals. The administration of remedies against epilepsy can be related to the phases of the moon, with the beginning of a new lunar cycle as the most propitious moment. The awareness of the patient—or, more often, the lack of it—is a significant detail, especially in the case of love potions. Fumigations are a common

43 See, for instance, the chapter on wondrous fermentations (*al-taʿfīnāt al-ʿağība*) in the *Kitāb Išrāsīm*, (MS Paris Ar. 2634 ff. 27v–35v and MS Paris Ar. 2635, pp. 83–90). 'Chapter on the fermentation that has a huge effect and on the extraordinary secret. The Egyptians said: if Indian peas flour is taken, kneaded with bull blood, stuffed in a vessel filled with bull urine, buried as mentioned for one day, then a beast will be generated from it. This has the head of flowers [?], the body of a bird, and its colour tends to red. When it is like this, give it ram blood to drink for four days, one *raṭl* every day. When you hear a rustling noise, seal the lid of the vessel with clay and close it, drill a small hole through it, fill the receptacle with old wine and *Is* [?] water, and then bury it in the manure for fourteen days. Then open it, purify the wine and the water that comes out of it, and you will obtain a yellow water. Then add water for a second time, when it is needed, and close the hole. Then put it in a moderately hot oven for a whole night, let it cool, and put it back in the manure for three days. Then open it—but only after you have rubbed your hands with lily and violet oil—and you will find a red worm in it. Then purify the water and pour some of it on the worm. Then grind it with water and let it precipitate from the 'cucurbit' (*qarʿa*) and from the alambic. Then store it, and this will make people blind. No wonder that when three hundred dirhams of melted lead are diluted with one ounce of it—after it has been melted for three times—turn into red gold of the highest quality. If some of it is given to a man to eat with his food in a suitable quantity, then he will die. If leprosy is rubbed with it for three days, then this will cure it. If a man struck by a paralysis enters a hot bath, and rubs himself with this, then he will immediately be healed' (see MS Paris Ar. 2635, pp. 85–87). For the *Kitāb Išrāsīm*, see Ullmann 1972, 382 and Coulon 2017. For a study of the processes of fermentation in magical literature, see Saif 2016; for the phenomenon of spontaneous generation in general, see Kruk 1990.

application and in the case of gynaecological applications the woman has to stand over the source of smoke, so that it can penetrate her womb (21.13). Sometimes, the medicament is administered via a specific medium: it is quite common to dilute it in wine, but there also are more peculiar ways like inserting it into an egg (8.25).

The chapter about the dog describes a procedure that may have been intended as an empirical diagnostic test. In order to understand whether a man is going to survive the bite of a rabid dog, one has to check his reflection in a mirror: if the mirror reflects the image of a dog, it means that the patient is doomed (8.17). Other examples are a pregnancy test based on the observation of lice in milk (95.2), the use of a feather to sort out which one of the two owl eggs has the faculty to remove unwanted hair (60.1), and the effect of kite gall on snakes tested in the basket of the snake charmer (58.5).

II.3.3 The purpose of the recipe

Every recipe aims to obtain some effect, and this text contains a wide range of them. These can vary a lot, from relieving a patient from an illness to the preparation of wondrous and probably amusing tricks. If a recipe mentions more than a single outcome, then these are usually related in some way. When a recipe is meant to cure a specific skin problem, such as freckles, it is likely that it may be used for treating other skin conditions (leprosy, pigmentation spots, impetigo, etc.)

To summarize, the recipe can be seen as the minimum structural component of the text, the smallest textual block conveying a coherent and enclosed segment of procedural knowledge. This unit works thanks to the interaction of three different components (ingredient, processing, and purpose), whose extension determines the length of the recipe itself. Recipes can reach a considerable length and complexity, as a consequence of the addition and multiplication of elements to any of its components. The formal approach to recipes adopted here helps us to explain how blocks were constructed up and transformed over time;[44] but the complexity of individual recipes cannot be used as evidence of any clear-cut chronological distinction between specific recipes. In other words, formal complexity alone does not demonstrate that the simplest recipes represent the oldest layer of the text.

III. The world of recipes: a thematic approach

The description of the formal structure of recipes, however, does not by any means fully exhaust their significance. Recipes do not simply convey a structured procedure; they also offer a vivid image of the readership's interests and tastes, and of many aspects of daily life and widely held beliefs. The purpose of the recipes describes the needs and wishes of those who read, copied and carried them out. This aspect can be especially appreciated in the purpose of the recipe. A relatively limited number of issues are dealt, if compared with that of the recipes. Below is a detailed description of the recipes' themes, whose distribution is recorded in the 'Thematic Index'.[45]

Absent from the *Manāfiʿ* of ʿĪsā ibn ʿAlī is a physiology that might explain the origin of the diseases and the properties of drugs. The traces of humoral physiology in the compendium are so scant that their presence could be merely accidental (52.25 with the pigeon excrement containing much hotness). Another element missing is any explicit reference to Islamic practices and beliefs. Although many recipes conclude with a pious invocation to the will of God, as *conditio sine qua non* for a successful result, this remains a superficial veneer. This also gives the impression that a light Islamic touch was enough for these materials to be fully accepted, although they might not always concur with Islamic precepts, for instance those concerning ritual purity. Only one manuscript mentions a Qur'anic verse, used as an invocation to calm a beast, and this too is easy to consider as a

44 For the notion of 'erratic block', see Ullmann 1978, 24.

45 When translating the recipes, I have tried to avoid anachronisms and retrospective projections of modern medical knowledge. The identification of ingredients is made on a lexocographical basis, and aims to give the reader an idea of the substance in question. For the most significant elements in the text, the choices of translation are recorded in the 'Glossary'.

material that entered the text in the course of its transmission, not least because it differs from the main stream of the *Manāfiʿ* recipes (20.17).

III.1 Diseases of the body, body parts and organs

Some diseases receive particular attention, as evidenced by their frequent appearance: illnesses of the internal organs (liver complaints, bladder stones, kidney complaints, heart palpitations, palsy, colic, etc.), skin diseases, eye diseases, swellings and tumours, haemorrhoids. It is known that skin and eyes are affected by a number of endemic diseases, still widespread in the Middle East, and also in the *Manāfiʿ* ophtalomological problems. Different manifestations of leprosy receive particular attention as well.[46] Various fevers are treated and classified on the basis of the frequency of their occurrence (tertian, quartan, etc.). Epilepsy has a special position along with insanity, etymologically connected to a devilish possession.

III.2 Sex and love

The topics of sex and love receive prominent attention, and the number of related recipes is considerable. Many of them deal with sexual potency, aiming to give men amazing power during coitus. They are somehow related to preparations that bind a woman to her lover in an exclusive way. Another possibility offered to would-be lovers is a potion that makes them visible only to the beloved one. In this field, prescriptions and purposes take on a somewhat different nuance with respect to gender. If a recipe is designed for both men and women, then there might be a difference in the outcome, which may also depend on their social class (1.25 and 1.26). The fear of being cheated on often goes hand in hand with sensual love and so, by placing the appropriate animal part under a woman's head while she is asleep, a man can obtain a full disclosure of everything she has done (9.23).

III.3 Reproduction and birth

The issue of human reproduction follows as a logical implication of the previous subject. Several recipes meant for sexual potency also offer help in conceiving. Both fertility and sterility can be induced. In most cases, it seems to be a unilateral male decision, since the awareness and the will of the woman are never mentioned. Moreover, if a woman gets pregnant, several pharmacological interventions are possible to interrupt the pregnancy and abort the child. On the other hand, in case of a difficult pregnancy, an unwanted miscarriage can be avoided and the foetus protected. The delivery can be eased or induced under difficult circumstances; as can the expulsion of a dead foetus from the womb.

III.4 Sleep and insomnia

Sleep can be either induced or prevented with the use of various preparations. There are cases in which the text suggests that prolongued wakefulness is meant to be imposed as an unpleasant condition. In this collection of recipes, several solutions are offered to cope with troubled and agitated sleep, especially when it afflicts children. Only one recipe mentions a procedure to induce nightmares (35.2).

---

46 In a number of cases, it seems that leprosy is equated with those skin diseases that provoke a similar decay of the epidermis, for instance vitiligo or black spots.

III.5 Cosmetic

Treatments for beauty and aesthetic improvement are another relevant topic and, mainly, relate to the skin and hair. Several recipes describe the preparation of ointments that removes freckles and unsightly spots from the face or the whole body. The hair can be made shinier and more beautiful, and its colour can be changed. The possible colours are limited to black and white: white hair can be turned black, and vice versa. More than a dyeing process, one is left with the the impression that the change is of a different nature, i.e. that it is an expression of spite or animosity, or a trick. Depilatory concotions can be prepared to remove superfluous hair from the body in general, or in particular from the area of the eye. Moreover, hair growth can also be induced in the hairless spots left by alopecia. A few recipes deal with the female figure, in particular with the breasts, offering a solution to prevent their excessive growth and for preserving their youthful shape (1.45).

III.6 Nature, husbandry, agriculture and hunting

Domestic animals are not only a source for ingredients, they also are counted among the beneficiaries of the recipes, and the protection of domestic animals is one of the main purposes of such preparations, for example, to ensure the safe return of cattle and beasts of burden to their stable, to calm them when they are afraid, and to heal them when afflicted by a number of diseases (1.39 and 38.16). As for the birds that live in close contact with humans, pigeons and their lofts have to be kept safe from predatory animals so that the birds can multiply; while the hunting hawk has to be kept healthy and well fed, so that its plumage may shine. A few recipes mention fishing, suggesting ways to attract water animals to the surface so as to catch them more easily (18.4). Much less numerous are the beneficial effects for plants and other agricultural activities. Among the rare cases, there is a recipe that explains how to protect vines from a particular parasite (5.18), and another one explaining how to induce a fig tree to bear fruit outside its season (21.10). Dealing with nature and animals also means knowing the hidden tensions and attractions that affect living beings. Though these might better pertain to other kinds of properties, the *Manāfiʿ* of ʿĪsā ibn ʿAlī contain a number of remarks on antipathies. Antipathies affect both domestic and wild animals, they may run between two animals (scarab and gazelle, 10.7 and 10.8), between an animal and a substance (cat and rose oil 30.6, and cat and rue water 30.7), or between and animal and a plant (lion and oak, 2.34).

III.7 Vermin and obnoxious animals

Other animals pester the daily existence of humans, in particular insects and rodents. Primarily fumigations, but also other actions, are carried out in order to drive away scorpions, bugs, lice, snakes, rats and all the other animals that are troublesome to mankind or domestic animals. Some recipes target a particular kind of vermin, for instance in the case of the prescription suggesting the placing of a lion skin among other textiles in order to protect them from moths (2.27).

III.8 Crafts

Only a few examples of craftsmanship can be found among the great number of ʿĪsā ibn ʿAlī's recipes. For instance, a long procedure for obtaining splinterproof glass (16.13). There are also recipes to treat different materials, from wool (100.2 and 110.10) to precious stones (22.19 and 22.31), and for the preparation of an invisible ink (104.13).[47] Recipes like these could have been addressing a particular professional category, but some of them could also be intended as targeted tricks.[48]

III.9 Tricks

A significant number of the recipes describe different kinds of tricks and pranks. They remind us of the *Paignia*, those tricks of *magie amusante* well attested to in Anassilaos of Larissa, in the pseudo-Democritean tradition, and in other Greek authors.[49] Several magic lanterns, whose wick has been soaked in a particular substance or mixture, create different illusions: people with the head of a dog or headless, women undressing and dancing around, a room entirely made of silver, even endless farting. Other tricks are meant to make fun of a particular professional category. For instance, those fumigations capable of shattering all the items in a glass shop (103.4), or those for splitting the membranes of drums and tambourines (3.7 and 3.8). Professional guilds may also avail themselves of these tricks, with mischievous and deceitful intentions: thieves carry with them a dog's tongue so that dogs will not bark at them (8.20), while street tricksters used to prepare an ointment to bring about an allegedly supernatural resistence to fire (108.2).[50] There are also commercial tricks, like the one to lower the price of an animal at the moment of the purchase by making appear the animal sick (93.9). If we are to believe the accompanying comments to the recipe, turning black hair white was also considered an amusing trick (50.2).

III.10 At court

The most detailed descriptions of antidotes and ways of detecting poisons always appear in connection with a courtly environment. This is explicit in the remarks about how kings and sovereigns used to carefully store these precious substances and objects in their treasures (42.3). Another issue strictly related to a courtly environment is the use of expedients or tricks to enter the court, and to ensure the king has a benevolent disposition. These practices also produce as a side effect a generalized love and admiration for the user, including the love of all women. The other side of this coin is represented by enmity, legal quarrels, verbal disputes, and the way to triumph over an adversary in such situations.[51]

III.11 Evil eye and black magic

The evil eye and the hideous effects of black magic are very concrete issues in the scenario offered by the recipes of ʿĪsā ibn ʿAlī. A man can protect himself from these supernatural attacks using a number of phylacteria and ointments. Some of them offer a form of protection against evil spirits and demons. A related therapeutical topic is the use of a prescription to darken blue eyes, in the inauspicious case that a baby is born with them, since blue eyes were—and still are—considered a powerful source of the evil eye. Some recipes, however, offer

---

47 See Raggetti 2016, 324.

48 See the following paragraph.

49 See Hershbell 1987, 7–8, and Martelli 2011, 99–114.

50 In a variant reading, this practice is associated with devils.

51 These materials are probably textual relics from the past, perhaps even an echo of the Babylonian *Egalkura* incantation, as I discuss in the forthcoming article 'Tricks to enter the court. Amulets, Rulers, and Social Distress', proceedings of the BabMed Workshop *Patients and Patrons* (Eisenbrauns). As for the connection with the ancient tradition, for instance in the case of the fat between the eyes of the lion (2.2), we can find in Pliny the Elder a remark on the Oriental origin of this unreliable remedy: 'The frivolous lies of the magicians assert that persons who are anointed with lion's fat, will more readily win favour with kings and peoples; more particularly when the fat has been used that lies between the eyebrows of the animal-a place, in fact, where there is no fat to be found!' (*Nat. Hist.* XXVIII.25). See Pliny 1963, 63–64.

more active interaction with the supernatural world. For instance, by applying a particular ointment on the eyes, it becomes possible to see the world of *ǧinns* and to interact with them (30.3).

IV. The edition

IV.1 Introduction to the edition

The description of the structure of ʿĪsā ibn ʿAlī's *Manāfiʿ* highlights a number of features that deeply affect the critical work on the text.[52] A text like this—with the recipe as minimal textual unit, arranged in chapters devoted to a single animal, and whose chapters follow an order that sketches a classification—is prone to being transmitted by a fluid tradition.[53] The fluidity manifests itself at different levels, and clearly emerges from the collation of the manuscript witnesses: a different number of chapters, a different number of recipes in the chapter, different formulations of the same recipe, an abundance of variant readings in the various manuscript witnesses.

The huge number of variants and the fluid development of the tradition, together with the early date of composition and the considerable time gap between this and the manuscript tradition, are all elements that make it impossible to reconstruct a form of the text that is close to the author's version.

In spite of this discouraging premise, the critical work on the text remains necessary. In this scenario, the edition becomes the occasion to display the development of the tradition, trying to explain the mechanisms that influenced it, rather than an attempt to reconstruct a version close to the unattainable original.[54]

The physical limits of a paper edition—instead of a digital one—and the necessity to cope with the limited space of the page, have also influenced the definition of the editorial approach.

In a fluid textual tradition like the *Manāfiʿ* of ʿĪsā ibn ʿAlī, it is not easy to find 'errors'. In order to sort out and group the manuscript witnesses, contextually relevant variants and structural features are often the only clues. Shared traits in the structure (the addition of a specific chapter or a shared lacuna, for instance) represent the strongest clue. In a fluid tradition, the variants are not alternatives in the reconstructrion of an original, rather they are complementary in the development of the tradition and in its philological reconstruction. A great number of these variants are carriers of meaning, relevant information and peculiar interpretations of the text. These meaningful variants deserve to be considered differently than other variants that only produce 'background noise', without really surrendering any important information. These variants, moreover, are valuable in the context of the whole textual tradition, rather than in isolation.[55]

As an easy solution to this problem, one could choose one manuscript witness, a so-called best manuscript. This decision results from the assumption that one manuscript is better than the other ones. Basing this choice on more or less reasonable criteria (date of the manuscript, length and therefore alleged completeness of the text, even readability) would not save us from a huge loss of material and information.[56]

On the other hand, it must be said that this rich variety easily strays into a chaotic and entangled mass, in which it is easy to get lost and lose courage. To spare first the editor and then the reader from such a predica-

52 The problematic aspects, in other words, are not simply due to the circumstances of the transmission, but to the nature of the work. These reason are instrinsic, rather than accidental. See Varvaro 1999

53 See Trovato 2014, 155–160.

54 Jan Just Witkam constructively warned against the fanatical search for an archetype in many Arabic textual traditions, see Witkam 1986 and Witkam 2013. On the other hand, in terms of scholarly practice he has shown that it is of fundamental importance to examine all the manuscript witnesses available, and to look at them with the eye of a historian.

55 The words of Alberto Varvaro are illuminating apropos the value of variability and its manifestation: 'The awareness of the very fertile variability of medieval and modern texts does not by any means imply unbrindled enthusiasm for variability as such. To begin with, Medieval variability (variance) is never the simultaneous presence of variants, but rather of the instability of a text in different locations, environments, and times. There has never existed a simultaneous competition of variants except in the margins of the *editiones variorum*. Moreover, neither variability nor its absence constitute value; they are only to be considered circumstances. As textual critics, we look insted for meanings and values'. See Varvaro 1999, 57.

56 On the importance of a complete *recensio*, see Bausi et al. 2015, 336.

ment, the variants must be looked at from a different perspective, in which the idea of an original text remains marginal. The primary sources agree on the fact that, in the 9th century, there lived a physician named ʿĪsā ibn ʿAlī and, among other things, he wrote a book on the useful properties of animal parts. Although some details remain unknown, and the information given by the sources might be not completely genuine, there is no reason to doubt the author's existence or his prestigious position in his time. That version of the text is, however, to be considered beyond our reach.

The image of the broken vase that has to be reconstructed from its fragments can be used to describe the state of this textual tradition, and the difficulties that the critical work on it encounters. In the 9th century, ʿĪsā ibn ʿAlī shaped a collection of useful properties, the original vase whose form we can guess in some detail. The fragments that have been handed down to us come from vases whose fashion was inspired by the original, but that were also freely reshaped in the course of centuries, with the introduction of additional elements or simplification of the form. The uncritical glueing of these fragments would only create a wildly eclectic hybrid. The aim of this edition is to collect and display all of them in an ordered and rational way, stressing their formal connection, so that the history of the textual tradition can be told and its contents made available.

So, after a complete collation of these large and varied materials, I opted for a division of the manuscript witnesses into three families, whose ties must be looked for in the order of chapters and recipes, their style, and in some *loci critici* where particularly meaningful structural variants can be found. Consequently, the edition is constructed in three different columns, representing the three branches (a), (b), and (c). In this way, visible parallels and gaps in the textual tradition are immediately detectable. One manuscript has been chosen to represent the textual tradition of each branch.[57] The choice fell upon the more inclusive in terms of contents—in other words, the longest text—and it was oriented by the pragmatic approach to this fluid tradition. The manuscripts chosen to carry the banner of each branch are not the best ones, but rather the most suitable and practical witnesses to the fluid tradition in all its richness.

The variants from the other manuscripts are given in the positive apparatus, whose structure mirrors the three branches of the tradition. In many instances, it was necessary to note in the apparatus the whole recipe, as attested to by another witness, either because the formulation is completely different, or because its syntactical arrangement did not allow for a more syntetic display of the variants.

IV.1.1 Order of the chapters

As for the order of the chapters, the choice has been strongly oriented by the implicit classification of animals that can be detected in all the manuscript witnesses. However, the order of the chapters in the edition is not exactly mirrored by any extant manuscript; rather, it is the result of an inclusive edition. The reason for the anomalous position of a chapter in a particular manuscript or branch is not always clear. The impression is that it may depend more on the innovation of a specific witness, rather than on the general fluidity of the order of the chapters in the textual tradition. To varying degrees, all the manuscript witnesses show oddities in terms of chapter order. In the making of the edition, I have decided to give some of the chapters a different position to the one they have in the manuscript. All these interventions are clearly marked in the 'Appendix', where the chapter order of the edition is matched with that of the manuscripts, by means of a synoptic table. The replacement of the chapters is, of course, a hypothesis based on the general idea of a formal structure of the work impressed by the implicit classification of the animals. The chapters are progressively numbered, and the edition of the *Manāfiʿ* counts one hundred and ten of them. The chapter numbers are an addition to the edition.

The degree of variance that may affect the level of the chapter finds an example in ch. 34, which is devoted to a curious pair of animals, the jackal and the chamois. Here, paleography is responsible for the co-presence of the jackal (*ibn āwā*) and the chamois (*arwī*). The implicit classification suggests that probably the 'right' animal here is the jackal. In the manuscript tradition of the text, however, this paleographically problematic reading generated different results. Branch (c) has two distinct headings followed by two clusters of recipes, respective-

57 Here I use the expressions branch, family and group of manuscripts practically as synonyms. The preference for branch is determined by the fact that it better conceptualizes, in concrete, the tripartite structure of the edited text.

ly associated with the jackal and the chamois (in other words, the more inclusive version); branch (b) has only the section on the chamois, whereas branch (a) has the chapter heading *ibn āwā* ('jackal') and is followed by the recipes that, in (b) and (c), are associated with the chamois. In the edition, this case is represented by a single chapter with the two inextricably related entries.

The case of the jerboa and the pig (chs 6 and 7) could be handled differently, because the the two different clusters of recipes remained distinct, and only one witness of branch (b) had put them together in the same chapter.

IV.1.2 Order of the recipes

In the edition, the recipes of each chapter are numbered progressively. In the critical apparatus, it is possible to see whether a recipe is omitted by other manuscripts of the same branch. The apparatus also informs the reader of cases when the manuscript chosen to represent a certain branch lacks the recipe. In this case, two possibilities are given. If the recipe is attested to in at least one of the other two branches, then it enters the text, and the apparatus tells the reader that the text of that particular recipe is taken from another manuscript of the same branch. If, instead, the recipe is attested to only as a singular feature of one manuscript, which has not been chosen to represent the branch, then the text of the recipe is given in the apparatus as an addition by a particular witness, together with a summary of its contents.[58]

The order of the recipes in the edition has been enstablished by a comparison of the relative position they have in the different manuscript witnesses. This is basically an internal and empirical criterion, but it relies on the fact that the order of the recipes in the manuscripts is quite stable. If a recipe, or a cluster of them, has a peculiar position in one of the manuscripts that diverges from the general trend, then this is indicated in the apparatus, by giving its position in relation to the other recipes in the edition.

IV.1.3 Parallel recipes: variants and positional value

This formal approach, adopted to determine the sequence of the recipes in the edition, raises a more general question about the possibility of comparing materials in a fluid tradition. As said, from the collation it emerges that these recipes were transmitted in a fairly stable order. It is not easy to guess why, in some instances, a recipe, or a cluster of them, appears in a different position. This change in the order, however, cannot simply be described as the result of a whim: almost any change in a formal frame requires a will and a plan behind it, though this may remain unknown to its modern readers.

In the case of added recipes, they usually share either the distinctive ingredient or a purpose with the one with they are are juxtaposed.

Then, when the focus moves to the recipes displayed in parallel, on the same line—and therefore considered not just as comparable materials, but relatively free variants of the same text—the issue of the degree of congruence emerges. To what extent can two or more recipes be considered as equivalent, i.e. a variant of the same procedural text, rather than different preparations? Since variants may emerge in each of the three components that construct a recipe (distinctive ingredient, processing of the ingredients, and aim), and in more than one simultaneously, the result is a bewildering number of possible combinations. Nevertheless, their position in the text is a strong clue to their analogy, which allows us to compare materials that, usually, are tricky objects of comparison, if one is only looking for an exact correspondence in the wording. The inclusive criterion applied here, next to their positional value, considers that one common element in one of the three parts of the recipe is already enough to consider them akin. In other words, when it comes to establishing a parallelism between two or more recipes, the specific contents and the position weigh more than the wording.

The wealth of variants is the result of the fluid tradion, in which the re-writing of a textual unit is a normal practice. Moreover, there is no end to the addition or omission of elements and this phenomenon was also possibly influenced by the readability of a particular *Vorlage*, the degree of creativity and literacy of single copyists,

58 This formal difference in the presentation and annotation of the text is an editorial choice that allowed for the sifting of singular additions of the particular manuscripts.

his expertise, the availability and the familiarity with supplementary ingredients, etc. Many other hypothesis can be formulated about the generation of variants, but what can be surely inferred from the textual tradition is that, in the fluidity of the process of copy and transmission, both trivial and relevant variants accumulated and interwove, becoming complementary rather than alternative. A further step in the direction of the definition of a more complex system of textual affiliations can be taken only after a similar formal comparison with other related works is carried out, not only on short textual samples, but on a larger scale that includes entire compendia.

To recapitulate, the methodological approach devised for this edition allows two or more recipes to be considered as variants of the same procedural text, insofar as their position in the text and at least one of their three structural components remain the same.

The edition is as inclusive as possible, aiming to display the rich variety of this textual tradition.[59] All the interventions on the composition of the text are recorded, with a view to leaving as little room as possible for eclectism: at any moment, the reader can easily check the position of a particular chapter or recipe in the general picture of the textual tradition. The thematic analysis offers the possibility to evaluate the single recipes, and peculiar connections between distinctive ingredients and purposes (see 'Thematic Index').

The position of a chapter or of a particular cluster of recipes is also important for grouping the manuscript witnesses. The chapters on the sheep (ch. 21) and the goat (ch. 22), for instance, see a small cluster of four recipes in different positions. The manuscripts of branches (a) and (b) record them as recipes based on sheep ingredients, whereas the witnesses to branch (c) include them in the subsequent chapter on the goat. Such fluctuations are also present in the lexical ambiguities generated by animal names that can be generically applied to small cattle. Nevertheless, it provides a significant clue to structural relationships between manuscripts. The phenomenon of recipes that fluctuate from one chapter to another is attested to more than once, favoured by the affinity between the animals dealt with, like the wild cow and the buffalo (23.3 and 29.1), the mantis and the bedbug (89.4 and 92.3), or the sandgrouse and the vulture (45.8 and 46.1).

IV.2 Variants and linguistic features

An edition is a compromise between fidelity (to the author, to the manuscript witnesses and the text they transmit, to an alleged archetype) and legibility of the edited text, a compromise that the editor makes with the prospective readership of the edition in mind.[60] I have opted for an edition form that offers a tendencially normalized Arabic in order to reach a larger readership. At the same time, I have paid attention to preserving—in the apparatus or, in particular cases, in the edition—those linguistic features that might be relevant for a deeper linguistic study of this text, and of technical literature more generally.

In the context of an open recension like the *Manāfiʿ*, the copyst may decide to give the text a different formulation, which he finds more appealing, without affecting at all the meaning (e.g. second or third person singular, active or passive formulation of the sentence). The background noise of the orthographical variants and the different syntactic formulations of the recipes is loud. Some orthographic elements that produce this background noise have been normalized, since a different choice would have impared the readability of the edited text, without preserving any other relevant linguistic information (orthography of the *hamza*, *tāʾ marbūṭa* and *hāʾ*, *yāʾ* and *alif maqṣūra*). The alternance between emphatic and non-emphatic (ḍ – d, ṣ – s), interdental and non-interdental letters (ḏ – d, ṯ – t) in the spelling of the same word is normalized in the edition, but the record of relevant ortographic variants is recorded in the apparatus and in the glossaries.[61]

Together with the open recension, the linguistic peculiarities of middle and mixed Arabic gave the copyist a huge set of variants (orthographical, lexical, syntactical), and he was guided in their choice by many different

59 See Trovato 2014, 155–160.
60 See Varvaro 2012, 44–47.
61 See Varvaro 2012, 94 and Bausi et al. 2015, 345.

needs and reasons.[62] In general, these deviations from the standard can be regarded either as a conscious intention to mix registers for the sake of style, or as the result of a lack of familiarity with the contents, or sometimes a simple slip of the pen. In any case, an unintentional deviation from the standard might also be a trace of the influence of spoken language on orthography. For this reason, it remains important to record these relevant features as linguistic documents of the witness that contains them.

IV.2.1 Typology of the variants

As anticipated, the large degree of variation produces a huge number of equally acceptable readings: these do not offer any genealogical information, but carry with them meaningful knowledge.

In the great wealth of variants, it is still possible to stress some trends in terms of their character and genesis. The distinctive ingredient can vary in an associative way: the brain (*dimāġ*) can alternate with marrow (*muḫḫ*), which may be considered as a synonym for the anatomical notions about the the nervous system. A similar shift of meaning may happen between the penis (*qaḏb*) and the tail (*ḏanab*), where the sexual organ of some animals is placed; or between the saliva (*luʿāb*) and the foam (*luġām*) of a camel (20.10); or, like in the case of the deer (12.15), between the quite specific hooves (*aẓlāf*) and the more general extremities(*aṭrāf*). An interesting case (22.29) is one in which the variation features an organ on one side (*minfaḫa*), and an entire periphrasis on the other (*man aḫaḏa muḫḫ*).

A complex list of supplementary ingredients rarely remains stable, and its elements vary from one manuscript witness to another, revealing omissions and additions (12.2). A variant concerning the name of a simple drug may consist of a quite lengthy explanation and collection of synonyms (20.9 and 26.1).

Sometimes, an apparently negligible variant (singular/plural, or the addition of a pronoun) can give a completely different flavour to the recipe. For instance, a procedure that aims to confer a man with a particular appeal, is very different to saying that his woman or all women will find him irresistible (76.2). In other cases, a variant offers a different perspective on the same object: a mound of earth can be described as an anthill, or as the sign of a molehill (10.11).

These variants acquire a particular meaning when they do more than create an equivalent and basically synonymic expression. That is, when a paleographical similarity leads to a semantic ambiguity in the specific field of medicine and pharmacology.

As already seen for ch. 34, a paleographical ambiguity may affect entire chapters. In the case of ch. 82, all the manuscripts show an irregular and uncertain dotting. The majority opts for the reading *ǧirdawn* (large rat), the others go for *ḥirdawn* (lizard), suggesting the former as a more familiar name. On the other hand, the position of the chapter rather suggests that it should be read as lizard, and the edition follows this positional line.

As for the distinctive animal ingredient, the brain (*dimāġ*) and the blood (*damm*) are interchangeable. One of the names used for the herbivorous dung (*ḫaṯan*, and its different plurals) can alternate with *ḥašan*, 'bowels' or 'intestine' (15.17). Other ingredients show this kind of variation: (12.20) safflower (*qirṭim*) and alfalfa (*qurṭ*) with a third and more banal reading that may emerge on the side (*qirāṭ*); and (15.5) Indian hemp (*šahdānǧ*) and fumitory (*šāhtraǧ*). Pitch (*zift*) and oil (*zayt*) are not hard to confuse either (21.18), while honey (*ʿasal*) is just one dot away from being red like washing (*ġusl*) (15.4). It is striking how one of the manuscripts from branch (b)—MS Istanbul Saray Ahmet 2083—always uses *zaybaq* (quicksilver) instead of *zanbaq* (lily).

Two verbs used frequently in the recipes—that is, *saḥaqa* (to grind) and *saqā* (to give to drink) frequently alternate (22.26). In respect of hair, the paleographical similarity concerns the verbs *nabata* (to grow) and *natafa* (to pluck out), which have entirely opposite meanings.

Much rarer are cases—often connected to unusual ingredient names—in which none of the readings preserve a plausibly correct form. Only in one case, that of gum ammoniac (13.15), has it been possible to reconstruct the ingredient, whereas a question mark remains over the names of remedies and electuaries that are impossible to identify (3.21 and 10.9).

62 See Lentin and Grand'Henry 2008; Zack and Schippers 2012.

Similar phenomena are attested to in connection to diseases. The characterization of a swelling (8.9) can vary from warm (*ḥarr*) to acute (*ḥadd*). Laboured breathing (*buhr*) and the skin disease called (*bahaq*) can generate a similar kind of variant too (24.2). The shift from hotness (*ḥarāra*) to impetigo (*ḥizāza*) represents another example.

The processing phase offers a case that occurs very often with the verbs that mean 'to mix, dilute'. The frequency of this phenomenon is high, but the different forms are irregularly distributed in the manuscript tradition. The origin of the variants remain partially unclear, and it is possible to propose more than one reason for their genesis. The forms attested to in the tradition include the verb *ḏāba/yaḏūbu* and the verb *dāfa/yadūfu*.[63] Both generate a number of variants that may depend on both paleographical similarity and influence of the spoken language. The verb *ḏāba* is also attested to as *dāba*, which Wehr describes as a form derived from *ḏāba* seen mostly in modern Egyptian Arabic.[64] The verb *dāfa*—which specifically refers to the moistening of medicines or perfumes—also appears as *ḏāfa*, which Lane describes as a dialectal variant.[65] Another variant associated to this second verb is *ḍāfa/yaḍīfu*, which, in its fourth form, means the adding of something to something else. More rare, but still present, is the variant *ḍāba/yaḍību*. In sum, the origin of these variants can be connected with different and non-mutually exclusive causes: a paleographic similarity and the consequences of defective writing, the semantic closeness of the forms, influence of spoken language in the written realization. Considering the complex nature of these variants, largely attested to in technical texts, the edition preserves them as they appear in the manuscripts.

Sometimes, the genesis of the variant crosses the border of the recipe as textual unit, and the collation shows that, often, two recipes are merged into one (for instance, 8.20–21 and 15.21). Usually, two recipes are attracted to each other by a shared element, the distinctive ingredient or purpose (26.5), in a homoteleuton that also involves contents next to forms.

V. The manuscript witnesses and the branches of the tradition

The literature on *Manāfiʿ* and other properties is vast and largely unexplored. The materials, moreover, are quite repetitive in nature, creating the impression of being at the forefront of a tradition 'where everything is similar but nothing is the same'.[66]

In order to be included in the recension, a manuscript witness has to have the introduction (preferably mentioning the author's name), the contents have to be arranged by animal, and it must deal with useful properties. Exploring the standard repertories, I was able to collect seven manuscript witnesses.[67] I have omitted all the indirect tradition, or better, all the other texts in which a certain recipe appears. The exploration of these materials are the subject of my ongoing research interests and intentions.

Already in the collation phase, the great fluidity of the materials required the development of a specific approach, mainly based on practical and empirical instances. From the synoptic overview of the manuscripts emerged a need to present more than one text in the edition. It has not been possible to establish among the witnesses those relations that are usually shaped in a *stemma codicum*. Nevertheless, on the basis of the aforementioned common structural features, the manuscript witnesses have been divided into three different groups. They represent three different recensions of the text, or three different branches of the tradition, at least as they

63 Lane 1863, I 933.

64 Wehr 1979, 343.

65 Lane 1863, I 988.

66 Special thanks to Remke Kruk, who shared with me this aphoristic formulation that so precisely depicts the circulation of the 'science of properties'.

67 See Brockelmann 1943, 267 and Brockelmann 1937, 417; Sezgin 1970, 377; Ullmann 1972, 21–22. The autoptic examination of manuscripts and the research in different libraries have made an important contribution to the bibliographical research. The text attributed to ʿAlī ibn ʿĪsā (the ophtalmologist) in the Chester Beatty catalogue, in fact turned out to be a copy of Ibn Buḫtīšūʿ's book on animal properties, see Arberry 1964, 3. On the other side, during a research period in Cairo at the National Library, I was struck by a title on animal properties attributed to Ibn Sīnā, which turned out to be a misattributed copy of ʿĪsā ibn ʿAlī's *Manāfiʿ*.

are attested to by the extant manuscript witnesses. Manuscripts belong to the same branch when they share, firstly, formal features (disposition of chapters and recipes) and, secondly, similarities in terms of formulation.

V.1 Branch (a)

(S) MS Istanbul Şehid Ali Pasha 2096, 181 ff., 7 ll. per page.

Some blocks of folia are in disorder and some are missing, possibly as a result of a new binding given to the manuscript. This hypothesis, however, cannot be checked against quire numbers. The foliation was added after the misplacement. There are no catchwords, and the correct order of the folia had to be reconstructed on the basis of the text and the average order of its entries in the rest of the tradition. This manuscript is a particularly rich copy: it is written in *nasḫ* script, largely vocalized, just a few lines per page and ample margins. The title page is written in gold letters outlined in black and vocalized in blue—the chapter headings are written in the same fashion—the text of the introduction is framed by a blue rule-border. The text on this first folio, however, is more of a descriptive subtitle. The title page is missing, but it is plausible to imagine it decorated with a squared panel containing a medallion. This manuscript was probably one of those copied in the Mamluk barracks as school exercises. This institutional training system seems to have counted the sciences of nature among its interests.[68]

The subtitle page gives the following information about the work and the author: *Kitāb maǧmūʿ ḫawāṣṣ min aʿḍāʾ al-ḥayawānāt taʾlīf al-šayḫ al-ḥalīm al-awḥad ʿAlī bin ʿĪsā al-mutaṭabbib bi-madīnat al-Andalus* ('Collection of the occult properties from the parts of animals, the author is the clement the unique ʿĪsā ibn ʿAlī the medical practitioner, in the city of al-Andalus'). The attribution Andalusian origins to the author is unique and can be explained as an attempt to place the author, whose name revealed little, in the most prestigious location for Mediaeval Islamic medicine.

(B) MS Berlin Pet. II 244 (Ahlwardt 6240), 91 ff., 10–11 ll. per page.[69]

Written in a plain *nasḫ* script by a book hand, the text is partially vocalized. The front page has a simple carpet decoration in black, dark blue and red. There is no title on the front page, only the name of the author (*ʿAlī bin ʿĪsā al-mutaṭabbib*). The text is framed by a black double line, chapter headings are inscribed in a rectangular cartouche. The beginning of the recipes is marked either by rubrics, or by a bolder script. From f. 40 onwards the decoration, the rubrics and the frame are incomplete.

V.2 Branch (b)

(T) MS Istanbul Saray Ahmet III 2055/1, 55 ff. (1r–54r), 15 ll. per page.

Written in an elegant *nasḫ* script by a professional book hand, largely vocalized. A title is given in the recto of the first folio: *Kitāb mā fī al-ḥayawān wa-baʿḍ ḥikāyāt min al-ṭibb*. This one is probably a partial transcription of the longer title given in red at the beginning of the text (f. 1v): *Kitāb mā fī al-ḥayawān wa-baʿḍ ḥikāyāt min al-ṭibb min al-manāfiʿ mimmā yaǧmaʿuhū ʿĪsā ibn ʿAlī al-mutaṭabbib* ('Book about the Useful Properties of Animals and Some Stories of Medicine Collected by ʿĪsā ibn ʿAlī, the Medical Practitioner'). Then follows a list of the chapters,[70] more numerous than the actual chapters that are attested in the manuscript (See 'Appendix'). Chapter headings are either rubricated or marked by a red stroke over them: a small *hāʾ* (ﻫ) marks the end of the recipes. The text shows corrections and annotations that may be by the same hand. The first chapter, on man, is

---

68 As I discuss in a forthcoming article 'Rolling Stones Do Gather: MS Istanbul Aya Sofya 3610 and Its Collection of Mineralogical Texts', the Proceedings of the workshop *The Emergence of Multiple-Text Manuscripts*, held in Hamburg in November 2016.

69 See Ahlwardt 1893, 505–506.

70 At the end of the list, the chapters are said to be one hundred and twenty three but, in fact, they are less numerous (see 'Appendix').

interpolated with a long Aristotelian passage on the description and classification of animals. The text has a number of lacunae that suggest that parts were already missing in the *Vorlage*.

(W) MS Wien 1481/2 (ff. 134v–145v), 15 ff., 21 ll. per page.[71]

Written in a clear *nasḫ* book hand. The first line of f. 134v gives a rubricated title: *Kitāb manāfiʿ al-ḥayawānāt*. This is followed by a list of all the chapters that were supposed to be included in the text. However, there are only thirteen chapters (see 'Appendix'), out of a much longer list given in the manuscript. Chapter headings and some incipts of recipes are rubricated. The text is incomplete, ff. 146–149 show a melange of incantations and magical prescriptions always related to animals that, however, do not belong to the work of ʿĪsā ibn ʿAlī. The codex is a multiple-text manuscript that also contains a hippiatric work of the 14th century.

(G) MS Gotha 67/2 (ff. 32v–61v), 30 ff., 15 ll. per page.[72]

Written by a book hand in a plain *nasḫ*, sporadically vocalized. The chapter headings are written in a bolder script. A dot inscribed in a circle is used to mark the end of a recipe and the beginning of the following one. The same hand indexed the text, by systematically adding the purpose of the corresponding recipe in the outer margins. This manuscript shows a consistent gap in the contents, i.e. chapters 38–63 do not appear (see 'Appendix'). Among the witnesses of this branch of the tradition, G is the only one that does not have the initial list of chapters. Other formal aspects, however, resultedin its inclusion in this branch. The *Manāfiʿ* represents the second of two units in a multiple text manuscript. The first contains a text on the use of animal substances in agriculture, with a small addition of various properties arranged by purpose.

V.3 Branch (c)

(L) MS Leipzig 770 (ff. 2r–45v), 45 ff., 15 ll. per page.[73]

Written by a book hand in a plain and regular *nasḫ*. The title page gives the following title and description for the book in a spear-shaped arrangement: *Kitāb durrat al-ġawāṣṣ ʿalā al-manāfiʿ [wa] al-ḫawāṣṣ, min manāfiʿ al-waḥš wa-l-ṭayr wa mā ḏaḫarahū al-mulūk mimmā lā yuṭlaʿu ʿalayhī* ('Book of the Pearls of the Diver about the Useful and Occult Properties of Wild Animals, Birds, and the Highest Things that the Kings Recorded'). The codex is a multiple text manuscript. On the second line of f. 45v another text begins, in which other recipes are arranged by vegetal simple drugs. From f. 52r onwards the text is arranged by disease *a capite ad calcem*. The second text ends on f. 71r, with a spear-shaped colophon dating the copy to the year 1074 H. (1663–64 AD).This manuscript contains the longest version of the text.

(C) MS Cairo Dār al-Kutub, *Ṭibb Taymūr* 205, 31 ff., 23 ll. per page.

Written by a book hand in a cursive *nasḫ*, sporadically vocalized. The title page gives the following title and description for the book, arranged in the form of a spear: *Kitāb durrat al-ġawāṣṣ ʿalā al-manāfiʿ [wa] al-ḫawāṣṣ, min manāfiʿ al-waḥš wa-l-ṭayr wa mā ḏaḫarahū al-mulūk mimmā lā yuṭlaʿu ʿalaihi al-ġayra min asrār al-ḥikmat wa-fawāʾid al-ǧumla* ('Book of the Pearls of the Diver about the Useful and Occult Properties of Wild Animals, Birds, and the Highest Secrets of Wisdoms and all the Advantages that the Kings Recorded'). The chapter headings have their own dedicated line and are written in a bolder script (from the black-and-white reproduction it is

---

71 See Flügel 1865, 550–551.

72 See Pertsch 1878, 121–122.

73 See Vollers 1906, 249–250. This manuscript has been digitased by the Refaya Project and is available online: <https://www.refaiya.uni-leipzig.de/servlets/solr/select?fl=*&sort=ihsinvent+asc&q=%2BobjectType%3A%22islamhs%22+-ihsstatus%3A%22STAT0001%22+%2BallMeta%3Avollers&mask=search_form_islamhs_simple.xed&XSL.lastPage.SESSION=%2Fsearch_form_islamhs_simple.xed&version=4.5&start =562&fl=id,returnId&rows=1&XSL.Style=browse&origrows=25> (last accessed 11 February 2018).

not possible to see whether these were rubricated as well). In ff. 30v–50r there is a second text containing recipes arranged by illness and purpose, rather than by animal.[74]

74 It is significant to observe, in particular in branch (c), how the text of the *Manāfiʿ* used to circulate in association with one or more text that offered a different perspective on the properties. L and C are also very close in terms of wording, though L includes a higher number of recipes and chapters.

Bibliography

Ahlwardt, W. 1893. *Verzeichniss der arabischen Handschriften der königlichen Bibliothek zu Berlin*. Fünfter Band. Berlin.

Álvarez Millán, C. 1994. *Kitāb al-Muŷarrabāt. Libro de las experiencias médicas*. Madrid.

Álvarez Millán, C. 2010. “The case history in medieval Islamic medical literature: *Tajārib* and *Mujarrabāt* as source”. In: *Medical History* 54. 195–214.

Arberry, A. J. 1964. *The Chester Beatty Library. A Handlist of The Arabic Manuscripts*, vol. 7. Dublin.

Bausi, A et al., 2015. *Comparative Oriental Manuscript Studies. An Introduction*. Hamburg

Bos, G. 2009. “Maimonides on Medicinal Measures and Weights”. In: *Aleph* 9/2, 255–276

Brockelmann, C. 1943. *Geschichte der arabischen Literatur. Erster Band*. Leiden.

Brockelmann, C. 1937.*Geschichte der arabischen Literatur. Erster Supplementband*, Leiden.

Contadini, A. — 2008. ‘The Zoological-medicinal Material in the Arcadian Library Manuscript’. In: Ch. Burnett (ed.) *Ibn Baklarish's Book of Simples*. Oxford. 133–159.

Coulon, J.Ch. 2017. *La Magie en terre d'islam au Moyen Âge*. Paris

Dorpmueller, S. 2005. *Religiose Magie im »Buch der probaten Mittel«. Analyse, kritische Edition und Übersetzung des* Kitāb al-*Muǧarrabāt von Muḥammad ibn Yūsuf as-Sanūsī (gest. Um 895/1490)*. Wiesbaden.

Eamon, W. 1985. “Book of Secrets in Medieval and Early Modern Science”. In: *Sudhoffs Archiv* 69. 26–49.

Eisenstein, H. 1991. *Einführung in die arabische Zoographie*. Berlin.

Encyclopedia of Islam, New Edition, 1960–2002. Leiden (online edition).

Fani, S. 2013. *Le arti del libro secondo le fonti arabe originali. I ricettari arabi per la fabbricazione degli inchiostri (sec.* IX–XIII*): loro importanza per una corretta valutazione e conservazione del patrimonio manoscritto*. PhD dissertation, Napoli.

Flügel, G. 1865. *Die arabischen, persischen und türkischen Handschriften der kaiserlich-königlichen Hofbibliothek zu Wien*. Wien.

Frazer 1906–15. J.G. Frazer, *The Golden Bough*, 12 vols. London.

al-Ǧāḥiẓ, Abū ʿUṯmān ʿAmr ibn Baḥr 1965. *Kitāb al-ḥayawān*, 7 vols. Edited by ʿAbd al-Salām Muḥammad Hārūn. Cairo.

Hershbell, J.P. 1987. “Democritus and the Beginning of Greek Alchemy”. In: *Ambix* 34, 5–20.

Ibn abi ʿUṣaybiʿa, 1884. *ʿUyūn al-anbāʾ fī-ṭabaqāt al-aṭibbāʾ*. Herausgegeben von August Müller. Königsberg.

Ibn al-Nadīm 1872. *Kitāb al-Fihrist*. Herausgegeben von Gustav Flügel, 2 Bände. Leipzig.

Ibn al-Nadīm 1970. The *Fihrist* of al-Nadīm: a tenth century survey of Muslim culture, 2 vols. Edited and translated by Bayard Dodge. New York.

Ibn al-Qifṭī, 1903. *Taʾrīḫ al-ḥukamāʾ*. Herausgegeben von Julius Lippert. Leipzig.

Ibn Qutayba, ʿAbdallāh ibn Muslim 1949. “The Natural History Section from a 9th Century ‘Book of Useful Knowledge’, the *ʿUyūn al-aḫbār* of Ibn Qutayba”. Edited by L. Kopf and F.S. Bodenheimer. Leiden.

Kahl, O. 2002: *Sābūr Ibn Sahl. Small Dispensatory*, Leiden/Boston.

Käs, F. 2012. *Die* Risāla fī l-Ḫawāṣṣ *des Ibn al-Ǧazzār*, Wiesbaden.

Kraus, P. 1942. *Contribution à l'histoire des idées scientifiques dans l'Islam. Jābir et la science grecque*, vol. 1, Paris.

Kruk, R. 1990. “A Frothy Bubble: Spontaneous Generation in Medieval Islamic Tradition”. In: *Journal of Semitic Studies* 35, 265–82.

Kruk, R. 2001: ‘Timotheus of Gaza *On Animals* in the Arabic Tradition’. In: *Le Muséon*, 114. 355–87.

Laurenti, R. 1985. ‘La questione Bolo-Democrito’. In: *L'atomo fra scienza e letteratura*. Genova, 75–106.

Lane, E.W. 1863. *An Arabic-English Lexicon*, 8 vols. London

Leclerc, L. 1980. *Histoire de la Médicine Arabe*, 2 vols. Rabat.

Lehmhaus, L. and Martelli, M. 2017 (eds). *Collecting Recipes. Byzantine and Jewish Pharmacology in Dialogue*. Berlin.

Lentin, J and Grand'Henry, J. (eds.) 2008. *Moyen arabe et variétés mixtes de l'arabe à travers l'histoire*. Louvain-la-Neuve.

Lloyd, G. 1979. *Magic, Reason and Experience*. Cambridge.

Lloyd, G. 1983. *Science, Folklore and Ideology*. Cambridge.

Martelli, M. 2011. *Pseudo-Democrito. Scritti alchemici con un commento di Sinesio. Edizione critica del testo greco, traduzione e commento*. Paris/Milano.

Meyerhof, M. 1931. “ʿAlî at-Tabarî's “Paradise of Wisdom”, one of the oldest Arabic Compendium of Medicine'. In *Isis* 16. 6–54.

Muth, R. 1954. *Träger des Lebenskraft. Ausscheidungen des Organismus im Volksglauben der Antike*. Wien.

Pertsch, W. 1878. *Die orientalischen Handschriften der Herzoglichen Bibliothek zu Gotha*, vol 3.1. Gotha.

Pliny the Elder, 1963. *Natural History*, vol. 8. Translated by W.H.S. Jones. London/Cambridge, Massachussets

Raggetti, L. 2015. 'The ‚Science of Properties' and its Transmission'. In: J.C. Johnson (ed.), *In the Wake of Compendia: Infrastructural Contexts and the Licensing of Empiricism in Ancient and Medieval Mesopotamia*. Berlin, 159–176.

Raggetti, L. 2016. “*Cum Grano Salis*. Some Arabic Ink Recipes in Their Historical and Literary Context”. In: *Journal of Islamic Manuscripts* 7, 294–338.

Rosenthal, F. 1947. *The Technique and Approach of Islamic Scholarship*. Rome.

Ruiz Bravo-Villasante, C. 1980: *Libro de las utilidades de los animales*, Madrid.

Ruska, J 1912. *Das Steinbuch des Aristoteles mit literargeschichtlichen Untersuchungen nach der arabischen Handschrift der Bibliothèque Nationale*. Heidelberg.

Saif, L. 2016. "The Cows and the Bees: Arabic Sources and Parallels for Pseudo-Plato's *Liber vaccae* (*Kitāb al-Nawāmīs*)". In: *Journal of the Warburg and Courtauld Institutes* 79, 1–48.

Sauvaire, M.H. 1884a: "Matériaux pour servir a l'histoire de la numismatique et de la métrologie musulmanes. Deuxieme partie—poids". In: *Journal Asiatique* 8/3, 368–445.

Sauvaire, M.H. 1884b: M.H Sauveire, "Matériaux pour servir a l'histoire de la numismatique et de la métrologie musulmanes. Deuxieme partie—poids (suite)". In: *Journal Asiatique* 8/4, 307–321.

Sauvaire, M.H. 1885: "Matériaux pour servir a l'histoire de la numismatique et de la métrologie musulmanes. Deuxieme partie—poids (fin)". In: *Journal Asiatique* 8/5, 498–506.

Schopen, A. 2006. *Tinten und Tuschen des arabisch-islamischen Mittelalters*. Göttingen.

Sezgin, F. 1970. *Geschichte des arabischen Schrifttums*, vol. 3, Leiden.

Siggel, A. 1951. *Decknamen in der arabischen alchemistischen Literatur*. Berlin.

al-Ṭabarī, ʿAli b. Rabbān 1928. *Firdausu'l-Ḥikmat or Paradise of Wisdom*. Edited by. M.Z. Siddiqi. Berlin.

Thorndike, L. 1923. *A History of Magic and Experimental Science*, vol. 1. New York.

Totelin, L. 2009. *Hippocratic Recipes. Oral and Written Transmission of Pharmacological Knowledge in Fifth- and Fourth-Century Greece*. Leiden/Boston.

Trovato, P. 2014. *Everything You Always Wanted to Know about Lachmann's Method. A Non-Standard Handbook of Genealogical Textual Criticism in the Age of Post-Structuralism, Cladistics, and Copy-Text*. Padova.

Ullmann, M. 1970. *Die Medizin im Islam*. Leiden/Köhln.

Ullmann, M. 1972. *Die Geheimwissenschaft im Islam*. Leiden.

Ullmann, M. 1978. *Islamic Medicine*. Edinburgh.

Ullmann, M. 2002. *Wörterbuch zu den griechisch-arabischen Übersetzungen des 9. Jahrhunderts*. Wiesbaden.

Varvaro, A. 2012. *Prima lezione di filologia*, Roma/Bari.

Varvaro, A. and Cherchi, M. 1999. "The "New Philology" from an Italian Perspective". In: *Text* 12, 49–58.

Vollers, K. 1906. *Katalog der islamischen, christlich-orientalischen, jüdischen und samaritanischen Handschriften der Universitäts-Bibliothek zu Leipzig*. Leipzig.

Wehr H. 1979. *A Dictionary of Modern Written Arabic*, edited by J. Milton Cowan. Wiesbaden.

Wellmann, M. 1928. *Die Physika des Bolos Demokritos und der Magier Anaxilaos aus Larissa*. Berlin.

Witkam, J.J. 1988. "Establishing the stemma: fact or fiction?". In: *Manuscripts of the Middle East* 3, 88–101.

Witkam, J.J. 2013. "The Philologist's Stone. The Continuing Search for the Stemma". In: *Comparative Oriental Manuscript Studies Newsletter* 6. 34–38.

Wüstenfeld, F. 1840. *Geschichte der Arabischen Ärzte*. Göttingen.

Zack, L and Schippers, A. (eds.) 2012. *Middle Arabic and Mixed Arabic. Diachrony and Synchrony*. Leiden/Boston.

Manuscripts

(S)	MS Istanbul Şehid Ali Pasha 2096
(B)	MS Berlin Pet. II 244 (Ahlwardt 6240)
(T)	MS Istanbul Saray Ahmet III 2055
(W)	MS Wien 1481/2
(G)	MS Gotha 67/2
(L)	MS Leipzig 770
(C)	MS Cairo Dār al-Kutub, *Ṭibb Taymūr* 205

Conspectus siglorum

[...]	addidi
add.	addidit
om.	omisit

Edition and translation

	a	b	c
*	بسم الله الرحمن الرحيم الحمد لله رب العلمين وصلواته على سيدنا محمد واله وصبحه وسلم	بسم الله الرحمن الرحيم وما توفيقي الا بالله كتاب ما في الحيوان من المنافع مما عنى يجمعه عيسى ابن علي المتطبب	بسم الله الرحمن الرحيم وبه نستعين الحمد الله الحكيم المنان الديان الذى خلق الانسان وعلمه البيان وشرفه على سائر الحيوان والظهره بلطيف الامتنان على ما اودع من الحكمة فيما سيذكر من الحيوان والصلاة والسلام على اشرف آمل آنف من عبد مناف وبعث من ولد عدنان ونعت بدلائل الاعجاز القرآن وعلى اله واصاحبه ما تعاقب الجديدان
**	قال شيخ الامام ندرة الزمان علي بن عسى المتطبب رحمه الله تعالى هذا كتاب قد جمعته وجمعت فيه جميع اعضاء الحيوانات مما وجدته منفردا في كتب الفلاسفة المتقدمين والعلماء الاولين مثل هرمس واقليدس وبقراط وغيرهم من العلماء المتقدمين والذين عنوا بهذا الشأن والنظر فيه	قال مؤلف هذا الكتاب اني لم اجد له نسخة وانما جمعتُه من كتب متفرّقة للحكماء الاوائل مثل هرمس ودامقراطيس وغيرهما من الفلاسفة الذين عنوا بهذا الشأن	وبعد فهذا الكتاب جمعه فيه الامام العلامة ابو الحسن علي بن عيسى المطبب فرائد القوائد وعقائد القلائب مما ادخره الحكماء وانه من تجربته به العلاماء قيمته من المال انفس ويضاهي بحسنة الانفس وانتخبه ذامقراطيس وهرمس وغيرها ممن عنا هذا الشأن

* (a) وسلم] اجمعين B | S has a subtitle, probably completing the missing title page: كتاب مجموع الخواص من اعضاء الحيوانات تأليف الشيخ الحليم الأوحد علي بن عسى المتطبب بمدينة اندلس رحمه الله وغفر لكتابه وقاريه ولمن نظر فيه ولسائر المسلمين اجمعين امين يا رب العلمين S
(b) وما توفيقي...المتطبب] بسم الله الرحمن الرحيم بالله استفتح وبه استنجح وعليه اتوكل وبه استعين وهو حسبي ونعم الوكيل ولا قوة الا بالله العلى العظيم W; كتاب منافع الحيوانات. نبدا بعون الله تعالى بكتاب الحيوان وما فيها من المنفعة G
(c) وبه...الجديدان] بسم الله الرحمن الرحيم واسياله الاعانة والتوفيق الحمد الله الحليم المنان الديان الذى خلق والداء والدواء بلطيف الامتنان. اودع في كل شيء حكمته وخلق الانسان علمه البيان والصلاة والسلام على شرف الرسل سيد ولد عدنان وعلى اله واصابحه ما تعاقب الجديدان C

** (a) رحمه الله تعالى] *om.* B | جمعتُه] *om.* B | جميع] جمع B | هرمس] هرير B | واقليدس] وافلندس B | وبقراط] وابقراط B | وغيرهم] وغير B | المتقدمين] الاوّلين B | والذين عنوا بهذا الشأن والنظر فيه] *om.* B
(b) متفرّقة] كثيرة G; كثير W | الاوائل] *om.* W | من الفلاسفة] *om.* G
(c) العلامة] *add.* والطبيب الفهامة C | وانه من تجربته] واتقن مجربت C | قيمته من المال انفس ويضاهي] مما يضاهي C | وانتخبه] انتخبه الايمة من علماء C | ذامقراطيس] كابقراط C | *add.* هذا الفن C | عنى] اعتنى C

Introduction

	a	b	c
*	In the name of God the Merciful the Compassionate. Praise be to God, Lord of the worlds, His Prayer and Peace upon our Lord Muḥammad, his Family and His Companions.	In the name of God the Merciful the Compassionate, I have no success but in God. Book of the useful properties found in animals, collected by ʿĪsā ibn ʿAlī the medical practitioner.	In the name of God the Merciful the Compassionate. In Him we seek help, Praise be to God, the Perfectly Wise the Benefactor the Judge, who created the man, taught him eloquence, and honoured him over the rest of the animals, and with kindness showed him the gratitude, in conformity with the wisdom that is preserved in what we will mention about the animals. Prayer and Peace be upon the Noble that descended from ʿAbd Manāf, he came from the progeny of ʿAdnān and characterised the Qur'an with proofs of inimitability, [Prayer and Peace] on Him and his Companions, as long as the succession of days and nights will last.
**	The master, unique man of the time, ʿĪsā ibn ʿAlī the medical practitioner—may God be pleased with him—said: 'I composed this book and I have collected in it all the parts of animals that I found scattered in the books of the ancient philosophers, and of the first wise men, like Hermes, Euclid, Hippocrates, and other ancient learned men who dealt with this subject, and researched it.	The author of this book said: 'I did not find an original copy of this book, but I just composed it anew from different books of the first wise men, like Hermes, Democritus, and other philosophers who dealt with this subject.	Now then, in this book were collected by the most erudite master, Abū al-Ḥasan ʿAlī ibn ʿĪsā the medical practitioner, the gems of the benefits and the doctrines of the hearts that the wise men preserved, that is what comes from the experience of the learned men—its value comes from the wealth of the spirits, and imitates the beauty of the spirits—Democritus, Hermes, and other authors who dealt with this issue and investigated this field of knowledge.

***	*om.*	ووجدت في بعض هذه الكتب من المنافع التي قصدنا لجمعها اشياء خارجة عن هذا الغرض داخلة في باب الرقاء والعزائم ولم نر ندخلها في هذا الكتاب لشناعتها	*om.*
****	وجعلت هذا الكتاب ابوابا على كل باب منه اسمه منعته ومنفعته ثم نذكر كل حيوان منه ليكون ذلك اسهل وابين لمن نظر فيه والله الموفق للصواب	وقد صنّفت هذا الكتاب ابوابا وجعلت وعلى كل باب عددا ليسهل طلب ما يريد منه ولعله يكون قد خلط بالمنافع التي فيه اشياء من جنس ما قلنا بذئا فينبغى لك ايها الناظر في هذا الكتاب ان تعرف الغرض الذي قصدنا في جمعنا ما جمعنا فيه وتبسط بالعذر فيما يلقاك منه مما مخالف الغرض ويعلم ما ينال من قصد هذا الشأن من التعب والنصب وذلك يسير في جنب ما يحاوله من المنافع للناس	وترجم عنه بعد التجربة والبيان ومرتبة برتبها يسهل النظر فيه ويوضع معانيه والله الحق الاعانة على التهذيب وعليه توكلت واليه انيب

*** (b) من المنافع التي] *om.* G | قصدنا] *om.* G; قصدت W | لجمعها] *om.* G | الرقاء والعزائم] والرقاء العزائم G | ولم نر ندخلها] ولم ار ادخالها G W | لشناعتها] *om.* G; لاستعانتها W

**** (a) ونعته] ولغته B | ذلك] *om.* B

(b) صنّفت] جعلت G; وضعت W | هذا الكتاب] له G | وجعلت...منه] ليسهل طلب ما يراد منه وجعلت له عدد المنافع التي وصفها على الحواشي ايسهل W | ولعله...بذئا] ذلك G | بذئا] *om.* G | لا عن تعمدنا W | بذئا وذلك *add.* W | ايها الناظر في هذا الكتاب] *om.* W | مما مخالف الغرض] منه بخالف غرضك G; فيما خالف غرضنا W | ويعلم...والنصب] *om.* G | هذا الشأن] مثله W | والنصب] *om.* W | وذلك...للناس] *om.* G; الذي من منافع من يومّله من كتب في هين وذلك W يلحق الناس الذي سقى اظافير نفسه يصح له تلك الوكيل او الغلام وازداد له حبا وبُصاق اانسان من لدغ الهوي

(c) وترجم] واخبروا C | والبيان] بالبيان C | ومرتبة...انيف] حسان ابواب على ورتبه الانسان منافع يذكر فيه وبدأ الحيوان من انواع منافع من C

***	*om.*	In some of these books on the useful properties that we considered for the present collection; in the chapter on charms and spells, I found things outside its main purpose, but I did not want to include them in this book for their hideousness.	*om.*
****	I divided this book into chapters, every chapter has its name, its coherence and its usefulness; then I mentioned every single animal so that it will be easier and clearer for the one who looks in it, and God is the One who grants what is right.'	I compiled this book in ifferent chapters, and I assigned numbers to every chapter in order to ease the search of what one may want from it. Perhaps, however, some of the things of the kind that we defined loathsome have already mixed with the useful properties. So you should know, oh you who search in this book, the purpose that we have tried to achieve in our composition, and the sincere apology for anything extraneous to this purpose that we have laid in front of you, and to know the inconvenience and the problematic aspects that may derive from the consideration of this topic. This is, however, a small thing if compared to the useful properties that are here given to the people.'	It was translated from this following the experience, the explanation, and the order of its arrangement, in order to ease the search inside it, and to explain its meanings. God is the Truth, the Help for the rectification, in Him we put our trust, and to Him we will return.

١. الانسان

	a	b	c
	ذكر منافع اعضاء ابن ادم	الانسان	باب منافع الانسان
1.1	يؤخذ ضرس انسان ميت يجعل على الضرس الوجع يسكن وجعه باذن اللّه تعالى	لوجع الضرس يؤخذ ضرس انسان ميت يعلق على من به وجع الضرس فيسكن باذن الله تعالى	اذا أخذ ضرس الانسان وعلق على من يشتكي وجع الضرس ابرأه
1.2	للناسور في الانف يؤجد عظم الميّت يحرق حتى يصير رمادا ثم تخلط معه صبر ويحشي الناسور فيبرأ باذن اللّه تعالى	للناسور في الانف يؤخذ عظم الانسان الميت يحرق بالنار حتى يصير رمادا ثم يسحق ويخلط معه صبر يحشّي به الناسور وينفخ منه في الانف يبرأ	واذا أخذ وسحق وخلط بصبر ونفخ في الانف الذي في الناسور ابرأ
1.3	للبياض في العين يؤخذ حيات بطن الانسان فتجففت ويُسحق سحقا ناعما ويكتحل بها من في عينه بياض فيذهب باذن اللّه تعالى	للبياض في العين يؤخذ حيات الجوف فتجفف وتدق ويكتحل بها من بياض العين يبرأ	اذا أخذ الحيات الذي تظهر من بطن الانسان وجففت وسحقت ناعما واكتحل بها من بعينه بياض ابرأه
1.4	الآكلة في جميع البدن يؤخذ سذاب يابس ويدر على الأكلة فتبرأ باذن اللّه تعالى	للآكلة يؤخذ رجيع الانسان يابسا يخلط معه سذابا يابس ويدر على الآكلة يبرأ ان شاء الله تعالى	*om.*

1: (b) انسان] صفات منافع الانسان T
In W the section on 'Man' is at the end of the chapter, هذا منافع ما في الانسان ان شاء الله تعالى
1.1: (a) على الضرس] على صاحب الضرس B
(b) لوجع الضرس...فيسكن] ضرس الانسان الميت يعلق على من به وجع الضرس فيسكن W
(c) وجع الضرس] وجع اسنانه C
1.2: (a) للناسور في الانف] *om.* B | ثم تخلط] ويجعل B | ويحشي الناسور] ويجعل في الانف الذي فيه الناسور B | فيَبرأ] يبرا B
(b) للناسور...يبرأ] وعظم الانسان اذا حرق ثم سحق رماده وخلط معه صبر حشى به الناصور ونفخ منه في الانف الذي فيه النصاور W | *om.* G
(c) واذا اخذ...ابرا] لحم بني ادم واذا حرق وسحق وخلط بصبر ونفخ منه في الانف الذى في الناسور ابرأه C
1.3: (a) *om.* B
(b) للبياض...يبرأ] وحيات بطن الانسان يجففت ويدق ويكتحل بها البياض العين فيذهب W | *om.* G
(c) الانسان] الادمي C | بياض ابرأه] بياض من الجدري ابرأه C
1.4: (a) *om.* B
(b) للآكلة...يبرأ] رجيع الانسان يسحق ويخلط معه شراب يابس ويدر عليه الآكلية تبرأ W | *om.* G

1. Man

	a	b	c
	Exposition of the useful properties of the parts of the man	**The man**	**Chapter on the useful properties of the man**
1.1	Molar tooth of a dead man: if it is taken and placed on the aching molar tooth, then its pain will subside, with the permission of God, may He be exalted.	Against the pain of the molar: if the molar of a dead man is taken and hung on the man suffering from an aching molar, then it will cease, with the permission of God, may He be exalted.	Molar of a dead men: if it is taken and hung on the man suffering from the pain of a molar, then this will cure him.
1.2	Against the fistula in the nose: if the bone of a dead man is taken, burnt until it becomes ash, then mixed with aloe and stuffed inside the fistula, then this will heal, with the permission of God, may He be exalted.	Against the fistula in the nose: if the bone of a dead man is taken, burnt on the fire until becomes ash, then ground, mixed with aloe, stuffed inside the fistula, and blown inside the nose, then this will be cured.	And if it is taken, ground, mixed with aloe and blown inside the nose affected by a fistula, then this will be cured.
1.3	Against the glaucoma of the eye: if the worms that come out from the abdomen of a dead man are taken, dried, finely ground and rubbed on the eye of the man affected by glaucoma, then this will go away, with the permission of God, may He be exalted.	Against the glaucoma in the eye: if the worms of the belly are taken, dried, ground, and rubbed on the eye affected by glaucoma, then this will cure it.	If the worms that come out from the abdomen of man are dried, finely ground, and rubbed on the eye affected by glaucoma, then this will cure it.
1.4	Against the gangrene that affects the entire body: if some dry rue is taken and put on the eruption, then this will heal, with the permission of God, may He be exalted.	Against gangrene: if human excrement is taken when it is dried, pounded and melted with dry rue and applied on the eruption, then this will heal.	*om.*

1.5

اذا أخذ رجيع بن ادم وجفف وسحق وعجن بخل وعسل وطليت به الآكلة بريت اذا طليت به الخوانيق التي في الحلق برئت

وان أخذ من رجيع انسان يابس يسحق ويخلط ويعجن بعسل وطلى به الحلق نفع من الخانوق وكذلك ان نفخ منه في الحلق يابسا نفع من الخانوق

وان أخذ من رجيع الانسان يابسا فيسحق ويخلط معه خلّ خمر وعسل ويطلى به الحلق الذي يكون فيه الآكلة او الخوانيق فتزول باذن اللّه يعالى

1.6

اذا أخذ ضرس انسان وعظم الجناح الايمن من الهدهد ووضع تحت رأس النائم لم ينتبه ما دام تحته

يؤخذ ضرس الانسان وعظم جناح الهدهد الايمن فيجعل تحت رأس الانسان فلا يزال نائما حتى ينزع ذلك من تحت رأسه

يؤخذ ضرس ميّت وعظم جناح الهدهد فيجعل تحت رأس النائم فلا يزال نائمًا حتى تزعها من تحت رأسه

1.7

شعر ابن ادم اذا علق على من يشتكي الشقيقة برئ

شعر الانسان اذا علق على من يشتكي شقّ رأسه سكن الوجع

شعر الانسان اذا علّق على من يشتكي الشقيقة في دماغه فتسكن باذن اللّه تعالى

1.8

واذا بل الشعر بالخل ووضع على عضة الكلب ابرأها

والشعر ايضا اذا بل بالخل ووضع على عضة الكلب نفع من ساعته وبول الانسان اذا صب على عضة الكلب نفع

وشعر الانسان اذا بل بخل خمر وجعل على عضّة الكلب الكلب نفعه باذن اللّه تعالى

1.9

اذا أخذ من دم الحجمة او الفصادة او الرعاف وترك في الماء في اناء فخار اربعين يوما وجد فيه تمثال بني ادم فيجعل ذلك التمثال في دقيق شعير سبعة ايام يخرج ويذبح فيسيل منه دم اذا خلط هذا الدم شيء من خمر عتيق

للمحبة اذا أخذ من دم الحجمة او الرعاف ويجعل ذلك الدم في فخارة ويترك اربعين يوما فيؤجد فيه مثل الانسان فيجعل ذلك المثال في دقيق الشعير سبعة ايام فخذه بعد ذلك واذبحه وخذ

دم الانسان ان اأخذ وجعل في وعاء فخار وطين رأسه ويدفن في اي شيء اربعين يوما ثم يخرج الوعاء فتأخذ الدم يصير بمثال ابن ادم فيجعل ذلك التمثال في دقيق سبعة ايام ثم يؤخذ فيذبح فيسيل منه دم فخذ ذلك الدم فاخلط معه شيء من خل خمر خالص

1.5: (a) فتزول] فتبرأ B

(b) وان أخذ...الخانوق] زبل الانسان يابس ناعما فيسحق ويخلط ويعجن يعسل ويطلي به الخلق من داخل فيبرأ من الحوانيق W | وكذلك...الخانوق] وكذلك ان نفخ فيه بغير W | om. G

(c) اذا أخذ رجيع بن ادم وجفف] رجيع الانسان اذا جفف C | بريت] ابرأها C | In C other three recipes are added: the first with the tooth of a man against the toothache سن الانسان اذا علق على السن الوجع اسكنه; the second with the tooth of a man to induce sleep وان وضع تحت رأس انسان نائم زاد نومه; and the third involving fumigations with human hair to turn something yellow شعر الانسان اذا بخر به شيء صفره وغير لونه.

1.6: (b) يؤخذ] *om.* W | فيجعل] تجعل W | ينزع] يرفع W | ذلك من تحت رأسه] *om.* W

1.7: (a) *om.* B

(b) This recipe is attested only in W and G

(c) الشقيقية] الشقيقية اي صداع الراس *add.* C | برئ] ابرأه C

1.8: (b) شعر الانسان] واذا بُل شعر W; والشعر ايضا G | نفع] نفعه W; من ساعته add. G | وبول...نفع] *om.* W G

(c) بالخل] بالخل البصل *add.* C

1.9: (a) This recipe is attested only in B

(b) للمحبة...فانه يحبك] *om.* W G

(c) اذا أخذ من دم الحجمة] دم الانسان اذا أخذ من الحجمة C | وترك في الماء في اناء] وجعل في اناء C | وجد] ظهر C | في دقيق شعير] في دقيق من دقيق الشعير C | يخرج] ثم يخرج C | لاحد من ذكر] لاحد ذكر C

1.5	Human excrement: if it is taken when it is dried, ground, mixed with wine vinegar and honey, rubbed on the throat affected by gangrene or suffocation, then these will cease, with the permission of God, may He be exalted.	Dry human excrement: if it is taken, ground, melted, kneaded with honey, rubbed on the throat, this will cure the suffocation; and likewise, if it is blown dry inside the throat.	Human excrement: if it is dried, ground and kneaded with vinegar and honey, rubbed on the throat affected by gangrene or a feeling of breathlessness, then these will be cured.
1.6	If the molar of a dead man and the bone from a hoopoe's wing are taken, placed under the head of a sleeping man, then he will keep sleeping as long as they remain under his head.	If the molar of a man and the bone from the right wing of a hoopoe are placed under the head of a man, then he will keep sleeping until this is removed from underneath his head.	If the molar tooth of a man and the bone of the right wing from a hoopoe are taken and placed under the head of a sleeping man, then he will not wake up as long as they remain under him.
1.7	Hair of a man: if it is hung on the man suffering from migraine in his brain, then this will subside.	Hair of a man: if it is hung on the man suffering from migraine, then the pain will subside.	Hair of a man: if it is hung on the man suffering from migraine, then he will heal.
1.8	Hair of a man: if it is moistened with wine vinegar and applied on the bite of a rabid dog, then this will be useful against it, with the permission of God, may He be exalted.	The hair, again: if it is moistened with vinegar and applied on the bite of a dog, willthis be instantly useful against this; the urine of a man is effective too, if poured on the bite of a dog.	If the hair is moistened with vinegar and applied to the bite of a dog, then this will cure it.
1.9	Man blood: if it is taken and put in a pottery vessel, then its opening is covered with clay and buried somewhere for forty days; then take out the vessel with the blood inside, which in the meanwhile has turned into the effigy of a man, take this effigy and put it in the flour for seven days, take it out and slaughter it, then the blood will run from it. Take this blood, mix it with some pure wine vinegar and give it	For love: if the blood from cupping or from a nosebleed is taken, put in a vessel, and left there for forty days, then the figurine of a man can be found inside it; put this figurine in some wheat flour for seven days, then take it out, slaughter it, and take the blood that runs from it, mix it with wine, and give it to drink to	If the blood from cupping or blood-letting or the blood from a nose-bleed is left in water inside a pottery vessel for forty days, then the effigy of a man can be found inside it; put this effigy in some wheat flour for seven days, take it out, slaughter it and then the blood will run from it. If this blood is mixed with a bit of old wine, given to someone—man or

وتسقيه لاحد من ذكر او انثى فعل في المحبة ما لا يكاد بغير عنه

ما يسيل من دمه فاخلطه بخمر اسقه من شئت ذكر كان او انثى فانه يحبك

واسقيه لبن شيت ذكرا او انثى فانه يحبك حبا شديدا

1.10

وان خلط من ذلك الدم بشيء من دهن ورد خالص عتيق ودهن به انسان وجهه كان مقبولا عند السلاطين والامر او عظماء الناس وفعله عجيب جدا

وان طرحتَ ذلك الدم الذي يخرج من التمثال في دهن ومسحتَ به وجهك كان نافعا للسلطان ولكل حاجة فانها تقضي

وان أخذت من ذلك الدم وخلطت معه دهن زنبق ودهنت وجعل كنت مقبولا عند الملوك والسلاطين وجميع بني ادم

1.11

دم بن ادم اذا عجن بدقيق الحلبة وماء السذاب والعسل وطليت به قرحة تكون في البدن خصوصا التى بالساقين والرطبة المايية التى تسيل الدم تبرأ باذن الله تعالى

وان أخذ دم انسان اذا احتجم يعجن به دقيق حلبة وماء سذاب والعسل وطلى على كل قرحة تكون في الجسم وخاصة الساقين والقروح التي يسيل منها الماء نافع ان شاء الله تعالى

دم الانسان يؤخذ ويعجن بدقيق الحلبة ويرطّب بماء السذاب عسل النحل ويطلي كل قرحة [...]

المرأة والصبيان

1.12

اذا أخذ دم الحيض من امرأة جارية بكر وخلط بخمر عتيق واكتحل به في عينه بياض ابرأه

يؤخذ دم حيض المرأة لم يلمسها رجل يخلط معه المنى ويحتكل به للبياض الذي في العين فانه يبرأ

يؤخذ دم حيضة المرأة البكر فيخلط معه خمر ويحتكل به من في عينه بياض فانه يبرأ باذن الله تعالى

1.13

خرقة دم الخيض اذا علقت على مؤخر سفينة لا يدخلها ريح ولا زوبعة

خرقة الحيضة تعلّق في موخر السفينة لا يقربها ريح ولا زوبعة

يؤخذ خرقة دم الحيضة فيعلق على مؤخر السفينة فلا يدخلها الريح عاصف ولا زوبعة

1.10: (a) This recipe is attested only in B
(b) *om.* G W
(c) بشيء من دهن] بشيء بدهن C | مقبولا] مقبولا عند كل احد *add.* C | عند السلاطين] عند السلطان C | والامر او عظماء الناس] الاكابر C | وفعله] وله فعل C
1.11: (a) *om.* B
(b) وان أخذ...نافع] دم الانسان من حجامة اذا عجن به دقيق حلبة ورطّب بماء الشراب الطري وشيء من عسل وطلى على كلّ قرحة تكون في الجسد جاصة في الساقين حلبه ورطبه وابرأ ذلك W; دم حجامة الانسان او دم رعاف اذا عجن به دقيق حلبة ورطب بماء السذاب الرطب مع العسل وطلي به القروح التي تكون في الجسد جميعة الرطب واليابس نفع نفعا جيدا G
(c) دم بن ادم...تبرأ] دم بن ادم اذا عجن بدقيق الحلبه وماء الفنجل وهو السداب والعسل وطليت به القروح التي تكون في البدن خصوصا الذى تكون بالساق ابرأه وكذلك تذهب الرطوبة الماية C
1.12: (a) *om.* B
(b) يؤخذ] *om.* W G; حيض المرأة] حيضها W | لم يلمسها] لم يكونوا مسهّل W; لم يلمسها] لم يمسّها G | للبياض] البياض W; الذي في العين] om. W G | فانه يبرأ] فيبرأ W G
(c) اذا أخذ] *om.* C | امرأة] *om.* C | وخلط] اذا خلط C | في عينه] بعينيه C
1.13: (a) ولا زوبعة] *om.* B
(b) تعلّق] اذا علّقت W G

	to drink to whomever you desire—either man or woman—then this person will love you passionately.	whomever you desire, either man or woman, and this person will love you.	woman—to drink, then this will do for love what cannot be achieved by any other mean.
1.10	If you take this blood, mix it with lily oil and rub it on the body, then you will be welcome in the presence of kings, sultans and of all the people.	If you add the blood that comes out of this figurine to some oil and rub your face with it, then this will be useful for an audience with the sultan and for any other need, in fact the need will be satisfied.	If this blood is mixed with some pure rose oil and a man rubs it on his face, then he will be welcome in the presence of sultans, princes, and the mighty people, and its effect is really amazing.
1.11	Man blood: if it is taken, kneaded with fenugreek flour, moistened with rue water and rubbed on every kind of ulcer [...]	Human blood from cupping: if it is taken, kneaded with fenugreek flour, rue water, and honey, then rubbed on any kind of ulcer that affects the body, especially the legs, then this will be useful, God willing.	Blood of a man: if it is kneaded with fenugreek flour, rue water and honey, rubbed on the ulcers that affect the body, especially the ones on the legs and the moist ulcers from which the blood flows, then these will heal, with the permission of God, may He be exalted.
	–	**Woman and Children**	–
1.12	Menstrual blood of a virgin: if it is taken, mixed with wine and rubbed on the eyes of a man affected by glaucoma, then this will heal, with the permission of God, may He be exalted.	Menstrual blood of a woman, who has not yet been touched by a man: if it is mixed with some sperm and rubbed on the eyes against the glaucoma, then this will heal.	Menstrual blood of a virgin maiden: if it is taken, mixed with old wine and rubbed on the glaucoma of the eyes, then this will cure it.
1.13	If a piece of cloth soaked in menstrual blood is taken, hung on the stern of a ship, then neither a violent wind nor a storm will damage it.	If a piece of cloth from the menstruation is hung on the stern of a ship, then neither the wind nor a storm will damage it.	If a piece of cloth soaked in menstrual blood is hung on the stern of a ship, then neither the wind nor a storm will damage it.

1.14	زبل الانسان نافع من جميع السموم القاتلة شربا ومن نهش الافاعى القاتلة	*om.*	*om.*
1.15	شعر الانسان اذا بخرت به اذا تحت امرأة منعها من انتفاخ الرحم	*om.*	*om.*
1.16	دهنه اذا أخذ وهو حار حين يخرج من الزق وطلى به السرطان ابرأه	*om.*	*om.*
1.17	اذا صاب المرأة وجع السرة تأخذ خرقة الحيض وتحرقها حتى تصير رمادا ثم تأخذ من ذلك الرماد جزء ومن الكثوث جزء ويذاب بماء فاتر ويطلي به حول السرة تبرأ وان اصابها ذلك عند النفاس سكن ذلك	المرأة اذا اصابها وجع السرة عند النفاس يؤخذ خرقة حيضها فتحرق ويؤخد منها ومن دمها جزء ومن الكشوث اليابس جزء ويذاب بماء فاتر ويطلي به المكان فيسكن الوجع باذن الله	واذا اصاب المرأة وجع في السرة عند النفاس فتأخذ خرقة الخيضة فتخرقها حتى تصير رمادا ويؤخذ من رمادها جزء ومن الاكشوث العراقي جزء ويداف الجيع بماء فاتر ويُطلي به مكان الوجع باذن الله تعالى
1.18	لبن الجارية البكر اذا شربه انسان مع عسل فتت الحصاة وادر البول	لبن النساء اذا شرب مع الشراب والعسل فتّت الحصاة	يؤخذ لبن امرأة فيخلط معه العسل والخمر العتيق ويسقي لمن به الحصاة ولبول الرمل
	—	الصبي	—
1.19	اذا ولد الطفل ازرقا رضعه لبن حبشية فانها تذهب تلك الزرقة	اذا ولد الصبي ازرق العين فارضعته حبشية سبعة ايام صار اشهل وذهبت الزرقة من عينيه	اذا ولد الصغير اشهلا ازرقا فيسقي لبن حبشية سبعة ايام فيذهب من عينه الزرقة باذن الله تعالى

1.14: (c) *om.* C

1.15: (c) *om.* C

1.16: (c) *om.* C

1.17: (a) السرة] الصر S | السرة] الظهر B | ويؤخذ] وخذ B | الاكشوث] الكشوَث B | ويداف] وتطلق B | الوجع] الوجع فيذهب عنه *add.* B
(b) السرة] الضرس T | فيسكن الوجع...فيسكن الوجع] ويؤخذ خرقة حيض المراة التي اصابها وجع في سرّتها عند النفاس فيحرق الخرقة ويؤخد من رمادها جزء ومن الكسوب اليابس جزء ويضاف بماء فاتر ويطلي به مكان الوجع فيسكن W; المرأة اذا اصابها وجع الضرس عند النفاس يؤخذ خرقة حيضها فتحرق ويؤخد منها ومندمها جزء ومن الكشوث اليابس جزء ويذاب بماء فاتر ويطلي به المكان فيسكن الوجع باذن الله G
(c) تأخذ] فتأخذ C | حتى] الى ان C | ويطلي به حول السرة] ويطلي بها السرة C | تبرأ] فانها تبرا C | سكن ذلك] فيسكنه C

1.18: (a) فيخلط] تخلط B | ولبول الرمل] فيذهب عنه وببول الرمل *add.* B
(b) الشراب والعسل] الشراب او السذاب G | الحصاة] الحصاة من المثانة W; حصاة المثانة G
(c) لبن الجارية...وادر البول] لبن الجارية اذا شربه من به الحصاه مع شي من عسل فتت الحصاة وادر البول C | In C another recipe is added, with woman milk to dissolve the stones in the bladder: لبن المراة من شربه مع مبن حليب فتت الحصاة من المثانة.

1.19: (a) أشهلا ازرقا] ازرقا اشهلا B | من عينه الزرقة] الزرقة من عينيه B
(b) اشهل] اسهل W G | وذهبت الزرقة من عينيه] *om.* W G
(c) In C this recipe is after 1.20 | اذا ولد...الزرقة] اذا كانت عين الطفل زرقا عند الولادة ارتضعه من فتات حبشة اذهب الزرقة C

1.14	*om.*	*om.*	Human excrement is useful against all the deathly poisons and the bite of a deadly viper.
1.15	*om.*	*om.*	Hair of a man: if it is fumigated under a woman, then this will prevent the swelling of the womb.
1.16	*om.*	*om.*	His grease: if it is taken warm, as it comes out from the skin, and rubbed on a cancer, then this will cure it.
1.17	If a woman happens to have umbilical pain at the moment of the delivery, take a piece of cloth soaked with menstrual blood, burn it until it becomes ash, take one part of its ash and one part of Iraqi clover dodder, mix everything with lukewarm water and rub it on the aching part, with the permission of God, may He be exalted.	If a woman happens to have umbilical pain when she breathes, take a piece of cloth soaked with menstrual blood, burn it, take one part of it and one of her blood, one part of dry clover dodder, mix it with warm water and rub it on the part, then the pain will cease with the permission of God.	If a woman happens to have umbilical pain, take a piece of cloth soaked with menstrual blood, burn it until it becomes ash, take one part of its ash, one part of clover dodder, liquefy it with lukewarm water and rub it around the umbilicus; and if it happens at the moment of the labour, then this will calm the pain.
1.18	Woman milk: if it is taken, mixed with honey and old wine, and then given to drink to a man suffering from [bladder] stones and sand in his urine, then this will be useful.	Woman milk: if it is drunk with wine and honey, then this will dissolve the bladder stones.	If a man drinks the milk of a virgin maiden with honey, then this will dissolve the [bladder] stones and will make his urine flow more easily.
	–	**Child**	–
1.19	If a baby has deep-blue eyes, he has to be given the milk of an Abyssinian woman for seven days to drink, then the blue will leave his eyes, with the permission of God, may He be exalted.	If a child is born with blue eyes, then an Abyssinian woman should nurse him at her breast for seven days, then the blue will turn to black.	If a child is born with blue eyes, he should be breast-fed with the milk of an Abyssinian woman, then this blue colour will go away.

1.20	يؤجد رجيع المولود ساعة يولد فيجفف ويسحق ويكحل به صاحب البياض والغشاوة على العين فيبرأ باذن الله تعالى	رجيع الصبي حين يولد اذا جفف وكحّل البياض في العين نفع منها وينفع من الغشاوة في العين ايضا	رجيع الطفل عند الولادة يجفف ويسحق ويكتحل من بعينه بياض يبرأ
1.21	يؤخذ قلفة الصغير عند ختانه فتجفف ويسحق ويخلط معها مسك خالص وتسقي لمن بدأ في الجذام فيفق عنه باذن الله تعالى	قلفة الصبيان تجفّف وتدق وتخلط ما شيء من مسك ويسقي من به الجدام فيقف ولا يزيد	قلف الصبيان المطهرين اذا اجففت وسحق وخلطت بمسك وشربه صاحب البرص والجذام وقعه
1.22	وان احرقت ويسقي منها صاحب البرص يبرأ باذن الله تعالى	وان احرق ودق وسقي من به برص وشرب بعده الماء وقع ولم يزدد	واذا احرقت ويسحقت وشربها من به البرص اذهبه
1.23	يؤخذ رجيع الانسان العتيق قدر ربع مثقال يسحق ويسقي لمن به القولنج وكان ابلغ	للقولنج يؤخذ رجيع الانسان قدر حمصة ودق فيذاف بخل حادق ويسقي من به القولنج يبرأ باذن الله تعالى	رجيع ابن ادم اذا اسحق واذيب بماء فاتر ابرأ القولنج لوقته وان اذيب بالخل فابلغ
1.24	يؤخذ رجيع الانسان وهو سخن كما يخرج ويخلاط معه خمر يوجر به الدابة التي بها الحمر فيزول باذن الله تعالى	لحم الدواب يؤخذ رجيع الانسان حارا وتوجر الدابة منه ويخلط مع خمر وتوجر به الدابة فان الخمر يذهب من قوته ومن ساعته	رجيع الانسان وهو حار حين يظهر يخلط بخمر ويسعط به الدابة الممغولة تبرأ لوقته

1.20: (a) ويكحل] ويكتحل B | على العين] om. B
(b) رجيع الصبي...في العين] رجيع الصبي حين يولد تجفّف وتكتحّل به البياض في العين ويقلعه ونفع الغشاوة في العين W | In T and W another recipe is added, with evaporated child urine, said to be included in the 'chapters on the art (alchemy)' بول الصبي يصاعد فيدخل في ابواب الصنعة.
(c) يجفف ويسحق ويكتحل] اذا جفف وسحق وكتحل C | يبرأ] برأه C
1.21: (a) ختانه] الختان B | لمن بدا في الجذام] في بدن الخدام B
(b) قلفة الصبيان ...ولا يزيد] قلفتي الصبي اذا جمع; W بول الصبي يجفّف ويدق ويخلط معها شيء من مسك وتسقي منه من ابتداء به الجدام فلا يزيد; G وجفف ودق وخلط بشيء من مسك وسقي من بدأ به الجذام فانه ليقف ولا يزيد
(c) وشربه صاحب البرص والجذام] وشربها من به برص او جذام C | وقعه] add. وقعه وزال البرص C
1.22: (a) يبرأ] فيبرأ B
(c) om. C
1.23: (a) قدر] مقدار B | فيزول عنه] وكان ابلغ B
(b) للقولنج...يبرأ] ورجيع الانسان يسحق ويؤخذ منه قدر حمصة فتضاف بالخل حالمض ويسقي منه من به القولنج واسر البول أي رجيع كان من رجيع الناس W | اذا أخذ من رجيع الانسان والصبي قدر حمصة ودق واذيف بخل خالس وسقى صاحب القولنج برئ G
(c) أبرأ] ذهب C
1.24: (b) لحم الدواب...ومن ساعته] ورجيع الانسان اذا; W رجيع الانسان ايضا حارا اذا خلط مع جزء الحرث الحمير والدواب دهن حمره من ساعته; G أخذ حارا كما يخرج وخلط مع خمر واوجرت منه الدابة ذهب عنها الحمر من ساعته
(c) رجيع الانسان...لوقته] واذا اخذ رجيع الانسان حين يطهر وهو حار وسعط به الدابة الممغولة ابرأها C

1.20	Excrement of a baby: if it is taken when he is just born, dried, ground and rubbed on the eyes of the man suffering from glaucoma and cataract, then he will heal, with the permission of God, may He be exalted.	Excrement of a baby: if it is taken when he is just born, dried and rubbed on the eye, this will be useful for the eye and for the cataract as well.	Excrement of a baby: if it is taken when he is just born, then is dried, ground and rubbed on the eyes of a man suffering from glaucoma, then he will heal.
1.21	Foreskin of a baby: if it is taken at the moment of his circumcision, dried, ground, mixed with pure musk and given to the man who has just contracted elephantiasis to drink, then he will recover, with the permission of God, may He be exalted.	Foreskins of babies: if they are dried, pounded, mixed with some musk and given to drink to the man who is affected by elephantiasis, then this will cease and will not increase.	Foreskin of babies: if they are dried, pounded, mixed with musk and drunk by the man suffering from leprosy and elephantiasis, then these will cease.
1.22	And if it is burnt and given to drink to a man affected by leprosy, then this will heal, with the permission of God, may He be exalted.	And if it is burnt, ground, and given to drink to a man affected by leprosy—and he drinks water after it—this will cease and will not increase.	And if it is burnt, ground and drunk by a man affected by leprosy, this will make it cease.
1.23	Man excrement: if one quarter *miṯqāl* of it is taken, ground and given to drink to a man suffering from colic, then this will be even more effective.	Against colic: if the measure of a chickpea of excrement from an adult or from a child is taken, pounded, mixed with sour vinegar and given to a man suffering from colic to drink, then he will heal, with the permission of God the Highest.	Human excrement: if it is taken, ground, liquefied with lukewarm water, then this will instantly cure colic. And if it is liquefied with vinegar, this will be even more effective.
1.24	Man excrement: if it is taken—and it should be warm as in the moment in which it comes out—melted with wine and given to a beast which suffers from erysipelas, then this will cease, with the permission of God, may He be exalted.	Against the suffering of the beasts, human excrement: if it is taken warm as they come out, melted with wine and given to a beast, then this will make the erysipelas cease instantly.	Human excrement: if is taken warm as it comes out, is melted with wine and inhaled by the beasts suffering from abdominal pain, then this will cure them instantly.

1.25	اذا اسقيت المرأة وسخ قدميك احبتك حبا شديدا وان شربت وسخ قدميها أحببتها حبا سديدا	وان اسقت المرأة وسخ قدميها لانسان احبها وكذلك الرجل اذا اسقاها وسخ رجليه	وسخ رجل بني ادم اذا غسلت بالماء وشربه انسان حبك حبا شديدا وكذلك المرأة اذا فعلت ذلك
1.26	اذا اردت ان ينصحك خادمك في خدمته فقلم اظفارك الجميع واحرقهم واسقيهم له في شيء من خمر او بماء فانّه ينصحك ويحبّك حبا عظيما ويواظب علي خدمتك وكل من شرب من تلك احبّك حبا شديدا	وان اردتَ ان ينصح لك خادمك فقص اظفارك كلها واحرقها بالنار واسقه إياها وكل من سقيتَ منه من جميع الناس احبك حبا شديدا	اذا قلمت اظفارك بالمقلوب وحرقتهم واسقيتهم لمن تريد حبك حبا مفرطا وكان من شرب من ذلك اثر فيه
1.27	*om.*	بصاق الانسان ينفع من لدغ الهوام	*om.*
1.28	*om.*	عظم الانسان الميت اذا علق على من به الحمى الربع ينفع نفعا بينا	*om.*
1.29	*om.*	للحمى الربع والمثلثة يكتب في رقاع ان كانت ربعا يكتب في رقاع اربعة وان كانت مثلثة يكون في ثلاثة وان كانت يومين قطّعت اثنين وان كان يوما تكتب واحدة نافع ان شاء الله تعالى	*om.*
1.30	*om.*	بول الانسان اذا غلى النار وطلى به النقرس سكن وجعه وضربانه	*om.*

1.25: (b) *om.* W | In G another recipe is added, with the dirt from the feet diluted in wine to induce pregnancy: اذا اردت ان تحبل المرأة فاسقها وسخ قدميك في نبيذ اغيره ومن الاشربة وهي لا تعلم فانها تحبل.
(c) وسخ رجل...ذلك] غسالة اليدي الانسان ورجليه اذا شرب احد فعل المحبة امرا عجيبا C
1.26: (a) اظفارك الجميع] جميع اظفارك B | ويواظب...شديدا] *om.* B | In B another recipe is added, with human saliva to cure the stings of the hornets: اذا الطخت لسعة الزنبور بريقك فانه يزول المها
(b) وان اردت...حبا شديدا] اذا الطخت لسعة الزنبور بريقك فانّه يزوّل المها W | In W another recipe is added, to increase the flow of milk during the lactation: وقلة اللبن تسقي المرأة من كل يوم من بزر الرطبة مدقوقا في كل يوم وزن درهم ونصف يشرب ايام فيكثر اللبن ويغزر ان شاء الله تعالى
(c) اذا قلمت...اثر فيه] قلامة الاظفارك اذا احرقت وشربها احد فعل في محبة ايضا فعلان غريبا C
1.27: (b) بصاق] بزاق T | *om.* W | In G another recipe is added, with human urine against the deadly poisons: بول الانسان اذا شرب نفع من السموم المهلكة.
1.28: (b) عظم] بول T | *om.* W
1.29: (b) Qur'an 73:15 ('Indeed, We have sent to you a Messenger as a witness upon you just as We sent to Pharaoh a messenger') follows this recipe | *om.* W G
1.30: (b) بول الانسان...والضربان] بول الانسان اذا غلى النار وعلى به النقرس سكن وجعه وضربانه W | بول الانسان اذا غلى على النار وطلى به صاحب النقرس رجله نفعه G

1.25	If you give the dirt from your feet to a woman to drink, then she will love you passionately; and if you drink the dirt of her feet, then you will love her passionately.	If a woman gives the dirt from her feet to a man to drink, then he will love her; and the same happens with a man, if he gives the dirt from his feet to drink to her.	If you wash the dirt from human feet with water and someone drinks this, then he will love you passionately. And it is the same for the woman, if she does so.
1.26	If you want that your servant is well disposed towards you during his service, clip all your nails, burn them and give him them to drink with some wine or water, then he will be well disposed towards you, will deeply love you, will be constant in his service; and everyone who drinks this will deeply love you.	If you want that your servant is well disposed towards you, clip all your nails, burn them in the fire, and give them to drink; then anyone who drinks it will deeply love you.	If you cut your nails the upside-down, burn them and give them to drink to the one whose love you deeply desire, since this potion will leave a sign inside him.
1.27	*om.*	Human saliva is useful against the sting of harmful insects.	*om.*
1.28	*om.*	Bone of a dead man: if it is hung on the a man suffering from quartan fever, then this will be really useful to him.	*om.*
1.29	*om.*	Against quartan and tertian fever write on a slip of paper: write ‘four’ if it is a quartan fever, write ‘three’ if it is a tertian fever, if it is a fever that comes every two days write ‘two’, and if a fever comes everyday write ‘one’, and this will be useful, God willing.	*om.*
1.30	*om.*	Urine of a man: if it is boiled on a fire and rubbed on the feet of a man suffering from gout, then this will be useful to him.	*om.*

§			
1.31	اذا اردت ان يحبك انسان فاغسل جيت قيمصك واسقيه من ماء وهو لا يعلم فانة يحبك حبا شديدا	وان اردت ان يحبك انسان فاغسل جيب قميصك بالنبيذ واسقيه اياه وهو لا يعلم فانه يحبك ويكرمك	اذا اردت ان يحبك انسان فاغسل جيب قميصك واسفه وهو لا يعلم فهو يحبك ويكرم عليه الاكرام
1.32	اذا اردت يجتمع في برج الحمام خذ رأس انسان ميت يكن له مده وادفنه في ذلك البرج فانه يجتمع عليه الحمام من كل مكان	وان كان لك برج حمام واردت ان يكثرون ويزيدون فادفن جمجمة ميت قديم	اذا اردت ان يكثر الحمام في البرج فادفن في رأس انسان ميت ويكون له مدة زمان قد مات فانه يكثر فيه الحمام
1.33	لبن الجارية الحبشية اذا خلط بشىء من دهن الزنبق وسعط به صاحب الفالج واللوقة ابرأه لوقته ومقدار السعوط منه وزن قيراط للرجل وللطفل ورن حبة ويخلط معه في بعض الاوقات عنزروت ابيض ويقطر في العين للحمرة تبرأ	للقوة والفالج قضيب الانسان يسعط بلبن جارية حبشية وان وضع معه شىء من زنبق مضرّب حتى يختلط ويسعّط به الرجل وزن قراط والصبي وزن حبتين	يؤخذ لبن حبشية ويخلط معه دهن زنبق وعنزروت ويسعط به صاحب اللقوة في الوجه فانه يبرأ باذن اللّه تعالى
1.34	*om.*	ويذاف ايضا بعض الاوقات على قدر الاحتمال كندس وعروق كندس من كل واحد جزء ويسحق ويذاف في اللبن ويقطّر عليه الزنبق ويسعط به فانه نافع ان شاء الله تعالى	*om.*
1.35	*om.*	لوجع الضرس يؤخذ عظم انسان ميت فيمرّ به على الضرس فيسكن	للمغل اذا امغلت الدابة تاخذ عظم ميت وتسحقه سحقا ناعما ويذيبه بماء حار وتسقه للدابة فتبرأ باذن اللّه تعالى

1.31: (b) *om.* W | وان اردت] اذا اردت G | بالنبيذ] بنبيذ G | ويكرمك] *om.* G
(c) ماء] ماية L
1.32: (a) ويكون] *om.* B | فانه يكثر فيه الحمام] *om.* B
(b) وان كان...ميت قديم] ومكثرة الحمام يدفن في برج الحمام جمجم من كل مكان C
(c) اذا اردت...مكان] رأس الميت من بني ادم اذا وضع في برج الحمام اجتمع اليه الحمام صاحب الفالج *add.* B
1.33: (a) الوجع] وة ميت قد يمت الوجع W; واذا دفنت جمجمة قديمة في برج الحمام كثر الحمام G
(b) للقوة...مضرّب] واذا كان بانسان فالج او لقوة يؤخذ لبن W; وللقوة وفالج يسعط بلبن جارية حبشية برجيع جارية مع شىء من زنبق مضروب مختلط جارية حبشية مع شىء من زنبق يضرب G
(c) لوقته] *om.* C | وزن قيراط للرجل وللطفل ورن حبة] للرجل قيراط وللطفل وزنة حبة C | ويخلط...تبرأ] *om.* C
1.34: (b) ويذاف...فانه نافع] وللقوة يؤخذ لبن الجارية الحبشية ويذاف فيه كندس وعروق من كل واحد جزء ويسحق ويذاف في اللبن ويقطر عليه الزنبق ويسعط منه صاحب اللقوة W | ويذاف ايضا بعض الاوقات على قدر الاحتمال] وللقوة يؤخذ لبن الجارية الحبشية ويذاف فيه G | الزنبق] الزبيق T
1.35: (a) للمغل...فتبرأ] اذا امغلت دابة فخذ عظم ميت اسحقه وضيفه بما حار واسقيه للدابة فتبرأ W | *om.* G
(b) انسان] *om.* W | به] *om.* W | فيسكن] فيسكن وجعه الذي يشتكي W | *om.* G

1.31	If you want that a man loves you, wash the pocket of your shirt and give him the water to drink—but he should not be aware of it—then he will love you, and honours will be bestowed upon him.	If you want that a man loves you, wash the pocket of your shirt with wine and give it to drink to whomever you desire—but he should not be aware of it—then he will love you.	If you want that a man loves you, wash the pocket of your shirt and give him the water to drink—but he should not be aware of it—then he will love you passionately.
1.32	If you want that the pigeons multiply in the pigeon house, bury there the head of a man who died a long time ago, then this will make the pigeons multiply.	If you have a pigeon house and you want that the birds multiply and increase in it, then bury there the skull of a man who died long ago.	If you want to gather pigeons in a pigeon house, take the head of a man who died a long time ago, bury it in this pigeon house, then the pigeons will gather there from every direction.
1.33	Take the milk of an Abyssinian woman, mix it with lily oil and sarcocolla, make it inhale to a man suffering from facial paralysis, then he will recover, with the permission of God, may He be exalted.	Against paralysis and facial paralysis: take the penis of a man, make it inhale with the milk of an Abyssinian woman; give it with some lily oil, whipped until it is well mixed, then let the man inhale one carat of it, or two grains for a child.	Milk of an Abyssinian girl: if it is mixed with some lily oil and inhaled by a man suffering from paralysis and facial paralysis, this will heal him; the correct amount for inhalation is one carat for a grown man, and one grain for a child; and if it is mixed with a few ounces of white sarcocolla and applied in drops in the inflamed eye, then this will cure it.
1.34	*om.*	Also mixed with a few ounces of hellebore and roots—in the sufficient amount, one part of each oneground and mixed with the milk, with the addition of some lily oil in drops and inhaled, then it will be useful, God willing.	*om.*
1.35	Against an upset stomach: if the stomach of an animal is upset, take the bone of a dead man, pound it into a fine powder, liquefy it with warm water and give it to that beast to drink, then this will recover, with the permission of God, may He be exalted.	For the pain of a molar: if the bone of a dead man is taken and passed over the aching tooth, then the pain will cease.	*om.*

1.36

اذا أخذ الكاشم ودق ناعما واذيب ببول الصبيان لم يبلعوا الحلم ويسقي الدابة المغلة بريت [فتبرأ] لوقتها

وللقولنج الدواب يؤخذ كف كاشم يسحق ناعما ويضاف ببول صبي ويوجر الدابة فانها تبرأ

وايضا للملغة يؤخذ كاشم فيدق دقا ناعما ويخلط معه بول صبي صغير ويُسقي للدابة فتبرأ باذن اللّه تعالى

1.37

اذا اردت لا يقرب المرأة احد غيرك خذ من اطراف شعرها واحرق حتى يصير رماد ثم اجعل منه على رأس الاحليل عند الجماع فلا يستطيع غيرك هذا عجيب

وان اردت ان لا يقرب المرأة غيرك احدا فتأخذ ما تسرّحه من رأسها من شعرها فاحرقه ودقه دقا ناعما وذره على رأس الاحليل وجامعها به

اذا اردت ان لا يقرب المرأة احد غيرك فخذ من شعرها وقت ما تسرحه فاحرقه واسحقه ثم اجعله على الاحليل عند الجماع فلا يقرب احد غيرك

1.38

يؤخذ من منى الرجل جزء ومن الزنبق جزء ويخلطا وسعط صاحب اللوقة ثلاثة ايام متواليات يبرأ

للقوة منى الرجل ومن الزنبق من كل واحد جزء يخلطان جميعا ويسعّط به على الريق ثلاثة ايام فانه يبرأ باذن الله تعالى

يؤخذ من منى الرجل جزء من دهن الزنبق جزء ويخلط الجميع ويسعط به صاحب اللقوة ثلاثة ايام متواليات يبرأ باذن اللّه تعالى

1.39

رجيع الانسان اذا حرق وسحق ناعما وخلط بملح اندراني وشىء من حنظل وخلط الجميع ونفخ في الدابة الذي بها بياض برأت

للبرص في العين من الدواب يؤخذ رجيع الانسان يابسا فيحرق ويسحق سحقا ناعما ويخلط مع شىء من ملح اندراني ومسك وينفخ في عين الدابة ينقطع البياض ويذهب باذن الله تعالى

يؤخذ رجيع الانسان يابسا فيسحق ويخلط معه ملح اندراني وقليل حنظل وينفخ في عين الدابة التي بها البياض فزول وينفع ايضا للطرفة في عين الدابة

1.36: (a) وايضا للملغة] *om.* B | فيدق دقا ناعما] يدق ناعما B
(b) فانها تبرأ] للقولنج... فانها تبرأ] وللقولنج الدواب يؤخذ كف كاشم يسحق ناعما ويضاف ببول صبي ويوجر الدابة فانها تبرأ W | *om.* G
(c) *om.* C

1.37: (a) يقرب] يمكن B
(b) وان اردت...وجامعها به] وان اردت ان المرأة غيرك فخذ ما يسقط من شعر رأسها اذا سرحته فاحرقه وخذه ناعما وذره على رأس احليلك وجامعها W | *om.* G
(c) In C this recipe is after 1.41 | اذا اردت...مليح جدا] تستطع لم يبق مرأة وجامع الاحليل رأس على منه وجعل رمادا وصار احرق اذا المرأة شعر اطراف — corrected reading: اذا اردت...مليح جدا] اطراف شعر المرأة اذا احرق وصار رمادا وجعل منه على رأس الاحليل وجامع مرأة لم يبق تستطع غيره وهو عجيب جدا C | In C another recipe is added, against the inflammation of the eye, واذا حلط معه انزرون ابيض وقطر منه في العين ازال ما بها من الحمره.

1.38: (a) ويخلط الجميع] ويخلطان B | يسعط به] يتوسّط بها B | يبرأ] فانه يبرئ B
(b) للقوة...فانه يبرأ] وللقوة يؤخذ من مني الرجل جزء ومن الزنبق جزء يخلطان ويسعط به على الريق ثلاثة ايام يبرأ G | *om.* W
(c) In C this recipe is after is 1.41 | يؤخذ من منى الرجل] منى الرجل اذا أخذ منه C

1.39: (a) حنظل] حني فتل S | فيسحق] يسحق B | التي بها البياض فزول] *om.* B | ايضا للطرفة] *om.* B
(b) للبرص...ويذهب] ولبرص العين من الدواب يؤخذ رجيع الناس فيجفف ويسحق ناعما ويخلط معه ملح اندراني ومسك وينفخ في عين الدابة فيَقلع البياض W; رجيع الانسان اذا اخذ يابس واحرق وسحق ناعما وخلط معه شىء من ملح اندراني ومسك ونفخ في عين الدابة قلع البياض وبغير مسك يقلع البياض ايضا G

1.36 Against an upset stomach, again: Mediterranean moon carrot, pounded into a fine powder, mixed with the urine of a baby and given to drink to the animal, then this will recover, with the permission of God, may He be exalted.

Against the colic of an animal: if a handful of Mediterranean moon carrot is taken, ground into a fine powder, mixed with the urine of a child and given to the animal, then it will recover.

If the Mediterranean moon carrot is taken, ground into a fine powder, liquefied with the urine of children who have not reached puberty, and given to the animal suffering from an upset stomach with oil to drink, then this animal will instantly recover.

1.37 If you want to be the only one who can approach a woman, in the moment in which it is cut, take her hair, burn it and grind it, then apply this on the outer opening of the urethra at the moment of coitus, then nobody but you will approach her.

If you want to be the only one who can approach a woman, in the moment in which it is cut, take the hair that falls from her head, burn it, pound it finely, and place it on top of the outer opening of your urethra and have sexual intercourse with her.

If you want to make it so that only you can approach a woman, take the extremities of the hair, burn it until they become ash, place it on top of the outer opening of urethra at the moment of coitus, then nobody but you will be able to touch her, and this is amazing.

1.38 If one part of human semen and one part of lily oil are taken, melted and a man suffering from facial paralysis inhales it—the same quantity for three days—then he will recover, with the permission of God, may He be exalted.

Against facial paralysis: if one part of human semen and one part of lily oil are taken, mixed and inhaled on an empty stomach for three days, then this will cure it.

If one part of human semen and one part of lily [oil] are taken, a man suffering from facial paralysis inhales it—the same amount for three days—then he will recover.

1.39 Dried human excrement: if it is taken, ground, mixed with rock salt and a bit of colocynth, applied on the eye of a beast affected by the glaucoma, then this will disappear; it is also useful against the inflammation that causes lachrymation in the eyes of the beasts.

Against the whiteness in the eye of an animal: if the dry excrement of a man is taken, burnt, ground into a fine powder, mixed with a bit of rock salt and musk, and applied on the eye of an animal, then this will make the glaucoma disappear.

If one part of human semen and one part of lily [oil] are taken, a man suffering from facial paralysis inhales it—the same quantity for three days—then he will recover.

1.40

بصاق الانسان اذا طلى به الثآليل على الريق ابرأها وقلعها وكذا دم التيس

om.

om.

1.41

منى الانسان اذا أخذ وهو حار وطلى به برص غيره ابرأه

وللبرص يطلي موضعه بالمنى الحار فانه يذهب باذن الله تعالى

يؤخذ منى الرجل وهو حار يطلي به البرص فيزول باذن اللّٰه تعالى

1.42

بول الصبي قبل البلوغ اذا جعل في اناء وحمى على النار وأخذت صوفة وغمست فيه وطلى بها العين التي بها ورم احمر برأت بقدرة الله تعالى

بول الصبيان الذين لم يبلغوا الحلم يسخن على النار ويؤخذ سفنجة فيغمس فيه ويكمّد به العين الورامة من الرمد والحمرة فيبرأ ويسكن باذن الله

بول صبي لم يبلغ الحلم او صغير فيسحق على النار ودهن به العين الوارمة المحمّر لوجعه فتسكن باذن اللّٰه تعالى

1.43

اذا أخذت شيئا من ابوال الصبيان وجعلت في قدر نحاس وطبخته ينقد فاذا ننقد جففه واخلط به ملح الطعام واسحقه بالماء الزعفران واجعله في بوندقة واوقد عليه فلنة يذوب كما تذوب الفضة فاجعله بسبيكة وحكه على المسن بالماء والمسك واكحل به العين التي عليها البياض فانها تبرأ وتقلع البياض وهو مجرب والحكماء يسمون الجوهر النفيس الذي لا قيمت له

وقال بعض الحكماء يؤخذ بول الصبي ويجمع في قدر نحاس ويطبخ حتى ينعقد ثم تركه الى ان يجفّ ثم يسحق ويخلط ملحا ويعجن بالماء الزعفران ويتركه في بوطقة من ايلي واوقد عليه بالجمر حتى يدور فاذا داب مثل الفضة وسبكه حله بالماء واخلط معه شيء من مسك وانحل به البياض العتيق والحديث يقلعه ان شاء الله تعالى وكان القدماء يسمونه لجودته ونفعه الجوهر الذي لا ثمن له

قال بعض الحكماء بول الصبي فجمعه في وعاء نحاس وغلاه على النار حتى ينعقد ثم جفف واخلط معه ملح وزعفران وجعله في بوندقه ثم اوقد عليه فانه الرصاص ثم يأخذه ويحلّه بالماء ويخلط معه شيئا من مسك ويحتكل به صاحب البياض في العين فيجلوه باذن اللّٰه تعالىوكان المتقدمين يسمونه الجوهر النفيس وهذا اعلى ما يكون

1.40: (c) الثآليل] التواليل L | الثآليل] اياما التواكيل موضع C | وكذا دم التيس] وكذلك يفعل دم التيس C

1.41: (a) يطلي به] اذا طلى B | ذهب عنه] فيزول B

(b) In T, G, and W this recipe is after 1.38 | فانه يذهب] فيذهب W | وللبرص...فانه يذهب] واذا طلى البرص بالمنى الحار ذهب G

(c) *om.* C

1.42: (a) صبي لم يبلغ] الصبي الذي لم يبلغ B | فيسحق] يسحق B | ودهن] يدهن B | فتسكن] تسكن B

(b) يبلغوا] يبلغ W | يسخن] يسحق W | فيغمس] فتغمس W | به] بها W | فيبرأ] om. W | بول الصبيان...ويسكن] بول صبي لم يبلغ الحلم او صغير فيسحق على النار ودهن به العين الوارمة المحمّر لوجعه فتسكن باذن اللّٰه تعالى G

(c) برأت] برأها C

1.43: (a) قال بعض الحكماء] *om.* B | فجمعه] وحطّه B | حتى ينعقد ثم جفف] *om.* B | وزعفران] وزعفرانا واعقده بعد ذلك *add.* B | يأخذه] فتأخذه B | فيجلوه] فيجليه B | In B another recipe is added, to stop the flow of milk, يؤخذ حلبه تدق وتعجن بالماء وتلطخ به ثدى المرأة فان لبنها ينقطع.

(b) وقال بعض الحكماء...يقلعه] وحكى بعض العلماء في بعض كتب الصنعة انه أخذ بول الصبيان في قدر نحاس وطبخه حتى انعقد ثم قلاه فلما جف سحقه وخلط معه ملحا وعجنه بالماء الزعفران في بُودقة طين من بئر ايلي ثم وقد عليه بالحمر فذاب كما يدوب الفضة ثم يسكنه وكان يحله بالماء ويخلط معه شيئا من مسك ويكحل به البياض الجديد والعتيق من غير اذاء للعين ويلقط الحمرة والورم W; بول الصبيان في قدر نحاس وطبخ حتى ينعقد فاذا جفّ سحقه مع شيء من ملح وعجنه بالماء الزعفران وصيّره في توبقة من طين ايلي ثم يوقد عليه بالجمرفانه يدور كما تدور الفضة ثم يسكبه لحاله ويخلط معه شيء من مسك واكتحل به البياض العتيق والحديث فيقلعه من غير أذي للعين G | وكان القدماء] *om.* W | لجودته ونفعه] الجوهر الدوائى W | الذي] *om.* W

(c) اذا أخذت شيئا من] *om.* C | وجعلت] *om.* C | ينقد] تعقد C | واسحقه] وسحق C | واجعله] وجعل C | عليه فلنة] *om.* C | التي] الذي C | البياض] البياض من الجدري C | فانها تبرا وتقلع البياض وهو مجرب] قلع البياض وابرأها C | والحكماء...لا قيمت له] وهو الذي يسموه الحكماء الجوار النفيس C

1.40	*om.*	*om.*	Man saliva: if it is rubbed on the warts, then this will cure and erase them; the blood of the billy goat has the same effect.
1.41	Human semen: if it is taken when it is warm, and rubbed on a leprous part, then the leprosy will disappear, with the permission of God, may He be exalted.	Against the leprosy: the part affected by it has to be rubbed with warm semen, and then it will disappear, with the permission of God, may He be exalted.	Human semen: if it is taken while it is warm and rubbed on a leprous part, then this will change its colour and will cure it.
1.42	Urine of a boy who has not yet reached puberty, or of a baby: if it is ground on the fire and rubbed on a swollen eye against the pain, then this will calm it, with the permission of God, may He be exalted.	Urine of a boy who has not reached puberty: if it is warmed on the fire, then a sponge is taken, soaked in it, and applied as a hot compress on a swollen eye due to ophtalmia and inflammation, then this will heal and the pain will be calmed, with the permission of God.	Urine of a boy before puberty: if it is put in a vessel, heated on the fire, then a woollen cloth is taken and soaked in it, then the eye affected by the red swelling should be rubbed with it, then this will heal it by the power of God, may He be exalted.
1.43	Some wise man said that child urine should be collected in a vessel, boiled on the fire until it thickens, then it should be dried and mixed with salt and saffron and made into pills, then set it on fire, and this is lead; then one of them should be taken, dissolved in water, mixed with a bit of musk and rubbed on the eyes of a man suffering from glaucoma, then the eye will be cleared up. The ancient man used to call it 'the precious substance'.	Some wise men said: take the urine of some boys in a copper cooking pot, cook it until it thickens; then leave it until it dries, pound and mix it with some salt and knead it with saffron water; leave it in a melting pot, kindle the embers under it until it moves in circles; when it has a circular movement like silver when is melted, dilute it with water, and mix it with a bit of musk; it can be used to dissolve and remove both the chronic and the recent glaucoma, God the Highest willing. The ancient men used to call it 'the priceless substance'.	Take the urine of some boys, put it in a copper cooking pot, cook it until it thickens; once it has thickened, dry it, mix it with cooking salt, pound it with saffron water, make it into pills and place it on fire, it will liquefy as the silver does, then give it the shape of a bar and rub it on an old man with water and musk, and rub it on an eye affected by glaucoma, then this will heal it and remove it: this has been tried out. The wise men call this 'the precious substance that has no equal'.

1.44	يؤخذ لبن جارية يذاب فيه شيء من زغفران بيسير من لعاب السفرجل ويقطر في العين يسكن الوجع والضربان ويزيل البثرة	وللرمل والبثر في العين يؤخذ لبن جارية ويضاف اليه شيء من زعفران وحب السفرجل ويفتّر قليلا ويقطر في العين فيسكن الوجع والضربان باذن الله تعالى	يؤخذ لبن السوداء فيذاف فيه شيء من زعفران وحب السفرجل ويفتر على النار ويقطر في العين التي يكون فيها البثرة والرمد العتيق فانه يبرأ باذن اللّه تعالى
1.45	اذا اردت ثدى المرأة يبقي قائما لا ينكسر ابدا فخذ من دم حيضة الجارية اول حيضها واطل به رؤوس النهود فانها لا ينكسر	علاج يمنع ثدى الجواري والابكار ان يكبر يؤخذ اول دم يخرج من الجارية البكر اذا حاضت فيمسح به حلمتي الصبية فان ثديها لا يكبران	*om.*
1.46	وان مسح جبهة كبش في شحم تمساح لم يقدر ينطحن كبش كلب البحر	*om.*	*om.*
1.47	اذا اكتحل احد بمرارته اذهب بياض العين	*om.*	*om.*
1.48	واسنانه من جانب الايمن يقوي الجماع	*om.*	*om.*
1.49	وكل عين تنفع الم العين	*om.*	*om.*
1.50	دم الحيض وهو حار طرى اذا الطحت به العين ازال ما بها من الحمر والورم	لضربان في العين يؤخذ دم حائض طري يلطخ به العين من خارجها فيسكن الضربان	*om.*

1.44: (a) *om.* B
(b) والبشر في العين] *om.* W G | ويضاف] فيذاف . G | ويفتّر قليلا] *om.* W | فيسكن] يسكن G | In T an incantation is added, against the inflammation of the eye: رقية للرمد الم ترء الى ربك كيف مدّ الظل ولو شاء لجعله ساكنا الى اخر الآية ثم تقول اسكن ايها الوجع كما سكن عرش الرحمن.
(c) البثرة] البترة L C | يؤخذ لبن...البثرة] لبن جارية اذا اذيب فيه شيء من زغفران مع شيء من يسير الزعفران بلّ من لعاب السفرجل وقطر في العين سكن الوجع والضربان وازال البثرة C
1.45: (b) علاج يمنع] *om.* G | الجواري] *om.* W | والابكار] *om.* G | ان يكبر] ان يكبران G | فان ثديها لا يكبران] فان ثديها لا يكبر W; فانه لا يكبر G
(c) اذا اردت...ينكسر] قائدة السمن دم حيضة الجارية اول حيضها اذا لطخ به العين زار ما بها من الحمرة والورم C
1.46: (c) *om.* C
1.47: (c) *om.* C
1.48: (c) *om.* C
1.49: (c) *om.* C
1.50: (b) في العين] العين W G | يلطخ] فيلطخ W; تلطخ G | من خارجها] من خارج W G | فيسكن] يسكن G | الضربان] جميع ذلك W; *om.* G
(c) *om.* C

1.44	If the milk of a black woman is taken, mixed with a bit of saffron and a grain of quince, heated on a fire and applied in drops to the eye affected by pustules and chronic inflammation, then these will heal, with the permission of God, may He be exalted.	Against the inflammation and the pustules in the eye: if the milk of a maiden is taken, mixed with some saffron and a grain of quince, warmed a little and applied in drops in the eye, then the pain and the pangs will cease.	Milk of a maiden: if it is taken, mixed with a bit of saffron and of the mucilage from a quince, applied in drops in the eye, then the pain and the pangs will cease, and the pustules will disappear.
1.45	*om.*	The remedy which prevents the breasts of the girls and of the virgins from growing: if the first menstrual blood of a virgin is taken when it appears for the first time, rubbed on the breasts of a young girl, then they will not grow.	If you want that the breasts of a woman remain as they are without being damaged, take the blood from the first menstruation of a girl, rub it on the top of the breasts, and then they will not be ruined.
1.46	*om.*	*om.*	If the forehead of the ram is wiped with crocodile fat, then the ram will not be able to fight with the shark.
1.47	*om.*	*om.*	If the eyes of a man are rubbed with its gall, then the glaucoma will disappear.
1.48	*om.*	*om.*	His teeth from the right side give power to the coitus.
1.49	*om.*	*om.*	Every eye is useful against the pain of the eyes.
1.50	*om.*	Against the pain of the eyes: if some fresh menstrual blood is taken and spattered on the eye from the outside, then the pain will cease.	Menstrual blood: if it is taken while it is warm and fresh, and it is is spattered on the eye, then the irritation and the swelling will subside.

1.51	*om.*	دواء للتسمن يؤخذ شحم الوز فدقه ويخلط معه بورقا وكمونا كرمانيا ودقق القمح ثم يلقم منه دجاجةً حتى تسمن فمن أكل من تلك الدجاجة سمن حتى يضيق جلده عليه	اذا اردت ان تسمن المرأة خذ شحم اوزة انثى واخلط معها من البورق والكمون الكرماني ودقيق الحلبة ودق ذلك جميعا وبلعه لدجاجة سوداء تسعة ايام متوالية ثم اذبحها واطعمها فكل من أكل من ذلك يسمن سمنا عظيما من ذكر او انثى
1.52	يؤخذ حلبة تذاف وتعجن بالماء ويلطخ به ثدى المرأة فان لبنها ينقطع	لقطع لبن المرأة يؤخذ الحلبة فتدق ويعجن بالماء وتضمد به الثدى فان اللبن ينقطع	اذا اردت ان تقطع لبن المرأة خذ شيء من حلبة واسحقها واعجنها بالماء واطل بها ثدى المرأة يسقطع اللبن
1.53	اذا اردت ان يدر لبن المرأة فتأخذ حنطة تدق وتذاف بزيت وتاخذ صوفة يكون لونها ازرق وتلق على عود وتغمس في ذلك الزيت والطخ بها رأس الثدى فيدر اللبن باذن اللّٰه تعالى	واذا انقطع اللبن ويقعد في الثدى فيؤخذ خنطلا فيدق ويذاف بزيت وتلف صوفة على عود وتكون لون السماء ويلطخ بها رأس الثدى فيدر اللبن	وان اردت ازداده ودق حنطة واعجنها بالزيت وخذ صوفة زرقاء لفها على عود واغمسها في الزيت واطل بها رأس الثدى يدر اللبن
1.54	اذا اردت ان تخرب دار عدوك فخذ عظم ابن ادم فادفنه في داره فانها تخرب يتثت شمله	*om.*	*om.*
1.55	*om.*	وان كان اللبن قليلا واحبت ان يكثر لبنها ويزيد فاسقها في كل يوم بزر الحلبة يدر لبنها باذن الله تعالى	*om.*

1.51: (b) دواء للتسمن] وللسمن W G | الوز] الورل W; الودك G | ثم يلقم] واطعمه G | تلك] هذه W; *om.* G | عليه] *om.* W | فمن…عليه] ثم أكلها G
(c) تسمن المرأة] ذلك C | ودق ذلك جميعا] ودق الجميع C | تسعة ايام] سبعة ايام C | واطعمها] وكل من لحمها واشرب مرقتها C | يسمن سمنا عظيما] سمن C | من ذكر] ذكرا كان C
1.52: (a) *om.* B
(b) يؤخذ] *om.* W | فتدق] يدق W; ناعما *add.* G | ويعجن] ويعجنها W | وتضمد به] ويضمدها W | فان اللبن] فانه W | In W another recipe is added, to stop the flow of milk, ولقطع اللبن وعقده في الثدي يؤخذ حنظل مسحوق يدق بزيت تلف الثدى فان اللبن ينقطع.
(c) تقطع] قطع C
1.53: (a) فتأخذ] فخذ B | تدق] دقها ناعما B | وتداف] وضفها B | وتأخذ] وخذ B | صوفة يكون لونها ازرق] صوفة زرقاء B | وتلق] وتلق B | وتغمس] واغمسها B | ذلك] *om.* B
(b) واذا انقطع اللبن…فيدر اللبن] ولقطع اللبن وعقده في الثدى يؤخذ حنظل مسحوق يدق بزيت تلف على صوفة على عود وتكون الصوفة بلون السماء ويلطخ رأس الثدى فيدر اللبن المنعقد وبالله نستعين وعليه نتوكّل ونستعين في التوفيق لما عرضناه W; ومما يدرّ اللبن يؤخذ حنظل يدق ويذاف بزيت ولفّ صوفة على عود وتكون الصوفة مثل لون السماء ولطخ رأس الثدى من ذلك فانه يدر اللبن G
(c) صوفة زرقاء] صوفة من صوف ازرق C | يدر] فانه يدر C
1.55: (b) وان كان اللبن…يدر لبنها] *om.* W | ومما يكثّر اللبن ان تسقي المرأة كل يوم بزر الرطبة مدقوق وزن درهم ونصف بشراب G

1.51	*om.*	Remedy for fleshiness: if the fat of a goose is taken, pounded, mixed with natron, cumin and corn flour, then fed to a hen for some days until it gets fat, then the one who eats this hen will become fat to the point that his skin will become too tight for him.	If you want that a woman becomes fleshy, take the fat of a female goose, mix it with natron, cumin and fenugreek flour, pound everything together and make a black hen swallow it up—the same quantity for seven days—then slaughter it and feed it to the woman, then everyone—man or woman—who eats this will become extremely plump.
1.52	Take some fenugreek, dissolve it and knead it with water, spatter the breats of the woman with it, and then her milk will stop.	To stop [the flow of] milk in a woman: take some fenugreek, grind it into a fine powder, knead it with water and bandage the breasts with it, and then the milk will stop.	If you want to stop the milk of a woman, take some fenugreek, grind it, knead it with water and rub it on her breasts, then the milk will stop.
1.53	If you want that the milk of a woman flows copiously, take some common wheat, pound it, mix it with oil, take a blue woollen cloth and hang it on a branch and soak it in this oil, spatter it also on the breasts, and then the milk will flow copiously, with the permission of God, may He be exalted.	If the flow of milk has stopped and the milk has coagulated in the breasts, some colocynth has to be taken, ground, mixed with oil, wrapped in a woollen cloth around a branch—the wool should have the colour of the sky—and the breasts have to be spatteredwith this, then the milk will flow copiously.	If you want to increase the flow of milk, pound some common wheat, knead it with oil, take a blue woollen cloth and wrap it around a branch, soak it in oil and rub it on top of the breasts, then the milk will flow copiously.
1.54	If you want to destroy the house of your enemy, take the bone of a man, bury it in his house, then this home will be destroyed and its parts dismembered.	*om.*	*om.*
1.55	*om.*	If there is only little milk and you want to increase it, then give her fenugreek seeds everyday, and the milk will flow copiously, with the permission of God, may He be exalted.	*om.*

٢. الاسد

	a	b	c
	ذكر منافع اعضاء الاسد	الاسد	باب منافع الاسد
2.1	*om.*	*om.*	جلد الاسد يزيل الحمى والجلوس عليه ويذهب البواسير والنقرس
2.2	يؤخذ الشحم الذي بين عيني الاسد فاذنه بدهن ورد ويدهن به وجهه من تريد فانه يكان مهابا عند الملوك والسلاطين وجميع الناس	اذا أخذ الانسان من شحم الاسد الذي بين عينيه فذوّبه بدهن ورد ومسح به وجهه اهابه كل من راه	شحم الاسد الذي بين عينيه واذنه اذا اذيب بدهن ورد ومسح به انسان وجهه كان مهابا عند كل من يراه وهو قبول عند السلطان
2.3	واذا أخذ شحم الاسد وجعل في الماء الذي يشربوا منه الدواب او بخّر به فلا يقربوا منه ابدا	شحم الاسد ان يبخّر او وضع منه في موضع ترده الدواب لشرب الماء لم يشرب من ذلك الموضع	[شحم] الاسد اذا جعل في الماء لا تقربه الدواب
2.4	اذا اسرجت سراجين أحدهما بشحم الاسد والاخر بشحم كبش ابلق وجعلتَ كل واحد منهما ناحية ويكون قريب فانهما يجتمعان السراجين وهذا مليح عجيب	واذا اسرجت سراجين احدهما بشحم الاسد والاخر بشحم الكبش ووضعت كل واحد بقريب من الاخر التقيا	اذا اسرجت سراجين احدها من دهن الاسد من دهن الكبش وفرقت بينهما فانهما يجتمعان
2.5	*om.*	*om.*	[و]اذا شرب منه حبتين باوقية لبن البقر منع الشيب

2.1: (c) *om.* C

2.2: (a) يؤخذ...وجميع الناس] الشحم الذى يكون بين عيني الاسد اذا أخذه انسان واذابه مع دهن ورد ودهن به وجهه كان مهابا عند الملوك وجميع الناس B

(b) اذا أخذ...كل من راه] شحم الاسد بن عني الاسد يذوب بدهن ورد ويمسح الرجل به وجهه هأبه كل من راه W | الانسان] *om.* G | عينيه] عيني الاسد G | فذوّبه] وذوّبه G | اهابه] هابه G

(c) السلطان] الملوك C

2.3: (a) يشربوا] تشرب B | او بخّر به فلا يشربوا] *om.* B

(b) شحم الاسد] *om.* G | يبخّر او وضع] وضع W | بخّر G | في] om. G | ترده] يرده W | يشرب من ذلك الموضع] ايضا يشرب من ذلك الماء ولم رده W | تقربه الدواب G

(c) [شحم] الاسد اذا جعل] اذا جعل شحم الاسد C | لا تقربه] لم تقربه C

2.4: (a) ابلق] بلق B | ويكون قريب فانهما يجتمعان السراجين] قريب من صاحبه فان السراجين يجتمعان B

(b) *om.* W | أسرجت] سرّج G | ووضعت...التقيا] وكانا قريبان التقيا جميعا G

(c) اذا اسرجت...يجتمعان] اذا اسعلت سراجا من دهن الاسد وسراجا من دهن الكبش وفرقت بينهما تلاقيا جميعا W

2.5: (c) منه] منه وزن احد *add.* C

2. Lion

	a	b	c
	Exposition of the useful properties of the parts of the lion	**The lion**	**Chapter on the useful properties of the lion**
2.1	*om.*	*om.*	The skin of a lion makes the fever disappear, and sitting on it cures the haemorrhoids and the gout.
2.2	If the fat which is between the eyes of the lion is taken, mixed with rose oil and rubbed on the face of whomever you want, then he will be respected by kings, sultans and all the other people.	If the man takes the fat which is between the eyes of the lion, liquefies it, and rubs it on his face, then everyone who sees him, will respect him.	Fat which is between the eyes and the ears of a lion: if it is liquefied with rose oil; then a man wipes it on his face, then he will be respected by everyone who sees him, moreover, he will be welcomed by the sultan.
2.3	Lion fat: if it is taken, put in the water from which the beasts drink, or it is used for fumigations, than the animals will not approach the place anymore.	Lion fat: if it is fumigated or placed in which the beasts go to drink, then these beasts will not drink there anymore.	Lion fat: if it is put in the water, then the other beasts will not approach it.
2.4	If two lanterns—one of the two with the fat of a lion, while the other with the fat of a ram—are lit and put side by side, one close to each other, then the two lanterns will join, and this is witty and amazing.	If two lanterns—one with the fat of a lion, the other with the fat of a ram—are lit and put next to each other, then they will join.	If two distinct lanterns are lighted—one of them with the fat of a lion, the other with the fat of a ram—then they will join.
2.5	*om.*	*om.*	If two grains of it are drunk with one ounce of cow milk, then this will prevent him from becoming white-haired.

2.6	[اذا] شرب منه دانقا مع حبتين كافور لم يراه احد الا احبه محبة شديدة	*om.*	*om.*
2.7	شحم الاسد اذا دق وخلط معه ثوم ومسح به جسد ابن ادم لا يقربه تمساح بقدرة الله تعالى	وان دق انسان شحم الاسد بالثوم ومسح به وجهه وجسده لم يقربه شيء من السباع	شحم الاسد اذا دقّ بالثوم وطلى به انسان بدنه فلا يقربه التمساح ولا شيء من دواب البخر
2.8	لحم الاسد اذا طبخ واكل نفع من الفالج والريح والبارد والاسترخاء ايضا	لحم الاسد اذا أكل ينفع من الفالج والاسترخاء	ولحم الاسد اذا أكل مشويا نفع من الفالج
2.9	[مرارة] الاسد اذا اذيبت بالعسل وطليت به الخنازير بزيت لوقتها خصوصا التي في الحلق	واذا خلط بالعسل وطلى بالخنازير التي في العين ذهبت بها	يؤخذ مرارة الاسد فتخلط بالعسل النحل واطلِ به الخنازير التي يكون في الحَلق وفي سائر البدن فانها تبرأ باذن الله تعالى
2.10	[مرارة] الاسد اذا اديبت بالبزر قطونة وشربها من به اليرقان برئ بقدرة الله تعالى	وكذلك اذا سقى منها صاحب اليرقان وزن دانق بماء بزر قطوناء الرطب او المنقوع نفعه	مرارة الاسد اذا اذيبت وشرب منها صاحب اليرقان ذهب عنه باذن اللّه تعلى وان شربت المرارة المذكورة بماء البزر قطوناء فكان أبلغ
2.11	كبد الاسد اذا شويت وأكلها من به وجع الكبد برئ	*om.*	يؤخذ كبد الاسد تشوي ويسحق ناعما ويسقي منها صاحب وجع الكبد فيبرأ باذن اللّه

2.7: (a) *om.* B

(b) واذا دق...يعر له] وشحم الاسد اذا سحق معه ثوم ومسح به انسان جلده لم يعرض له W | وان دق انسان شحم الاسد بالثوم ومسح به وجهه وجسده لم يقربه G

(c) *om.* C

2.8: (b) منع] نفع W | ينفع G | والاسترخاء] لانه يسخن البدن *add.* W G

(c) In C this recipe is after 2.10

2.9: (a) يؤخذ] *om.* B | فتخلط] تخلط B | بالعسل النحل] بعسل نحل B | واطلِ] ويطلى B | الحلق وفي سائر] *om.* B

(b) واذا خلط] ومرارة الاسد تخلط W; مرارة الاسد اذا خلطت G | العين] العنقَ W G | ذهبت] فتذهب W

(c) In C this recipe is after 2.10 | بزر قطوناء] بزر قطونة C | لوقتها خصوصا التي في الحلق] برد ابرأتها سرعة C

2.10: (b) مرارة الاسد] وكذلك G | بزر قطوناء] منقوع *add.* W; الرطب او المنقوع نفعه *add.* G

(c) بالبزر قطونة] بماء بزر قطونا C | برئ] براه C

2.11: (a) يشوي] تشوي S

(c) *om.* C

2.6	*om.*	*om.*	If a man drinks one *dāniq* of it with two grains of camphor, then no one will see him, except for the one who loves him passionately.
2.7	Lion fat: if it is ground with garlic, and a man rubs it on his body, then neither a crocodile, nor other sea animals will approach him.	If a man pounds the fat of a lion with garlic, wipes his face and body with it, then no wild animal will touch him.	Lion fat: if it is ground, mixed with garlic, and a man wipes his body with it, then no crocodile will approach him, for the power of God, may He be exalted.
2.8	Lion meat: if it is eaten roasted, it will be useful against the paralysis.	Lion meat: if it is eaten, it will be useful against the paralysis and muscle weakness.	Lion meat: if it is cooked and eaten, then it will be useful against paralysis, wind, coldness, and the weakness of the muscles.
2.9	Lion gall: if it is taken, mixed with honey, rubbed on the scrofula that affects the throat and the rest of the body, then this will heal.	Lion gall: if it is mixed with honey, and rubbed on the scrofula which affects the eye, then this will disappear thanks to this.	Lion gall: if it is liquefied with honey, and rubbed on the scrofula together with some oil, then this will disappear, especially that particular kind that affects the throat.
2.10	Lion gall: if it is liquefied and the man suffering from jaundice drinks it, then he will heal, with the permission of God, may He be exalted; and if the gall in question is drunk with black psyllium water, this will be even more effective.	Likewise, if it is given to drink with dark psyllium, it will be useful to the man suffering from jaundice.	Lion gall: if it is mixed with black psyllium, and a man suffering from jaundice drinks it, then this will heal, for the power of God, may He be exalted.
2.11	Lion liver: if it is taken, roasted, minced finely, and fed to a man with liver complaint, then this will heal him, with the permission of God, may He be exalted.	*om.*	Lion meat: if it is roasted, and fed to a man suffering from liver complaint, then he will heal.

	(a)	(b)	(c)
2.12	*om.*	كبد الاسد نافع من وجع الكبد اذا سقى منه درهم وصرّفه	[ايضا] شويت وسحقت وشرب منها صاحب وجع الكبد وزن درهم بشراب عتيق برئ
2.13	*om.*	*om.*	مرارة ايضا اذا مزخت بسمن بقر واكتحل بها من بعينه بياض ابرأه وابرأ البهق الاسود طلى
2.14	*om.*	*om.*	اذيبت بدهن زنبق وطلى بها الوجه قضيت حاجته
2.15	خصية الاسد تشقّ وتملح وتجفف ويؤخذ منها ربع مثقال ومن المصطكي جزء ومن البورق جزء ويسحق الجميع يُلت بدهن الزنبق ويسقي منها صاحب وجع الجوف وزن درهم بماء حار فينفعه من كل وجع الجوف والفوالنج والريح والبواسير ووجع الاحشاء	خصية الاسد اذا ملحت مع ملح وبورق احمر ومصطكى وجففت وسحقت ولتّت بزنبق نفعت من جميع اوجاع الجوف ومن المغص والقولنج والبواسير والزحير ووجع الرحم ويشرب بماء حار على الريق	[خصية] الاسد اذا لتت ببورق ومستكا وجففت وسحقت وخلطت بدهن زنبق وشرب منها وزن درهم بماء خيار نفعت من علل الجوف والمغص والقولنج والزحير والبواسير ووجع الاحشاء
2.16	يؤخذ خصية الاسد اليمنى تجففت وتسحقت وشرب منها انسان ينقطع نسله وان اكلها مشوية كان كذلك	اذا جففت في الشمس وسحقت وسقى منها وزن دانق بماء ورد اورثت العقر	[خصية] الاسد اليمنى اذا جففت وسحقت وشرب منها انسان وزن درهم بماء ورد فانه يصير عقيما وينقطع نسله وان اكلها مشوية كان اجود
2.17	*om.*	*om.*	[واذا] أكلها نيه لحمت الولد باذن الله

2.12: (b) من وجع] لوجع W | منه درهم وصرفه] منها وزن درهم بنبيذ تمّ الضربان W | كبد الاسد...وصرفه] *add.* W كبد الاسد اذا شرب منها وزن درهم بنبيذ نفع من وجع الكبد والضربان G
(c) [ايضا] شويت...برئ] كبد الاسد اذا شويت وأكلها من به وجع الكبد بوزن درهم بخمر عتيق ابرأه C
2.13: (c) In C this recipe is after 2.32 | مزخت] اذيبت C | بقر] البقر C | وابرأ لهق الاسود طلى] وابرأ لهق الاسود C
2.14: (c) In C this recipe is after 2.32 | اذيبت...حاجته] واذا اضيف اليها بدهن زنبق وطليت بها اليد ووجه في حاجة قضيت C
2.15: (a) كل وجع] جميع علل B
(b) وجففت] ثم جففت W | بزنبق] بزيبق W G | من جميع اوجاع الجوف] من اوجاع البطن جميعا G | ومن المغص...على الريق] *om.* G
(c) مصطكى] مستكا C
2.16: (a) يؤخذ] *om.* B | تجففت وتسحقت] اذا جففت وسحقت B | ينقطع] انقطع B
(b) اذا جففت] وخصية الاسد ايضا اليمنى W; خصية الاسد اليمنى G | في الشمس] *om.* W G | وسقى] وشرب G | اورثت] ولدت W; اورث G | العقر] من الرجال فلا تحبل لهم وان اكل منه مشوية حسّمت الولد واورثت العقر ايضا *add.* W; وكذلك اذا أكلت مشوية *add.* G
(c) *om.* C
2.17: (c) *om.* C

2.12	*om.*	The liver of the lion is useful against the liver complaint, if it is drunk in the quantity of one dirham, and this will make it cease.	And also, if it is roasted, ground, and a man suffering from liver complaint drinks one dirham of it with some old wine, then this will heal.
2.13	*om.*	*om.*	The bile again: if it is mixed with cow fat, and rubbed on an eye affected by glaucoma, then this will cure it; and this will also cure the black vitiligo.
2.14	*om.*	*om.*	If, instead, it is liquefied with lily oil, and rubbed on the face, then one's needs will be satisfied.
2.15	If the testicle of a lion is split, salted, dried and one quarter *miṯqāl* of it is taken with one part mastic and one part natron, everything ground, kneaded with lily oil; if one dirham of it is given to a man suffering from abdominal pains to drink with warm water, then this will be useful against every pain in the abdomen, colic, wind, haemorrhoids and the bowel complaint.	Lion testicle: if it is seasoned with salt, red natron and mastic, then dried, ground, kneaded with lily oil, then this will be useful against all the pains of the abdomen, for gripes and colic, haemorrhoids, dysentery, and the pains of the uterus, if drunk with warm water on an empty stomach.	Lion testicle: if it is mixed with natron and mastic, dried, ground and liquefied with lily oil, this will be useful against the diseases of the abdomen, gripes, colic, dysentery and bowel complaints, if drunk with one quarter dirham of cucumber water.
2.16	Lion right testicle: if it is taken, dried, ground and given to a man to drink, then this will cut off his offspring; and if it is eaten roasted, it will be even more effective.	If it is dried in the sun, ground and drunk in the quantity of one *dāniq* with rose water, then this will cause sterility.	Right testicle of lion: if it is ground, and a man drinks one dirham of it with rose water, then he will become sterile and his offspring will be cut off. And if it is eaten roasted, this will be even better.
2.17	*om.*	*om.*	If, instead, it is eaten, then this will form the child, with the permission of God.

	(a)	(b)	(c)
2.18	*om.*	*om.*	زبله اذا علق على امرأة لم تحمل ابدا ما دام عليها
2.19	*om.*	*om.*	[واذا] بخر به في الحمام وقع الضراط على من يشمه
2.20	*om.*	*om.*	[وان] طلى به النمش اذهبه
2.21	يؤخذ لحم الاسد وشحمه وكبده فيدق الجميع ويطبخ بماء الجرجير ويلقي عليه عسل نحل وفلفل وسنبل الطيب من كل واحد جزء ويسقي منه صاحب وجع البدن وزن درهم بماء حار فيبرأ باذن الله تعالى	لحم الاسد وكبده وشحمه يدق رطبا ويطبخ بماء الجرجير ويلقي فيه عسل وفلفل وسنبل ويسقي منه وزن مثقال بماء حار ولمن به وجع في كبده يبرأ باذن الله تعالى	[لحمه] وشحمه وكبده يدق الجميع ويطبخ بماء الجرجير ويلقي عليه سنبل وقرنفل ويسقي منه لصاحب وجع الكبد وزن مثقال برئ
2.22	يؤخذ دم الاسد ويلطخ راس من به السرطان فيبرأ باذن الله تعالى	دم الاسد للسرطان يلطخ فيدهن به	*om.*
2.23	دماغ الاسد اذا يذاب على النار ويخلط معه دهن الزنبق ويقطّر منه في الاذن القليلة السمع فتبرأ	دماغ الاسد يذاب بزنبق ويقطّر منه في الاذن الثقيلة السمع فيجود دشمعها	دماغ الاسد اذا اذيب بدهن الزنبق وقطر منه في الاذن المحروشة الموجوعة ازال طرشها وابرأ المها
2.24	*om.*	واذا اذيف بزيت عتيق ودهن به الاختلاج الذي يكون في الجسد والارتعاش نفع	*om.*

2.18: (c) زبله] زبل الاسد C
2.19: (c) وقع الضراط على من يشمه] فمنشمه اخذه الضراط C
2.20: (c) النمش] القوب والنمش *add.* C
2.21: (a) فيدق] يدق B | ويطبخ] *om.* B | فيبرأ] يبرأ B
(b) يدق] يُسحق بالجمع W; اذا دُق G | ويلقي] وطرح G | وفلفل] مع فلفل G | ويسقي] وشرب G | وزن] *om.* G | ولمن به وجع في كبده يبرأ] نفع من وجع الكبد G
(c) *om.* C
2.22: (a) ويلطخ] فيلطخ B | من به] *om.* B | فيبرأ] فانه يزول عنه B
(b) دم الاسد...فيدهن به] دم الاسد جيد للسرطان يلطخ عليه يذهب W; دم الاسد اذا طلى به السرطان اذهبه G
(c) This recipe is attested only in C
2.23: (a) اذا يذاب] يذاب B | على النار] *om.* B | الزنبق] زنبق B | فتبرأ] تبرا B
(b) يذاب] اذا اذيف G | بزنبق] بزيبق G | فيجود دشمعها] حد سمعها G
(c) *om.* C
2.24: (b) واذا اذيف] دماغ الاسد يذوب W; الدماغ ايضا اذا اذيف G | بزيت عتيق] بزيبق عتيق S | ودهن] ويدهن W | الاختلاج الذي يكون في الجسد والارتعاش] الارتعاش الذي يكون في الجسد والاختلاج G | نفع] *om.* W; اذهبه G

2.18	*om.*	*om.*	Its excrement: if it is hung on a woman, then she will not get pregnant as long as this remains on her.
2.19	*om.*	*om.*	If it is fumigated in the bath, the man who smells it will break winds.
2.20	*om.*	*om.*	If it is rubbed on the discoloured spots, then these will disappear.
2.21	Lion meat, its fat and its liver: if these are taken, everything minced and cooked with rocket water, some honey, pepper and nard are added to it—one part of each one—then one dirham of it is given to a man suffering from abdomen pain to drink with warm water, then he will heal, with the permission of God, may He be exalted.	Meat, liver, and fat of lion: if they are minced fresh, cooked with rocket water, with the addition of some honey with pepper and hyacinth, then given in the quantity of one *miṯqāl* with warm water to someone suffering from liver complaint to drink, then this will cure him, with the permission of God, may He be exalted.	Lion meat, its fat and liver: if they are minced together, cooked with rocket water, with the addition of some hyacinth and cloves, and given to a man suffering from liver complaint to drink, then he will recover.
2.22	Lion blood: if it is taken, spattered on the head of the man affected by cancer, then he will recover, with the permission of God, may He be exalted.	Lion blood: it is useful for cancer, if spattered and rubbed on it.	*om.*
2.23	Lion brain: if it is liquefied on the fire, mixed with lily oil and applied in drops inside the ear with little hearing, then this will cure it.	If it is liquefied with lily, and applied in drops inside the ears that are hard of hearing, then their hearing will be improved.	Lion brain: if it is liquefied with lily oil, and applied in drops in an inflamed and painful ear, this will cure its pain.
2.24	*om.*	The brain, again,: if it is liquefied with lily and used as ointment against the tremors and the convulsions of the body, then these will cease.	*om.*

§			
2.25	دم الاسد اذا اذيب بخل عنصل ودهن ورد وطل به الجسد ووضع منه على الجبين نفع من الوسواس العارض من المرة السوداء والشربة منه وزن نصف درهم ويسعط ايضا طباشير وزن قراط بدهن بنفسج	ومخ الاسد للوسواس العارض في المرة السوداء يذاب بخل عنصل ودهن ورد ويُطلي به الجسد ويوضع منه على الرأس ويُسقي منه مثقال مع وزن نصف مثقال طباشير بماء البرساء يشرب باردا او يسعط منه ايضا بهذا العلة وزن قراط بدهن بنفسج	يؤخذ مخ الاسد فيذاف بخل عنصل ودهن ورد واطلِ به الرأس والجسد فانه ينفع من الوسواس العارض من السوداء
2.26	جلد الاسد اذا خلط بعسل وملح وطلى به الحلق ابرأه من الخنازير والورم	دم الاسد يسحن مع شيء من عسل وملح ومُر ويطلي على الخنازير والنزلات التي تكون في البدن وخاصة في الرقبة	يؤخذ دم الاسد ويلقي عليه شيء من ملح وعسل ومُر ويذاف الجميع واطلِ به الخنازير التي تكون في الرقبة والورم الحاس وجميع القروح التي يكون في الساقين فتبرأ الجميع باذن الله تعالى
2.27	رجيع الاسد اذا شددت فيها الثياب لم تقربها السوس	جلد الاسد اذا جعل في ثياب لم يقربها السوس	جلد الاسد اذا شدت في الثياب او القماش فلا يقربها السوس ابدا
2.28	واذا جعل في اوافي الغلة لم يقربها السوس ايضا	*om.*	*om.*
2.29	*om.*	وان جعل جلد الاسد مع غيره من الجلود تساقط شعر تلك الجلود	جلد الاسد اذا خلط مع جلد غيره تأثر جميع وبره
2.30	*om.*	ولاحتباس الطمث والمغص الشديد يدهن به المرأة مراق بطنها وتحمل منه صوفة لضعف البصر نافع	*om.*

2.25: (a) يؤخذ] *om.* B | فيذاف] يضاف B | بخل عنصل] بخل عسل B | واطلِ] ويطلي B | الرأس والجسد] الجسد والرأس B
(b) في المرة السوداء] من السوداء W | ويوضع] ويضع W | البرساء] البرسه T | البرساء] القربه W | ومخ الاسد...بدهن بنفسج] مخ الاسد اذا اذيف بخل عنصل ودهن ورد وطلى به الجسد والراس وشرب منه وزن مثقال ونصف مثقال طباشيرية بماء العرينه باردا وسعّط منه ايضا بدهن بنفسج اذهب الوسواس العارض من المرة السوداء G
(c) *om.* C
2.26: (a) يؤخذ] *om.* B | ويلقي] فيلقي B | ويذاف] ويضاف B | واطلِ] ويطلي B | والورم الحاس] والورم لطبي B | الجميع] *om.* B
(b) تكون] *om.* W | دم الاسد...في الرقبة] دم الاسد اذا سحق مع عسل وملح ومُر وطلى به النزلات والخنازير التي تجمع في البدن نفعه G
(c) جلد الاسد] *om.* C | بعسل] بعسل نحل C
2.27: (b) اذا جعل] تخبه W
(c) رجيع الاسد...السوس] جلد الاسد اذا وضع منه شي في ثياب لم تعت C
2.29: (a) This recipe is attested only in B
(b) وان صيّر...الجلود] صير هذا الجلد مع جلد غيره من السباع تساقط وبر تلك الجلود W | وان صيّر] وان خعل G | غيرها] غيره G

2.25	Lion marrow: if it is taken, mixed with red squill vinegar and rose oil, rubbed on the head and the body, then this will be useful against the occasional obsession due to the black gall.	The marrow of the lion is useful against the occasional obsession due to the black gall: if it is mixed with red squill vinegar and rose oil, then rubbed on the body and the head, given to drink in the quantity of one *miṯqāl* together with half *miṯqāl* of gypsum with lebbek water to be drunk cold; or also inhaled against this disease, with one carat of violet oil.	Lion blood: if it is mixed with red squill vinegar and rose water, rubbed on the body and applied on the forehead, then this will be useful against the occasional obsession due to black gall; half dirham of it can be drunk, and also inhaled with one carat of gypsum together with violet oil.
2.26	Lion blood: if it is taken, a bit of salt is added to it, everything mixed together, and rubbed on the scrofula that affects the neck, the suppurative swelling, and all the ulcers of the legs, and this will cure everything.	Lion blood: if it is mixed with some honey, salt, and myrrh, then rubbed on the scrofula and the phlegm which affects the body—and especially the neck—[it will be useful].	Lion skin: if it is mixed with honey and salt, rubbed on the throat, then this will cure the scrofula and the swelling.
2.27	Lion skin: if it is tied to cloths or textiles, then the moths will not approach them.	Lion skin: if it is put among cloths, then the moths will not approach them.	Lion excrement: if it is tied to the cloths, then the moths will not approach them anymore.
2.28	*om.*	*om.*	If it is placed among the cereals, then the moths will not approach them anymore.
2.29	Lion skin: if it is mixed with other skins, it will affect the fur of all the other ones.	If the skin of a lion is placed among other skins, then the fur on these other skins will fall out.	*om.*
2.30	*om.*	Against the retention of the menstruation and the intense gripes: the belly of the woman has to be rubbed with it, and she has to carry it in a woollen cloth; it is also useful for the weak eyesight.	*om.*

2.31	بول الاسد اذا شمته الكلاب هربوا منه	بول الاسد اذا شمته الكلاب فرت منه	بول الاسد اذا شمته الكلاب هربت
2.32	وان اردت ان تبغض الشراب لمن لا يصير عنه فاسفه من رجيع الاسد في الشراب وهو لا يعلم فانه يبغضه بغضا شديدا والله اعلم	وان اردت ان يبغض انسان الشراب فاسف من رجيع الاسد ورن دانق وهو لا يعلم	بول الاسد اذا سقيته لمن لا يبغض عن الخمر فانه لا يقربه ابدا
2.33	*om.*	والاسد يخاف من الديك الابيض ومن والفأرة	*om.*
2.34	اذا اردت ان تغلب الاسد فاضرب قوائمه بشيء من خشب السنديان فانه يخاف منك و لا يقبل بك ابدا المخ ولا يبرح من مكانه والله اعلم	وان مسح قوائم الاسد الحاشرة السيّد وان يتحرك من مكانه حذرا	واذا اردت ان يخاف الاسد فضربه بعود من السنديان فانه لا يتحرك ابدا

2.31: (a) This recipe is attested only in B

2.32: (a) وان اردت...شديدا] رجيع الاسد اذا جعل في شراب فمن شربه يبغض شربه B

(b) وان اردت...لا يعلم] وبعض الشراب يسقي من رجيع الاسد وزن دانق من شراب فيبغض الشراب من لايصبر عنه W

(c) بول الاسد...لا يقربه ابداً] رجيع الاسد اذا شرب من لم يقدر يصير علو الخمر فانه يكره ولايرجع بقربه بعد ذلك C

2.33: (b) This recipe is attested only in W and G

2.34: (a) This recipe is attested only in B

(b) This recipe is attested only in W

(c) واذا اردت...يتحرك ابدا] واذا ضربت الاسد بعود من السنديان فانه لا يتحرك ابدا ويهابك اذا زال C

2.31	If the dogs sniff the urine of a lion, then they will flee from it.	If the dogs sniff the urine of a lion, then they will run away.	If the dogs sniff the urine of a lion, then they will flee.
2.32	If you want that drinking wine becomes hideous to someone who uses to drink, let him drink lion excrement with wine—but he should not be aware of it—then he will hate it as if it were poison, and God knows best.	If you want that someone hates drinking wine, then give him one *dāniq* of lion excrement in wine to drink, but he should not be aware of it.	Lion urine: if it is given to drink to someone who does not hate wine, then he will never touch it again.
2.33	*om.*	Lions are afraid of white roosters and mice.	*om.*
2.34	If you want to defeat a lion, hit its legs with a piece of oak wood: it will be frightened, will not approach you anymore and it will not be able to move from the place where it is, and God knows best.	If all the legs of the lion are rubbed with [?], the lion will move with caution from its place.	If you want to frighten the lion, hit it with an oak branch, then the lion will not move anymore.

٣. الذئب

	a	b	c
	ذكر منافع اعضاء الذئب	الذئب	باب منافع الذئب
3.1	رأس الذئب اذا علق في برج الحمام لم يقربه نمس ولا هرّ ولا شيء يؤذيه	رأس الذئب اذا علق في برج الحمام لم يقربه نمس ولا سنور ولا شيء يؤذي الحمام	رأس الذئب اذا علق في برج الحمام لم يقربه نمس ولا ذئب ولا سنور ولا ما يؤذيه
3.2	كعب الذئب الايمن اذا علق على الرأس الرمح وحمله انسان واجتمعوا جماعة بالارماح لم يصلوا اليه	كعب الذئب الايمن اذا علق على الرأس رمح واجتمع عليه جماعة رماح لم يصلوا اليه	كعب الذئب الايمن اذا علق على رمح واجتمعت على ذلك الرمح جميع الرماح لاتصل اليه
3.3	مرارة الذئب يذاف بدهن ورد ويطلي به الرجل حاجبيه وفي الكفّة الايمن فلا يراه احد الا احبّه ولا امرأة الا تبعته	مرارته اذا اذيفت بدهن ورد ودهن به الرجل حاجبية احبته المرأة اذا مشى بين يديها	مرارة الذئب اذا اذيبت بدهن الورد ودهن الرجل حاجبيه كان محبوبا لمن يراه خصوصا عند النساء فلا تراه امراة الا احبته
3.4	يؤخذ مرارة الذئب فتخلط بشيء من الورس واطلِ به الوجه فانه يذهب البرش النمش والكلف وجميع الطبوع التي في الوجه	مرارة ايضا اذا خلط مع ورس وطلى به الوجه اذهب بالبروشة والنمش	مرارة الذئب اذا خلط معها ورس مسحوق ودلك به الوجه اذهب الوضح
3.5	خصية الذئب اليمنى حففها واسحقها واذيفها بزيت مغسول واجعل في صوفة وتحتمل به المرأة فانها تسكن عنها شهوة الجماع	*om.*	اذا اردت ان تسكن غلمة المرأة خذ خصية الذئب اليمنى وجففها واخلطها بزيت وتحمل المرأة منه قراط في قطنة فانه سكن عنها ذلك

3.1: (a) ولا هر] ولا نمر ولا هر B
(c) نمس…يوديه] قط نمس ولا ذيب C
3.2: (a) انسان] للاسان B | واجتمعوا] واجتمعت عليه B | بالارماح] الرماح B | اليه] عليه B
(b) رماح] بالرماح W | اليه] اليه ما دام ذلك الكعب معلّق على رمحه *add.* W
3.3: (a) يذاف] تضاف B
(b) *om.* W
(c) مرارة الذئب] مرارته C | اذيبت] اذيف C | ودهن] ودهن به C
3.4: (a) يؤخذ] *om.* B | واطلِ به] ويطلي بها B | فانه يذهب البرش النمش] فانها تذهب النمش B | وجميع الطبوع] وجميع الافات B
(b) *om.* W
(c) ورس] ورص L | مرارة الذئب] *om.* C | ورس] ورص L | ودلك] ودهن C | اذهب الوضح] الوضح اذهبه C
3.5: (a) This recipe is attested only in B | واذيفها] وضيفها B
(b) *om.* W
(c) اذا اردت ان تسكن غلمة المرأة خذ] *om.* C | وجففها واخلطها] جففت وسحقت وخلطت C | وتحمل…فانه] التي بها غلمة اي قوة طلب الجماع C

3. Wolf

	a	b	c
	Exposition of the useful properties of the parts of the wolf	**The wolf**	**Chapter on the useful properties of the wolf**
3.1	Wolf head: if it is hung on a pigeon house, then neither an ichneumon, nor a cat, or anything harmful will approach it.	Wolf head: if it is hung on a pigeon house, then neither an ichneumon, nor a cat or anything harmful to pigeons will approach it.	Wolf head: if it is hung on a pigeon house, then no ichneumon, wolf, cat, or anything harmful will approach it.
3.2	Wolf right anklebone: if it is hung on the top of a spear and carried in this way, then all the other spears will stay tight without interlocking.	Wolf right anklebone: if it is hung on the top of a spear, then all the other spears will stay tight next to this one without interlocking.	Wolf right anklebone: if it is hung on the top of a spear, then all the other spears will stay tight, close to this one.
3.3	Wolf gall: if it is mixed with rose oil, rubbed on the eyebrow and on the palm of the right hand, then everyone will love this man and every woman will follow him.	Its gall: if it is mixed with rose oil and anointed on the eyebrow, then a woman will fall in love with that man when he passes in front of her.	Wolf gall: if it is liquefied with rose oil and anointed on the eyebrow, then the man will be loved by everyone who sees him, especially the women, and every woman will love him at first sight.
3.4	Wolf gall: if it is taken, mixed with some curcuma and rubbed on the face, then the spots, the freckles and the discoloured spots will go away, and also all the other marks that can be found on the face.	Its gall again: if it is mixed with curcuma and rubbed on the face, the spots and the freckles will go away.	Its gall again: if it is mixed with ground curcuma and rubbed on the face, then the leprosy will go away.
3.5	Wolf right testicle: if it is dried, ground, mixed with washed oil and put in a woollen cloth and a woman carries it, then her desire of coitus will be calmed.	*om.*	If you want to quench the lust of a woman, take the right testicle of the wolf, dry it, mix it with oil and the woman should carry one carat of it in a cotton cloth, then this will calm her down.

عين الذئب اليمنى اذا علقت على انسان لم يخف لصا ولا سارقا ولا أذى	عين الذئب اليمنى من علقها عليه لم يخف لصّا ولا سبعا	من علق عليه عين الذئب اليمنى فلا يخاف لصّا ولا سارقا ولا سبعا ولا شيئا مما يخاف منه	3.6
جلد الذئب اذا يبخره حانوت من يصنع الدف تفتقت جميع الدفوف	وان دخن الدكان الذي يعمل فيه الدفوف بجلد ذئب تشققت	جلد الذئب اذا بخر به حانوت من يدبغ الدفوف انشقت جميعها	3.7
واذا عمل من جلدها طبلا وضرب في عسكر لم يبق طبل والا شق	وان اتخذ طبلا جلد ذئب فضرب به عسكر تشققت الطبول التي فيه	وان عمل طبلا من جلد ذئب ثم ضربت به في عسكر تشققت الطبول ذلك العسكر جميعها	3.8
خصية الذئب اذا شققت وشتت بملح وشونيز وشرب منها صاحب وجع الخاصرة والجنب نفعه	خصية الذئب اذا شقت وملحت بسعتر وملح وسقى منها صاحب وجع الخاصرة بماء الجرجير وزن مثقال نفعه	خصية الذئب تملح بملح ودقيق الشعير ويسقي منها صاحب وجع الخاصرة فانه يبرأ باذن الله تعالى	3.9
om.	وهو ايضا نافع لذات الجنب اذا شرب بماء حار وعسل	وهو ايضا نافع لذات الجنب اذا شربت بماء حار	3.10
دم الذئب اذا خلط بدهن ورد ودهن جوز وقطر في الأذن الموجوعة ابرأها ونفع من الصمم	دم الذئب اذا اذيف بدهن الجوز وقطّر في الأذن نفع من الصمم	دم الذئب اذا اخلط بدهن ورد ودهن جوز وقطّر في الاذن الثقيلة السمع والصمم فتبرأ باذن الله تعالى	3.11

3.6: (a) فلا] فانه لا B | ولا سبعا ولا شيئا مما يخاف منه] *om.* B
(b) *om.* W
(c) لصا ولا سارقا] ولم يهب سارقا ولا قاطع الطريق C
3.7: (b) وان دخن...تشققت] وجلد الذئب اذا دخل به حانوت رجل يعمل الدفوف التي تلعب بها النساء تشقّقت الدفوف والطبول التي فيه W
(c) يبخره] وضع في C | الدف] الدفوف C | تفتقت جميع الدفوف] شققها C
3.8: (a) ذلك] في ذلك الذي B
(b) *om.* W
(c) وضرب] وضرب عليه C | والا شق] الا وقد تشقق C
3.9: (a) بملح] بشيء من الملح B | ويسقي] ويسحق ويسقي B | فانه] *om.* B
(b) خصية الذئب...نفعه] خصية الذئب اذا اشرحت وملّحت بملح وسعتر ويسقي منها مثقال بماء الجرجير نفع من وجع الخاصرة W
(c) خصية الذئب] واذا أخذ خصوة الذيب C | وشونيز] وشعير C | نفعه] نفعه نفعاً جيدا C
3.10: (a) *om.* B
(b) وهو ايضا نافع لذات الجنب] وينفع ذات الجنب W
3.11: (a) وقطّر] ويقطر B | الثقيلة السمع] *om.* B | فتبرأ] تبرأ B
(b) دم الذئب...الصمم] وذنب الذئب ينفع من الصمم اذا اضيف بدهن الجوز وقطر في الأذن W
(c) خلط بدهن] خلط به دهن C | ابرأها] برأها C

3.6	The man who hangs the right eye of a wolf on his person will not be afraid of thieves, raiders, beasts of prey, or anything that used to frighten him.	Wolf right eye: the one who hangs it on his person will not be afraid of thieves or beasts of prey.	Wolf right eye: if it is hung on a man, then he will not be afraid of thieves, raiders, or anyone who may harm him.
3.7	Wolf skin: if it is used to fumigate a shop in which tambourines are tanned, then this will split each and every one of them.	If a shop in which tambourines are made is fumigated with the skin of the wolf, then the instruments will split.	Wolf skin: if it is used in the fumigation of a shop where tambourines are made, it will undo the sewing of all the tambourines.
3.8	If a drum is made with the skin of a wolf, and beaten among an army, then this will split all the drums of the army.	If a drum made of wolf skin is taken and beaten in the midst of an army, then it will split the drums that are there.	If a drum is made of its skin and beaten among an army, then no drum will split there.
3.9	Wolf testicle: if it is seasoned with salt and barley flour, given to a man suffering from waist pain to drink, then he will heal, with the permission of God may He be exalted.	Wolf testicle: if it is split, seasoned with wild thyme and salt, then given to a man suffering from waist pain with one *miṯqāl* of rocket water to drink, this will be useful to him.	Wolf testicle: if it is split, spattered with salt and fennel flower and drunk by a man suffering from waist pain and pleurisy, then this will be useful for him.
3.10	And this is also useful against pleurisy, if drunk with warm water.	And this is useful also against pleurisy, if drunk with warm water and honey.	*om.*
3.11	Wolf blood: if it is mixed with rose oil and nut oil, applied in drops in the ear that is hard of hearing or deaf, then this will heal, with the permission of God may He be exalted.	Wolf blood: if it is mixed with nut oil and applied in drops inside the ear, then this will be useful against deafness.	Wolf blood: if it is mixed with rose oil and nut oil and applied in drops inside an aching ear, then this will cure it, and will be useful against deafness.

3.12

لحم الذئب وشحمه وطحاله اذا دق مع قلب الجوز وطبح بماء الكرفس والعسل النحل مع شيء من ورس وخولنجان وفلفل ابيض ودار فلفل أخذ متساوية وشربه صاحب الملايل بالماء المردقوش ابرأه

لحمه وشحمه وطحاله اذا دق في الجوز ثم طبخ بماء الكرفس والعسل مع شيء من خولنجان وورس وفلفل ابيض من كل واحد جزء ثم اسقي منه صاحب المليلة وبماء المرزنجوش

يؤخذ لحم الذئب وشحمه وطحاله فيدق الجميع ويخلط معه قلب الجوز ويطبخ بماء الكرفس والعسل ويلقي عليه ورس وخولنجان وفلفل من كل واحد جزء واطمعه لمن يكون بلبيد الخاطر كثير النسيان بماء المزرنحوش فانه يفهم

3.13

دماغ الذئب اذا اذيب بماء السذاب والزيت وطلى به الجسد نفع من العلل الظاهرة والباطنة

دماغه اذا اديف بماء السذاب والزيت ودهن به الجسد نفع من كل علة ظاهرة وباطنة [من البرد]

دماغ الذئب يداف بماء السذاب الاخضر والزيت الخالص ويدهن به الجسد فينفع من كل علة ظاهرة وباطنة

3.14

واذا غسل بعسل وخل وشرب بماء حار في الحمام ابرأه من وجع الرية

دماغ ايضا اذا غلى بعسل وشرب بماء حار في الحمام نفع من وجع الرية

دماغ اذا غلى بعسل وشرب بماء حار في الحمام نفع لوجع الرية

3.15

مخ الذئب اذا اذيب بماء الحضض المكي وطلى به الاورام التي في الاهان برأه

مخه اذا اذيف بماء الحضض وطلى به ورم اللهاية نفعه

مخ الذئب يذاف بماء الحضض المكي ويلطخ به الورم الذي يكون في اللهاة فتصلح باذن الله تعالى

3.16

[رية] الذئب اذا جفف وسحقت مع ورد احمر وطبخ بلبن حليب وشربه صاحب الربو ابرأه

ريته اذا جففت وسحقت مع كثيراء وطبخت بلبن حليب وسقى منها صاحب الربو نفعه

رية الذئب اذا جففت وسحقت بشيء من الكثيرة الحمراء وطبخت بلبن حليب من شاة حمراء وسقى منه صاحب الربو على الجوف والخفقان والرجيف نفع باذن الله تعالى

3.12: (a) يؤخذ] om. B | فيدق] يدق B | لمن] للذي B | الخاطر] om. B | المزرنحوش] المزرنكوش B

(b) وطحاله اذا دق في الجوز] وهنجاله يدق الجميع في جاون W | طبخ] يطبخ W | مع شيء من خولنجان وورس] وتخلط معه وريش W | اسقى منه صاحب] يسقي من به W | وبماء المرزنجوش] بماء المر والمروزرنجوش W

(c) أخذ متساوية] اجزاء متساوية C

3.13: (a) يذاف] يضاف B | ظاهرة وباطنة] om. B

(b) دماغه...[من البرد] دماغ الذئب يضاف بماء الشراب وزيت فيدهن به الجسد فينفع من كل علة ظاهرة وباطنة في البدن من البرد W

3.14: (a) om. B

(b) دماغ ايضا...وجع الريّة] دماغ الذئب اذا غلى بعسل نفع من وجع الرية اذا شرب بماء حار في الحمام W

3.15: (a) يذاف] يذاب B | الحضض] الحصص B | فتصلح] om. B

(b) مخه...نفعه] مخ الذئب اذا يضاف بماء الخصيص ويحل به اللهات من ورمها فيبرأ W

(c) اذيب] اذيف C | الحضض] الحضض C | برأه] ابرأها C

3.16: (a) وسقي] ويسقي B | الربو علي الجوف] الرجعة B | نفع] نفعه B

(b) ريته] ورية W | كثيراء] الكبر W

(c) ورد] قرد C

3.12 Wolf meat, its fat and its spleen: if they are taken, everything minced with the heart of a nut, cooked with celery water and honey, curcuma, galangal and pepper are added to it—a part of each one—and given to a man with an incoherent mind and a lot of forgetfulness to eat together with marjoram water, then he will understand and remember.

Its meat, its fat and its spleen: if they are minced in a nut, then cooked with celery water, honey and some galangal, curcuma and white pepper—one part of each one—then it should be given to a man suffering from feverish heat with marjoram water to drink, [then it will be useful].

Wolf meat, its fat and its spleen: if they are minced with the heart of a nut, cooked with celery water and honey, with a bit of curcuma, galangal, white pepper and long pepper, in the same amount, and drunk by a man suffering from feverish heat, along with marjoram water, then this will cure him.

3.13 Wolf brain: if it is mixed with green rue water and pure oil, anointed on the body, then this will be useful against every illness, manifest or hidden.

Its brain: if it is mixed with rue water and oil, anointed on the body, then this will be useful against every illness, manifest or hidden, that is due to coldness.

Wolf brain: if it is liquefied with rue water and oil and rubbed on the body, then this will be useful against both manifest and hidden illnesses.

3.14 Brain: if it is boiled with honey and drunk with warm water in the bath, then this will be useful against the lung complaint.

Its brain, again: if it is boiled with honey and drunk with warm water in the bath, then this will be useful against lung complaint.

If it is washed with honey and vinegar and drunk with warm water in the bath, this will cure the lung complaint.

3.15 Wolf marrow: if it is mixed with Meccan lycium water, spattered on the swelling of the uvula, then this will cure it, with the permission of God may He be exalted.

Its marrow: if it is mixed with lycium water and rubbed on the uvula, then it will be useful for it.

Wolf marrow: if it is mixed with Meccan lycium water and rubbed on the swelling, then this will cure it.

3.16 Wolf lung: if it is dried, pounded with a bit of red goat's thorn, cooked with the milk of a red sheep and given to a man suffering from asthma of the heart, palpitation and convulsions to drink, then this will be useful for him, with the permission of God may He be exalted.

Its lung: if it is dried, pounded with goat's thorn, cooked with milk and given to a man suffering from asthma to drink, it will be useful for him.

Wolf lung: if it is dried, pounded with a red rose, cooked with milk and drunk by a man suffering from asthma, this will be useful to him.

3.17	ناب الذئب وقطعه من جلده وعينه اليمني اذا احملها الانسان معه غلب جميع من يخاصمه وكان محبوبا عند الناس	انيابه وجلده وعينيه اذا حمله الانسان غلب خصمه وكان محبوبا الى الناس	انياب الذئب اذا حملها مع جلده وعينه انسان غلب جميع من يخاصمه وكانت له وجاهة عند من يراه
3.18	زبل الذيب اذا حل بالماء ورس به مكان الزرع لا ينبت	زبل الذئب اذا بل بالماء وتضخ على قراح الذي بزرع الحبوب لم ينبت فيه شخمة التي يقال لها اسدا القطائ	[زبله] اذا اذئب بالماء ورس في المكان الذي تريد ان تزرعه فلا يطلع فيه شحرة التي يقال لها اسد الفار التي تمنع الزرع الظهور
3.19	ذنب الذئب اذا علق على مداود البقر فانها لا يقدر ياكل شيئا	ذنب الذئب اذا علّق على من ودّ البقر لم يقدران يعفل شيئا ما دام معلّق عليه يعنى المدود	ذنب الذئب اذا علق على مداود البقر منعها الأكل
3.20	زبل الذئب اذا اذيب بالعسل وسقى منه صاحب القولنج سكن عنه باذن الله تعالى	زبله اذا سحق مع شيء من فلفل وعجن بعسل منزوع الرغوة ولعق منه من به القولنج نفعه	زبل الذئب اذا جففت وسحق بالعسل المنزوع والرغوة ابرأ صاحب القولنج وسهل جوفه
3.21	كبد الذئب اذا جفّفت وسحقت واخلط معها معجون يقال له ابابا [؟] نفع من وجع الكبد	كبد الذئب ينفع من اوجاع الكبد ويخلط في معجون يدعى ابا ياميا	كبد الذئب اذا جففت وخلطت بمعجون يقال له ياساما [؟] فانه ينفع من وجع الكبد
3.22	قصيب الذئب اذا اكل مشويا نفع عند الجماع	قضيبه اذا أخذ وشوى في القدر وقطّع مضغ قطعة قطعة هيّج الجماع	قضيب الذئب اذا شوى وأكل منه حال الجماع وزن حبة فانه يقوي على الجماع

3.17: (a) معه] *om.* B
(b) انيابه] انياب الذئب W | الانسان غلب خصمه] الانسان معه غلب خصمه W | محبوبا الى الناس] محبيبا عند الناس W
(c) انياب...يراه] انياب الذيب وجلده وعينيه اذا حملها انسان غلب كل من حاصمه وكانت له وجاهة عند كل من يراه C
3.18: (a) This recipe is attested only in B
(b) This recipe is attested only in W
(c) تريد ان تزرعه] يريد تزعزعه او يزعزعه C | الزرع الظهور] الظهور واذا سحق بالعسل المنزوع الرغوة ابرأ صاحب القولنج *add.* C
3.19: (a) فانها لا يقدر] فلا يقدروا البقر B
(b) This recipe is attested only in W
(c) مداود] معالق C
3.20: (b) زبله...نفعه] زبل الذئب المسحوق مع شيء من فلفل اذا عجن بعسل منزوع الرغوة ولعق منه منه صاحب القولنج نفعه نفعا بينا وهذا مجرب W
(c) For this recipe in C, see 3.18
3.21: (a) ابايا] ابایاسا B
(b) This recipe is attested only in W
(c) ياساما] باساما C | فانه ينفع] نفع C
3.22: (b) قضيبه...الجماع] وخصية الذئب تشوي في الفرن وتقطع وتمضع منه قطعة فتهيّج الجماع مجرب W
(c) شوي] شويته C | وأكل] ووضعت C | يقوي] قويت C

3.17	Wolf canine tooth, a piece of its skin and its right eye: if a man carries them with him, then he will defeat anyone who disputes with him, and will be loved by the people.	Its canine tooth, its skin and its eyes: if a man carries them, then he will defeat his adversary and will be loved by the people.	Wolf canine teeth: if a man carries them with him, then he will defeat all his adversaries, and will be loved by everyone who sees him.
3.18	Wolf excrement: if it is diluted in water and a field is spattered with it, then it will not be fertile.	Wolf excrement: if it is moistened with water and spattered on a ploughed field prepared for the grain, then the dark matter, called *asad al-Qaṭā'i*, will not grow there.	Its excrement: if it is liquefied in water and spattered in the place where you want that something grows, then the kind of soot called *asad al-fār* [?] which hinders the cultivations, will not grow there.
3.19	Wolf tail: if it is hung on the manger for the cows, they will not eat anything.	Wolf tail: if it is hung on a man who feeds the cows, then they will not do anything as long as the manger remains hung on them.	Wolf tail: if it is hung on the cow mangers, it will prevent the cows from eating.
3.20	Wolf excrement: if it is liquefied with honey and given to a man suffering from colic to drink, then this will calm it, with the permission of God may He be exalted.	Its excrement: if it is ground with a bit of pepper, kneaded with honey without foam and licked by a man suffering from colic, then it will be useful for him.	Wolf excrement: if it is dried, ground with honey without foam, it will cure a man suffering from colic, and will purge him.
3.21	Wolf liver: if it is dried, ground and mixed with an electuary called *ayāyā* [?], this will be useful against the liver complaint.	The liver of a wolf is useful against liver complaint, if it is mixed with an electuary named *abā yāmiyā*.	If the liver of a wolf is dried and melted with an electuary called *yāsāmā* [?], then this will be useful against the liver complaint.
3.22	If its penis is eaten roasted, this will be useful at the moment of coitus.	If its penis is taken, roasted in a cooking pot, cut in pieces and chewed piece by piece, then this will excite coitus.	Wolf penis: if it is roasted and one grain of it is eaten at the moment of coitus, then this will give power to the coitus.

§	(a)	(b)	(c)
3.23	*om.*	قضيبه ايضا اذا أخذ فعقد على اسم امرأة لم يقدر احد عليها حتى تُحل ذلك العقد منه	*om.*
3.24	ناب الذئب اذا علق على انسان لا يخاف من الذياب	ومن علق عليه نابه لم يخف منه	من علق عليه ناب الذئب فانه لا يخاف من الذياب
3.25	[مرارة] الذئب اذا خلطت بشيء من مسك وسعط به المصروع في رأس كل هلال مرة لا يقربه الجنون ولا يعارضه صرع	مرارة اذا أخذ منها وزن دانق وخلط مع حبة مسك وسعّط به المصروع في رأس كل هلال نفعه	مرارة الذئب اذا خلط معها شيء من مسك وسعّط بها المصروع في كل هلال فانه يبرأ
3.26	مرارة الذئب اذا يكتحل بها من بعينيه غشاوة ابرأها	مرارته ايضا اذا اكتحل منها نفع من الماء الذي في العين ومن الغشاوة	مرارته اذا يكتحل بها من في عينه الغشاوة او ماء فانه يبرأ باذن الله تعالى
3.27	[مرارة] اذيبت بعسل وطلى الاحليل حال الجماع لا يشتهي بعده جماع غيره ولها تاثيرة في المحبة	ومرارته ايضا اذا اذيف منها بعسل وماء وطلى به الذكر وقت الجماع فانها تحبك حبا شديدا	*om.*
3.28	[اذا] اذيبت بعسل وطلى به الاحليل حال الجماع لا يشتهي بعده جماع غيره ولها تاثيرة في المحبة	مرارة الذئب يذاف بشيء من عسل ويطلي بها الاحليل عند الجماع فانه يهيّج المرأة	مرارة الذئب يذاف بشيء من عسل ويطلي بها الاحليل عند الجماع فانه يهيّج المرأة شيء عظيم

3.23: (b) *om.* W

3.24: (a) لا يخاف] لم يخف B

(b) نابه] ناب الذئب W | منه] ذيبا W

(c) علق على انسان] علقه عليه احد C | لا يخف] لم يخف C

3.25: (b) مرارة اذا أخذ] مرارة الذئب ان أخذ W | مع حبة مسك] معه وزن حبة مسك W | المصروع] صرع W | رأس] *om.* W | نفعه] نفعه وقام مقام السلبا *add.* W

(c) لا يقربه الجنون ولا يعارضه صرع] زال عنه الصرع ولا يعتر به الجنون C

3.26: (a) *om.* B

(b) مرارته...الغشاوة] ومرارة الذئب يكتحل بها مِن ضعف البصر والماء في العين والغشاوة فيهدا ان شاء الله تعالى W

(c) This recipe is attested only in C, after 3.28

3.27: (b) *om.* W

(c) به] بها C | ولها] ولذلك C

3.28: (a) *om.* B

(b) *om.* W | يذاف] يضاف G

(c) *om.* C

3.23	*om.*	Its penis, again: if it is taken and tied in the name of a woman, than no one will have power over her until the knot of the penis is untied.	*om.*
3.24	The one who hangs its tooth on his person will not be afraid of wolves.	The one who hangs its tooth on his person will not be afraid of wolves.	Wolf tooth: if it is hung on a man, then he will not be afraid of wolves.
3.25	Wolf gall: if it is mixed with a bit of musk and an epileptic man inhales it—at every new moon—then he will be cured.	Wolf gall: if one *dāniq* of it is taken and mixed with a grain of musk, inhaled by an epileptic man at the new moon, then this will be useful for him.	Wolf gall: if it is mixed with a bit of musk and inhaled by a man—once at the new moon—then neither insanity nor epilepsy will touch him.
3.26	Its gall: if it is rubbed on an eye affected by cataract or by water, then this will be cured, with the permission of God may He be exalted.	Its gall again: if it is smeared on the eye, it will be useful against the water in it and against the cataract.	Wolf gall: if it is rubbed on an eye affected by the cataract, then this will cure it.
3.27	*om.*	Its gall again: if it is mixed with honey and water and rubbed on the penis at the moment of coitus, then the woman will love you passionately.	Its gall: diluted with honey and rubbed on the outer opening of the urethra at the moment of coitus, and, after this, she will not desire any other man, and this will influence her love.
3.28	Wolf gall: if it is mixed with some honey and rubbed on the outer opening of urethra at the moment of coitus, then this will greatly excite the woman.	Wolf gall: if it is mixed with some honey and rubbed on the outer opening of urethra at the moment of coitus, it will excite the woman.	Mixed with honey and rubbed on the outer opening of urethra at the moment of coitus, it will not let the woman desire any other man, and this will have an influence on her love.

٤. الضبع

	a	b	c
	ذكر منافع اعضاء الضبع	الضبع	باب منافع الضبع
4.1	جلد الضبع اذا امسكه انسان معه لم ينبح عليه الكلاب	جلده اذا امسكه انسان لم تنبح عليه الكلاب	جلد الضبع اذا حمله انسان لا ينبح عليه كلب
4.2	مخاليب الضبع اليمنى تقلعهم بيدك اليسار وعلّقها عليك فكل من ابصرك من الناس احبّك	*om.*	مخلابه اذا قطعت بيدك اليسرى وعلقته عليك احبك كل من راك من الناس حبا شديدا
4.3	*om.*	مرارته يكتحل بها من ضعف البصر والماء في العين	*om.*
4.4	عين الضبع تقلع [وتنقع] في الخل وتشال من الخل فتجعل تحت فص خاتم حديد فان من تختّم بذلك لم يخف سحرا ولا مكروها ولا أذي باذن الله تعالى	عين الضبع اليمنى تقلع وتنقع في خل سبعة ايام ثم اجعلها تحت فض خاتم والبسه فانك لا تخاف سحر ولا شيء من الاشياء	عين] الضبع اذا قلعت ونقعت في خل جديد ورفعت منه وجففت وجعلت تحت فض خاتم ولبسه انسان لا يخاف سحرا وشيئا مكروها
4.5	وان علمت بانسان مسحور فاغسل ذلك الخاتم بماء واسقه ذلك الماء اياه فيذهب عنه السحر باذن الله تعالى	وان علمت ان بانسان سحر فاغسل الخاتم بالماء واسقه اياه فيذهب عنه	واذا عملت انسانا به سحر فاغسل الخاتم بالماء واسقه لمن به السحر فانه يذهب عنه السحر

4.1: (a) اذا] ان B | انسان] الانسان B
(b) الكلاب] كلب W
4.2: (a) تقلعهم] تقطعهم B | اليسار] اليسرى B
(c) مخلابه...حبا شديدا] مخلاب الضبع الايمن اذا قطعها احد بيده اليسر وعلقها عليه نال حبا من جميع من الناس وكان مقبولا W
4.3: (b) مرارته] مرارة الضبع W | العين] العين فجلوه ويقوّيه add. C
4.4: (a) تقلع] تنقع B | وتشال من الخل] om. B | فتجعل] ومجعل B | فان من...ولا أذي] فمن حمله لا يخاف سحرا ولا مكرا ولا اذي B
(b) خل] خل خمر W | اجعلها] تخرج W | والبسه...الاشياء] يلبس لمن يخاف السحر والعين فلا يخاف ان يشيبه من ذلك شيء W
(c) عين الضبع] عين الضبع اليمنى C | قلعت] اخذت C | ورفعت منه وجففت وجعلت] ثم جففت ووضعت C | وشيئا] او لا C
4.5: (a) *om.* B
(b) علمت] علم W | فيذهب عنه] ويذهب عنه العين والسحر *add.* C
(c) واذا عملت انسانا به سحر فاغسل] واذا كان بانسان سحر اغسل C | يذهب عنه السحر] يزول عنه C

4. Hyena

	a	b	c
	Exposition of the useful properties of the parts of the hyena	**The hyena**	**Chapter on the useful properties of the hyena**
4.1	Hyena skin: If a man carries it with him, then the dogs will not bark at him.	Its skin: if a man carries it in his hand, then the dogs will not bark at him.	Hyena skin: if a man carries it in his own hand, then no dog will bark at him.
4.2	Hyena right claws: if you clip them with your left hand and hang them on your body, then everyone who sees you will love you.	*om.*	Its claws: if you clip its claws with your left hand and hang them on your body, then everyone who sees you will love you passionately.
4.3	*om.*	Its gall: if it is applied on the eye whose eyesight is weak or has the cataract [it will be useful].	*om.*
4.4	Hyena eye: if it is pulled out, macerated in vinegar, set under the stone of an iron seal [ring], then the one who wears this ring will not be afraid of any magic, its hideous effects or anything that can harm him, with the permission of God, may He be exalted.	Hyena eye: if you pull it out, macerate it in vinegar for seven days, set it under the stone of a seal [ring] and wear it, then you will not be afraid, neither of magic nor of anything else in the world.	Hyena eye: if it is pulled out, macerated in new vinegar, preserved, dried and set under the stone of a seal [ring], then if a man wears it, he will not be afraid, neither of any magic nor of any of its hideous effects.
4.5	And if you know that a man is bewitched, wash this seal with water, and give him the water to drink, then the magic will leave him.	And if you know that a man is bewitched, wash this seal with water and give him the water to drink, then the magic will leave him.	And if you know that a man is bewitched, wash this seal with water, and give this water to the bewitched one to drink, then the magic will leave him.

4.6	وان أخذت يد الضبع اليمنى وشيئا من جلده حال الحياة وعلق ذلك على من يريد الدخول على السلاطين فانه يعظم امره ويهابه وتقضي حاجته	يد الضبع اليمني بجلدها تقطع وهي حية اذا اعلقت على انسان ودخل على السلطان او على من احبب قضيت حوائجه	يؤخد جلد الضبع ويده اليمنى تعلق على من يريد الدخول على السلطان ولا يخاف وتقضي حاخته
4.7	واذا اردت تعلم صحة ذلك خذ معك صبيا لم يبلغ الحلم واخفي تلك اليد وادخل الصبي معك على السلطان فانه يري كان على [فم السلطان] خاتم	*om.*	واذا اردت ان تعلم ان هذا صحيح فخذ معك عصفورا لم يبلغ الحلم وادخله معك الى ذلك السلطان فترى على فم السلطان لجاما
4.8	رأس الضبع اذا جعل في برج الحمام فانها تكثر فيه	رأس الضبع اذا جعل في برج حمام كثر ذلك	*om.*
4.9	واذا عسرت الولاده على المرأة فارها يد الضبع اليمنى ثم ضعها تحت رجلها فانها تلد سريعا	واذا عسر على المرأة ولادتها فضع يد الضبع اليمنى تحت قدميها فانها تلد	اذا عسر على المرأة الولادة فعلق عليها يد الضبع اليمنى فتلد من ساعتها باذن الله تعالى
4.10	الفخذ الايمن من الضبع الذكر اذا حرق وسحق بزيت ودهن به دبر الرجل المخنث من بُغاء ابرأه وازال ما به	*om.*	*om.*
4.11	فخذ الضبعة الانثى وشواها جيدا وسحمها بزيت او لا زيت ودهن به دبر	*om.*	*om.*

4.6: (a) يؤخد] *om.* B
(b) In G this recipe is after 4.3
(c) وان أخذت] *om.* C | وشيئا] مع شيء C | السلاطين...حاخته] السلطان نال منها به وانقضت حاخته W
4.7: (a) عصفورا] صغيرا B | الى ذلك] على ذلك B | على فم السلطان لجاما] على فمه اللجام B
(b) In G this recipe is after 4.3
(c) لم يبلغ الحلم] دون البلوغ C | واخفي] واخق C | يرى] ترى C | خاتم] لجام C
4.8: (b) جعل] صير W | كثر ذلك] كثر فيه الحمام W
(c) كثر فيه الحمام] فانها تكثر C
4.9: (c) الفخذ الايمن من الضبع الذكر] فخذ الضبع الايمن الذكر C | حرق] احرق C | دبر الرجل] دبر المخنث C
4.11: (c) *om.* C

4.6	Hyena skin and right paw: if they are hung on a man who wants a hearing with the sultan, then he will not be afraid and his requests will be fulfilled.	Right paw of hyena and its skin, cut while still alive: if you hang it on a man and he has a hearing with the sultan, or with a lover, then his requests will be fulfilled.	If you take the right paw of the hyena and a bit of its skin while it is alive, hang this on the one who wishes to have an audience with the sultans, and then this will make him more important, he will be respected, and his need fulfilled.
4.7	If you want to verify that this is true, take with you a boy who is not yet pubescent, let him come with you in the presence of the sultan, then you will see a seal on the mouth of the sultan.	*om.*	If you want to verify that it is true, take with you a boy who is not yet pubescent, hide that paw and let the boy come with you in the presence of the sultan, then he will see a seal on the mouth of the sultan.
4.8	*om.*	Hyena head: if it is placed inside a pigeon house, then the pigeons will multiply.	Hyena head: if it is placed inside the pigeon house, then the pigeons will multiply there.
4.9	If a woman has difficulties in giving birth, then the right paw of a hyena shall be hung on her, and she will instantly give birth, with the permission of God, may He be exalted.	If a woman has difficulties in giving birth, put the right paw of a hyena under her feet and then she will give birth.	If a woman has difficulties in giving birth, show her the right paw of a hyena and put it under her feet, then she will instantly give birth.
4.10	*om.*	*om.*	Right leg of a male hyena: if it is burnt, ground with oil and, anointed on the backside of a man who is effeminate because he wants to be this way, this will cure him and change this condition.
4.11	*om.*	*om.*	Take a female hyena, roast it well, ground it with or without oil, anoint the back of a straight man with it, then this will turn him into an effeminate man.

			الرجل السليم من هذا آلد احدث به وصار مخنث
4.12	خصية الضبع تملح تسلق وتطعم لصاحب وجع الكبد والصفار يبرأ باذن الله تعالى	خصيته اذا ملحت بملح ورمان وشرب منها وزن مثقال بماء حار نفع من وجع الكبد والصفار	خصية لضبع اذا ملحت بملح ورماد وشرب منها مثقال بعسل نفع من وجع الكبد والصفار
4.13	*om.*	*om.*	دم الضبع اذا نتف الشعر واكتحل به منع نبت الشعر في العين
4.14	يؤخذ مرارة الضبع جزء من الدار فلفل جزء ويخلط الجميع ويسقي لصاحب الزحير الخراطة ورمي الدم فيبرأ باذن الله تعالى	مرارته اذا شرب منها جزء ومع وزن مثقال من دار فلفل نفع من الزحير	مرارة الضبع اذا سحقت بدار فلفل وشرب منها صاحب الزحير ورمى الدم ابرأاه سريعا
4.15	دم الضبع يذاف بدهن ورد ويطلي به الجسد فيذهب بالسحر وعين السوء والنطرة الردية باذن الله تعالى	دمه اذا اذيف بدهن ورد وطلى به الجسد نفع من السحر والنظرة	*om.*
4.16	*om.*	شحمه اذا ادهن به انسان واراد اخذ النمر قوى عليه ولا يوده بشىء	*om.*
4.17	يؤخذ لحم الضبع وشحمه وطحاله وكبده ثم يطبخ الخميع في طنجير حتى ينهر ويلقي عليه ماء الجرجير ومن الورس	لحمه وشحمه وطحاله وكبده يطبخ خميعا بماء ويسحق ويلقي عليه عفص وشب وورس من كل واحد جزء ويخلط جيدا ويشرب منه مقدار بندقة بماء	*om.*

4.12: (a) تسلق] تشوي B | والصفار] والعسار B
(b) *om.* W
(c) In C this recipe is after 4.13 | بعسل] *om.* C | نفع من] من نه C | والصفار] نفعه نفعا جيدا *add.* C
4.13: (c) دم الضبع...في العين] دم الضبع اذا اكتحل من في عينيه شعرة منع انباتها C
4.14: (a) جزء] بجزء B | جزء] *om.* B | ويخلط] يخلط B | ورمى] ونزف B
(b) مرارته...من الزجير] خصية الضبع تشرب منها جزء مع وزن مثقال من دار فلفل ينفع من الزحير جدا W
(c) صاحب] من به C | سريعا] *om.* C
4.15: (a) فيذهب...الردية] يذهب عنه السحر والعين الردية B
(b) *om.* W
4.16: (b) *om.* W
4.17: (a) This recipe is attested only in B
(b) لحمه وشحمه...والحديث] لحم الضبع وشحمه وطحاله يطبخ الخميع بماء ويدق ويلقا عليه حرمل وعفص وورس وشب من كل واحد جزء ويخلط ناعما ويشرب منه مثقال او مقدار بندقة بماء الجرجير مقدار جر عتيق في فينفع من السعال العتيق والحديث W

4.12	Hyena testicle: if it is salted, boiled, and fed to a man suffering from liver complaints and yellow bile, then he will recover, with the permission of God, may He be exalted.	Its testicle: if it is seasoned with salt and pomegranates and drunk with one *miṯqāl* of warm water, then this will be useful against the liver complaint and the yellow bile.	Hyena testicle: if it is seasoned with salt and ash and one *miṯqāl* of it is drunk with honey, this will be useful against liver complaint and the yellow bile.
4.13	*om.*	*om.*	Hyena blood: if it is rubbed on the area from which hair has been pulled out, this will prevent the growth of hair on the eye.
4.14	Hyena gall: if one part of it is taken with one part of long pepper, everything mixed up and given to a man affected by acute dysentery with blood to drink, then he will be cured, with the permission of God, may He be exalted.	Its gall: if it is drunk with one *miṯqāl* of long pepper, this will be useful against dysentery.	Hyena gall: if it is ground with long pepper and drunk by a man suffering from dysentery with blood, this will heal him instantly.
4.15	Hyena blood: if mixed with rose oil and rubbed on the body, then this will void the effects of magic and evil eye, with the permission of God, may He be exalted.	Its blood: mixed with rose oil and rubbed it on the body, will be useful against magic and evil eye.	*om.*
4.16	*om.*	Its fat: if a man rubs his body with it, when he wants to hunt a cheetah, then he will defeat it and will not be harmed at all.	*om.*
4.17	Hyena meat, its fat and its spleen: if they are cooked in a casserole until they are well done, one part of rocket water and one part of pure curcuma are added to it, and given	Its meat, its fat, its spleen and its liver: if they are cooked with water and minced, with the addition of nutgalls, alum and curcuma, one part of each one, and if one pill is swallowed with two bowls of rocket	*om.*

	الحالص جزء ويسقي لصاحب السعال الشديد فيذهب عنه	الجرجير في جرعتين نفع من السعال العتيق والحديث	
4.18	لسان الضبع اذا مسكه انسان معه لم تنبح عليه الكلاب ولا شيء من الوحوش	لسانه ان امسكه انسان لم تنبح عليه الكلاب	لسان الضبع اذا كان مع انسان لم ينبح عليه كلب
4.19	واذا اردت ان يكون الصبي ذكيا سريع الفهم والتعليم فخذ قلب الضبع ومنخره الايسر فعلّقها عليه	واذا اردت ان يكون الصبي ذكيا سريع التعليم لا يعمل فيه سحر فعلق عليه قلب الضبع مع منخره الايسر	اذا اردت ان يكون الصبي ذكيا سريع الفهم لا يعمل فيه سحر خذ قلب ومنخره الايسر وعلقهما عليه بشعر الضبع الذي يكون حول العينه
4.20	شعر الضبع من حول جفن عينيه ويحرق بزيت ويدهن به دبر الخنث فيتوب عمّا كان عليه	عر الضبع الذكر الذي حول فخذه يؤخذ فيحرق ويسحق بزيت ويدهن به دبر رجل مخنّث فانه يقطع عنه	*om.*
4.21	*om.*	وان أاخذ شعر الضبع الانثى فاحرق وسحق بزيت وطلى به رجل غير مخنث استحال ودعا الى نفسه	*om.*
4.22	*om.*	خرء الضبع اذا احرق وخلط مع دهن آس ودهن به الموضع الذي تريد النبات الشعر فيها نبت وكذلك يفعل خرو الكلب	*om.*

4.18: (a) مسكه] حمله B | ولا شيء من الوحوش] *om.* B
(b) لسانه...الكلاب] ولسان الضبع من امسكه معه او أخذه بيده لم ينبح عليه الكلاب ولم توذيه W
(c) اذا كان مع] اذا حمله C
4.19: (a) واذا اردت...فعلقها عليه] قلب الضبع ومنخره الاسير من علقه عليه زاد في الحفظ والفهم B
(b) واذا اردت...الايسر] ولذكاء الصبيان وتعليمهم سرعة يؤخذ قلب ضبع او منخره الأيسر فعلّقها في ذراع الصبي W
(c) خذ] *om.* C | ومنخره...حول العينة] قلب الضبع ومنخره الايسر اذا علقا على صبي جاد اذا اردت ان يكون الصبي ذكيا سريع الفهم لا يعمل فيه سحر فهمه وصار من الاذكياء W
4.20: (a) جفن] اجفان B | ويحرق بزيت] ويربب بالزيت B | عما كان] عما هو B
(b) الذكر الذي حول] ذكر اذا كان فخذه مما حول W | به دبر رجل] بذلك الزيت رجل W | يقطع عنه] انقطع عنه ما به W
4.21: (b) الانثى] *om.* W | ودعا] وعاد W
4.22: (b) خرء الضبع...فيها نبت] وخرؤ الضبع يحرق ويخلط بدهن الاسد ويدهن به الموضع الذي يريد أن ينبت الشعر فينبت W | In W other three recipes are added, one with hyena fat against the pains due to the cold والضبع الصحيح اذا أخذت صحيحة وطبخت و أخذت من دسمها ودُهن به من يشتكي من السرياح والاوجاع الباردة فانه ينفعه; the second for an Indian electuary: مَعجون يقال الفقطارغاز وهو هندي وقد ينحل من الضبع دواء; and the third with part of its liver against the cataract وزيادة كبد الضبع تخذ منه كحل ينفع للغشاوة في العين من لايبصر بالليل.

	to a man suffering from a severe cough to drink, then this will cease.	water, then this will be useful against both chronic and occasional cough.	
4.18	Hyena tongue: if a man carries it with him, then the dogs will not bark at him, nor will any other wild animal.	Its tongue: if a man carries it with him, then the dogs will not bark at him.	Hyena tongue: if a man carries it with him, then not a single dog will bark at him.
4.19	If you want that a boy becomes clever, quick in thinking and learning, take the heart of a hyena and its left claw and hang them on him.	If you want that a boy becomes clever, quick in learning and free from any magic, hang the heart of hyena on him, along with its left claw.	If you want that a boy becomes clever, quick in learning and safe from any magic, take the heart of a hyena and its left claw, hang them on him along with the hair that is around the eyes of the hyena.
4.20	If the hair that grows around the eyelids of a hyena is burnt with oil, and the back of an effeminate man is rubbed with it, then he will repent of his faults.	Hair of a hyena which grows around its eyelids: take them and burn them with oil, then rubbed on the back of an effeminate man, then this will prevent him from acting in this way.	*om.*
4.21	*om.*	If the hair of a female hyena is taken, burnt, ground with oil and rubbed on a man who is no longer effeminate, this will change his condition and he will return to his previous state.	*om.*
4.22	*om.*	Hyena excrement: if it is burnt and mixed with myrtle oil, rubbed on the areas where you want the hair to grow, then it will grow. Dog excrement has the same effect.	*om.*

4.23	*om.*	مرارته يشرب منها وزن درهم بماء السنبل المغلي المصفي فينفع من الاستسقاء الطبلي	*om.*
4.24	مرارة الضبع تذاب ويلقي عليها حب بلسان وزعفران وسكبينج ودرونج من كل واحد جزء ويسحق الجميع ناعما ويلقي عليه المرارة ويكتحل به من في عينيه غشاوة او ضعف النظار يبرأ	مرارته ايضا تأخذ مع زعفران من كل واحد مثقالين وبلسان وماء الرازيانج وسكبينج من [كل] واحد مثقال يخلط الجميع في الهاون ويحكل به من ضعف البصر	*om.*

4.23: (b) الطبلي] ودم الضبع اذا تلي عليها مصنافا بدهن ورد وهو فاتر *add.* W

4.24: (a) In B another recipe is added, with hyena testicles to increase the sexual pleasure: يؤخذ خصى الضبع يجفف ويسقي ويلقي عليه دهن السمسم ويطلي به الاخليل عند الجماع فانك ترا عجبا ولا تمكن من تفسها احدا غيرك.
(b) مرارته...البصر] العين في الذي الماء ليزول به ويكتحل ذلك يخلط جزء واحد كل من ولسان النعناع وعصارة الديك ومرارة الضبع ومرارة W

4.23	*om.*	One *dirham* of its gall, drunk with boiled and purified hyacinth water, will be useful against the drum-shaped dropsy.	*om.*
4.24	The gall of hyena, liquefied with the addition of one grain of balsam of Mecca, saffron, Persian giant fennel and leopard's bane—one part of each one—everything finely ground and rubbedet on the eye afflicted by cataracts or weak eyesight, then this will heal.	Its gall again: taken with saffron—two *miṯqāl* of each one—with balsam of Mecca, fennel water and Persian giant fennel—one *miṯqāl* of each one—everything mixed in a mortar, then this should be rubbed on the eye of the man suffering from weakness of the eyesight.	*om.*

٥. الدب

	a	b	c
	ذكر منافع اعضاء الدب	الدب	باب منافع الدب
5.1	شحمه اذا اذاب الانسان وجهه كان فهيما عارفا عاقلا حفظان لكل ما علم له	شحمه اذا اذيب ومسح به انسان وجهه كان قيما حافظا لكل ما يتعلمه ويقرأه	شحم الدب اذا اذابه به انسان ومسح به وجهه كان فهيما عالما عاقلا
5.2	مرارة الدب تجفّف وتسحق ويخلط معها فلفل ويطلي بها على داء الثعلب فينبت فيه الشعر	مرارته اذا سحقت مع شيء من فلفل وطلى به على الموضع الذي داء الثعلب نبت فيه الشعر	مرارة الدب اذا سحقت وخلط معها شيء من فلفل ويطلي بها المواضع التى يكون فيها داء الثعلب فانه ينبت فيه الشعر
5.3	مرارة الدب اذا شرب منها دانقين بعسل وماء حار صاحب البواسير وصاحب الارياح الغليظة فيبرأ باذن الله	مرارته ايضا اذا شرب منها وزن دانقين بعسل وماء حار للربو او للبواسير او طرد الرياح والناصور	اذا شرب من مرارة الدب دانقين بعسل وماء حار نفع صاحب الربو والبواسير وطرد الارياح الغليظة
5.4	*om.*	*om.*	قضيبة اذا شوى في الفرن ومضغ منه قطعة هيج الجماع
5.5	*om.*	*om.*	مرارة الدب اذا سحق معها فلفل وطلى به مواضع ذاء الثعلب نبت الشعر
5.6	شحم الدب يحشي به الباسور العتيق فينفعه باذن الله تعالى	شحمه اذا طلى به الباسور وحشى موضعه منه اذهبه	واذا اذيب شحمه وحشى به النسور نفعه

5.1: (a) شحمه...علم له] شحم الدب اذا اذابه انسان ومسح به وجهه صار فهيما B
(b) *om.* T W
(c) كان فهيما عالما عاقلا] نال من الفهم امرا عجيبا وكان عالما عاقلا C
5.2: (a) بها] به B | فيه] *om.* B
(b) *om.* T | مرارته...الشعر] مرارة الدب تسحق مع فلفل ويطلي على الموضع الذي فيه داء الثعلب فينبت الشعر W
(c) سحقت] جففت C | ويطلي بها] وطلى به C | التى يكون فيها] *om.* C | فانه ينبت] انبت C
5.3: (a) مرارة...فيبرأ] مرارة الدب اذا شرب منها دانقين ينفع البواسير وطرد الرياح الغليظة B
(b) om. T | مرارته ايضا اذا شرب] مرارة الدب يشرب W
(c) من مرارة الدب] احد منها C | بعسل وماء حار] بماء حار وعسل C | الربو والبواسير وطرد] والبواسير وطرد C
5.4: (c) *om.* C
5.5: (c) *om.* C
5.6: (b) *om.* T | شحمه...اذهبه] يؤخذ شحم الدب فحشي به الناصور فيبرأ W
(c) In L and C this recipe is after 5.13 | واذا اذيب...نفعه] شحم الدب اذا حشا منه الناسور نفع نفعا جيدا W

5. Bear

	a	b	c
	Exposition of the useful properties of the parts of the bear	**The bear**	**Chapter on the useful properties of the bear**
5.1	If a man rubs his face with its fat, then he will be clever, intelligent and he will remember everything that is taught to him.	Its fat: if it is liquefied and a man wipes it on his face, then he will remember everything that is taught and read to him.	Bear fat: if it is liquefied and a man rubs it on his face, then he will be intelligent, clever and smart.
5.2	Bear gall: if it is dried, ground, mixed with pepper and rubbed on the alopecia, then this will make the hair grow there.	Its gall: if it is ground with a bit of pepper and rubbed on the areas affected by alopecia, then the hair will grow there again.	Bear gall: if it is ground, melted with a bit of pepper and rubbed on the areas where there is alopecia, then the hair will grow there.
5.3	Bear gall: if two *dāniq* of it are drunk with honey and warm water by a man affected by haemorrhoids or by viscous winds, then he will recover, with the permission of God.	Its gall, again: if two *dāniq* of it are drunk with honey and warm water, this will be effective against asthma, haemorrhoids, or as treatment of the winds and the fistula.	If two *dāniq* of bear gall are drunk with honey and warm water, this will be useful to a man affected by asthma, haemorrhoids, and the emission of viscous winds.
5.4	*om.*	*om.*	Its penis: if it is roasted in a baking oven, and a morsel of it is chewed, then this will excite the coitus.
5.5	*om.*	*om.*	Bear gall: if it is ground with pepper and rubbed on the areas affected by alopecia, this will make the hair grow.
5.6	Bear fat: if it is stuffed inside a chronic fistula, this will be useful against it, with the permission of God, may He be exalted.	Its fat: if it is rubbed on the fistula and stuffed inside it, then this will make it subside.	If its fat is liquefied and stuffed inside a fistula, then this will be useful against it.

5.7	دم الدب اذا جفف واكتحل به نفع من الشعر في العين وذهبها	دمه اذا نتف الشعر الذي في العين ثم اكتحل منه فلا ينبت ابدا	دم الدب يجفف ويسحق ويكتحل من في عينيه الشعر فلا ينبت ابدا
5.8	لحم الدب وشحمه وكبده يسحق الجميع ويطبخ بماء السذاب ويلقي عليه بورق وسمن بقري خالص ويسقي للمراه التي قد انحبس عليها وان [...] وجع الارحام والمغص الشديد ودهن به مراق بطهنا نفعها نفعا شديدا بليغا باذن الله تعالى	لحمه وشحمه وكبده يسحق جميعا جميعا ثم يطبخ بماء السذاب ويلقي عليه بورق وسمن بقر واسقى منه صاحب وجع الارحام وينفع لاحتباس الطمث والمغص الشديد يدهن به المرأة مراق بطنها وتتحمّل منه بصوفة	يؤخذ لحم الدب وكبده وشحمه فيطبخ الجميع ويلقي عليه بورق وسمن بقري ويطعمه المرأة التي يحتبس عليها الطمث ويأخذها وجع المثانة والمغص الشديد ويذهب منه مراق بطنها وسُرّها فتبرأ باذن الله تعالى
5.9	*om.*	مرارة الدب وعسل غير منزوع الرغوة مدخّن من كل واحد جزء يجمعان ويكتحل به	*om.*
5.10	*om.*	ومن أخذ شعرا من الدب وقرأ عليه لا يصدعون عفنها ولا ينزفون ثم وضع ذلك الشعر على اذنه وهو يشرب النبيذ لا يسكر ما دام ذلك الشعر على اذنه	*om.*
5.11	دماغ الدب يذاب بشيرج ويطلي به المليلة فانه نافع له	دماغه اذا اذيف بدهن شيرج وطلى به صاحب المليلة جسده نفعه	يؤخذ دماغ الدب يذاب على النار والق عليه شيرج وطري وأطل به بدن صاحب الحمى الصالبة والمليلة فتزول عنه باذن الله تعالى

5.7: (a) ينبت ابدا] يعود ينبت B
(b) دمه...ينبت ابدا] دم الدب جيد للشعر الذي ينبت في العين اذا نتف واكتحل به فلا ينبت ابدا W
(c) In L and C this recipe is after 5.13 | نفع من] ازال C | من العين] في العين C | وذهبها] *om.* C
5.8: (a) يؤخذ] *om.* B | فيطبخ] يطبخ B | بقري] البقر B | يحتبس عليها] يحدث لها B | المثانة] الشنه T | وسرّها] وسرعها B
(b) *om.* T | لحمه...بصوفة] لحم الدب وشحمه وكبده يسحق الجميع ويطبخ بالشراب ويلقا عليه بورق وسمن بقر واسقي منه لوجع الارحام والاحتباس الطمث والمعر الشديد يدهن به المراة مراق بطنها وتتحمّل به لضعف البصر C
(c) In L and C this recipe is after 5.13 | وشحمه] *om.* C | يسحق الجميع ويطبخ] وسحق طبخ C | ويسقي للمرأة] وشربته المرأة C | وجع الارحام] واعتراها وجع الرحم C | ودهن به...بليغا] *om.* C
5.9: (b) مرارة الدب] مرارة دب W | ضعف البصر] *om.* W | منزوع الرغوة] يؤخذ مرارة دب وعسل غير مدخّن من كل واحد جزء ويجمعان ويكتحل به W
5.10: (b) *om.* W G
5.11: (a) والق] ويلقي B | شيرج...فتزول عنه] بدهن الشيرج ويطلي بدن صاحب المثلثه والحمى الصالبة فتزول B
(b) دماغ الدب] دماغه G | يذاف] *om.* W; اذا اديف G | ويطلي] وطلى G | المليلة جيد] المليلة جيدة G | صاحب المليلة جسده نفعه W; صاحب المليلة جسده نفعه G
(c) In L and C this recipe is after 5.13 | يذاب] اذا اذيب C | ويطلي...نافع له] نفعه ودهن به من به الملآئل C

5.7	Bear blood: if it is dried, ground and rubbed on the eye with hair, then the hair will never grow again.	Its blood: if the hair is removed from the eye, and its blood is rubbed on it, then the hair will never grow again.	Bear blood: if it is dried and rubbed on the eye, it will be useful against the hair and will remove it.
5.8	Bear meat, its liver and its fat: if they are cooked, some natron and cow fat are added to them, then this is fed to the woman who has a retention of menstrual blood; this will be good also for the pain of worn out skin and acute cramps; if rubbed on the flow of her womb, it will cure her, with the permission of God, may He be exalted.	Its meat, fat and liver: if they are ground into a fine powder, cooked with rue water, with the addition of natron and cow fat, given to a woman suffering from womb pain to drink, it will be useful also against the retention of the menstruation and the acute cramps; the woman should anoint the flow of her abdomen with it and carry this in a woollen cloth.	Bear meat, its fat and its liver: if they are ground into a fine powder, cooked with rue water, with the addition of natron and pure cow fat, then given to a woman who suffers from menstrual retention, abdomen pains and acute gripes to drink, and rubbed on the flow of her abdomen, this will be very useful and effective, with the permission of God, may He be exalted.
5.9	*om.*	Bear gall and smoked honey whose foam has not been removed—one part of each—mixed and applied on the eye [will be useful].	*om.*
5.10	*om.*	If one takes the hair of a bear—without pain or bleeding—and recites over it 'they will not cause its decay, nor they will dry out'; then he places this hair behind his ear when he drinks wine, and then he will not get drunk, as long as the hair remains behind his ear.	*om.*
5.11	Bear brain: if it is taken, liquefied on the fire, some sesame oil is poured into it to soften it, and rubbed on the body of a man suffering from constant fever and feverish heat, then these will go away, with the permission of God, may He be exalted.	Its brain: if it is mixed with sesame oil and rubbed on the body of a man suffering from feverish heat, it will be useful against this.	Bear brain: if it is liquefied with sesame oil and rubbed on feverish heat, then this will be useful against this.

5.12	واذا ربط على الفخذ الايمن كانت اقوى في الجماع جدا	مرارة الدب اذا ربطتها على فخدك عند النوم فانك تجامع ما شئت ولا يضرك شيء	مرارة الدب تجفف وتربطها علي فخذك الايسر عند الجماع فانك تجامع ما شئت ولا يضرك وهو مليح عجيب
5.13	اذا أخذت عين الدب اليمنى وجففت وعلقت على من يفزع في النوم فانه لا يخاف ولا يفزع ما دامت معلقه عليه	عين الدب اليمنى اذا جففت وعلقت على الطفل لم يفزع في نومه	عين الدب علقت على من يفزع في نوم فلا يضرّه شيء ولا يفرع
5.14	مخ الدب يذاب بماء السذاب المغلى ويدهن به رأس صاحب البرسام والصداع يبرأ باذن الله تعالى	مخ الدب يذاف بماء السذاب الحار ويدهن به رأس من به البرسم يبرأ باذن الله تعالى	مخ الدب يداف بماء السذاب ويدهن به صاحب البرسام فيزول عنه باذن الله تعالى
5.15	*om.*	شحمه اذا اذيب وخلط معه رماد وعجن بزيت وطلى به الحاجبين نبت فيهما الشعر	يؤخذ شحم الدب يزيت بزيت ويطلي به الحاجبين فينبت فيهما الشعر ويغلظهم ويحسّنهم وهو مليح
5.16	واذا أخذ من مرارة الدب مقدار حمصة واذيب في تسعة اواق خل خالصا وشرب تجب الجماع وقوى عليه	مرارة الدب مقدار حمصة تذاف في مقدار تسع اواق طلا ويشرب يهيج الجماع مجرب	مرارة الدب مقدار حمصة تضاف في طلاء خالص ويسقي منه الانسان فانه يقوي في الجماع ويهيج المرأة شيء عظيم

5.12: (a) يضرّه شيء ولا يفرع] يفزع ولا يضرة شيء B
(b) مرارة الدب ... شيء] وللجماع يؤخذ مرارة الدب فيربطها عند النوم على الفخذ الايمن W | مرارة الدب اذا ربطتها] واذا اردت الجماع فاربط G | فخذك] فخذك اليمنى G | جدا] *om.* G
(c) واذا ربط...جدا] *om.* C | مرارة...يضرك] مرارة الدب اذا جففت وربطها احد في فخذه الايمن عند الجماع راى العجب من كثرته C
5.13: (a) وهو مليح عجيب] *om.* B
(b) عين الدب اليمنى] *om.* W; عينه اليمنى G | لم] *om.* G | في نومه] من نومه W
(c) In L and C this recipe is after 5.13 | اذا أخذت] *om.* C | وجففت] اذا جففت C | وعلقت] وعلق C | فانه...معلقه عليه] ذهب عنه الفزع ما دامت عليه C
5.14: (a) يذاف] يضاف B | صاحب البِرسام] الراس الذي به البرسام B | فزول عنه] يبرأ B
(b) مخ الدب] مخه G | يذاف] يضاف W; اذا اديف G | السذاب] الشراب W | ويدهن] *om.* W; ودهن G | من به البرسم] من قام من البرسام فيها W; من قد قام من البِرسام G | يبرأ] *om.* W; نفعه G
(c) يذابَ] اذا أذيب C | ويدهن] ودهن C | صاحب] من به C | يبرأ] ابرأه C
15.15: (a) يؤخذ] *om.* B | بزيت] يضاف B | فينبت] تنبت B | فيهما...مليح] *om.* B
(b) شحم الدب] شحمه G | يذوب ويخلط] اذيب وخلط G | ويعجن] وعجن G | ويطلي] وطلى G | الحاجبان] الحاجبين G
15.16: (a) This recipe is attested only in B
(b) مرارة...مجرب] واذا أخذت مرارة الدب مقدار حمّصة فاضفته في تسع اواق طلى وشربته هيج الجماع وزاد فيه جيد مجرب W; مرارته اذا اديف منها مقدار حمّصة في تسع اواقي طلى وشرب جامع ما شاء G
(c) واذا أخذ...حمصة] مرارة الدب اذا أخذ من قدر الحمصة C | واذيب] واذبتها C | اواق] اواقي C | تجب الجماع] يهيج الجماع C

5.12	Bear brain: if it is taken, liquefied on the fire, some sesame oil is poured on it to soften this, and rubbed on the body of a man suffering from constant fever and feverish heat, then these will go away, with the permission of God, may He be exalted.	Bear gall: if you tie it on your leg while sleeping, then you will have sexual intercourse with everyone you want, and nothing will harm you.	If someone ties it to his right leg, then he will be really more powerful in the coitus.
5.13	If the eye of a bear is hung on the man who is afraid in his sleep, then nothing will harm him and he will not be afraid again.	Bear right eye: if it is dried, and hung on a child, then he will not be afraid during his sleep.	If the right eye of a bear is dried, hung on a man who is afraid during his sleep, then he will not be afraid as long as this remains on him.
5.14	Bear marrow: if it is mixed with rue water and anointed on a man affected by pleurisy, this will leave him.	Bear marrow: if it is mixed with warm rue water and rubbed on the head of a man affected by pleurisy, then he will be cured, with the permission of God, may He be exalted.	Bear marrow: if it is liquefied with boiled rue water and rubbed on the head of a man affected by pleurisy and headache, then he will be cured, with the permission of God, may He be exalted.
5.15	Take the fat of a bear, add some oil to it and rub it on the temples, then the hair will grow there, will be strong and nicer, and this is witty.	Its fat: if it is mixed with ash, kneaded with oil and rubbed on the temples, this will make the hair grow there.	*om.*
5.16	The measure of one chick-pea of bear gall, mixed with pure liquid pitch and given to a man to drink, will give him power during the coitus, and will excite the woman. very much.	If the measure of a chick-pea of its gall is mixed with nine ounces of liquid pitch and drunk, then this will excite the coitus: this has been tried out.	If the measure of a chick-pea of bear gall is taken, liquefied with nine ounces of pure vinegar and drunk, then the coitus will be bound to happen, and this will give it power.

5.17	اذا اردت المرأة لا يقربها احد غيرك تأخذ خصية الدب فتسقها وتجفّفها واسحقها وتذيفها بدهن ورد وامسح به راحتك اليسرى وامسح بها على فؤادها فانك لا تخاف عليها ابدا وهو عجيب ومليح	اذا اردت ان لا يمس المرأة غيرك فخذ خصية دب شقها وجففها ثم يسحق بدهن شيرج وادهن به راحتك اليسرى واجعلها على فؤادها فانه حرزها من الرجال فلا تخاف عليها	*om.*
5.18	اذا اردت ان تطرد الدود من الكرم تأخذ شحم الدب تدهن به المنجل الذي تقطع به العود فلا يقرب الشجر الدود واياك ان تقرب المنخل الى جسد ابن ادم فانه يهلك	شحم الدب ان دهن به منجل الزبار الذي يزبر الاكرم فانه يطرد الدباب من الكرم واياك ان يصاب ذلك المنخل شيئا من جسد الانسان فانه ان اصابه قتله	واذا اردت ان تطرد الدود من الكرم فخذ شحم الدب وادهن به المنخل الذي تعمل به عود الكرم فلا يقربه الدود وايا ان تقرب المنجل الى بدن بن ادم فانه ان اصابه قتله
5.19	شحم الدب اذا دهنت به جسد الكلب تجنّن والله اعلم	وان دهنت به كلبا جنّ	واذا دهنت رأس الكلب اعمى
5.20	*om.*	وكذلك شحم الضبع وعلاجه ان يغسل بماء الكمون المغلى	شحم الدب يجنن وكذلك السنبل اذا شمه القط الذكر تجنن

5.17: (a) المرأة لا يقربها] المرأة ان لا يقرب B | فتسقها] تسقّها B | وتذيفها] وتذيبها B | وامسح] وادهن B | فؤادها] فؤاد المرأة B
(b) *om.* W G
5.18: (a) تدهن] وادهن B | تقطع به العود] يكون تكسح به العود B | الشجر الدود] الشجرة دود B
(b) *om.* W | شحم الدب... قتله] شحمه اذا دهن به منخل القضب وقضب به طرد الدود من ذلك الكرم وايا كان تصيب المنجل شيء من بدن انسان فان اصابته قتله G
(c) به المنخل] به الة التعنيب اي المنخ *add.* C | الذي تعمل...قتله] الذي تقطع به اطراف العنب فانه لا يقربه الدود C
5.19: (c) اعمى] تجن C
(b) وان... جنّ] شحم الدب ان دهن به كلب وجنّ وكذلك يفعل بالكلاب W; شحمه اذا دهن به كلب جنّ G
5.20: (b) وكذلك شحم الصبع] *om.* T; شحم الصبع ايضا W | وعلاجه] فعلاجه واذا اخلط الكلب وجن W; وعلاج الكلب G
(c) شحم الدب يجنن] *om.* C | وكذلك...تجنن] وكذا السنبل اذا سمه القط الذكر تجنن C | In C a remark about the effect on the man is added: واذا اصاب احدا من بني ادم قتله

5.17	If you want that no one but you is able to approach a woman, take the testicle of the bear, split it, let it dry, pound it and mix it with rose oil, wipe it on the palm of your left hand and wipe her heart with it, then you will never be worried about her again, and this is amazing and witty.	If you want that no one but you is able touch a woman, then take the testicle of a bear, split it, dry it, ground it with sesame oil, and rub it on your left palm and wipe it on her heart, then this will protect her from other men, and you will not worry about her.	*om.*
5.18	If you want to drive the vermin away from the vine, take the fat of a bear, rub it on the sickle used to cut the branches, then no vermin will approach the plants; but beware, if the sickle gets close to the body of a man, then he will die.	Its fat: if the sickle used to trim the vines is greased with it, then it will drive the vermin away from the vine; but if the sickle touches a human body, then this will kill the man.	If you want to drive the vermin away from the vine, take the fat of a bear, grease the sickle used to cut the branches of the vine with it, then no vermin will approach it; but if the sickle gets close to the body of a man, then he will die, if he has been touched.
5.19	Bear fat: if it is rubbed on the body of a dog, then this will drive it insane, and God knows best.	If you anoint a dog with its fat, then this will drive it insane.	And if the head of a dog is anointed with it, then this will make it blind.
5.20	*om.*	The fat of the hyena has the same effect. Its cure: the dog should be washed with boiled cumin water.	The fat of the bear drives insane; hyacinth likewise, if smelled by a male cat, this will drive him insane.

٦.اليربوع

	a	b	c
	ذكر منافع اليربوع	اليربوع	—
6.1	دم اليربوع يطلي به الشعرة التي تنبت فتقلعها ولا تنبت ابدا	دم اليربوع يؤخذ فيطلي به على موضع الشعر الذي ينبت في الجفون بعد ما ينتف فيذهب باذن الله تعالى	—
6.2	يؤخذ اليربوع يذبح ويؤخذ دمه فيطلي به الجسد الذي يطلع فيه الشعر فلا ينبت ابدا والله اعلم	*om.*	—

(b) اليربوع] الخنزير واليربوع G, see Ch. 7
6.1: (a) تنبت] تنبت في العين *add.* B | ولا] فلا B
(b) يؤخذ] *om.* W | في الجفون] في العين W | بعد ما] بعد ان W; دم اليربوع...فيذهب] دم اليربوع يطلي به الشعرة التي تنبت فتقلعها ولا تنبت ابدا G
6.2: (a) فيطلي] يطلي B | يطلع] ينبت B | فلا] فانه لا B

6. Jerboa

	a	b	c
	Exposition of the useful properties of the jerboa	**The jerboa**	—
6.1	Jerboa blood: if it is rubbed on the growing hair, than it will never grow again.	Jerboa blood: if it is taken and rubbed where the hair grows on the eyelids—after that it has been plucked out—this will make it disappear.	—
6.2	If a jerboa is taken, slaughtered, its blood is taken and rubbed on the hairy parts of the body, then the hair will never grow there again, and God knows best.	*om.*	—

٧. الخنزير

	a	b	c
	ذكر منافع اعضاء الخنزير	الخنزير	باب منافع الخنزير
7.1	عظم الخنزير يحرق ويسحق ويحشي به موضع الناسور فيبرأ باذن الله تعالى	عظم الخنزير يحرق ويسحق ويحشي به الباسور	عظم الخنزير اذا احرق وسحق وحشا به النسور فانه يبرأ باذن الله تعالى
7.2	اذا اردت الرجل يطلق زوجته فالطخ باب بيته بدم خنزير وشحمه مثل الصليب وتقول جعلت هذا الدم ليطلّق فلان ابن فلانه فلانه بدهن كادي ويقطّر في الاذن فيسكن باذن الله تعالى	واذا اردت ان يطلق الرجل امرأته فليلطخ باب داره بدم خنزير مثل صليب وقل جعلت هذا الدم في هذا الموضع ليطلّق فلان ابن فلانة لفلانة بنت فلانة	*om.*
7.3	عظم الخنزير يعلّق على من يشتكي الحمى تذهب عنه	عظم الخنزير يعلق على من به حمى الربع تذهب باذن الله تعالى	*om.*
7.4	اذا رايت انسانا مهزولا ولا يكون به علة السل فاطعمه لحم خنزير فالقى عليه دهن جوز فانه يبرأ باذن الله تعالى	واذا رأيت الباز مهزولا وخفت ان يكون به سدد فاطعمه لحم الخنزير بدهن الجوز يبرأ	واذا رأيت انسانا مهزولا ووخفت ان يكون به علة السل فاطعمه خنزير مغلي بدهن جوز فانه يسمن حتى يكاد ينفلق

(b) In G the jerboa and the pig are in the same chapter, see Ch. 6

7.1: (a) موضع] *om.* B | فيبرأ] ايبرأ B

(b) ويسحق] *om.* W | الباسور] الباسور فيبرأ *add.* W | عظم الخنزير...الباسور] عظم الخنزير يحرق ويحشي به الباسور فيبرأ G

(c) يبرأ] ابرأه C

7.2: (a) الرجل] الرجل ان *add.* B | باب بيته] بابه ثلاثة ايام B | بدهن كادي ويقطّر في الاذن] om. B | فيكون ذلك وهو عجيب] فيسكر C

(b) *om.* W G

7.3: (b) تذهب] فيذهب W | عظم الخنزير...تذهب] وان علق عظمه على من به حمى الربع برئ G

7.4: (a) فالقي] مقلئ ياقي B

(b) عظم الخنزير...تذهب] واذا طعم الباز المهزول لحم الخنزير بدهن الجوز سمن وبرا من السل W | انسانا] الباز G | سل] سدد G

(c) ووخفت] وخشيت C | به علة] به مرض قد اعتراه C | خنزير] لحم خنزير C | جوز] لوز حلو C | حتى يكاد ينفلق] جدا C

7. Pig

	a	b	c
	Exposition of the useful properties of the parts of the pig	**The pig**	**Chapter on the useful properties of the pig**
7.1	Pig bone: if it is burnt, ground, and stuffed inside the fistula, then this will heal, with the permission of God, may He be exalted.	Pig bone: if it is burnt, ground, and stuffed inside the fistula [this will cure it].	Pig bone: if it is burnt, ground, and stuffed inside a fistula, then this will heal, with the permission of God, may He be exalted.
7.2	If you want that a man repudiates his wife, spatter the door of his house with pig blood and its fat, drawing a cross and saying: "I put this blood so that so-and-so son of so-and-so repudiates a certain woman". With pandang oil applied in drops in the ear, then it will calm [the pain], with the permission of God, may He be exalted.	If you want that a man repudiates his wife, spatter the door of his house with pig blood, drawing a cross and saying: "I put this blood so that so-and-so son of so-and-so repudiates so-and-so daughter of so-and so".	*om.*
7.3	Pig bone: if it is hung on a feverish man, then the fever will cease.	Pig bone: if it is hung on someone affected by quartan fever, then this will cease, with the permission of God, may He be exalted.	*om.*
7.4	If you see that someone is emaciated without being affected by consumption, feed him with pork meat, with the addition of some nut oil and then he will recover, with the permission of God, may He be exalted.	If you see that a man is emaciated, and you are afraid that he is affected by consumption, feed him with pork meat and nut oil.	If you see that someone is emaciated and you are afraid that he is affected by consumption, feed him with pork boiled with nut oil, and then he will become fatter and fatter, to the point of bursting.

7.5	واذا أخذ شحم الخنزير واذيب وطلى اسافل قدمي الذي به السحر والجنون فانه يبرأ	شحم الخنزير يذوب ويدهن به قدميه او قدم من شئت فلا يصيبه سحر ولا جنون	*om.*
7.6	مرارة الخنزير اذا اذيبت ببول عند اسود وسعط بها المجنون في رأس كل هلال مرة واحدة برئ	*om.*	*om.*
7.7	لبن الخنزير وعصارة الكراث النبطي سحق ويغلي على النار ويدهن به صاحب وجع المثانة يبرأه	يؤخذ لبن حليب وشحم خنزير وعصارة كراث نبطي يغلي على النار ويحقن به لورم المثانة	يؤخذ لبن خنزير ويخلط معه ماء الكراث النبطي ويحقن به صاحب وجع المثانة وبرد الكلى فيزول باذن الله تعالى
7.8	مرارة الخنزير اذا اذيبت ببول عبد اسود وسعط بها المجنون في رأس كل هلال مرة واحدة برئ	مرارة الخنزير تداب ببول ويسعّط به المجنون يفرّ منه كل ريح سوء	مرارة الخنزير اذا تذاف ببول صبي اسود ويسعّط به المجنون الذي يصرع في كل اوان فانه يبرأ باذن الله تعالى
7.9	*om.*	زبل الخنزير يطلي به الدبيلة تبرأ	*om.*
7.10	لبن الخنزير اول ما تلد اذا شربه صاحب الجذام اوقفه	ولبن الخنزير اذا رضع منه صبي اصابه الجذام وهو سال	لبن الخنزير اذا شربه صغير تجذم

7.5: (b) شحم الخنزير...ولا جنون] شحم الخنزير يدوب ويدهن به قدمي من يخاف عليه السحر والجنون فلا يصيبه W | شحم الخنزير] شحمه G | يذوب] اذا اذيب G | ويدهن] *om.* G | قدميه او قدم] القدمين G
(c) واذا أخذ] *om.* C | وطلى] وطلى به C | الذي به] من به C | والجنون] او جنون C | فانه يبرأ] ابرأه C
7.6: (c) الكراث] الكرات C | سحق ويغلي] اذا غلى C | ويدهن] وادهن C | صاحب] من به C | يبرأه] برئ C
7.7: (a) فيزول] يبرأ B
(b) يؤخذ] لوجع المثانة *prae.* W; لورم المثانة *prae.* G | يغلي] om. W; يسحق الجميع G
(c) سحق ويغلي] اذا غليا C | ويدهن به صاحب] وادهن به من به C | يبرأه] برئ C
7.8 (a) تذاف] تصاب B | يصرع] يفزع B | فيزول] يبرأ B
(b) om. W | مرارة الخنزير] مرارته G | تداب] اذا اذيفت G | ببول] ببول العبيد *add.* G | ويسعّط] وسعط G | يفرّ منه كل ريح سوء] نفعه G
(c) In C this recipe is after 7.5 | اذا اذيبت ببول] اذا جعلت معها بول C | المجنون] من برأسه جنون C | برئ] *om.* C
7.9: (b) زبل الخنزير] زبله G | يطلي] اذا طلى G | تبرأ] فيبرأ W; برئت G
7.10: (a) This recipe is attested only in B
(b) ولبن الخنزير] لبنه G | اذا رضع] يرضع W; ارضع G | صبي] الصبي W | اصابه] فيصيبه W | وهو سال] السيال W; وهو لبن سايل لا يجمد G
(c) لبن الخنزير اول ما تلد] واذا أخذ منه عند ما تلد C | اذا شربه] وشرب منه C | اوقفه] ابرأه C

7.5	*om.*	Pig fat: if it is liquefied and anointed on the feet of a man, then he will not be taken by magic or insanity.	Pig fat: if it is liquefied and rubbed under the feet of the man taken by magic or insanity, then he will heal.
7.6	*om.*	*om.*	Pig gall: if it is diluted with urine when it becomes black, inhaled by the insane man—once at the beginning of every month—then he will heal.
7.7	If the milk of pig is taken, mixed with some wild leek water, administered as a clyster to the man suffering from bladder complaint and kidney coldness, then these will cease, with the permission of God, may He be exalted.	Against the swelling of the bladder: if some cow milk is taken together with pig fat, and the sap of wild leek, everything ground on the fire and then administered as a clyster [it will be useful].	Pig milk and the juice of wild leek, if they are pounded and boiled on the fire, then anointed on the man suffering from bladder complaints, this will heal him.
7.8	Pig gall: if it is diluted with the urine of a black child, inhaled by the insane man who has continuous epileptic seizures, then this will cure him, with the permission of God, may He be exalted.	Pig gall: if it is mixed with the urine and it inhaled by the insane man, then this will put every evil spirit to flight.	Pig gall: if it is liquefied with the urine of a black servant and inhaled by the insane man—once at the new moon—then this will cure him.
7.9	*om.*	Pig excrement: if they are rubbed on the bubo, then this will subside.	*om.*
7.10	If a child drinks the milk of the pig, then he will contract elephantiasis.	Pig milk: if a baby is fed with it, then he will contract suppurative elephantiasis.	Pig milk, from the first time it gives birth: if it is drunk by a man affected by elephantiasis, then this will cease.

7.11	دماغ الخنزير اذا جعل في اناء فخار سبعة ايام فانه يدود اذا جفف ذلك الدود وسحق ناعما وخلط بعسل وشربه صاحب وجع الجوف ابرأه	دماغ الخنزير يصير في اناء سبعة ايام يدود فيؤخذ من ذلك الدود ويسحق ويخلط مع شيء عسل واسقها من شئت فمن شرب منه سكن جوفه	يؤخذ دماغ الخنزير ويصيره في اناء فخار فانه يدود فخذ ذلك الدود فجفّف واسحقه بعسل واسقه لصاحب وجع الجوف فيبرأ باذن الله تعالى
7.12	اذا خشى الانسان من المشى في ثلج ان تسقط اصابعه فليذيب [شحمه]	شحم الخنزير ينفع من انتشار اصابع اليدين والرجلين العارض من الثلج والبرد الشديد	يؤخذ شحم الخنزير فيذاب ويدهن به اطراف من قد سقطت اصابعه من الثلج فانه يمسك اطرافه
7.13	شحم الخنزير [يذاب] بالنار ويطلي به يديه ورجليه فانه يامن من ذلك	ونفع ايضا من الشقاق والعَرَن الذي في ارجل الدواب	*om.*
7.14	وينفع من رخو المثانة وقطار البول	اذا اطعم مثانة الخنزير مشوية لمن يبول كثيرا نفعه او يسقي اظلاف خنزير محرقة	مثانة الخنزير اذا طبخت وأكل منها صاحب وجع الكلى ومن يبول في فراش فانه يبرأ باذن الله تعالى وان أكلت مشويا كان ابلغ والله اعلم

7.11: (a) ويصيره] وتصبه B | فخذ] فتأخذ B | فجفف واسحقه بعسل] فتجفف ويسحق ناعما واخلط ببول B | الجوف فيبرأ] الخرق يبرأ B
(b) *om.* W G
(c) صاحب] من به C
7.12: (a) يؤخذ شحم...اطرافه] اطرافه لسقوط الاصابع من الثلج يؤخذ شحم الخنزير يذاب وادهن به اطراف صاحب ذلك المرض فانه يسبك B
(b) ينفع] ينتفع W | اليدين والرجلين العارض من] *om.* W | الشديد] *om.* W | شحم الخنزير...الشديد] في الأصابع في التثلج به ودهن اذيب اذا شحمه اليدين فالرجلين نفعه G
(c) اذا خشى الانسان] اذا خاف احد C
7.13: (b) واذا اذيب ودهن به نفع] واذا اذيب ودهن به نفع W; ونفع ايضا من G | ارجل] رجل W
(c) ذلك] *add.* ذلك المرض للشقاق الذي في رجل الخيل C
7.14: (a) فراش فانه يبرأ] فراشه B
(b) ويطعم...ينفع] اذا اطعم مثانة الخنزير مشوية W; وللبول الكثير يطعم مثانة الخنزير اهلي مطبوخة او شقاء اطلاق الخنزير برئ محرقة ان شاء الله تعالى لمن يبول كثيرا نفعه او يسقي اظلاف خنزير محرقة G
(c) وينفع...البول] مثانة الخنزير اذا شويت وأكلها من يبول في الفراش ابرأه C

7.11	Take the brain of the pig, put it in a ceramic vessel and it will produce worms, then take these worms, dry them, grind them with honey, and give this to a man suffering from abdomen pain to drink, and then he will heal, with the permission of God, may He be exalted.	Pig brain: if it is put in a vessel for seven days, it will produce worms; if this worms are taken, pounded, mixed with some honey, and given to whomever you want to drink, then this will calm his abdomen.	The brain of the pig, if it is put in a ceramic vessel for seven days, will become worms; once these worms are dried, finely ground, melted with honey and drunk by a man suffering from abdomen pain, then this will cure him.
7.12	Pig fat: if it is taken, liquefied, and rubbed on the extremities of the fingers that have already fallen for the ice, then this will make the extremities adhere again.	Pig fat is useful against the occasional spreading of the intense frost and the cold on the finger.	If a man is afraid that walking on the ice will provoke the fall of his fingers, then he should liquefy its fat.
7.13	*om.*	It is also useful against the lacerations and against that particular ulcer that affects the legs of the animals.	Pig fat: if it is melted on the fire and rubbed on his hands and feet, then this will protect him.
7.14	Pig bladder: if it is cooked and eaten by the man suffering from kidney complaints and by the man who urinates in the bed, then this will cure them, with the permission of God, may He be exalted; and if it is eaten roasted, then this will be even more effective.	And feed its bladder to the man who urinates during the night [in the bed].	It is also useful against bladder prolapse and urine dripping.

٨. الكلب

	a	b	c
	ذكر منافع اعضاء الكلب	الكلب	باب منافع الكلب
8.1	ناب الكلب اذا علق على من عضّه الكلب برئ باذن الله تعالى	ناب الكلب اذا علق على عضة الكلب سكن وجعه	ناب الكلب اذا علق على من عضه الكلب الكلب لم يضر ذلك
8.2	ناب الكلب اذا علق على الصبي عند خروج اسنانه فانها تخرج من غير الم ولا وجع	واذا علق ناب الكلب على الصبي وقت خروج الاسنان خرجت اسنانه بغير الم ولا وجع	واذا علق على الصغير عند الطلوع يخرج اسنانه سهلها خرجت من غير الم يعتر به ولا وجع منه
8.3	ناب الكلب اذا علق على صاحب اليرقان نفعه	واذا علق على من به اليرقان الظاهر نفعه	واذا علق على من به اليرقان الظاهر زال عنه
8.4	انياب الكلب اذا علقت على انسان لم تنبح عليه الكلاب	وان حمل انسان معه ناب الكلب لم تنبح عليه كلب	وان حمله انسان لم ينبح عليه كلب
8.5	ناب الكلب اذا علّق على من يتكلم في منامه فلا يعود يتكلّم	واذا كان الانسان يتكلم في نومه يعلق عليه فانه لا يتكلم في نومه	اذا علق على من يتكلم في نومه لم يعد يتكلم في نومه
8.6	منفحة الكلب تذاب بلبن كلبة ويسقي لمن عضّه الكلب الكلب نفعه ذلك	انفحة الكلب الصغير يشرب لعضة الكلب	انفحة الكلب اذا يسقت لمن عضه الكلب الكلب ابرأه

8.1: (a) اذا] *om.* B | برئ] *om.* B
(b) ناب الكلب] نابه G | اذا] *om.* W | على عضة الكلب] على من عضه الكلب G; على سرته عضة الكلب W | سكن] سكن عنه *add.* G | وجعه] الوجع G; وجعها W
(c) الكلب الكلب] الكلب السعر C
8.2: (a) ناب] هذي ناب B | خروج] الخروج B | الم ولا وجع] وجع ولا الم B
(b) ناب الكلب] *om.* G W | وقت...وجع] تخرج اسنانه بغير الم G; يخرج اسنانه يسهل خروجها بلا الم W
(c) This recipe is attested only in C
8.3: (b) الظاهر] *om.* W
(c) اليرقان] مرض اليرقان C
8.4: (b) كلب] الكلاب G | *om.* W
(c) وان] واذا C | لم ينبح] لم يكد ينبح C | كلب] ابدا كلب ليلا ولا نهارا *add.* C
8.5: (a) منامه] نومه B
(b) واذا...عليه] وان علق على من يتكلم في نومه G; واذا علق على من يتكلم في نومه W | فانه لا يتكلم] لم يتكلم G; لا يتكلم W
(c) في نومه] *om.* C
8.6: (a) ذلك] *om.* B
(b) انفحة الكلب] انفحته G | الصغير] *om.* G | يشرب لعضه الكلب] اذا شرب منها لعضه الكلب نفعه G; يشرب لمن عضه الكلب الكلب نفعه W
(c) يسقت لمن] شربها من C

8. Dog

	a	b	c
	Exposition of the useful properties of the parts of the dog	**The dog**	**Chapter on the useful properties of the dog**
8.1	Dog fang: if it is hung on the man bitten by a dog, then this will recover, with the permission of God, may He be exalted.	Dog fang: if it is hung on the bite of a dog, then this will calm the pain.	Dog fang: if it is hung on the man bitten by a rabid dog, then this will not harm him.
8.2	Dog fang: if it is hung on the child when his teeth are coming out, then they will come out without any pain or ache.	Dog fang: if it is hung on a child at the moment in which his teeth come, then his teeth will come out without any pain or ache.	If it is hung on a small child at sunrise, then his teeth will come out easily, and they will come out without any pain.
8.3	Dog fang: if it is hung on the man suffering from jaundice, then this will be useful to him.	If it is hung on the man suffering from manifest jaundice, then this will be useful to him.	If is hung it on the man suffering from manifest jaundice, then this will make it cease.
8.4	Dog fangs: if they hung on a man, then the dogs will not bark at him.	Dog fang: if a man carries it with him, then no dog will bark at him.	If a man carries it, then the dogs will not bark at him.
8.5	Dog fang: if it is hung on the man who talks in his sleep, then he will not talk again.	If a man uses to talk in his sleep, and the fang of a dog is hung on him, then he will not talk in his sleep.	And if it is hung on the man who talks in his sleep, then he will not talk again in his sleep.
8.6	Dog rennet: if is mixed with the milk of a bitch, and given to the man bitten by a rabid dog to drink, then this will be useful to him.	Rennet of a small dog: to be drunk against the bite of the dog.	Dog rennet: if it is given to the man bitten by a rabid dog to drink, then this will cure him.

8.7	اذا كان في جوف المرأة ميت وتعسر عليها ولا فاسقها لبن الكلب تضعه سريعا	واذا عسر على المرأة الولادة او كان في بطنها ولد ميت فاسقها من لبن كلبة وعسل وشراب من كل واحد جزء بالسواء يخلط الجميع وتشربه يسهل عليها الولادة	اذا عسر على المطلقة الطلق ومات الولد في جوفها فاسقها لبن كلبة مخلوطا بعسل وشراب فترميه سريعا باذن الله تعالى
8.8	لبن الكلبة اذا خلط بعسل وشيء من خمر صرف وشربته من تعسر ولدها نزل من غير اذى ولا مشقة	*om.*	*om.*
8.9	[رجيع] الكلب اذا سحق ويعجن بماء الكزبرة وطلى به الاورام الحادة انفشت	زبل الكلب اذا سحق وعجن بماء الكزبره ويطلي به الاورام نفعه	زبل الكلب اذا سحق وعجن بماء الكسفرة الخضراء فشّ جميع الاورام الحادّة وفتحتها
8.10	وسخ اذن الكلب اذا دهن به قتيلة واوقد في مصباح جديد بين جماعة راو وجوههم كوجوه الكلاب	وسخ الكلب ان أخذ منه واخلط منه بريق حالص عملت فتيلة قطن واشعلت نظر كل من في مجلس رأس الكلب	وسخ اذن الكلب يؤخذ ويوقد منه قتيلة في سراج جديد وأوقدها بين جماعة فانه يروا وجوههم كوجوه الكلاب وقيل كرؤوس الكلاب وهو عجيب
8.11	وسخ اذن الكلب اذا دهن به قتيلة واوقد في مصباح جديد بين جماعة رأوا وجوههم كوجوه الكلاب	يؤخذ خرؤ الكلب ويذاف بعد ان يحرق بدهن اس ومرارة تيس ويطلي على رأس الاقرع ينبت الشعر ولداء الثعلب	لدوء الثعلب خرئ الكلب يحرق ويسحق ويذاف بدهن الآس ومرارة تيس ويطلي به مكان داء الثعلب فينبت فيه الشعر

8.7: (b) فاسقه] واسقها G; فشربت W | وعسل وشراب] مع عسل او شراب G; وغسل بشراب W | من كل واحد جزء] om. G | بالسواء] om. W | يخلط الجميع] يخلطان G; om. W | يسهل عليها الولادة] فانها تضع ما في بطنها G; والقى ما في بطنها add. W

(c) اذا كان...تضعه سريعا] لبن الكلبة اذا شربته من في جوفها جنيناي ميت ولد ويعسر ظهوره اسرع بظهوره C

8.8: (c) لبن الكلبة اذا خلط] واذا اختلط بعسل C | ولدها نزل من غير اذى ولا مشقة] الوللدة نزل الولد بلا مشقة له ولا ألمه C

8.9: (a) فشّ] فشّشت B | الحادّة] om. B

(b) زبل الكلب] زبله G | الكزبره] الكريره T; الكسفرة G | ويطلي] وطلي G W | الاورام] الورم الحار G; الاورام الحارة W | نفعه] نافع W

(c) In C this recipe is after 8.10 | سحق ويعجن] جفف وسحق C | انفشت] انفست C

8.10: (a) قتيلة] فيبل B | وأوقدها بين جماعة] قد امر جامعا B | فانه] فانهم B | وهو عجيب لداء الثعلب] om. B

(b) om. G W

(c) دهن به] دهنت منه C | واوقد] واوقدت C | وجوههم] وجوه بعضهم بعضا C

8.11: (a) خرء الكلب] يؤخذ زبل الكلب B | ويذاف] ويذاب B

(b) يؤخذ] om. G; ولد الثعلب W | ويذاف] واذيف G; مضاف W | بعد ان يحرق] اذا احرق add. G; محرق add. W | آس] الآس W | ومرارة تيس] om. W | ويطلي...الثعلب] نبت فيه الشعر وطلى به موضع القرع ينبت الشعر G; يطلي به على موضع القرع W

(c) الكلب [خرء] اي رجيعه وخرء الكلب add. C | احرق] حرق C | داء الثعلب] المواضع التي اعترها داء الثعلب C | انبت شعرها] انبت الشعر سريعا C

8.7	If the labour is difficult for the woman and the child in her womb has died, give her the milk of a bitch melted with honey and wine to drink, and then she will quickly deliver, with the permission of God, may He be exalted.	If the labour is difficult to a woman, or she has a dead child in her womb, give her the milk of a bitch with honey or wine to drink—one equal part of each one—everything is mixed, and she drinks it, then this will ease the delivery.	If there is a dead [foetus] inside the belly of the woman and this oppresses her, give her the milk of a bitch to drink, and then she will quickly expel it.
	om.	*om.*	Bitch milk: if it is mixed with honey and some pure wine, and the woman whose labour is difficult drinks it, then the baby will come out without any damage or laceration.
8.9	Dog excrement: if it is ground, kneaded with fumitory water, then this will cure all the acute swellings and will make them open.	Dog excrement: if it is ground, mixed with coriander water, and rubbed on the swelling, then this will be useful against it.	Dog excrement: if it is ground, kneaded with coriander water, and rubbed on the acute swellings, then this will make them discharge.
8.10	Dirt from the ears of the dog: if it is taken, a wick is lit with it in a new lantern, and this is lit among a group of people, then they will see their faces like dog muzzles; and it is also said like dog heads, and this is amazing.	Dog dirt: if it is taken, mixed with pure saliva, put inside a cotton wick and lit, then everybody in the room will see [the others with] the head of a dog.	Dirt from the ears of the dog : if a wick is greased with it, and lit in a new lantern among a group of people, then they will see their faces like dog muzzles.
8.11	Against alopecia, dog excrement: if it is burnt, ground, mixed with myrtle oil and ram gall, rubbed on the area affected by alopecia, then the hair will grow there.	Dog excrement: if it is mixed, after it has been burnt, with myrtle oil and ram gall, rubbed on the area affected by the ringworm, then the hair will grow there; this will also be useful against the alopecia.	Dog excrement: if it is burnt, mixed with myrtle oil and ram gall, and rubbed on the alopecia, then this will make the hair grow; and it is also useful for the head affected by ringworm, and thenthe hair will grow on it.

8.12	منفحة الكلب الصغير تذاف وتسقي لصاحب القولنج فتسه له باذن الله تعالى	انفحة الكلب يسقي منها مع مذافا بشراب لمن به القولنج يسهله ويحل الطبيعة	انفحة الكلب اذا شربها صاحب القولنج ابرأه
8.13	قردان اذن الكلب اذا أخذ ونقع في باطية النبيذ وفكل من شرب من ذلك النبيذ سكر سكرا شديدا	قردان الكلب اذا نقعت في نبيذ وسقى منه انسان سكر لحاله	قراد اذن الكلب اذا نقع في نبيذ وشرب منه جماعة اسكرهم جدا
8.14	*om.*	لبن الكلبة بيضاء اول بطن يؤخذ منه ثلاث اواق الكبريت الاصفر المحروق اوقيتين ومن العسل ثلاث اواق يخلط الجميع ويطلي به الرجل احليله في وقت الجماع فلا يجامع امرأة الا اقتصرت عليه ولا يصل اليها غيره	اذا أخذ لبن الكلبة بيضاء اول ولادتها والقي عليه كبريت اصفر وعسل اذا أخذ منه وزن مثقالين وطلى به الرجل احليله عند الجماع وجامع لم تستطع غيره ولم تحب سواة
8.15	اذا اردت ان تحل المعقود فخذ رأس الكلب وجلد السمك الذي يكون في البحر المالح ويبخر المعقود فينحل باذن الله تعالى	اذا اردت ان تحل المعقود فخذ رأس كلب وجلد سمكة فتبخره ثلاثة ايام ينحل عقده	اذا أخذ رأس خف الكلب وجلد سمكة ويخربه المعقود انحل

8.12: (a) منفحة] يؤخذ منفحة B | تذاف] تذاب B
(b) انفحة...الطبيعة] انفحة الكلب الصغير اذا شرب منها مع شراب نفع من القولنج G; انفحة الجرو وويسحق منها مصناف بشراب من به القولنج فيلين بطنه وتنحل W
8.13: (a) In B this recipe is after 8.15
(b) In G and W this recipe is after 8.14 | اذا نقعت] نقعته G; ينقع W | وسقى منه انسان] وسقيته انسانا G; ويسقي W | سكر لحاله] سكر G; فيسكر على المكان W
(c) In C this recipe is after 8.15
8.14: (b) In G and W this recipe is after 8.9 | اول بطن] *om.* G; اول ولادتها W | يؤخذ...غيره] أخذ منه مقدار ثلاث اواقي اول بطن تلده ومن الكبريت الاصفر المحروق اوقيتين فمن العسل ثلاث اواقي يخلط الجميع فاذا اراد المجامعة طلى به الرجل احليله وجامع فان المرأة لا يريد غيره ولا يقدر عليها احد غيره G; والقي عليه كبريت اصفر وعسل اذا أخذ منه وزن مثقالين وطلى به الرجل احليله عند الجماع وجامع لم تسنطع غيره ولم تحب سواه W
(c) اذا أخذ] *om.* C | بيضاء] *om.* C | والقى] اذا أخذ والقى C | وعسل] وعسل نحل C | اذا أخذ] أخذت C | وطلى] وطليت C | الرجل] *om.* C | احليله] الاحليل C | وجامعت] وجامع C | غيره] غيرك من الرجال C | سواة] سواك في الجماع add. C
8.15: (a) In B this recipe is after 8.16 | المعقود] العقود به B
(b) In G this recipe is after 8.9 | *om.* W | المعقود] المأخوذ G | خذ...عقده] فبخره بقحف رأس كلب مع جلد سمكة من ناحي بطنها ثلاثة ايام ينحل G
(c) اذا أخذ...انحل] رأس لكلب واخذ منه ومن جلد السمك ويخربه المعقود انحل عقده C

8.12	Rennet of a small dog: if it is mixed and given to the man suffering from colic to drink, then this will be relieved, with the permission of God, may He be exalted.	Dog rennet: if it given to drink to the man suffering from colic mixed with wine, then this will relieve it and purge the nature.	Dog rennet: if the man affected by colic drinks it, then this will cure him.
8.13	Fleas from the ears of the dog: if they are taken, and macerated in a wine pitcher, then everyone who drinks this wine will get extremely drunk.	Fleas from the ears of the dog: if they are macerated in wine and you give it to a man to drink, then he will get drunk.	Fleas from the ears of the dog: if these are macerated in wine, and a group of people drink from it, then this will make them extremely drunk.
8.14	*om.*	Milk of a white bitch at her first litter: if three ounces of it are taken, with two ounces of burnt yellow sulphur, and three ounces of honey, everything is mixed up, and the man rubs it on the outer opening of the urethra at the moment of coitus, then the woman will have no intercourse with him without being satisfied, and nobody else will have sexual intercourse with her.	Milk of a white bitch at her first litter: if some yellow sulphur and honey are poured on it, and a man takes two *miṯqāl* of it, rubs it on the outer opening of his urethra at the moment of coitus, and has sexual intercourse, then the woman cannot have other man but him, will love only him and nobody else.
8.15	If you want to untie the one who has been tied [by magic?], take the head the dog and the skin the fish that lives in salty water, fumigate the tied one with it and he will be untied, with the permission of God, may He be exalted.	If you want to untie the one who has been tied [by magic?], taken the head of a dog and the skin of a fish, fumigate him for three days, and its knot will be untied.	If the extremity of the paw of a dog is taken with the skin of a fish, and the one who has been tied [by magic?] is fumigated with it, then this will be untied.

8.16	اذا عضه الكلب الكلب وخاف من شرب الماء اذا عضه الكلب الكلب وخاف من شرب الماء اذا أخذ اصبعا من رجل الكلب اليمنى لم يضره بعد ذلك شيء ويقدم على شرب الماء	اعلم ان من عضّه كلب ويخاف عليه ان تكون كُلب فلا يشرب الماء الا ومعه اصبع رجل الكلب اليمنى فانه يبرأ	اعلم ان من عضّه الكلب الكلب وشرب الماء فانه يهلك فاذا أخذ منه اصبع من رجل الكلب اليمنى ما يضر ذلك بقدرة الله
8.17	اذا اردت ان تعلم [هل] يبرأ الانسان من عضة الكلب الكلب ام لا فاره المرآة فان رأى صورة كصورة الانسان فانه يبرأ وان راها كصورة الكلب فانه عسير البرء ربما يموت	وان اردت ان تعلم ان كان يبرأ من عضة الكلب ام لا فأره مرآة فان رأى فيها صورة انسان فليس عليه خوف وان رأى صورة كلب فانه يموت	واذا اردت ان تعلم انه قد برئ من عضة الكلب فان به مرآة فان رأى وجهه وجه ابن ادم فقد برئ وان رأى صورته صورة الكلب فانه يموت والله اعلم بذلك
8.18	[دم] الكلب البهيمي اذا خلط مع الكندر فمسكته الحامل وضعت ما في جوفها وما تمسكه حامل الا اسقطت جنينها	دم الكلب البهيم اذا خلط معه كندر وامسكته المرأة وهي حبلا حفظ ولدها من كل ريح سوء	دم الكلب السلاقي اذا خلط معه كندر ومسكه وبخر به المرأة حامل اسقطت
8.19	بول الكلب اذا أخذ يوم الاربعاء قبل طلوع الشمس او التراب الذي يبول عليه وعمل منه بنادق وعلقت على المحموم برئ بإذن الله تعالى وجل	يؤخذ من بول هذا الكلب يوم الارباء قبل طلوع الشمس والتراب [الذي يبول] عليه فيصير مثل البندقة ويعلّق على المحموم فانه يبرأ	يؤخذ بول الكلب السلاقي ويكون ذلك يوم الاربعاء قبل طلوع الشمس او من على التراب الذي يبول عليه فيصره مثل البندق ويعلقه على المحموم فانه يبرأ باذن الله تعالى

8.16: (a) *om.* B
(b) اعلم...الماء] من شرب الماء W | وقد علمتَ ان عضة الكلب يخاف عليه من الماء; G ويخاف على من عضه الكلب الكلب من شرب ماء فان...يبرأ] W فلا
اصبع رجل الكلب اليمني ما في اناء بزيت فيبرأ; G من اناء ينبغي ان يكون معه اصبع رجل الكلب اليمنى فلا يضره بعده W
(c) اذا...الماء] *om.* C | شرب الماء...اذا عضه] فيعلقه C اصبع من رجل الكلب الرجل اليمنى اذا خاف المسعور الذي عضه الكلب الكلب من شرب الماء
عليه فانه لا يخاف من شرب الماء ابدا ما دام عليه فائدة C
8.17: (a) *om.* B
(b) وان] واذا G; قال واذا W | كان يبرأ من عضة الكلب] *om.* W | فليس عليه خوف] فلا باس عليه G; برئ W | فانه يموت] فيموت G; لم يبرأ ويموت W
(c) هل] هل الكلب السعر حال من عقره *add.* C | فان] ان C | صورة كصوره الانسان] صورته فيها صورة الانسان C | كصورة الكلب] صورته فيها صورة كلب C
فانه عسير] فانه يكون عسير C |
8.18: (a) This recipe is attested only in B
(b) دم] مرارة W | وامسكته المرأة] وحملت المرأة G; ثم امسكته المرأة معها W | حبلي] حامل G | من كل ريح سوء] *om.* G | سوء] *om.* W
(c) الكندر] الكندر وهو الحصالبان الذكر *add.* C | فمسكته] ومسكته C | ما في جوفها] الولد سريعا C | اسقطت] جهدت C | جنينها] الجنين اي سقط *add.* C
8.19: (a) يوم الاربعاء] ويكون ذلك يوم الاربع B | من على] *om.* B | عليه] فيه B | فيصره] فجعل B | ويعلقه] وعلقه B
(b) يؤخذ من بول] من أخذ من بول G; يؤخذ بول للحمى W | هذا الكلب] الكلب البهيم G; هذا البهيم W | والتراب] مع التراب G W | مثل البندقة] بندفقة G;
مثل بندفة W | ويعلق] وعلقها G | فانه يبرأ] يبرأ G; فيسكن الحمى W
(c) وعمل] وعملت C | المحموم] من به الحمى الربع C

8.16 Know that when someone who has been bitten by a rabid dog drinks water, then he will die. However, if the fingers from the right paw of a dog are taken, then this will not harm him, for the power of God.

The one bitten by a rabid dog is afraid of drinking water, and if he drinks water from a vessel, there should be a finger from the right paw of a dog inside it, then it will not harm him thanks to this.

If a man has been bitten by a rabid dog, then he is afraid of drinking water: if a finger from the right paw of the dog is taken, then nothing will harm him thanks to this, and he will be able to drink water.

8.17 If you want to know whether he has recovered from the bite of the dog give him a mirror, if he sees his face as a human one, then he has recovered; if, instead, he sees his image as a dog, then he will die, and God knows best.

If you want to know whether he will recover from the bite of the dog or not, show him a mirror and if he sees the image of a man in it, then there is nothing to fear; if, instead, he sees the image of a dog, then he will die.

If you want to know whether a man will recover from the bite of a rabid dog or not, show him a mirror, and if he sees a human image in it, then he will heal; if, instead, he sees the image of a dog, then his recovering will be difficult, and he may die.

8.18 Blood of the hunting dog (*salūqī*): if it is mixed with incense, and the pregnant woman holds it and is fumigated with it, then she will lose her baby.

Blood of a black dog: if it is mixed with incense, and the woman carries it while she is pregnant, then her baby will be protected from every evil spirit.

Blood of a black dog: if it is mixed with incense, and the pregnant woman carries it, then she will deliver what is in her belly, and no pregnant woman holds it without losing her foetus.

8.19 Urine of the hunting dog (*salūqī*): if it is collected on a Wednesday before sunrise—or the dust on which the dog has urinated—and it is made into a compress and hung on the feverish man, then he will recover, with the permission of God, may He be exalted.

Urine of this dog: if it is collected on a Wednesday before sunrise, together with the dust on which it has urinated, then is made into a compress and hung on the feverish man, then he will heal.

Dog urine: if it is collected on a Wednesday before sunrise—or the dust on which it has already urinated—it is made into a compress and hung on the feverish man, then he will recover, with the permission of God, may He be exalted.

8.20

لسان الكلب الاسود اذا حمله انسان معه لم ينبح عليه كلاب

وان أخذ من لسان الكلب البهيم فحرز في خف انسان لم ينبح عليه كلب ما دام ذلك

يؤخذ قطعة من لسان كلب اسود فيجعل في حرز فكل من حمل ذلك الحرز لم ينبح عليه الكلاب وهذا اما يعملوه اللصوص

8.21

قراد الكلب الاسود اذا اخذ منه ثلاث وشيئا من شعره ثم اجعل الجميع في خرقه ناروس ثم جعلت الخرقه تحت باطيه النبيد فمن شرب منها سكره جدا

واذا أخذت من لسان الكلب الاسود ثلاثة ومن شعره ويجعله في خرقة ويجعله تحت جرة بنبيذ او خابئة والناس يشربون من ذلك النبيذ لم يبق احد الا سكر

يؤخذ قردان الكلب وشيء من شعره ويجعل الجميع في خرقة واجعلها في الباطية او الجرة فكل من شرب من ذلك النبيذ سكر سكرا كثيرا ولشرب منها خلق كثير سكروا وهذا عجيب

8.22

خرء الكلب الابيض اذا سحق وخلط بالكامخ الاحمر واكتحل به صاحب البياض من الجدري والرماد العتيق زال ذلك باذن الله تعالى

وللبياض الذي يكون في العين من الجدري والرمد يؤخذ من خرؤ الكلب الابيض يجفف في الشمس ويسحق ويخلط بكامخ احمر ويكتحل به من في عينه بياض مرة او مرتين او ثلاثا يبرأ باذن الله تعالى

للبياض في العين يوخذ خرؤ الكلب الذي يخراه ابيضا فيسحق ويخلط معه كامخ احمر ويكتحل به صاحب البياض في العين من الجدري والرمد فانه يبرأ باذن الله تعالى

8.23

اذا أخد من ذباب الكلب سبعا وطلى به وجه مرآة فكل من يرى وجهها يرى وجه الكلب

يؤخذ من ذباب الكلب سبع ذبابات فيدقهن ويطلي بهن وجه المرآة فلا ينظر اليها احد الا رأى وجهها وجه كلب

يؤخذ من ذباب الكلب سبع ذبابات فتحرقهم وتأخذ من دمهم ويطلي به وجه المرآة فكل من ينظر اليها يرى وجهها وجه الكلب

8.20: (a) فيجعل] فتجعل B | الكلاب] كلب B
(b) This recipe is attested only in G and W | وان اخذ...البهيم] لسان الكلب الاسود W | فحرز] يحرز W | ذلك] ذلك في خفه وهذا تفعله اللصوص كثيرا *add.* W
(c) كلاب] كلاب ابدا C

8.21: (a) باطية او جرة] الباطية او الجرة B | كثيرا] شديدا B | ولشرب منها خلق كثير سكروا وهذا عجيب] *om.* B
(b) واذا...ويجعله] وان أخذ ثلاث من قردان هذا الكلب مع شيء من شعره وجعل G; وان أخذ من ترد ان هذا الكلب ثلاثة وشيئا من شعره فجعلته في خرقة وجعلتها W | بنبيذ او خابية] نبيذ G; نبيذ وحابية W | والناس...سكر] وشرب من ذلك الا اسكره G
(c) *om.* W

8.22: (a) للبياض في العين] *om.* B | يخراه] خراه B | فيسحق ويخلط] فيجفف ويسحق ويخلط B | من الجدري] *om.* B | يبرأ] يذهب B
(b) وللبياض الذي يكون في العين من الجدري والرمد] *om.* G | يؤخذ...يبرأ] ومن أخذ من خرؤ الكلب اليابس الابيض وسحقه واخلطه بكامخ احمر واكتحل به من في عينه بياض من الجدري وغيره قرتين او ثلاثة برئ G; يؤخذ خرؤ الكلب الذي قد ابيضّ وجف في الشمس ويسحق ويخلط بكامخ احمر واكتحل بعينه بياض مرتين او ثلاث W
(c) وخلط] وطلى به بعد خلطه C | الاحمر...زال ذلك] الاحمر ظاهر العين واكتحل منه من اصابه الجدري في عينه ابرأه وقلع البياض حادث من الجدري C

8.23: (a) يؤخذ من ذباب الكلب سبع ذبابات] يؤخذ سبع ذبابات من ذباب الكلب B | دمهم] رمادهم B | المرآة] امرأة B
(b) In G this recipe is after 8.30 | يؤخذ...اليها] اذا اخذ من ذباب الكلب سبعة ودققهن وطلي به وجه انسان فلا ينظر اليه G | *om.* W
(c) اذا أخد من ذباب الكلب سبعا] ذباب الكلب اذا أخذت منه سبعًا ومرهتها C | وطلى به] وطليت بذلك C | امرأة] انسان C | يرى وجهها يرى] يراه يراه C

8.20 Piece of the tongue of the black dog: if it is taken, made into a pendant, then the dogs will not bark at anyone who carries it, and this is what thieves do.

If the tongue of a black dog is taken and kept like a pendant inside the shoes of a man, then the dogs will not bark at him until this remains there.

Tongue of a black dog: if a man carries it with him, then the dogs will not bark at him.

8.21 Dog lice and some of its hair: if they are taken, put them in a piece of cloth, and put in a pitcher or a jar, then everyone who drinks wine from there will get extremely drunk; and even if a lot of people drink from it, all of them will get drunk, and this is amazing.

One third of dog tongue and its hair: if they are taken, wrapped in a piece of cloth and placed under a jar or a cask of wine, and the people drink from it, then everybody will get drunk.

Fleas of a black dog and some of its hair: if they are take, and wrapped together in a piece of cloth under a pitcher of wine, then the one who drinks from it will get extremely drunk.

8.22 Against the glaucoma of the eye, the excrement of the dog has to be taken once they have become white, ground, melted with red brine, and rubbed on the eyes of the man affected by glaucoma provoked by smallpox and inflammation of the eye, and then this will heal, with the permission of God, may He be exalted.

Against the glaucoma in the eye provoked by smallpox and inflammation of the eye, excrement of the white dog: if it is taken, dried in the sun, ground, mixed with red brine, applied on the eye affected by glaucoma one, two or three times, then this will heal, with the permission of God, may He be exalted.

Excrements of the white dog: if it is ground, mixed with red brine and rubbed on the eyes of the man suffering from glaucoma provoked by smallpox and chronic inflammation of the eye, then these will cease, with the permission of God, may He be exalted.

8.23 Seven flies of the dog: if they are taken, burnt, their blood is taken and rubbed on the surface of the mirror, then everyone who looks at it will see the muzzle of a dog.

Seven flies of the dog: if they are taken, ground and rubbed on the surface of the mirror, then nobody will look at it without seeing their faces like the muzzle of a dog.

If seven flies are taken, rubbed on the surface of a mirror, then everyone who looks at its surface will see the muzzle of a dog.

8.24	اذا أخذ من قراد الكلب وعصره دمه طلى به مواضع الشعر فلا تنبت فيه شعرا ابدا	قردان الكلب اذا ذلك به موضعا ينتف منه الشعر لم ينبت فيه الشعر	يؤخذ قراد اذن الكلب تفجر ويؤخذ دمه ويطلي به الشعر الذي ينبت على الجسد فيزول عنه الشعر
8.25	خرء الكلاب اذا سحق ناعما وأخذ منه ربع مثقال وجعل في بيض برشت بها من انكسار البطن برئ	زبل الكلب الابيض يسحق وينحل ويؤخذ منه مقدار نصف مثقال ويجعل في بيض مشوى ويحسوه المبطون يحبس جوفه	اذا اردت تعصم صاحب الزحير الذي يسهل طبعه فتأخذ زبول الكلب الذي يخراه ابيضا فجففه واسحقه وخذ منه ربع مثقال واجعله في بيضة برشت وحشيه لصاحب الزجير والمسهول فانه ينفعه باذن الله تعالى
8.26	زبل الكلاب السلاق اذا جفف وسحق ونفخ منه في الحلق نفعه	وكذلك اذا سحق ونفخ في الخلق ينفع من الخوانيق واورام الخلق	وللخوانيق والورام في الحلق يؤخذ زبل الكلب السلاقي فيجفف ويسحق في الحلق فيزول الورم باذن الله
8.27	اذا اردت ان يخرج البازي القرنصة حسنا مليحا سالما من كل افة فاطعمه رجيع الكلب والخنانيص فانه يخرج كما ذكرت ويحسن ريشه	واذا اردت ان تخرج البازي من قرنصته منشوي الريش فاطعمه خرء الكلب والخنانيص فانه ينفعه ويحسّن ريشه	*om.*

8.24: (a) يؤخذ] *om.* B | الشعر] *om.* B
(b) ينتف] الذي نتف G; نتف W | لم يعد] لم ينبت G | فيه الشعر] *om.* G W
(c) اذا أخذ...شعرا ابدا] قراد الكلب اذا أخذ من دمه وقلعت الشعر التي تكون في عين انسان وطليت به مكان الشعر لم ينبت ابدا باذن اللهتعالى وجل W
8.25: (a) زبول] زبل B | خراه] يخراه B | واجعله] ويجعله B | برشت] تمرشت B | والمسهول] والسهول B
(b) زبل] خرؤ G W | الابيض] اليابس الابيض *add.* G | يسحق...جوفه] اذا سحق ونخل واخذ منه نصف مثقال وجعل في بيضة وتحسّاها المبطون امسك بطنه G; اذا يسحق وينخل ويؤكل مقدار نصف مثقال يجعل في بيض مشوى وتحشوه المبطون فجلس بطنه W
8.26: (a) وللخوانيق والورام في الحلق] *om.* B | ويسحق في] ويجعل يضاح B
(b) وكذلك...الخلق] *om.* G | زبل الكلب يطعم فقطريا ثلاثة ايام ينفخ في الحلق فيضع للخوانيق واورام الحلق W
(c) زبل الكلاب...نفعه] خرؤ الكلب اذا سحق ناعما وأخذ منه زنة ربع مثقال وجعل في بيضة برشت وشربها من به انكسار البطن برى فائدة C
8.27: (b) واذا...ريشه] واذا اطعمت الباري خرء كلب او حناء بيض خرج من قرنصته واستوي ريشه وحسن G | تحرج البازي] يحرج الباز W | الخنانيص] والحنابيض T | ريشه] الريش W
(c) كما ذكرت] احسن ما يكون C

8.24 Fleas from the ears of the dog: if they are split, their blood is taken and rubbed on the hair that grows on the body, then the hair will cease to grow there.

Dog fleas: if an area on which the hair grows is rubbed with this, then the hair will not grow there.

Dog fleas: if they are taken, the blood is squeezed out and rubbed on the areas with hair, then it will never grow again.

8.25 If you want to protect a man affected by a dysentery that loosens his bowels, take some dog excrement that has already become white, dry it, grind, take one quarter *miṯqāl* of it, and put it inside an egg to drink, let it sip to the man suffering from dysentery, and then this will be useful to him, with the permission of God, may He be exalted.

White excrement of the dog: if it is ground and sieved, half *miṯqāl* is taken and put inside an egg that is given to the man affected by constipation to drink, then this will make it cease.

Dog excrement: if it is ground finely, one quarter *miṯqāl* of it is taken and put inside an egg to be drunk by the man who has a constipation, then he will recover.

8.26 Against suffocation and the swelling of throat, excrement of hunting dog (*salūqī*): if it is taken, dried and ground inside the throat, then the swelling will subside, with the permission of God.

Likewise, if it is ground and blown inside the throat, then this will be useful against the suffocation and the swelling of the throat.

Excrement of hunting dog: if it is dried, ground and blown inside the throat, then this will be useful to this.

8.27 *om.*

If you have purchased a hawk with ugly feathers, then feed it the excrement of the dog and of suckling-pigs, then this will be useful to it, and its feathers will become beautiful.

If you want that the hawk comes out from the purchase nice and completely healthy under every aspect, feed him with the excrement of the dog and of suckling-pigs, then it will come out of it as said before, and its feathers will become beautiful.

8.28

اذا رميت الكلب حجر فغمسه في فمه ورماه خذ ذلك الحجر واسقه لمن شئت فانه يكثر ضحكه وصياحه الى ان يهلك من الصياح

واذا عض الكلب الحجر وارمي به فاجعل ذلك الحجر في شراب اي من شرب منه كان كثير الضحك والصياح

يؤخذ من الحجر الذي يعضه الكلب وترمي قدر حمصة تسحق وتنخل فمن شرب منها مقدار جرولة كان كثير الضحك والصياح

8.29

دم الكلب الماء لو اخلط بالكمون الكرماني ويسقي لمن به عسر البول ادره لوقته

ودم الكلب الماء يخلط بماء الكمون الكرماني ويشرب في الحمام فينفع في تقطير وعسر البول ويدر الطمث

لعسر البول يؤخذ كلب البحر فيخلط بماء الكمون ويسقيه لصاحب عسر البول في الحمام فانه يزول باذن الله تعالى

8.30

اذا اردت ان الانسان لا ينام فاسقه وسخ اذن الكلب سبعة ايام

وسخ اذن الكلب اذا سقيت منه انسانا لم ينم سبعة ايام

اذا سقيت انسانا وسخ اذن الكلب فانه لا ينام سبعة ايام

8.31

يد الكلب اليمنى اذا احرقت ودر رمادها على القروح الجذام الذي يسيل منه الماء الاصفر والقيح من اليدين والرجلين برئ باذن الله تعالى

دم الكلب المائي يدلك بكمون ويطرح على القروح التي يسيل منها الماء وغيره في الوجه ينفع ان شاء الله تعالى

[يد الكلب] وربما ينفع من القروح الرطبة في الجسد والجذام الذي يسيل منها الدم والماء الاصفر يؤخذ يد الكلب فتحرق حتى تصير رمادا ثم يسحق سحقا ناعما ويذر على ذلك المرض فتقطع الماء ويبرأ باذن الله تعالى

8.32

مخ الكلب الميت اذا طليت به الخنازير التي في الحلق والرقبة [ابرأه] باذن الله تعالى

مخ الكلب للخنازير التي تكون في الرقبة والحلق فتذهب بها ان شاء الله تعالى

مخ الكلب الميت اذا أخذ وهو ميت فيطلي به الجراح الذي في الحلق والخنازير الذي يخرج في جسد [ابن ادم نفع]

(b) واذا...والصياح] om. G | الحجر الذي يعضه الكلب ويأخذه بفمه ويرمي به اذا جعل في شراب وشرب منه انسان صار كثير الصخب والصياح W

(c) In L and C this recipe is after 8.30 | اذا رميت الكلب حجر] ومما يكثر الضحك ان ترمي حجر الى كلب C | فغمسه] فان غمسه C | واسقه] واسحقه واسق منه C | يهلك من الصياح] يكاد يبلغ الموت C

8.29: (a) فيخلط] يخلط B | الكمون] الكمون الكرماني B | ويسقيه] ويسقي B | يزول] فيزول عنه B

(b) This recipe is attested only in W

(c) In L and C this recipe is after 8.30 | لو] اذا C

8.30: (a) In I and B this recipe is after 8.26

(b) In T this recipe is after 8.27 | اذن] اذان G | اذا سقيت] اسقيت منه G | سبعة ايام] اياما G | om. W

(c) سبعة ايام] مدة سبعة ايام C

8.31: (a) وربما ينفع...ويبرأ] يؤخذ يد الكلب اليمنى يحرقت حتى تصير رمادًا يسحق سحقا ناعما ويدر منه على من به القروح الرطبة الجسد والجذام الذي يسيل منه الدم والما الاصفرفينفع تلك المرض ويبرأ B

(b) دم الكلب...ينفع] يد الكلب اليمنى اذا احرقت ودقت ناعما وذرّ منها على القروح الرطبة من الجذام وغيره والذي يسيل منها الماء نفعا بينا G; يد الكلب اليمنى يؤخذ رمادها يسحق ناعما ويدرّ منه على القروح الرطبة التي يكون من الجذام او على ما يعضّ على اصابع يديه وريجليه وعلى قروح يديه التي يسيل منها الماء اثر رطوبة في جهته وغيره ينفع نفعا بينا W

8.32: (a) اذا أخذ وهو ميت] om. B | فيطلي] اذا لطخ وطلى B | والخنازير] والجدري B

(b) مخ...بها] مخ الكلب اذا طلى به الخنازير التي في الحلق والرقبة ذهبت G; مخ الكلب الميت يلطخ على الخنازير التي في الحلق فيذهب W

8.28	Stone that has been bitten and expelled by the dog, the measure of a chick-pea: if it is taken, ground, and sieved, then the man who drinks one pebble will laugh and shout a lot.	When a dog bites a stones and expels it, put this stone in the wine, and then anyone who drinks from it will laugh and shout a lot.	When the dog spits out a stone, that it has first moistened in its mouth and then expelled; take this stone and give it to drink to whomever you want, then he will cry and shout to the point that he will die.
8.29	Against urine retention, the shark: if it is taken, melted with cumin water and given to the man suffering from urine retention to drink in the bath, and then this will cease, with the permission of God, may He be exalted.	Shark blood: if it is melted with cumin water, and drunk in the bath, then this will be useful against urine dripping and urine retention, and this will also make the menstruation flow abundantly.	Shark blood: if it is melted with cumin, and given to the man suffering from urine retention to drink, then this will immediately make the urine flow abundantly.
8.30	If a man is given some dirt from the ears of the dog to drink, then he will not sleep for seven days.	Dirt from the ears of the dog: if it is given to a man to drink, then he will not sleep for seven days.	If you want that a man cannot sleep, give him the dirt from the ears of the dog for seven days.
8.31	Dog paw: it may be useful against the wet ulcers on the body and the elephantiasis from which blood and yellow water flow: if the paw of the dog is taken, burnt until it becomes ash, then ground finely, and abundantly applied on this disease, then this will stop the water and it will cure him, with the permission of God, may He be exalted.	Shark blood: if it is mixed with cumin and applied on the ulcers on the face from which water and other things flow, then this will be useful, God, may He be exalted, willing.	Right paw of the dog: if it is burnt, its ash is applied on the ulcers of the elephantiasis from which yellow water and fester flow—especially from the hands and the feet—then this will heal, with the permission of God, may He be exalted.
8.32	Marrow of a dead dog: if it is taken when he is dead, rubbed on the wounds on the back of the throat and on the scrofula that comes out from the human body, then this will be useful against them.	Dog marrow, against the scrofula on the back and on the back of the throat, then this will make it disappear, God, may He be exalted, willing.	Marrow of the dead dog: if it is rubbed on the scrofula that affects the back of the throat and the neck, then this will cure it, with the permission of God, may He be exalted.

8.33	*om.*	ول الكلب اذا طلى به الثآليل قلعها الثآليل	بول الكلب اذا طليت به الثآليل التي تكون في الجسد اليدين والرجلين فانهم يذهبوا باذن الله تعالى
8.34	كبد الكلب اذا شويته واكله من عضه الكلب الكلب برئ	كبد الكلب اذا اشويت واكلها من عضة الكلب نفعه	يؤخذ كبد الكلب تشوي ويأكلها من عضّه الكلب الكلب يبرأ باذن الله تعالى
8.35	عيني الكلب الاسود اذا دفنها في حائط حانوت او دار او غير خرب ولا تقم ما دام فيها	عيني الكلب الاسود الميت اذا ادفنت في حائط دار خربت	اذا اردت ان تخرب دار عدوّك فادفن في حائطها عيني كلب اسود فانها تخرب ولا تعمر ابدا
8.36	شحم الكلب الاسود اذا اذيب وطليت به الخنزير اذهبها	شحم الكلب الميت اذا طلى به الخنازير التي في العنق ذهبت	يؤخذ شحم كلب اسود ميت يذاب ويطلي به على الخنازير فتزول باذن الله تعالى
8.37	شعر الكلب الاسود البهيمى اذا علق على المصروع افاق باذن الله تعالى	واذا أخذ من شعر كلب اسود كله وعلقته على من به وجع الرأس نفعه	اذا اردت ان يفيق المصروع فعلق عليه شعر كلب اسود فانه يفيق والله اعلم بالصواب

8.33: (a) طليت] طلى B | الجسد...يذهبوا] الجسد والبدن يذهبوا B
(b) This recipe is attested only in G and W | الثآليل] الثالول G; التواليل W
8.34: (a) يؤخذ] *om.* B | تشوي] اذا يشوي B | الكلب الكلب] الكلب B
(b) This recipe is attested only in G and W | اذا اشويت وأكلها] اذا وأكل مشويا W | من عضة الكلب الكلب نفعه] تنفع من عضة الكلب الكلب W
(c) *om.* C
8.35: (a) عيني] عين B
(b) This recipe is attested only in G and W | اذا ادفنت] ادفنان W | خربت] فخرب W
(c) دفنها] دفنتا C | خرب] خربت C | ولا تقم] ولا تعمره C | دام] دام ذلك *add.* C
8.36: (a) يؤخذ] *om.* B | كلب اسود ميت] الكلب الاسود الميت B
(b) This recipe is attested only in G and W | اذا طلى به] يلطخ على W | التي في العنق ذهبت] التي في الحلق فتبلاا خاصّة التي W
(c) اذهبها] ابرأها C
8.37: (a) يفيق] يفيق وينفع *add.* B
(b) واذا...نفعه] وان أخذ من شعر كلب اسود كيلجه وقطعت على المصروع خف عنه وجعه G; شعر الكلب اسود اذا نتف وعلق على المصروع نفعه وجفّ W

8.33	Dog urine: if it is rubbed on the warts on the body, on the hands, and on the feet, then these will disappear, with the permission of God, may He be exalted.	Dog urine: if it is rubbed on the warts, then they will be removed.	*om.*
8.34	Dog liver: if it is roasted and given to the man bitten by a rabid dog to eat, then he will recover, with the permission of God, may He be exalted.	Dog liver: if it is roasted and eaten by the one who has been bitten by the dog, then this will be useful to him.	Dog liver: if it is roasted and eaten by the one bitten by the rabid dog, then he will recover.
8.35	If you want to destroy the house of your enemy, bury the eyes of a black dog in its walls, then it will be destroyed, and will never be inhabited again.	Eyes of a black dog: if they are buried in a wall, then this will be destroyed.	Eyes of a black dog: if they are buried in the wall of a shop, or of a house, or of anyanother place, then this will be destroyed and will have no chance to stand as long as the eyes remain there.
8.36	Fat of a dead black dog: if it is liquefied and rubbed on the scrofula, then this will cease, with the permission of God, may He be exalted.	Fat of a dead dog: if it is rubbed on the scrofula that affects the neck, then this will disappear.	Fat of the black dog: if it is liquefied and rubbed on the scrofula, then this will disappear.
8.37	If you want that the epileptic man recovers, hang on him the hair of a black dog, and then he will recover, and God knows best.	If all the hair of the black dog is taken and hung on the man suffering from headache, then this will be useful.	Hair of the jet black dog: if it is hung on the epileptic man, then he will recover, with the permission of God, may He be exalted.

٩. الارنب

	a	b	c
	ذكر منافع اعضاء الارنب	الارنب	باب منافع الارنب
			قال الحكماء ان ذكورهم تصير اناث واناثهم تصير ذكور
9.1	وبر الارنب اذا بخّر به المحموم زالت عنه الحمى باذن الله تعالى	وبر الارنب اذا بخّر به اطراف البدن نفع من الحمى العارضة من شدة البرد	وبر الارنب اذا بخّر به المحموم اذهب عنه الحمى
9.2	*om.*	دم الارنب تبلّ به خرقة لقطع الدم تحشي به الموضع الذي قد قطع فيه سربان	*om.*
9.3	دم الارنب تبلّ به صوفة وتتحمل به المرأة فينقطع عنها الدم ويترك منه	دم حيض الارنب وانفحتها اذا شربتها امرأة حامل سهلت ولادتها	*om.*
9.4	ايضا على الجرح الذي يسيل منه الدم فينقطع باذن الله تعالى	*om.*	دم الارنب ايضا يجفف ويسحق ويحشي به الجراحات التي يسيل منه الدم فانه ينقطع باذن الله عز وجل
9.5	خصية الارنب ومنفحته اذا شربتها امرأة حامل ولدت غلاما وسهّل الله عليها الولادة	*om.*	خصية الارنب وانفحته اذا اذيب الجميع وشرب منه الحمل وضعت جنينها

(c) قال الحكماء ان ذكورهم تصير اناث وناثهم تصير ذكوره] *om.* C
9.1: (b) اذا بخّر به] اذا ما بخّر بها W | الحمى العارضة] *om.* W; الحصر العارض G
(c) وبر الارنب] *om.* C
9.2: (b) دم الارنب ... سربان] وَبَر الارنب يحشي به الموضع الذي يسيل منه الدم مثل السربان W
9.3: (a) تبلّ به] تبل منه B | به] بها B | ويترك منه] *om.* B
(b) امرأة حامل] المرأة الحامل زرقت ولدا ذكرًا W | سهلت ولادتها] ويسهل عليها الولادة W | *om.* G
9.4: (a) ايضا على الجرح] وتجعل ايضا في الجرح B | الذي] التي B
(c) This recipe is attested only in C, after 9.6
9.5: (a) غلاما وسهّل] غلاما فهيما ويسهّل B
(c) خصية] خصوة C | This recipe is attested only in C, after 9.6

9. Hare

	a	b	c
	Mention of the useful properties of the parts of the hare	**The hare**	**Chapter on the useful properties of the parts of the hare**
			The sages say that their males turn into females, and that their females turn into males.
9.1	Hare fur: if a feverish man is fumigated with it, then the fever will leave him, with the permission of God, may He be exalted.	Hare fur: if the hare is used to fumigate the extremities of the body, this will be useful against the occasional fever due to the intense cold.	Hare fur: if a feverish man is fumigated with it, than the fever will go away.
9.2	*om.*	Hare blood: if a piece of cloth is soaked in it, this will be useful to staunch the blood, stuffing it inside the place where the flow has already stopped.	*om.*
9.3	Hare blood: if a woollen cloth is soaked in it, and the woman carries it with her, then the [menstrual] blood will stop and leave her.	Menstrual blood of a hare: if a pregnant woman drinks it, then her labour will be easy.	*om.*
9.4	And it can also be applied on bleeding wounds, and then the bleeding will stop, with the permission of God, may He be exalted.	*om.*	Hare blood again: if it is dried, ground, and stuffed inside bleeding wounds, then this will staunch the blood, with the permission of God, may He be exalted.
9.5	Hare testicle and its rennet: if a pregnant woman drinks them, then her baby will be a boy, and God will ease her labour.	*om.*	Hare testicle and rennet: if they are liquefied together and drunk by a pregnant woman, then she will give birth.

9.6	دم الارنب اذا طلى به البهق الاسود غيّر لونه وازاله	دم الارنب اذا طلت امرأة او رجل به البهق الاسود في البدن غير لونه وقلعه	دم الارنب اذا طلى به البهق الاسود غيّر لونه وازاله
9.7	اذا تجبن اللبن في جوف الطفل تذاب منفحة الارنب بعسل وتسقي للطفل فانه يحلل اللبن من معدته	انفحة الارنب اذا شربها من يستكي من معدته مع شيء من عسل وخل نفعه	واذا اختبز اللبن في معدة الطفل يؤخذ منفحة الارنب فتحلّ بالماء ويسقي الطفل وان كانت بعسل كانت انفع
9.8	انفحة الارنب اذا اذيبت بشراب عتيق وشربها صاحب الحمى المثلثة وغيرها ذهبت عنه	وكذلك اذا شرب منه مقدار باقلاة بشراب صرف نفع من حمى الربع	منفحة الارنب اذا شرب منها صاحب الحمي المثلثة مقدار ربع مثقال فتزول عنه باذن الله تعالى
9.9	انفحة الارنب اذا خلط بختمية وزيت وطلى بها موضع النصل والشوكة فانه يخرج من بدن الانسان بغير الم	وكذلك اذا خلط معها خطمي وزيت ووضع على موضع في البدن فيه نصل نشاب او شوك واخرجه باذن الله تعالى	اذا اردت ان تخرج النصول من الجسد والشوكة فخذ منفحة الارنب وتذاف بزيت طيب والقى عليها شيئا من خطمية البيضاء واضرب الجميع والطخ مكان النصل والشوكة فيخرج باذن الله تعالى
9.10	انفحة الارنب اذا اذيبت بشراب عتيق وشربها صاحب الحمى المثلثة وغيرها ذهبت عنه	*om.*	منفحة الارنب اذا شرب منها صاحب الحمي المثلثة مقدار ربع مثقال فتزول عنه باذن الله تعالى
9.11	*om.*	وكذلك اذا سقى منها صبي لم يفزع في نومه	منفحة الارنب واذا سقيت منها لصبي يفزع في النوم يزول عنه الفزع باذن الله تعالى

9.6: (b) طلت امرأة او رجل به] W; طلى على اذا طلى به | G في البدن] من البدن W | غير لونه] *om.* G
9.7: (a) ويسقي] ويسقيها B | انفع] ابلغ B
(b) انفحة الارنب...نفعه] G انفحتها اذا شربت مع خل وعسل نفعت من اللبن الذي قد تجبّن في المعدة
(c) اذا تجبن...الارنب] C منفحة الارنب اذا تجبن اللبن في جوف الطفل تذاب المنفحة | In C the recipes 7-15 are after 9.15
9.8: (b) وكذلك] W; انفحة الارنب G ايضا | مقدار] قدر W G | صرف] *om.* G
9.9: (a) وتذاف] واضيفها B | فيخرج] يخرج B
(b) وكذلك] ايضا G | في البدن] *om.* G | نشاب] *om.* G | واخرجه] جذبه G
(c) انفحة الارنب] *om.* C | اذا خلط بختمية وزيت] خلطت بزيت وختميه C | فانه يخرج] فانها تخرج C
9.10: (a) منفحة الارنب] انفحة الارنب B | اذا شرب] يشرب B
(c) انفحة الارنب] *om.* C | اذيبت] اذيفت C | المثلثة] المربع C
9.11: (a) منفحة الارنب...الفزع] واذا سقيت منها صاحب الصبي الذي يفزع في نومه يبرا B
(b) وكذلك...في نومه] انفحة الارنب تنفع اذا سقى منها شيء يسير صبي يتفزع من نومه W | وكذلك] ايضا G

9.6	Hare blood: if it is rubbed on the black vitiligo, then this will change its colour, and make it disappear.	Hare blood: if it is rubbed on the black vitiligo that is on the body, this will change its colour and erase it.	Hare blood: if it is rubbed on black vitiligo, then this will change its colour and this will make it cease.
9.7	If the milk ferments in the stomach of a baby, take the rennet of the hare, dissolve it in water and give it to a child to drink; and if it is given with honey, it will be even more useful.	Hare rennet: if it is drunk by someone suffering from pain in his stomach, along with some honey and vinegar, then this will be useful.	If the milk curdles in the stomach of a baby, liquefy the rennet of a hare with honey, and give it to the baby to drink, then the milk in his stomach will be digested.
9.8	*om.*	Likewise, if the quantity of a broad bean of it is drunk with pure syrup, then it will be useful against the quartan fever.	*om.*
9.9	If you want to extract an arrowhead or a thorn from the body, take the rennet of a hare, mix it with good oil, add some white marshmallow, whip everything up, spatter this where the arrowhead or thorn is, and then it will come out, with the permission of God, may He be exalted.	Likewise, if it is mixed with marshmallow and oil, applied on the body where an arrowhead or thorn is, then this will remove it.	If the rennet of a hare is melted with marshmallow and good oil, rubbed on the area where an arrowhead or thorn has penetrated, then then they will come out of the body without any pain.
9.10	Hare rennet: if a man affected by a tertian fever drinks a quarter *miṯqāl* of it, then the fever will go away, with the permission of God, may He be exalted.	*om.*	Hare rennet: if it is liquefied with old wine and drunk by a man suffering from a tertian fever, then this will change this condition and will make the fever go away.
9.11	Hare rennet: if it is given to drink to a child who is scared during its sleep, then this fear will go away, with the permission of God, may He be exalted.	Likewise, if a child drinks it, then he will not be frightened during his sleep.	*om.*

9.12	اذا اردت ان تحمل امرأة سريعا فاسقها مقدار دناقين من منفحة الارنب فانها تحبل	وكذلك اذا سقيت منها المرأة التي لا تحمل حملت سريعا	واذا شرب منها امرأة عاقر فانها تحبل باذن الله
9.13	دماغ الارنب اذا أكله من يبول في الفراش ومن يبول كثيرا في سائر الايام نفعه باذن الله تعالى	*om.*	كبد الارنب اذا شرب منه من يبول في الفراش منعه
9.14	اذا اردت ان يسكن الارتعاش فاطعم صاحبه دانقين من مخ الارنب	دماغ الارنب اذا أكله من به الارتعاش نفعه واذا سقى بشراب لمن يسعل نفعه	واذا أكله صاحب الارتعاش سكنه
9.15	كبد الارنب اذا تجفف ويسحق ناعما وتذاف بماء الشاهترج وتسقي لصاحب وجع الكبد فيبرأ باذن الله تعالى	كبد الارنب اذا جففت وسحقت وشرب منها وزن درهم بماء الشهدانج نفع من وجع الكبد	كبد الارنب اذا سحق وشرب منه من به وجع الكبد بالشاهترج نفعه نفعا جيدا
9.16	زبل الارنب يذاف بخل خمر ويطلي به القوبة وهي الحزازة التي يكون في الجسد فتذهبها باذن الله تعالى	زبل الارنب يذاف بخل ويطلي به القوباء التي يكون في الجسد والنمش الذي يكون في الوجه فانه يزيل	*om.*
9.17	ويطلي ايضا الكلف والنمش الذي يكون في الوجه فيزول	زبل الارنب اذا اذيف بخل وطلى به النمش نفعه	كبد الارنب اذا اذيبت بخل خمر وطلى به الحكة والحرارة اذهبه وينفع ايضا للنمش والكلف الذي على الوجه والبدن يزيد في لونه ويحسنه

9.12: (a) منفحة] انفحة B | فانها تحبل] *om.* B
(b) وكذلك] انفحة الارنب W; ايضا G | سقيت] سقى W G | المرأة التي لا تحمل] المرأة لا تلقح W; امرأة لا تحبل G | حملت] حبلت G | سريعا] *om.* W G | In W another recipe is added, with hare fur to favour pregnancy: وبر الارنب يدق ويضاف بالعسل وتتحمل المرأة تأتي مضجعها فانها تحبل لو فتها ان شاء الله تعالى
(c) شرب] شربت C
9.13: (a) كثيرا] *om.* B
(c) كبد الارنب] دماغ الارنب C
9.14: (b) *om.* W | دماغ الارنب] دماغها G | واذا سقى بشراب لمن يسعل نفعه] *om.* G
9.15: (a) تجفف] يجفف B | وتذاف] وتذاب B | الشاهرج] الساهنرج B | وتسقي] ويسقي B
(b) الشهدانج] الشادانج T | كبد الارنب] ودماغ الارنب W; كبدها G | وسحقت] *om.* W G
(c) This recipe is attested only in C | بالشاهترج] بالشاهطرج C
9.16: (a) يذاف] يذاب B | القوبا] العقربا B | في الجسد فتذهبها] في البدن يبرأ B
9.17: (b) This recipe is attested only in G
(c) وينفع ايضا] ويقلع C

9.12	If you want that a woman gets pregnant quickly, give her two *dāniq* of hare rennet to drink, and then she will get pregnant.	Likewise, if a woman who is not able to get pregnant drinks it, then she will quickly get pregnant.	If a sterile woman drinks it, then she will get pregnant, with the permission of God.
9.13	Hare brain: if the man who urinates in the bed—or who urinates a lot during the rest of the day—eats it, this will be useful to him, with the permission of God, may He be exalted.	*om.*	Hare liver: if a man who urinates in the bed drinks it, then this will prevent him from doing so.
9.14	If you want to calm a tremor, then feed the man suffering from it with hare marrow.	Hare brain: if a man affected by tremor eats it, then this will be useful; it is useful if it is given with syrup to the man who coughs.	And if a man suffering from tremor eats it, then this will calm his tremor.
9.15	Hare brain: if it is dried, pounded into a fine powder, mixed with fumitory, and given to a man suffering from liver complaint to drink, then this will cure him with the permission of God, may He be exalted.	Hare liver: if it is dried, ground, and drunk with one dirham of Indian hemp water, it will be useful against the liver complaint.	Hare liver: if it is ground and drunk with fumitory by a man affected by liver complaint, then this will be very useful against it.
9.16	Hare excrement: if it is mixed with wine vinegar and rubbed on the tetter—that is a kind of impetigo that may affect the body—will make it go away, with the permission of God, may He be exalted.	Hare excrement: if it is diluted with vinegar and rubbed on impetigo on the body and on the discoloured spots on the face, then this will make them disappear.	*om.*
9.17	Also if it is rubbed on the freckles and the discoloured spots on the face, then they will disappear.	Hare excrement: if it is mixed with vinegar and rubbed on the discoloured spots, it will be useful against these.	Hare liver: if it is mixed with vinegar and rubbed on the scabies and the burnings, then this will make them go away; it is also useful against the discoloured spots and the freckles on the face and the body, this will improve its colour and make them appear nicer.

	(a)	(b)	(c)
9.18	زبل الارنب اذا علق على امرأة لم تحبل ابدا	وان شربت منها قليلا دفع عنها الطمث وينشف رطوبة الرحم تنشيفا مفرطا	كبد الارنب اذا علق على المرأة منعها من الحبل ما دام عليها
9.19	ضرس الارنب اذا علق على انسان يشتكي وجع الضرس يسكن المه باذن الله تعالى	ضرس الارنب ان علقه انسان على الجانب الذي يشتكي منه ضرسه سكن	ضرس الارنب اذا علق على من يشتكي وجع الضرس سكن وجعه
9.20	مرارة الارنب اذا شربها انسان لم يزل نائما واذا اردت ان تقيمه من نومه فاسقه خل خمر فيستفيق	مرارتها اذا شرب في شراب لانسان فانه لا يزال نايما	مرارة الارنب اذا شربها انسان لم يزل نايما فاذا اردت ايقاظ اسقه خلا حاذقا
9.21	*om.*	*om.*	خصيته تبرأ من السم القاتل طلا بها
9.22	*om.*	*om.*	وانفحته اذا جففت في الظل وخلطت بميك وسحقت نفعت البياض الذي في العين وابرأه
9.23	اذا اردت ان تخبرك المرأة بكل ما عملت فخذ شحم ارنب فاجعله في خرقة على اسمها واسم امها واجعله تحت رأسها وهي نائمة فتخبرك بكل ما صنعته وهذا عجيب مليح	شحم الارنب اذا أخذ باسم امرأة وامّها وجعل تحت رأس المرأة وهي نائمة لا تعلم تكلمت بكل شيء فعلت	[شحم] الارنب جعل في خرقة على اسم الشخص واسم امّه ومعه صوفة من كبش وجعل تحت رأس المرأة فانها تخبر بكل صنعته في حتى الجماع

9.18: (a) ابدا] *om.* B
(b) وان شربت...مفرطا] زبل الارنب اذا علقتها المرأة عيها لم تحبلوان حملت منه شيئا قليلا نشف رطوبة الرحم حتى لا تحيض W; وان علق زبل الارنب على المرأة لم تحبل G
(c) كبد الارنب] *om.* C
9.19: (b) ضرس الارن... يسكن وجعه] ضرس الارنب ان علق على الجانب الذي يشتكي من اضراسه سكن عنه وجع ضرسه و نفعه W; ضرس الارنب ان علقه انسان على الجانب الذي يشتكي منه ضرسه سكن G
9.20: (b) *om.* W G
(c) This recipe is attested only in C
9.21: (c) *om.* C
9.22: (c) *om.* C
9.23: (a) فاجعله] واجعله B | فتخبرك] فتخبر B | وهذا عجيب مليح] *om.* B
(b) شحم الارنب ...عملت] *om.* W | شحم الارنب اذا أخذ باسم امرأة وامّها وجعل تحت رأس المرأة وهي نائمة لا تعلم تكلمت بكل شيء فعلت G

9.18	Hare excrement: if it is hung on a woman, then she will never get pregnant.	If a woman drinks a bit of it, the menstruation will leave her, and this will absorb the moistness in the womb in a very strong way.	Hare liver: if it is hung on a woman, then this will prevent her from getting pregnant as long as it remains on her.
9.19	Hare molar: if it is hung on a man suffering from molar pain, this will calm his ache, with the permission of God, may He be exalted.	Hare molar: if it is hung on the side where there is an aching molar, then the pain will be relieved.	Hare molar: if it is hung on a man suffering from molar pain, then this will calm its pain.
9.20	If a man drinks the gall of a hare, then he will not stop sleeping; if you want to wake him up from his sleep, give him some wine vinegar to drink, and he will wake up.	Hare gall: if it is given to a man mixed in his drink, then he will not stop sleeping.	If a man drinks the gall of a hare, he will not stop sleeping; and if you want him to wake up, give him some acid vinegar to drink.
9.21	*om.*	*om.*	Its testicle is a remedy against the deadly poison, if rubbed on the body.
9.22	*om.*	*om.*	Its rennet, dried in the shade and mixed with *mīk* [?], is useful against the glaucoma of the eye, and will cure it.
9.23	If you want that a woman tells you everything she has ever done, take the fat of a hare, put it in a piece of cloth in her name and in the name of her mother, put it under her head while she is sleeping, and then she will tell you everything she did, and this is amazing and witty.	Hare fat: if it is taken in the name of a woman and her mother, put under the head of a woman while she is sleeping—but she should not be aware of it—then she will tell you everything she has done.	Take the fat of a hare, wrap it in a piece of cloth in the name of a woman and her mother, along with ram wool, place it under the head of the woman, and then she will tell you everything she has done, even about the sexual intercourse that she had.

9.24	خصية الارنب اذا أخذت وملحت بملح وكافور وورس وجففت وسحقت ناعما وسعط منها صاحب علة الانسان بوزن قراطين من لبن امرأة نفعه نفعا جيدا	خصية الارنب اذا ملحت بملح وكافور وورس وجففت وسعّط منها صاحب السِلّ وزن قراطين بلبن امراة نفعه	خصية الارنب اذا تملح بملح الطعام وشيء من كافور وورس فاذا جف سحقت ناعما وسعّط بنها صاحب علة الدق يزول عنه مرضه باذن الله تعالى
9.25	*om.*	مرارة الارنب تخلط مع دقيق حُوّاري وكُندُر وسذاب يابس مدقوق ومنخول ويلطخ على الجبين للصداع	*om.*
9.26	لحم الارنب وشحمه ودماغه اذا خلط الجميع ودق ناعما ويلقي عليه سذاب يابس وكمون كرماني ونطرون سلطاني وشرب منه صاحب الحمى وزن مثقال بعسل نحل ذهب عنه الحمى	لحم الارنب وشحمه يدق في هاون مع كف سذاب يابس وكمون كرماني وبطرون ويُرفع ويشرب منه وزن مثقال بمعلقة عسل مصفى للحمى المثلثة على الريق وقت ان يحسن بها	لحم الارنب وشحمه يخلط ويدق مع شيء من سذاب وكمون كرماني ونطرون سلطاني ويذاف الجميع بالعسل النحل ويشرب صاحب الحمى النافض وقت أخذها فتزول باذن الله تعالى
9.27	انفحة الارنب ودماغه اذا اذيب الجميع وطلى به مواضع الشعر فلا ينبت ابدا	شحم الارنب ودماغه يمنع ان ينبت اذا نتف من الموضع الذي يطلع عليه	مخ الارنب اذا طلى به الشعر حلقه ولا يطلع ابدا
9.28	انفحة الارنب اذا اذيبت بدهن بان وحملت منه ساعتها اذا اجتمعها الرجل لو كان لها سبعون سنة [حبلت]	الانفحة اذا اذيفت ببان خالص وتحملت به المرأة في صوفة حبلت	منفحة الارنب يذاف بدهن خالص وتحمّل بها المرأة فتحبل باذن الله تعالى

9.24: (a) تملح] ملحت B | فاذا جف] وجففت B | عنه مرضه] *om.* B
(b) وسعّط] يسعّط W | صاحب] لاصحاب W | بلبن امرأة] *om.* W
(c) ملحت بملح] أخذت وملحت بملح C | صاحب] اذا جعلت فيها ملح C | قراطين] من به C قراط
9.25: (b) مرارة الارنب] مرارتها G | تخلط] اذا خلط G | مع] معها G | ويلطخ] فيلطخ W; وطلى G | الصداع] اذهب الصداع G
9.26: (a) ويذاف] يذاب B | النافض] النافضة B | وقت أخذها] *om.* B
(b) يدق] ضاف W; اذا دق G | في هاون] *om.* WG | مع كف] مع جوز وكف G | ويرفع] ورفع G | للحمى المثلثة] لحمى المهلبة W | بها] مجيها W
9.27: (a) مخ الارنب...يطلع ابدا] مخ الارنب يذاب بدهن البان وتحمل بها المرأة فانها تحبل B
(b) شحم الارنب… يطلع عليه] مخ الارنب ودماغ الارنب يصبع الشعر ويمنعه من ان ينبت فيه الشعر ويطلي عليه W; مخ الارنب ودماغه اذا طلى به الموضع الذي نتف منه لم يَعُد G
(c) *om.* C
9.28: (a) *om.* B
(b) يذاف] تضاف W; اذيفت G | وتحملها] وتحمله W; وتحملت به G | بصوفة] في صوفة G | تحبل] فتحبل وللحبل مجرب W; حبلت G
(c) انفحة الارنب] مخ الارنب C | اذيبت] اذيب C | وحملت منه] وحملتها C | اجتمعها...سنة] جامعها ولو بلغ اربعين سنة C

9.24	Hare testicle: if it is seasoned with cooking salt, a bit of camphor and curcuma and, once it has dried, finely ground and a man suffering from a wasting disease inhales, then his illness will leave him, with the permission of God, may He be exalted.	Hare testicle: if it is seasoned with salt, camphor and curcuma, dried and inhaled by a man suffering from consumption—two carats of it with woman's milk—then it will be useful against this.	Hare testicles: if it is taken, seasoned with salt, camphor and curcuma, dried and pounded finely, then inhaled by a man suffering from phthisis—two carats of it with woman's milk—it will be very useful against this.
9.25	*om.*	Hare gall: if it is melted with gypsum powder, incense and dry rue, ground and sieved, then rubbed on the forehead, this will be against the headache.	*om.*
9.26	Hare meat and its fat: melted and minced with a bit of rue, cumin and *Sulṭānī* soda, then mixed with honey and drunk by the man affected by fever with shivers, in the very moment in which he contracts it, then this will make it go away, with the permission of God, may He be exalted.	Hare meat and its fat: ground in a mortar with a handful of dry rue, cumin and soda, preserved in a vessel and drunk, one *miṯqāl* of it with a spoon of purified honey against tertian fever, on an empty stomach, at the most convenient moment.	Hare meat, its fat and its brain: everything mixed up, finely minced with some dry rue, cumin and *Sulṭānī* soda, drunk by a feverish man—one *mitqāl* with honey—this will make the fever cease.
9.27	If the hair is rubbed with hare marrow, this will remove it and the hair will never grow back again.	Hare fat and its brain: they prevent the growth of the hair, if they are rubbed on the area where the hair grows.	Hare rennet and its brain: if they are mixed and rubbed on hairy areas, then the hair will never grow back again.
9.28	Hare rennet: if it is mixed with pure oil and carried by a woman, then she will get pregnant, with the permission of God, may He be exalted.	Its rennet: if it is mixed with pure ben oil and a woman carries it in a woollen cloth, then she will get pregnant.	Hare rennet: if it is mixed with ben oil and is carried by a woman at the very moment in which she has sexual intercourse with a man, then she will get pregnant, even if she were seventy years old.

9.29	*om.*	واذا اردت ينزعن النساء ثيابهن ويرقصن في البيت فخذ دم ارنب وتبل فيه فتيلة واسرجها في البيت فانه ليس يراه في البيت احد من النساء الا رقصت	*om.*
9.30	*om.*	[اذا] اردت ان تضرّط انسان فخذ بعر ارنب واكتب به على قميصة فانه يضرط	*om.*
9.31	اذا كانت المرأة عقيما تحبل فخذ ارنب انثى فاذبحها وخذ رحمها فاشويه للمرأة فانها تحبل باذن الله تعالى	واذا أخذت ريشا حاملا وشققت بطنها وأخذت رحمها وطبخته واطعمه لمرأة مع لحمها وجامعتها حبلت في تلك الليلة بامر الله تعالى	*om.*
9.32	اذا اردت ان تحبل بذكر فخذ رحم ارنبة وجففه واسحقه واسقه للمرأة فانها تحبل بغلام والله اعلم	واذا اردت ان تذكر المرأة فخذ الارنب فجففه واسحقه واسقه المرأة منه بنبيذ	واذا اردت ان تحمل المرأة فخذ رحم ارنب وجففه واسحقه واسقت منه فان ذلك نافع جدا ان شاء الله تعالى

9.29: (b) *om.* W | وتبل] واجعل G | في البيت] في وسط البيت G | فانه ...الا رقصت] فاي مرأة رأته نزعت ثيابها ورقصت G
9.30: (b) *om.* W | بعر] بعرة G | به] بها G | قميصة] قميصة ظرطي G
9.31: (a) *om.* B
(b) واذا أخذت...معها] يشق بطن ارنبٍ حامل ويؤخذ رحمها فيطبخ ويأكل من الارنب فاذا كان الليل نام الرجل W; وان اردت المرأة تحبل فخذ ارنب حامل فشقها فاخرج رحمها فاطبخه واطعمه المرأة فاذا كان الليل فجامعها G
9.32: (a) ارنبة] ارنب انثى B | للمرأة] المرأة B
(b) واذا] فان W; وان G | ان تذكرا المرأة] ان تحبل ذكر W; تحمل المرأة ذكرا G | جففه] وجففه G | المرأة منه بنبيذ] *om.* W; المرأة في نبيذ G
(c) رحم] حيا C | واسقت] واسقها. C | ذلك] *om.* C

9.29	*om.*	If you want that the women take off their clothes and dance in the house, take the blood of the hare, soak a wick in it, light it up in the house, then every woman in the house who sees it will undress and dance.	*om.*
9.30	*om.*	If you want that somebody starts to break winds, take the droppings of a hare and write with them on his shirt, then he will break winds.	*om.*
9.31	If you want that a sterile woman gets pregnant, take a female hare, slaughter her, take her womb and roast it for the woman, and then she will get pregnant, with the permission of God, may He be exalted.	If you take a pregnant hare, cut her belly open, take her womb, cook it, feed its meat to a woman, and have sexual intercourse with her, then she will get pregnant on that very night by divine decree.	*om.*
9.32	If you want that a woman gets pregnant with a boy, take the womb of a female hare, dry it, grind it and give it to the woman to drink, then she will get pregnant with a boy, and God knows best.	If you want that a woman gets pregnant with a boy, take the womb of a hare, dry it, pound it and give it to the woman with some wine to drink.	If you want that a woman gets pregnant with a boy, take the womb of a hare, dry it, grind it and give it to drink to her, and this will be very useful God, may He be exalted, willing.

١٠. الغزال

	a	b	c
	ذكر منافع اعضاء الغزالة	الغزال	باب منافع الغزال
10.1	بعر الغزال البري يداف بدهن ورد وريحان وهراس ويعلف به الرأس فانه يربي الشعر ويقويه ويحسنه ويلينه	بعر الغزال الري يسحق ويذاف بدهن الريحان يكثر الشعر ويلينه ويجوده	بعر الغزال البري يذاب بدهن الريحان فيقوي الشعر ويحسنه ويطوله ويقرره
10.2	اذا اردت ان تحبك المرأة حبا شديدا فخذ شحم الغزال فأذبيه واطل به الاخليل عند الجماع تحبك حبا شديدا	واذا أخذ انسان شحم الغزال وطلى به الاحليل في وقت الجماعة احبته	شحم الغزال البري اذا طلي به الاحليل عند الجماع فان المرأة تحب الرجل حبا شديدا ولا تكاد تفارقه
10.3	يؤخذ مرارة غزالة تداف ويلقي عليها عقارا يقال له خصى الثعلب وفلفل وبزر جرجير يعجن الجميع بعسل منزوع الرغوة وتتحمل المرأة منه في صوفة بمقدار دانق فان كانت الغزال ذكرا فانها تحبل بذكر وان كان انثى فتحبل بانثى	ويؤخذ مرارة الغزال وعقاب سمى خصى الثعلب وبزر الجرجير من كل واحد وزن مثقال او عسل او قيتين يسحق الادوية ويحل ويعجن بالعسل ويصبّ في قارورة وتأخذ من المرأة بصوفة ويواقعها زوجها فتحبل فان كان الغزال ذكر ذكرا او ان كان انثى ولدت انثى	مرارة الغزال وعقار يقال له خصى الثعلب وفلفل وبزر الجرجير من كل واحد وزن مثقال سحق الجميع مع مرارة ويعجن بعسل منزوع الرغوة ويجعل في اناء فاذا اردت ان تحبل المرأة فخذ من ذلك الدواء مقدار حمصة ودعها تتحمل به عند الجماع فان كان الغزال ذكر حملت بذكر فان كان الغزال انثى حملت بانثى

10.1: (a) البري] يذاف يذاب والنبطي لبري B | وهراس] وهواس S; om. B | ويعلف] ويدهن B | ويلينه] om. B
(b) البري] الذي T; البرّي والجبلي add. W | يسحق ويذاف] اذا اسحق واذيف G; يسحق ويضاف W | يكثر الشعر ويلينه ويجوده] فانه يربّي واستعمل في الرأس مرى الشعر ويقويه وينبته وتجوده W; الشعر والجودة G
(c) يذاب] اذا اذيف C | فيقوى...ويقرره] وحشى الشعر عزره وحسنه وطوّله C
10.2: (a) حبا شديدا] om. B | فاذبيه واطل] ذيبه واطلي B | تحبك] فتحبك B
(b) واذا...احبته] om. W | شحمه اذا دهن به الاحليل في وقت الجماع احبته المرأة G
(c) طلى] يطلي C | فان المرأة تحب الرجل حبا شديدا] لم تستطع المرأة غيره من شدة الحب له C
10.3: (a) غزالة تذاف] تذاب B | غزال B | وفلفل] om. B | بعسل] بعسل نحل B | وتتحمل] وتحمل B | المرأة منه...بانثى] المرأة مقدار دانقين في صوفة فان كانت الغزالة انثى فانها تحبل بانثى وان كان ذكرا فتحبل بذكر W
(b) This recipe is attested only in W
(c) مرارة الغزال...حملت بانثى] مرارة الغزال اذا خلطت بالخمر مع شيء من خصاء الثعلب وفلفل وجرجير وعجن بعسل منزوع الرغوة ونزل في اناء فاذا اردت ان المرأة تحبل خذ من ذلك قدر حمصة ودعها تتحمل بها عند طلب الجماع فان كان الغزال ذكرا حملت بذكر وان كان الغزال انثى حملت بانثى باذن الله تعالى اردع هذه الحكمة في هذه الواقعة W

10. Gazelle

	a	b	c
	Exposition of the useful properties of the parts of the gazelle	**The gazelle**	**Chapter on the useful properties of the gazelle**
10.1	Wild gazelle droppings: if they are mixed with rose oil, basil and white acacia, and applied on the head, then this will make the hair grow, will strengthen it, and make it nicer and softer.	Wild gazelle droppings: if they are ground, mixed with basil oil and applied on the head, then this will make the hair grow, and will be god for it.	Wild gazelle droppings: if they are mixed with basil oil, then this will strengthen the hair, will make it nicer, longer and stronger.
10.2	If you want that a woman loves you intensely, then take the fat of the gazelle, liquefy it, and rub it on the outer opening of the urethra at the moment of coitus, then she will intensely love you.	If a man takes the fat of the gazelle and rubs it on the outer opening of urethra at the moment of coitus, then [the woman] will love him.	Wild gazelle fat: if it is rubbed on the outer opening of the urethra at the moment of coitus, then the woman will intensely love the man, and she will not be able to part from him.
10.3	Gazelle gall: if it is taken, liquefied, a remedy called “fox testicle” is added to it, with pepper and rocket—kneaded without foam—this has to be carried by a woman, in the quantity of one *dāniq* in a woollen cloth, and then she will get pregnant with a boy; while, if the gazelle is female, she then will get pregnant with a girl.	Gazelle gall: if it is taken with a remedy called “fox testicle”, rocket seeds—one *miṯqāl* of each one—or honey or *qīṭīn* [?], ground and kneaded with the honey, and eventually poured in a long-necked flask; then the woman should carry it in a woollen cloth, her husband should take her: then she will get pregnant with a boy, if the gazelle is a male; while, if the gazelle is a female, with a girl.	Gazelle gall and a remedy called “fox testicle”, pepper and rocket seeds—one *miṯqāl* of each one—everything pounded with the gall, kneaded with honey without foam, and preserved in a vessel; then when you want that a woman gets pregnant, take this remedy—in the amount of a chick-pea—give her this to carry at the moment of coitus and, if the gazelle is a male, then she will get pregnant with a boy; if, instead, it is a female, then she will get pregnant with a girl.

10.4	دماغ الغزال اذا يداف بدهن ورد مغلى ويجعل عليه ماء لوز ابيض ويسقي لصاحب السعال برئ باذن الله تعالى	دماغه اذا اذيف بدهن الغار على النار حتى يغلي ويؤخذ منه مقدار جرعة فتذاف بماء الكمون وتسقي للسعال	دماغ الغزال اذا اذيب بدهن ورد وماء الكمون وشرب به صاحب السعال العتيق سكن عنه
10.5	دم الغزال يداف بماء الجرجير ويدهن به حبتين من يشتكي الصداع والحمى الصالب فتسكن عنه باذن الله تعالى	مخه اذا اذيف بماء الجرجير واغلى على النار وطلى به جسد صاحب المليلة برئ	دماغ الغزال اذا اذيب بالجرجير غلى على النار ودهن به جسد من يشتكي الصداع سكن باذن اله تعالى
10.6	منفحة الغزال فتداف بماء السذاب وشيء من زيت واطلى به اسنان فتنبت من غير الم ولا وجع ولا اذي	انفحة الغزال تضاف بماء السذاب وزيت ويطلي الصبي الذي يريد ان يخرج اسنانه فيخرج الوجع ولذلك انيابه	*om.*
10.7	*om.*	وان طرحت خنفساء حبة على الغزال مات	*om.*
10.8	وقال الحكيم الغزال القمر والخنفساء الرجل فاذا أخذت خنفساء وجعلتها على غزال يموت من ساعته	وان علقت خنفساء ميتة في خرقة على قرن الغزال ثم طرحت عليه خنفساء حية لم تضره ما دام ذلك عليه	واذا طرح على غزال حنفساء كبيرة فانها تموت من ساعتها واذا أخذت حنفساء صغيرة وجعلتها في خرقة و علقها على قرنه وطرحت عليه حنفساء كبيرة لم تضره

10.4: (a) *om.* B
(b) This recipe is attested only in G and W | دماغه...للسعال] وبوز شحرة الثعلب اجود دماغ الثعلب او الغزال يضاف بدهن الغار وغلى على النار ويؤخذ منه فيضاف بماء الكمون قد رخرقه ويشرب للسعال W
(c) In C this recipe is after 10.5 | (c) اذيب] اذيف C | وشرب به صاحب السعال العتيق] وشربه من به السعال قرح فيه C | سكن عنه] ازاله عنه C
10.5: (a) دم الغزال يذاف] دماغ الغزال اذا يذاب B
(b) This recipe is attested only in G and W, after 10.6 | مخه...برئ] مخ الغزال بماء الجرجير ويغلي ويدهن به حبي من به المليلة والمسلول فيبرأ W
(c) *om.* C
10.6: (a) فتذاف] تذاب B | وأطلى] ويطلي B | اسنان] اسنان الصغير B | ولا اذي] *om.* B
(b) This recipe is attested only in W
10.7: (b) This recipe is attested only in G
10.8: (a) وقال...من ساعته] قال الحكيم اذا اخذت خنفساة وجعلتها على غزال ماتت B
(b) This recipe is attested only in G and W | وان علّقت...ذلك عليه] واعلم ان الغزال العمل الحيف الرجل فاطرح خنفساة ميتة في خرقة علق عليها فبري الغزال ثم طرحت خنفساة لم تضره ما دامت ذلك عليه الخنفساة عليه لانه متى أخذت خنفساة حية طرحتها على الغزال لمات مكان والميته تمنع موته اذا علقت على قرنه W
(c) واذا طرح...من ساعتها] قال واذا طرحت على الغزال خنفساء كبيرة مات من ساعته C | واذا أخذت...تضره] *om.* C

10.4	Gazelle brain: if it is mixed with boiled rose oil, some white almonds water is added, and it is given to the man suffering from cough to drink, then he will recover, with the permission of God, may He be exalted.	Its brain: if is mixed with myrtle oil on the fire until it boils, then taken in the quantity of a mouthful—mixed with cumin water—and given to drink against the cough, [this will be useful].	Gazelle brain: if it is liquefied with rose oil and cumin water, then drunk by the man suffering from chronic cough, then will calm his cough.
10.5	Gazelle blood: if it is mixed with rocket water, and rubbed on the temples of the man suffering from headache and strong fever, then these will calmed, with the permission of God, may He be exalted.	Its marrow: if it is mixed with rocket water, boiled on the fire, and rubbed on the body of the man suffering from feverish heat, then this will cure him.	Gazelle brain: if it is liquefied with rocket, boiled on the fire and rubbed on the body of the man suffering from headache, then this will calm it, with the permission of God, may He be exalted.
10.6	Gazelle rennet: if it is mixed with rue water and some oil, rubbed on the teeth, then they will come out without any pain, ache, or harm.	Gazelle rennet: if it is mixed with rue water and oil, rubbed on the child whose teeth should come out, then these will come out without pain thanks to this.	*om.*
10.7	*om.*	If the scarab throws one of its balls at the gazelle, then this will die.	*om.*
10.8	The wise man said that the gazelle is like the moon, while the scarab is like the man: if the scarab is taken and placed on a gazelle, then it will immediately die.	If a dead scarab is hung on a gazelle horn in a piece of cloth, then a living scarab is thrown against the gazelle, then this will not harm it, as long as the dead scarab remains on it.	If a big scarab is thrown against a gazelle, then this will immediately die; while, if a small scarab is wrapped in a piece of cloth and hung on its horn and a big scarab is thrown at the gazelle, then this will not be harmed.

10.9	مرارة الغزال وعقّار يقال له باطس يداف الجميع بعسل وتتحمل به المرأة تحبل باذن الله تعالى	*om.*	*om.*
10.10	*om.*	*om.*	سن الغزال الذكر اول ما يلد اذا جعل تحت فص حاتم ذهب او فضة من لسانه من من وجع القولنج
10.11	ما يفشّ الاورام يؤخذ بعر الغزال ويسحق ويلقي عليه تراب بيت الخلد واعجنه بالخل واطل به الورم فتزول	بعره اذا أخذ منه جزء مع مثله تراب الخلد وعجنا بخل وطلى به الورم سكن باذن الله	بعر الغزال وتراب الخلد اذا أخذ من كل واحد جزء وعجن بالخل الحادق وطلى به الورم فانه ينفش
10.12	اذا اردت ان تخرج العلق من الحلق او الدود فتأخذ لسان الغزال تجففه وتسحقه ناعما وتبخر الحلق فان العلق يسقط من ساعته	لسانه اذا جفف وبخر به من في حلقه علق سقّط	اذا اردت ان تسقط العلق من الحلق بلا اذي خذ لسان الغزال جففه وبخر به من في فمه العلق يرميه سريعا
10.13	يؤخذ كعب الغزال يحرق ويسحق ويحشي به النصور فيذهب باذن الله تعالى	كعبه اذا احرق وسحق وحشى به الناصور اذهبه	خصية الغزال يحرق ويسحق ويحشي به النسور فانه يبرأ

10.9: (a) يذاف] يذاب B

10.10: (c) *om.* C

10.11: (a) ما يفشّ الاورام] *om.* B | ويسحق] *om.* B | بيت الخلد] بيت النملة B | واعجنه] ويعجن الجميع B | واطل] ويطلي B | الورم فتزول] الاورام تبرأ B
(b) This recipe is attested only in G and W | بعره...سكن] بعر الغزال وتراب الخلد وهو فارة عميا من كل واحد منها بالسوية ويعجن ويطلي به الورم فيسكنه W

10.12: (a) اذا اردت ان تخرج العلق من الحلق او الدود فتأخذ] *om.* B | تجففه وتسحقه] يجفف ويسحق B | وتبخر] وتبخر به في B | فان العلق يسقط] فيسقط العلق والدود B
(b) This recipe is attested only in G
(c) اذا اردت ان تسقط العلق من الحلق بلا اذى خذ] *om.* C | لسان...سريعا] لسان الغزال اذا جفف وبخّر به العلق الذي توعر في حلق الانسان او غيره رماه سريعا W

10.13: (b) This recipe is attested only in G and W | كعبه...اذهبه] لسان الطير يحرق ويحشي به موضع النصور W
(c) خصية الغزال] كعب الغزال C | يحرق ويسحق] اذا حرق وسحق C | فانه يبرأ] ابرأه سارعا C

10.9	If the gall of the gazelle and a drug called *bāṭis* [?], everything mixed with honey and a woman carries it, then she will get pregnant, with the permission of God, may He be exalted.	*om.*	*om.*
10.10	*om.*	*om.*	Tooth of the male gazelle: if it is taken as soon as it is born, put under the stone of a golden or silver seal, and then under the tongue of a man suffering from colic [it will be useful].
10.11	To make the swellings subside, gazelle droppings: if they are taken, ground, some dust from the mole's hole is added to it, kneaded with vinegar, and rubbed on the swelling, then this will subside.	Its droppings: if one part of it is taken with the same amount of mole's dust and rubbed on the swelling, then this will calm it with the permission of God, may He be exalted.	Gazelle droppings and the dust of mole, one part of each one: if they are kneaded with acid vinegar, and rubbed on the swelling, then this will make it subside.
10.12	If you want that either leeches or worms come out from the throat, take the tongue of the gazelle, dry it, grind it finely and fumigate the throat with it, then the leeches will immediately fall.	Its tongue: if it is dried and fumigated on the man who has a leech in his throat, then this will make it fall.	If you want that the leeches fall from the throat without any damage, take the tongue of the gazelle, dry it and fumigate with it the man who has leeches in his mouth, then he will immediately expel them.
10.13	Gazelle anklebone: if it is burnt, ground, and stuffed inside the fistula, then this will cure it, with the permission of God, may He be exalted.	Its anklebone: if it burnt, ground, and stuffed inside the fistula, then this will make it go away.	Gazelle testicle: if it is ground and stuffed inside the fistula, then this will cure it.

10.14

كعب الغزال اذا شتت بملح وورس وسندروس وسعد جبلي ودق الجميع وعمل في صوفة وحملته المرأة قطع النزيف عنها

خصية الغزال تمل ويخلط معها ورس وكندر وصعتر مدقوق يضاف بزيت ويبل به تمسكه المستحاضة معها وينفعه النزف

يؤخذ خصى الغزال يدقّ ويلقي عليه ورس وكندر وصعتر ويذاف الجميع بالزيت وتجعل على صوفة منه مقدار دانق وتتحمل به المرأة فينقطع نزف الدم

10.15

مرارة الغزال اذا خلطت بقطران وسذاب وشربها صاحب السعال بماء فاتر سكن عنه

مرارته اذا خلط معها قطران وملح مر وشرب منها صاحب السعال الذي يقذف القيح والدم جزء او بماء حار اذهبه

يؤخذ مرارة الغزال يخلط معها قطران وشيء من ملح ويسقي لصاحب السعال فسكن عنه باذن الله تعالى

10.16

مرارة الغزال اللطيف وكبده وشحمه اذا طبخ الجميع والقى عليه حلبة وسليخة وميعة وزروند احمر وجعل مثل البنادق وشرب منه كل يوم بندقة بماء حار كرر عن الفؤاد واذهب وجع الجوف والرية

لحمه وشحمه وكبده اذا طبخوا حتى يتهرّى ثم القى حلبة وكمون وصعتر جبلي وسليخة وسعد هندي وورد احمر ثم جعل مثل البنادق فهو جيد للربو والبهر ولوجع الرية والجنب اذا شرب منه بندقة بماء حار

للدود ووجع الرية يؤخذ لحم الغزال وشحمه وكبده فيطبخ الجميع حتى يتهرّى ويلقي عليه حلبة وسعتر شامي وورد عراقي وسعد كوفي يغلي الجميع حتى يبقي ويذهب الماء ويجعل مثل حب البندق ويسقي منه لصاحب وجع الرية فيبرأ

10.17

صوف الغزال اذا بخر منه انسان تسنخت عروقه لينها ونفعه جدا

بعره اذا بخّر به الانسان انقطع نتنه ورائحته

بعر الغزال اذا بخر به انسان قد سنخت عروقه نفعه ذلك والله أعلم بالصواب

10.14: (a) يدق] يذاف B | ويذاف] ويضاف B | وتجعل على صوفة منه] وتجعل منه على صوفه B | نزف الدم] النزيف B
(b) This recipe is attested only in W | وصعتر] وزعتر W
(c) كعب الغزال] مرارة الغزال C | وسعد جبلي] وسفرجل C | النزيف عنها] عنها النزيف C
10.15: (a) يؤخذ] *om.* B | فسكن عنه] يبرأ B
(b) This recipe is attested only in G and W | مرارته ...اذهبه] مرارت الغزال يخلط معها قطران وملح ويشرب منها صاحب السعال الذي يقدف الدم والقيح حرّا بماء حار اذهبه W
(c) مرارة الغزال اذا خلطت بقطران] واذا اخلطت بقطران C | بماء فاتر] *om.* C
10.16: (a) للدود ووجع الرية يؤخذ] *om.* B | فيطبخ] يطبخ B | عليه] عليهم B | وسعتر] وصعتر كوفي وسليحه B | يبقي] *om.* B | الرية فيبرأ] وجع الرية والجنب والربو كل يوم بندقة يزول B
(b) This recipe is attested only in G and W | لحمه...بماء حار] ولحم الطير وسكنجه وسعد هندي وورد احمر ثم يجعل مثل بنادق كان دواً للمبنى ووجع الرية والجنب شربته ببندقة بماء حار W
(c) مرارة الغزال] لحم الغزال C | وميعة] وسعد C | وشرب] ثم شرب C | بماء حار] بالماء C | كرر...والرية] اذهب الربوعن الفواد وجع الرية والجوف C
10.17: (a) سنجت] تشيخت B | نفعه ذلك] نفع B
(b) This recipe is attested only in G and W | الانسان] همسح انسان W | نتنه ورايحته] برئه W
(c) صوف] بعر C

10.14 Gazelle testicle: if it is minced, with the addition of curcuma, incense and wild thyme, mixed with oil and put—the quantity of one *dāniq*—in a woollen cloth that the woman has to carry with her, then this will stop her bleeding.

Gazelle testicle: if it is mixed with curcuma, incense, and ground wild thyme, mixed with oil and moistened with it, this is used to contain [the bleeding], and it will be useful against the bleeding.

Gazelle anklebone: if it is seasoned with curcuma, sandarac and mountain sedge, everything ground together, put in a woollen cloth that the woman has to carry, then this will stop her bleeding.

10.15 Gazelle gall: if it is taken, melted with tar and some salt, given to the man suffering from cough to drink, then this will calm the cough, with the permission of God, may He be exalted.

Its gall: if it is melted with tar, salt and myrrh, one part is drunk by the man suffering from the cough that makes him expectorate catarrh and blood—or with warm water—then this will stop the cough.

Gazelle gall: if it is melted with tar and rue, drunk by the man suffering from cough with lukewarm water, then this will calm the cough.

10.16 Against worms and lung pain, gazelle meat, its fat and its liver: if they are cooked until they are well done, with the addition of fenugreek, Syrian wild thyme, Iraqi rose and Kufic sedge, boiled altogether until the water has evaporated, made in pills and given to the man suffering from lung pain, then this will cure him.

Its meat, fat and liver: if they are cooked until they are well done, with the addition of fenugreek, cumin, mountain wild thyme, cassia, common galingale and red rose, and made in pills, then this will be good for asthma, breathlessness, lung pain and pleurisy, if one pill is taken with warm water.

The gall of a young gazelle, its liver and its fat: if they are cooked together with the addition of fenugreek, cassia, officinal storax and aristolochia, and made in pills; then one of them has to be taken every day with warm water—as long as you need it—then this will cure the abdomen and the pain of the lungs.

10.17 Gazelle droppings: if a man whose teeth are eroded at the root is fumigated with them, then this will be useful, and God knows best.

Gazelle droppings: if the man is fumigated with them, his putrid smell and odour will cease.

Gazelle wool: if a man whose teeth are eroded at the root is fumigated with it, then this will calm them, and will be very useful.

١١. الوعل

a

ذكر منافع اعضاء الوعل

b

الوعل

c

باب منافع الوعل

11.1

a: لوجع المثانة يؤخذ من لحم الوعل وشحمه ويدق الجميع حتى يختلطوا ثم يجعل عليها سعد كوفي وزعفران يطبخ الجميع بعسل نحل حتى ينعقد ويسقى منه صاحب وجع المثانة وزن مثقال بماء الكرفس ينفعه باذن الله تعالى

b: لحم الوعل وشحمه يدقان في هاون ويلقي عليه صبر وسعد وقرنفل وزعفران وعسل يخلط به خلطا نعيما ويسقي منه نصف مثقال بماء الكرفس لمن به الحصاة في مثانته ينفعه باذن الله تعالى

c: لحم الوعل وشحمه يدق الجميع ويعمل منه في طاجن نحاس صبر وسعد وزعفران وعسل بقدر الحاجة ويغلي على النار ويشربه صاحب الحصاة يفتت واذا استعمل مع ماء الكرفس منع قطار البول وفتت الحصاة

11.2

a: يؤخذ دماغ الوعل يخلط معه دقيق الكرسنة ويذاب بماء المردقوش ويشرب بماء حار في الحمام فينفع لصاحب الصفار

b: دماغ الوعل يخلط معه دقيق الكرسنة ويشرب بماء المرزنجوش حارا في الحمام لمن به الصفراء ينفعه

c: دماغه اذا خلط بدقيق الكرسنة وشرب بماء حار مع ماء المردقوش اذهب الصفار عن الوجه

11.3

a: يؤخذ مخ الوعل فيذاب على النار وتغمس في صوفة وتحمّل بها المرأة فينقطع عنها نزف باذن الله تعالى

b: ومخ الوعل جيد للمرأة التي بها نزف تحمل به في صوفة

c: مخ الوعل اذا جعل في صوفة وحملت المرأة قطع النزيف

11.1: (a) يختلطوا] يختلط B | سعد] صعد B
(b) In T this recipe is the last of the previous chapter (Ch. 10) | الوعل] الغزال T | يدقان] يسحقان W | في هاون] *om.* W | وسعد] وزعتر W | نعيما] جيدا W | نصف] وزن نصف W | لمن به الحصاة في مثانته ينفعه] فيفتت الحصا من المثانة W | لحم الوعل...ينفعه] لحمه وشحمه اذا سحقي في جرن والقي عليهما صبر وسعد وقرنفيل وزعفران وعسل وخلط ناعما ويسقي منه صاحب المثانة والحصاة وزن نصف مثقال بماء الكرفس G
(c) يدق] اذا دق C | ويعمل منه] وخلط معه C | وعسل] وعسل نحل C | بقدر الحاجة] *om.* C | ويغلي] وغلى C | ويشربه صاحب] وشرب منه من به C | يفتت] فتتها C | وفتت الحصاة] *om.* C
11.2: (a) ويذاب] *om.* B | فينفع] ينفع B
(b) الكرسنة] الاسنه W | المرزنجوش] المرونجوش W | لمن به الصفراء ينفعه] فيذهب بالصفار W | دماغ الوعل...ينفعه] دماغه اذا خلط معه دقيق الكرسنه وشرب منه صاحب الصُفار بماء المرزنجوش حار في الحمام نفعه G
(c) دماغه] دماغ الوعل C | حار] حار في الحمام C | عن الوجه] الذي يعتري الانسان C
11.3: (a) يؤخذ] *om.* B | فيذاب] يذاف B | نزف] نزول الدم B
(b) نزف] رق W | ومخ الوعل...صوفة] مخه اذا اتحمل به المرأة في صوفة نفعها من نزف الدم G
(c) وحملت] وحملتها C | قطع] قطع عنها C

11. Mountain Goat

	a	b	c
	Exposition of the useful properties of the parts of the mountain goat	**The mountain goat**	**Chapter on the useful properties of the mountain goat**
11.1	Against bladder complaint, mountain goat meat and its fat: if they are minced until they melt up, with the addition of Kufic sedge and saffron, cooked with honey until it thickens, then one *miṯqāl* of it is given to a man suffering from bladder complaint with celery water to drink, and this will be useful to him.	Mountain goat meat and its fat: if they are ground in a mortar, with the addition of aloe, sedge, saffron, cloves, and honey, mixed well and half *miṯqāl* of it is given with celery water to a man suffering from the stones in his bladder to drink, then this will be useful to him.	Mountain goat meat and its fat: if everything is ground and kneaded in a copper frying pan with aloe, sedge, saffron and honey—as much as you need—boiled on the fire and given to a man suffering from [bladder] stones to drink, then this will crumble them. Moreover, with celery water, this will prevent from urine dripping and will crumble the [bladder] stones.
11.2	Mountain goat brain: if it is mixed with vetches flour, liquefied with marjoram water and drunk with warm water in the bath, it will be useful to the man suffering from yellow complexion.	Mountain goat brain: if it is mixed with vetches flour and drunk with warm marjoram water in the bath, this will be useful to a man suffering from yellow bile.	Its brain: if it is mixed with vetches flour and drunk with warm water and marjoram water, then the yellow complexion will go away from the face.
11.3	Mountain goat marrow: if it is liquefied on the fire, used to soak a piece of cloth that a woman should carry with her, this will stop the loss of blood, with the permission of God, may He be exalted.	The marrow of mountain goat is good for a woman who is bleeding, if she carries it in a woollen cloth.	Mountain goat marrow: if it is put in a piece of cloth and carried by a woman, this will stop the loss of blood.

١٢. الايل

	(a)	b	c
	ذكر منافع اعضاء الايل	الايل	باب منافع الايل
12.1	قرن الايل اذا بخّر مع الكبريت الخفتاني الدار لم يبقا فيها شيء من الحيات ولا العقرب ولا شيء يوذي باذن الله تعالى	قرن الايل والكبريت اذا بخّر به البيت هربت منه سائر الحيات وسائر الذباب	قرن الايل اذا بخر به مع الكبريت طرد الذبيب من البيت وكل ذي سم
12.2	وكذلك خصى الايل اذا خلط معها شيء من صمغ الصناوبر ومرّ خالص وبخّر بها الدار المربيق فيها شيء يوذي من جميع الذبيب	وكذلك يفعل بخصيته اذا ملحت بملح ومر وصمغ صنوبر وبخر به موضع هربت منه الحيات وذبيب منه	خصوة الايل اذا جعل فيها ملح وصمغ ضوبر منع الذبيب ولا يوذي هناك الدبيب
12.3	[دم الايل] اذا خلط معه شيء من دقيق الكرسنة فعل مثل ذلك	دم الايل اذا خلط مع دقيق الكرسنة وبخر به الموضع فعل مثل ذلك	دم الايل اذا خلط بدقيق الكرسنة طرد الهوام
12.4	لوجع المفاصل واليدين والرجلين يؤخذ لحم الايل وشحمه يطبخ حتى ينهرا ويلقي عليه صبر ومر وملح وبورق من كل واحد جزء ويذيب الجميع بزيت خالص ويلطخ به جميع الجسد فينفعه باذن الله تعالى	لحم الايل وشحمه يطبخان ويدقان في هاون ويلقي عليه ملح ونطرون ومر وصَبِر ويذاف بزيت ويلطخ جسد من به وجع المفاصل فانه ينفع	لحم الايل وشحم اذا طبخ والقي عليه ملح ونطرون احمر وصبر واذيب بزيت ودلك به الحسد نفع من وجع المفاصل والرجلين نفعا جيدا

12: (a) الايل] الاريل B, in the whole chpater
(b) الايل] الاريل W, in the whole chapter
(c) الايل] الاريل L, in the whole chapter
12.1: (a) الدار مع الكبريت الخفتاني] به الدار مع الكبريت الحقاني B | العقرب] العقارب B
(b) قرن الايل] قرنه G | به] بها W | البيت] البيت او الموضع الذي فيه G W | هربت...الذباب] هربوا مع كبريت G; هربن منه W
(c) به] به البيت C | الكبريت] شيء من الكبريت C | طرد] انطرد C | سم] من الموضع الذي يبخر به فيه add. C
12.2: (a) صمغ الصناور] ضمغ B | المربيق] لم يبقي B
(b) صنوبر] صنوير T | وكذلك...منه] خصيته اذا ملحت بملح مع مر وصمغ الصنوبر G | يفعل] ينفع او ينعل W | بخصيته] بخصية الاريل W | وصمغ صنوبر] وصبر تجمع الصور W | وبخر...منه] وبخر بها البيت او الموضع هربن منه الحيات وكل شيء وكل ذيبب موذي W
(c) جعل فيها ملح] شتت بالملح C | الذبيب] الذبيب من المكان C | الذبيب] احدا ابدا C
12.3: (b) دم الايل...ذلك] اذا بخر بهم البيت هربوا ايضا الهوام G | دم الايل] دم الاريل وكذلك يفعل add. W | فعل مثل ذلك الموضع] البيت W
(c) طرد الهوام] وبخر به المكان طرد الهوام add. C
12.4: (a) يؤخذ والرجلين واليدين المفاصل لوجع] ينفع لوجع المفاصل B | فينفعه] om. B | جميع] om. B | ويذيب] ويرب B | ومر وملح] وملح ومر B | الوجع المفاصل] om. B
(b) لحم الايل] لحمه G | يطبخان...عليه] اذا اذقّا وطبخا ثم القي عليهما G; يطبخان ثم يدقان ويلقا عليهما W | ومر وصبر] وصبر ومر G W | ويذاف] واذيف W | فانه ينفع] نفعه G; فينفع نفعا بينا W | ذلك G; ويضاف ذلك W
(c) وصبر] وصبر سقطري add. C | بزيت] بالزيت C | المفاصل والرجلين] om. C

12. Deer

	a	b	c
	Exposition of the useful properties of the parts of the deer	**The deer**	**Chapter on the useful properties of the deer**
12.1	Deer horn: if it is fumigated inside the house with *Ḥiftānī* sulphur, then not a single snake will remain there, nor a scorpion or anything obnoxious, with the permission of God, may He be exalted.	Deer horn and sulphur: if the house it fumigated with these, then the snake and the flies will flee from it.	Deer horn: if it is fumigated with sulphur, this will chase the insects and every other poisonous animal away from the house.
12.2	Likewise, deer testicles: if they are melted with some pine resin and pure myrrh, then fumigated inside the house infested by any kind of obnoxious fly [this will cease].	Likewise, its testicles: if they are seasoned with salt, myrrh and pine resin, the house is fumigated with this, then the snakes and the flies will flee from it.	Deer testicle: if salt and pine resin are mixed with it, then this will prevent the flies from causing damage there.
12.3	Deer blood: if it is mixed with some vetches flour, it will have the same effect.	Deer blood: if it is mixed with some vetches flour, and the place is fumigated with it, then this will have the same effect.	Deer blood: if it is mixed with vetches flour, then this will chase the vermin away.
12.4	Against the pain of the joints, the hands and the feet, deer meat and its fat: if they are taken, cooked until they are well done, with the addition of aloe, myrrh, salt and natron—one part of each one—everything mixed with pure oil and spattered on all the body, then this will be useful, with the permission of God, may He be exalted.	Its meat and fat: if these are cooked, ground in a mortar, salt, soda, aloe and myrrh are added to it, mixed with oil, and spattered on the body of the man suffering from joints pain, then this will be useful to him.	Deer meat and its fat: if they are cooked and mixed with salt, red soda and aloe, liquefied with oil and rubbed on the body of the man suffering from joints and feet pain, then this will be useful to him.

12.5	لوجع الظهر والكلى يؤخذ شحم الايل ومخه فيذاب على النار ويجعل عليه قليل فلفل مسحوق وتمرخ به الظهر فيهدي باذن الله تعالى	شحم الايل ومخه نافع لكل ضربانه ووجع في الظهر والوركين اذا طبخ في قعر فيه الفلفل وتمرخ فيه	شحم الايل ومخه اذا اذيب والقي عليه فلفل ناعما نفع من وجع الظهر والوركين واذا مرخ البدن ودخل الحمام نفع نفعا بليغا
12.6	*om.*	*om.*	دماغ الايل اذا اذيب وطلى به الورم الحاسي نشبه
12.7	لورم الاسنان يؤخذ دماغ الايل يذاب على نار لينة ويمسح به لحم الاسنان الوارمة فيذهب ألمها باذن الله تعالى	دماغ الايل يحرق ويسحق ويعجن بشراب وصير منها على الاسنان ينفع من وجعها وضعفها	وينفع ايضا من من وجع الاسنان ويسكن الضربان ويخرج الصفراء والسوداء من الاسنان وينفع الوسوسة منها
12.8	قرن الايل اذا احرق وسحق وجعل منه شيء على الاسنان الوجعة وهي تتحرك فينفعها نفعا بليغا	قرنه اذا احرق وسحق وعجن بشراب ولطخ به الاسنان نفع من وجعها	قرن الايل ايضا اذا احرق وسحق ويقطع الصفرة من الاسنان والحفر التي فيها ويشد اصولها
12.9	*om.*	*om.*	واذا احرق الابيض منه بالخل وشربه من به طحال ابرأ
12.10	*om.*	*om.*	وجلده اذا علق على انسان لم ينم ما دام عليه
12.11	*om.*	*om.*	كتفه وذكره اذا اشد على العضد حرز من سائر الحيات

12.5: (a) فيذاب] يذاب B | قليل] *om.* B | فيهذي] يبرأ B
(b) الفلفل] العليل T | شحم الايل...فيه] نفعه G شحمه ومخه اذا طبخ بماء وتمرّخ من به وجع الظهر والوركين | ووجع في] ووجع يكون في *add.* W | اذا طبخ في قعد] اذا عقد في ماء W | فيه الفلفل وتمرخ فيه] ويطبخه بماء وتمرّخ به W
(c) شحم الايل ومخه] شحمه ومخه مخ الايل وشحمه C | فلفل] مسحوق ففل C
12.6: (c) نشبه] انفش C
12.7: (a) نار لينة] النار اللينة B | الوارمة] *om.* B | فيذهب ألمها] يذهب B
(b) دماغ الايل...وضعفها] نفعه الورم الحار به لطخ اذا دماغه G; به لطخ اذا الحارّة الاورام ينفع الاريل دماغ W
(c) ايضا] *om.* C | والسوداء] *om.* C | وينفع الوسوسة منها] *om.* C
12.8: (b) This recipe is attested only in G and W | قرنه...وجعها] وقرن الاريل محروق اذا اسحقه وعجنت بشراب وصبر منها على الاسنان نفع من وجعها وضعها W
(c) *om.* C
12.9: (c) *om.* C
12.10: (c) *om.* C
12.11: (c) *om.* C

12.5	For the pain of the back and of the the kidneys, deer fat and its marrow: if they are liquefied on the fire, with the addition of some ground pepper and rubbed on the back, then then it will be right, with the permission of God, may He be exalted.	Deer fat and its marrow: these are useful against every pang and pain in the back and in the legs, if it is cooked in a deep dish containing a bit of pepper, and rubbed on the body.	Deer fat and its marrow: if they are liquefied, with the addition of some fine pepper, then this will be useful against the pain of the back and of the legs. If the body is rubbed with this when the man comes out from the bath, then this will be even more effective.
12.6	*om.*	*om.*	Deer brain: if it is liquefied and rubbed on a suppurative swelling, then this will make it subside.
12.7	Against tooth swelling, deer brain: if it is liquefied on a light fire, then rubbed on the swollen gum, then the pain will cease, with the permission of God, may He be exalted.	Deer brain: if it is burnt, ground, kneaded with wine, and applied on the teeth, then this will be useful against their pain and their weakness.	It is also useful to the man suffering from tooth pain, it will calm the pangs, will remove the yellow and black matter, and will be useful against the obsession that derives from them.
12.8	Deer horn: if it is burnt, ground, and a little bit of it is put on the aching teeth—that are also moving—this will be effectively useful against it.	Its horn: if it is burnt, ground, kneaded with wine, and spattered on the teeth, then will be useful against their pain.	Deer horn, also: if it is burnt and ground, then this will remove the yellow matter from the teeth and their cavities, and it will strengthen their roots.
12.9	*om.*	*om.*	If the white part is burnt with vinegar and drunk by the man suffering from spleen complaint, then this will cure him.
12.10	*om.*	*om.*	Its skin: if it is hung on a man, then he will not sleep as long as this remains on him.
12.11	*om.*	*om.*	Its shoulder blade and its penis: if they are tied to the arm, then this will protect from some snakes.

12.12	*om.*	*om.*	قضيبته اذا شرب بعد ان جفف هيج الباه
12.13	*om.*	*om.*	دماغه كله او بعضه يمنع النوم
12.14	*om.*	*om.*	انفحته اذا اذيبت مع الخل تمنع السموم القاطلة مشروبا
12.15	اذا عسرت الولادة على المرأة يعلق عليها قرن الايل تلد سريعا باذن الله تعالى	وان علق قرن الايل على امرأة صعبت عليها الولادة وضعت شريعا	قرن الايل اذا علق على فخذ المرأة الفخذ الايمن اسرع النزول من تعسر عليها الولادة وهونت الطلق
12.16	لطرد البعوض والناموس يبخر البيت بقرن الايل واظلاف المعز فلم يقربه شيء من ذلك	فان بخر به مع ظلف عنز طرد البعوض	قرنه واطراف المغر اذا بخر به البيت طرد البعوض والناموس واذهب الهوام
12.17	للدود في الجوف يؤخذ قرن الايل فيحرق ويسحق ويسقي منه صاحب الدود بعسل فلا يبقي في جوفه دود ولا ما يُوذيه	وان احرق وسحق بشيرج ويطرح معه دار فلفل ابيض مسحوق يطرح على النار فاذا اكتحل به من بعينه الماء والغشاوة ينفعه نفعا جيدا	قرنه ايضا اذا احرق وسحق وخلط بعسل ولعقه انسان على الريق ارمي الدود الذي في جوفه كبارا او صغارا

12.12: (c) *om.* C
12.13: (c) *om.* C
12.14: (c) *om.* C
12.15: (a) اذا عسرت...سريعا] قرن الاريل واذا علق على امرأة عسرت عليها الولادة وصنعت سريعا B
(b) وان...شريعا] الولادة من عسر نفع من امرأة حامل على امرأة على قرنه واذا علق G; وجع بغير ولدت او تلد تريد امرأة على الاريل بقرون علقت وان W
(c) This recipe is attested only in C
12.16: (a) لطرد البعوض...من ذلك] الاريل اذا بخّر به البيت هرب منه البعوض والناموس [قرن] B
(b) فان...البعوض] قرنه اذا بخّر به البيت مع ظلف عنز هرب منه البقّ G | *om.* W
(c) اذا بخر] وبخر C
12.17: (a) للدود في الجوف] *om.* B | فيحرق] يحرق B | ولا ما] ولا شيئا B
(b) وان...جيدا] قرنه اذا احرق وسحق وشرب بعسل اخرج الدود من البطن G | قرون الاريل اذا احرقت وسحقت وشرب منها بعسل اخرج الدود من البطن W
(c) قرنه ايضا اذا احرق] قرنه ايضا اذا احرق C | بعسل] بعسل نحل C | ولعقه] ولعق منه C

12.12	*om.*	*om.*	Its penis: if it is drunk once dried, then this will excite the sexual desire.
12.13	*om.*	*om.*	Its brain, whole or just a part of it, will prevent from sleeping.
12.14	*om.*	*om.*	Its rennet: if it is liquefied with vinegar, then this will stop deadly poisons that one may drink.
12.15	If the a woman has difficulties in giving birth, the horn of the deer has to be hung on her, and then she will quickly give birth, with the permission of God, may He be exalted.	If the horn of the deer is hung on a woman who has a difficult labour, then she will quickly give birth.	Deer horn: if it is hung on the right leg of the woman, then this will speed up the labour, and will ease the labour pains.
12.16	To chase different kinds of mosquitos away, fumigate the house with deer horn and goat hooves, than no insect will approach it.	If it is fumigated together with a goat hoof, then this will chase the mosquitos away.	Deer horn and goat extremities: if the house is fumigated with these, then the mosquitos will be chased away, and the obnoxious insects will be expelled.
12.17	Against the worms inside the abdomen, deer horn: it has to be taken, burnt, ground and given with honey to the man who is affected by these worms to drink, then not a single worm will remain inside its abdomen, nor anything else that may harm him.	If it is burnt, ground with sesame oil, ground white long pepper is added to it, put on the fire, then applied on the eye of the man suffering from water [in the eye] and cataract, this will be very useful.	Its horn, again: if it is burnt, ground and melted with honey, and if a man licks it, then he will expel the worms—either big or small—that are inside his abdomen.

12.18

كبـد الايل اذا در عليـها دار فلـفل وجعلت على النار وأخذ ماؤها واكتحل به صاحب الغشاوة ومن بدا في عينيه وماء ازال ذلك عنه

يؤخذ كبد الايل يشوي حتى يشتوي ثم يجفف ويسحق ويتخذ منه برود ينفع من الغشاوة في العين ويزيل الماء ويحل البصر

للماء في العين والغشاوة يؤخذ كبد الايل يشرح وتدرّ عليه دار فلفل مسحوق ويجعل على جمر نار فاذا سرحا ماؤها فيكتحل به من في عينه غشاوة وبد وماء فيزول باذن الله تعالى

12.19

واذا شويت الكبد وسحقت واكتحل بها من في عينيه غشاوة ابرأها

وسحق الكبد الذكورة اذا جفف وتنخل وكحّل به من به غشاوة العين وظلمة البصر وبدر الماء نفعها

كبد الايل اذا جففت وسحقت يتخذ منها ذرور يكتحل به من في عينه غشاوة او ماء اصفر فيزول باذن الله تعالى

12.20

قضب الايل اذا جفف واحتفظ به واصاب انسان عسر البول او رياح القولنج فغسّله وسقاه ماء غسالته اطلق الاسر ونفع القولنج

قضيب الايل اذا جفف بالنار واحفض به فاذا اصاب انسان عسر البول او ارياح قولنج فاغسله واسقه مائه فانه ينطلق

للقولنج وعسر البول يؤخذ قضيب الايل فيجفف ويرفع فاذا اصاب الانسان قولنج او عسر البول فينقع القضيب في الماء ويسقي منه صاحب القولنج وعسر البول فيزول عنه باذن الله تعالى

12.18: (a) للماء في العين والغشاوة] *om.* B | يشرح] تشرحه B | ويجعل على...فيزول] ويتخذ منه حزود ويكتحل به صاحب الماء الاصفر في العين والغشاوة يبرأ B

(b) يؤخذ...البصر] كبده اذا شرّح وجعل فيها دار فلفل وفلفل ابيض مسحوق وشويت على النار فاذا شال ماؤها وكحل به من بعينيه الماء والغشاوة نفعها G; كبد الاريل تشرّح ويدر عليه دار فلفل ابيض مسحوق ويشوي فاذا استرخاء اكتحل تلك الرطوبة من بداسِر الماء في العين والغشاوة W

(c) وأخذ] من وأخذ *add.* C

12.19: (a) *om.* B

(b) This recipe is attested only in G and W | وسحق...نفعها] ويؤخذ الكبد اشوت فتجفف ويسحق ويتخذ منها برود ينفع من غشاوة العين وظلمة البصر وبدر فيها W

(c) This recipe is attested only in C

12.20: (a) للقولنج وعسر البول] *om.* B | فيجفف] يجفف B | اصاب] *om.* B | أو عسر] وعسر B | صاحب القولنج وعسر البول] صاحب عسر البول والقولنج B | عنه] *om.* B

(b) قضيب...ينطلق] قولنج فاغسله واسقه مائه فانه ينطلق W | فاذا اصاب] واصاب G | قضيبته اذا جفف وحفظ فاذا اصاب انسانا اشر او رياح او قولنج القولنج فغسّله وسقاه ما غسالته اطلق الاسر ونفع القولنج *add.* W

(c) واذا شويت...يبريه] قضيب الايل اذا وجفف ورفع الى وقت الحاجة فمن اصاب القولنج او عسر البول غسل ذلك القضيب بالماء وشربه ابرأه C

12.18 Against the water in the eye and the cataract, deer liver: it has to be taken, cut in slices, with abundant addition of ground long pepper, put on the embers and—once its water has evaporated—rubbed on the eye of the man affected by cataract and water as well, then all these will cease, with the permission of God, may He be exalted.

Deer liver: if it taken, roasted until it is well done, then dried, ground and its filing is taken, then this will be useful against the cataract in the eye, the flowing of water, and it will clear the eyesight.

Deer liver: if pepper is abundantly added to it, and it is put onto the fire, then its water is taken and rubbed on the eyes of the man affected by cataract and water in the eye, then these will cease.

12.19 Deer liver: if it is ground, its powder rubbed on the eyes affected with cataract or yellow water, then these will cease, with the permission of God, may He be exalted.

Ground stag liver: if it is dried, sieved, and applied on the man affected by cataract, obscuration of the sight and the flow of water [in the eye], then this will be useful to him.

Deer liver: if it is roasted, ground, and rubbed on the eyes of the man affected with cataract, then this will cure him.

12.20 Against colic and urine retention, deer penis dried and preserved; when someone is taken by colic or urine retention, the penis will be useful, if put in the water that should be given to the man suffering from colic and urine retention to drink, and then these will cease, with the permission of God, may He be exalted.

Deer penis: if it is dried with fire and reduced, then when a man has urine retention, winds and colic, wash the penis and give him its water to drink, and then he will be freed.

Deer penis: if it is dried and stored, and a man starts to suffer of urine retention, winds or colic, then the penis has to be washed and its water drunk, then this will be useful against the colic.

مخ الايل يغلي بدهن الغار ويخلط بماء القرط الاخضر مع شيء من عسل وشرب به صاحب القولنج وسعال العتيق وضيق النفس نفع جدا

مخ الايل يغلي بدهن الغار ويخلط معه ماء القرط وعسل واسقه للقولنج والسعال على الريق ينفع

12.21 يؤخذ مخ الايل فيذاب على النار ويلقي عليه من دهن الغار جزء ومن العسل جزء ومن القرط جزء الاخضر جزء ويسقي منه صاحب القولنج والسعال وضيق النفس فيبرأ باذنالله تعالى

12.21: (a) فيذاب] يذاب B | الاخضر] *om.* B | فيبرأ] يبرأ B
(b) مخ...ينفع] مخه اذا اغلي مع دهن الغار وخلط معه ماء القرط وعسل بماء حار وشرب منه صاحب القولنج وسعال على الريق نفعه G | واسقه] ويسقي منه W | ينفع] *om.* W
(c) القرط] القرطم C | وشرب به] وشربه C

12.21 Deer marrow: if it is liquefied on the fire, with the addition of one part of myrtle oil, one part of honey, one part of alfalfa and one part of vegetables, and if it is given to the man suffering from colic, cough and weakness of breath to drink, then he will recover with the permission of God, may He be exalted.

Deer marrow: if it is boiled with myrtle oil, mixed with alfalfa water and honey, and given against colic and cough on an empty stomach to drink, then this will be useful.

Deer marrow: if it is boiled with myrtle oil, melted with fresh alfalfa water and a bit of honey, then drunk by the man suffering from colic, chronic cough and weakness of the breath, then this will be useful to him.

١٣. الثعلب

	a	b	c
	ذكر منافع اعضاء الثعلب	الثعلب	باب منافع الثعلب
13.1	يؤخذ مرارة الثعلب تذاف بعسل ويجعل عليه كراويا ويشرب بماء حار في الحمام فينفع من وجع الجنب	مرارته اذا تذاف بعسل ويخلط معها كراويا ويشرب بماء حار تنفع من وجع الجنب	مرارة الثعلب تضاف بعسل ويخلط معها وكراويا ويؤخذ بماء حار لوجع الجنب
13.2	دم الثعلب اذا اخلط معه ملح وورس وجعل في الرأس نفع من القرع ويربي الشعر وينفع من جميع الالم في الرأس	ودمه نافع للقرع والحزاز في الرأس يخلط معه ملح وورس يلطخ على الرأس	ودمه نافع للقزع والحزاز في الرأس والآكل يخلط معه هذا الدم ملح وورس يطلي الرأس فيجود الشعر
13.3	يؤخذ لحم الثعلب وريّته فيطبخ ويخلط معه شحم عتيق ويأكل منه صاحب وجع المفاصل فيبرأ باذن الله تعالى	لحم الثعلب وشحمه يطبخ بزيت عتيق حتى ينهر ويقعد في مرقته من به وجع المفاصل من برد [نفعه]	لحم الثعلب وشحمه يطبخ بزيت عتيق ويدهن النقرس فيبرأ
13.4	يؤخذ شحم الثعلب فيذاف بدهن كادي ويدهن به النقرس فيذهب باذن الله تعالى	شحم الثعلب يذاف ويدهن به النقرس يبرأ	شحم الثعلب اذا اذيب بدهن الكادي ودهن به رجلا صاحب النقرس يبرأ

13.1: (a) يؤخذ] *om.* B | تذاف بعسل] تضاف بالعسل B | ويجعل] ويلقي B | كراويا] كراوية مسحوقة B | في الحمام] *om.* B | فينفع] ينفع B | من وجع] لصاحب وجع B
(b) تذاف] اذيف G | ويخلط معها] *om.* G | ويشرب...الجنب] وشربت نفع من وجع الجنب G | مرارته...الجنب] مرارة الثعلب تضاف بعسل ويخلط معها وكراويا ويؤخذ بماء حار لوجع الجنب W
(c) تذيب] تذاب C | مع كراويا] مع شيء من كراويا C | وتشرب] وشرب C | تنفع لذات] نفع ذات C
13.2: (a) اذا اخلط] يخلط B | وجعل في] يطلي به B | نفع...الرأس] الذي يكون خفيف الشعر فيكثر وينفع القرع وينبت الشعر B
(b) دمه...نفعه] دمه نافع للفزع والحزاز في الرأس والاكال يخلط معه ملح وورس يطلا الرأس فيجود الشعر W; دمه اذا خلط معه ورس وملح ولطخ به الرأس الاقرع وصاحب الحزازة في الشعر نفعه G
(c) للاقرع] لقرع C | والكلل] ولكل C
13.3: (b) الحم الثعلب] حمه G | مرقته] مرقتهم[1] G | ينهر ويقعد في مرقتهم] يتهرّا وقعد في مرقتهم G | برد] نفعه *add.* G | حتى...من برد] فيبرأ ويدهن النقرس W
(c) *om.* C
13.4: (a) يؤخذ...كأدي] شحمه يذاب على النار ويخلط معه دهن كادي B
(b) شحم الثعلب...يبرأ] *om.* W | شحمه اذا اذوب ودهن به النقرس برئ G
(c) شحم الثعلب] لحم الثعلب وريته C | يبرأ] ابرأه C

13. Fox

	a	b	c
	Exposition of the useful properties of the parts of the fox	**The fox**	**Chapter on the useful properties of the fox**
13.1	Fox gall: if it is taken, mixed with honey, with the addition of some caraway seeds, and drunk with warm water in the bath, this will be useful against the pain of the pleurisy.	Its gall: if it is melted with honey, mixed with caraway seeds and drunk with warm water, this will be useful against the pain of the pleurisy.	Fox gall: if it is mixed with honey, melted with caraway seeds and taken with warm water, it will be useful against the pain of pleurisy.
13.2	Fox blood: if it is melted with salt and curcuma, applied on the head, it will be useful against ulcer, it will make the hair grow; in general, it will be useful against all the pains of the head.	Its blood is useful against the ulcers and the impetigo on the head, if it is mixed with curcuma and salt, and spattered on the head.	Its blood is useful against the ulcers, the impetigo on the head and the gangrene, if this blood is melted with salt and curcuma, then rubbed on the head, and it will also be good for the hair.
13.3	Fox meat and its lungs: if they are cooked, melted with some old fat and fed to the man suffering from joints pain, then this will cure him, with the permission of God, may He be exalted.	Fox meat and its fat: if they are cooked with old oil until they are well done and the man suffering from joints pain due to the cold sits in this broth [this will be useful to him].	Fox meat and its fat: if they are cooked with old oil and rubbed on the gout, then this will cure it.
13.4	Fox fat: if it is mixed with pandang oil and rubbed on the gout, then this will make it cease, with the permission of God, may He be exalted.	Its fat: if it is liquefied and rubbed on the gout, then this will heal.	Fox fat: if it is mixed with pandang oil, and rubbed the feet of the man suffering from gout, then he will heal.

13.5	يؤخذ ناب الثعلب ويعلق على من يفزع في نومه فيذهب عنه الفزع باذن الله تعالى	ناب الثعلب يعلّق على الصبي الذي يفزع في نومه فيذهب ذلك عنه	وناب الثعلب يعلّق على الصبي الذي يفزع في نومه فلا يفزع ابدا
13.6	*om.*	*om.*	كليتي الثعلب مسكهما في يده لم ينبح عليه الكلب
13.7	*om.*	*om.*	شحم الثعلب ونابه حيث كان يجتمع اليه البرا[غيث]
13.8	شحمه اذا ذوّب وقطر في الاذن سكن وجعها	شحمه اذا ذوّب وقطر في الاذن سكن وجعها	شحم الثعلب اذا غلى على النار وقطر في الاذن الموجوعة الثقيلة السمع برئت
13.9	*om.*	خصيته ان دفعتها الى امرأة احبتك	وخصيته اذا جففتا تريد في الجماع والانعاظ اذا شرب منه وزن درهم بشراب
13.10	*om.*	*om.*	وزبله اذا سحق بدهن ورد يزيد في الجماع ما شاء ملل الاحليل في وقته
13.11	شحم الثعلب يطلي به عود ويترك في البيت فلا يبقي في البيت برغوث حتى يجتمعوا عليه	شحم الثعلب اذا طليت به شوكا او عودا او تركته في زواية البيت تعلق به البراغيث فتأخذه وتنقضه برا	واذا طلى شحمه على عود ووضع في البيت اجتمع اليه البراغيث وهو عجيب جدا

13.5: (a) يؤخذ ناب...الفزع] نابه اذا علق على صغير يذهب عنه الفزع B
(b) وناب الثعلب] نابه G | يعلّق] علق G | فيذهب ذلك عنه] اذهبه G; فلا يفزع ابدا W
(c) النوم] نومه C
13.6: (c) *om.* C
13.7: (c) *om.* C
13.8: (a) This recipe is attested only in B
(b)This recipe is attested only in G and W | شحمه] وشحم الثعلب W
(c) In L and C this recipe is after 12.10 | شحم الثعلب] شحم الثعلب وريته *add.* C | برئت] برئ ذلك C
13.9: (b) This recipe is attested only in G
(c) *om.* C
13.10: (c) *om.* C
13.11: (a) *om.* B
(b) شحمه...البراغيث] شحمه اذا طلى به عود وبقي في جابن البيت اجتمع عليه البراغيث G; شحمه يطلا به عود ويترك في جابن البيت فيلصق بها البراغيث فينفض عنه W

13.5	Fox canine tooth: if it is hung on the man who is frightened during his sleep, than the fear will leave him, with the permission of God, may He be exalted.	Fox canine tooth: if it is hung on the child who is frightened during his sleep, then this will leave him.	Fox canine tooth: if it is hung on a child who is frightened during his sleep, then he will never be afraid again.
13.6	*om.*	*om.*	If a man holds both the kidneys of the fox in his hand, then the dogs will not bark at him.
13.7	*om.*	*om.*	The fleas will gather on the fat of the fox and its canine tooth, wherever they are.
13.8	Its fat: if it is liquefied and applied in drops inside the ear, then this will calm its pain.	Its fat: if it is liquefied and applied in drops inside the ear, then this will calm its pain.	Fox fat: if it is boiled on the fire and applied in drops inside the aching ear that is hard of hearing, then this will cure it.
13.9	*om.*	Its testicle: if it is thrown towards a woman, then she will love you.	Its testicles: if they are dried, then they will give power to the coitus and to the erection, if one dirham of them is drunk with wine.
13.10	*om.*	*om.*	Its excrement: if it is ground with rose oil, this will increase the power of coitus, no matter how exhausted the urethra is.
13.11	Fox fat: if it is rubbed on a branch and this is left in the house, then not a single flea will remain there, to the point that all of them will gather on the branch.	Fox fat: if it is rubbed on a thorn or a branch and this is left in a corner of the house, then the fleas will stick to it, then you may take it and destroy it outside the house.	If its fat is rubbed on a branch and this is placed in the house, then the fleas will gather there, and this is really amazing.

13.12

من حمل كليتي الثعلب لم ينبح عليه الكلب

من حمل معه كلوتي ثعلب لم ينبح عليه الكلاب

ومن حمل معه كلى الثعلب لم ينبح عليه الكلاب

13.13

ذكر الثعلب اذا علق على من به صداع ابرأه لوقته

وذكر الثعلب يعلّق على من به صداع يسكن ان شاء الله تعالى

ذكر الثعلب يعلّق على من يشتكي الصداع فيزول عنه باذن الله تعالى

13.14

خصوة الثعلب اذا اعطيها للمرأة واكرمتك كراما عظيما

خصية الثعلب اذا اطعمتها امرأة احبتك واكرمتك

خصية الثعلب اذا أخذتها وشويتها واطعمها لمرأة احبك حبا شديدا

13.15

مرارة الثعلب اذا جعل معها وشق واذيبت بماء الكبرات النبطي ودهن زنبق وسعط به المصروع في شهر ثلاث مرات في كل عشرة ايام سقيه وهو اصلح واسهل الادوية

وللجذام يؤخذ مرارة الثعلب واشق من كل واحد جزء ويذاف بماء الكبريت وزنبق ويصعّد به من به جذام ثلاثة ايام في كل الشهر في كل عشرة ايام ويحمي من الخل والبقل ويمنع من الجماع فان جفت ان يشتد به نقي بدنه بمسهل

يؤخذ مرارة الثعلب واشق يذاب الجمع بماء القنبيط ودهن زنبق ويسعط به صاحب الفزع في الشهر ثلاثة ايام وامنعه من أكل الخل واللبن والسمك والجماع يبرأ

13.16

اسنان الثعلب اليمنى اذا علقها عليه من يشتكي وجع الاذن اليسرى ابرأ

اسنان الثعلب من ناحية اليمنى ينفع من به وجع الاذن اذا علقت عليه اليمنى لليمنى واليسرى لليسرى

انياب الثعلب تجفف وتسحق ناعما ويسقي منها صاحب وجع الاذن يبرأ

13.12: (a) *om.* B

(b) من حمل...الكلاب] كليتيه اذا حملا لم ينبح عليه الكلب G | كلوتي] كلوة W | لم] ثم W

(c) من حمل...الكلب] خصوتي الثعلب اذا علقت على انسان لم ينبح عليه كلب C

13.13: (a) ذكر الثعلب] ذكره B | فيزول عنه] يسكن B

(b) وذكر الثعلب...يسكن] ذكره اذا علق على من به صداع سكنه G | يسكن] فيسكن W

13.14: (a) خصية الثعلب...شديدا] اذا اعطيتها لامرأة احبتك حبا شديدا B

(b) *om.* G W

(c) This recipe is attested only in C

13.15: (a) This recipe is attested only in B

(b) مرارة الثعلب] مرارته G | واشق] واشح T; واسج G; واسح W | ويذاف] اذا اذيفا G; ويضاف W | الكبريت] الكزبره G | وزنبق] وزيبق T; زنبق مع G | في كل الشهر] في الشهر كل W | ايام] مرة نفعه *add.* G | ويحمي...بمسهل] وكحمه من اكل الخل والبقل وامنعه من الجماع وان جفتان يطول به الامر فاسهله بدواء G | او يمنع من] *om.* W | جفت ان يشتد به نقي بدنه بمسهل] مسهل حتى ينقي بدنه جففت او يزيد فانقص بريه كالدواء المسهل W

(c) واذيبت] واذيف C | به المصروع] به من يعتريه الصرع C | سقيه وهو اصلح واسهل الادويه] ايام مرة ابرأه وهو دواء نافع C

13.16: (a) This recipe is attested only in B

(b) من ناحية اليمنى] الميامن G; اليمنى W | ينفع...لليسرى] اذا علقت على من به وجع الاذن اليمنى سكن وجعها واسنانه المياسر اذا علقت على من به وجع الاذن اليسرى سكن G; اسنانه الميامن اذا علقت على من به وجع الاذن اليسرى سكن وجعها W

(c) اليمنى] *om.* C | علقها عليه] علقت على C

13.12	The dogs will not bark at the man who carries with him the kidney of a fox.	The dogs will not bark at the man who carries with him both the kidneys of the fox.	The dog will not bark at the man who carries with him the two kidneys of the fox.
13.13	Fox penis: if it is hung on the man suffering from headache, this will make it cease, with the permission of God, may He be exalted.	Fox penis: if it is hung on the man suffering from headache, then this will calm it.	Fox penis: if it is hung on the man suffering from headache, then this will instantly cure him.
13.14	Fox testicle: if it is roasted and fed to a woman, then she will passionately love you.	Fox testicle: if it is given to a woman to eat, then she will love and honour you.	Fox testicle: if it is given to a woman, then she will greatly honour you.
13.15	Fox gall and gum ammoniac: if they are liquefied with cauliflower water and lily oil, inhaled by the man who is scared—three times a month and he should be forbidden to eat vinegar, milk, fish and to have sexual intercourse—then he will recover.	Against elephantiasis: if fox gall and gum ammoniac—one part of each one—is mixed with sulphur water and lily, inhaled by the man effected by elephantiasis—three days every month, every ten days—forbid him from eating vinegar and herbs, and forbid him to have sexual intercourse; if it is dry, then the purification of the body with a purgative will be more intense.	Fox gall: if some gum ammoniac is added to it, then it is liquefied with Nabatean sulphur, water and lily oil, and inhaled by the epileptic man—three times per month, every ten days—he should be given this to drink and then he will be fine, and this is the best and easiest of drugs.
13.16	Fox canine teeth: if they are dried, finely ground and given to the man suffering from earache to drink, then he will recover.	Fox teeth from the right side are useful against earache, if they are hung one the man, the right [teeth] for the right side and the left ones for the left side.	Its right teeth: if they are hung on the man suffering from earache in the left ear, then this will cure him.

13.17	خصية الثعلب اليمنى تجفّف وتسحق ويسقي منها صاحب برد الكلى ووجع المثانة بماء التمر يبرأ	*om.*	خصوة الثعلب اليمنى تجفف وتسحق وتسقي لصاحب وجع الكبد بماء اغلى فيه ثمر فانه ينفع لبرد الكلى وتقطير البول ويزيد في الباه
13.18	*om.*	رية الثعلب تجفـفت وتسحق ويسقي منها وزن درهم بماء ثمر الصرفان مقدار كأس يزيد في الباه ويسخن الكلى	*om.*
13.19	مرارة الثعلب تضاف بماء قشر الجوز الاخضر وماء السلق مغليان ويغسل بهم الوسخ الذي في البدن فانه يزول	يؤخذ من مرارة الثعلب وزن درهم ومن ماء قشر الجوز الرطب وماء العليق المغلى المصفى من كل واحد جزء تذاف فيه المرارة وتلطخ على الموضع الوسح القبيح يتغير لونه	مرارة الثعلب وماء قشر الجوز الاخضر وماء السلق المغلى يذاب الجميع ويطلي به الوضح الفاصح وهو البهق الابيض اي البرص فانه تزيله
13.20	زبل الثعلب يسحق ويذاب بدهن ورد ويطلي به الاحليل عند الجماع فانه يقوي الشهوة	وزبل الثعلب يذاف بدهن ورد ويطلي به الاحليل في وقت الجماع فانه يزيد في الشهوة ويعين على الحبل	زبل الثعلب يذاف بدهن ورد ويطلي به الاحليل عند الجماع فانه يقوي الشهوة
13.21	ان اردت ان تخبر برج الحمام ويهربوا منه فعلق فيه رأس الثعلب فلا يبقي فيه طير	واذا اردت ان تخرب برج حمام وتهرب الطيور منه فاجعل رأس ثعلب فانه لا يبقي فيه طائرا	رأس الثعلب اذا وضع في برج الحمام اخربه واذهب الطيور منه

13.17: (a) This recipe is attested only in B

(c) خصوة الثعلب...في الباه] خصوة الثعلب تجفف وتسحق وتسقي لصاحب وجع الكبد بماء اغلى فيه ثمر فانه ينفع لوجع الكلا وتقطير البول وازاده الباه C

13.18: (b) ريته...الكلى] رية الثعلب تجفّفت وتسحق ويسقي منه وزن درهم فمن به الربو الشديد بماء الشويز المقشّر المصفا مقدار كأس يزيد في الباه وسسحق الكلى G | بماء ثمر الصرفان] فمن به الربو الشديد بماء الشويز المقشّر المصفى W

13.19: (a) This recipe is attested only in B

(b) يؤخذ...لونه] وزن درهم مرارته مع ماء قشور الجوز الرطب واء العليق المغلى المصفى من كل واحد حبة تذاف فيه المرارة ويلطخ به البرص غيّر لونه وقلعه G | ومرارة الثعلب] ومرارة الثعلب W | درهم ومن] فيما W | العليق] الغار W | من كل واحد جزء] اجزاء متساوية W | تذاف فيه المرارة] *om.* W | وتلطخ] ويخلط | الموضع] *om.* W

(c) This recipe is attested only in C

13.20: (a) This recipe is attested only in B

(b) *om.* G | يذاف] يسحق ويضاف W | فانه يزيد في الشهوة] ويزيد الشهوة W

(c) يذاف] اذا اذيب C | ورد] الورد C | ويطلي] وطلى C | عند] حال C | فانه يقوي الشهوة] قواه وقوى الشهوة C

12.21: (a) This recipe is attested only in B

(b) رأس ثعلب] في برج *add.* W | فانه لا] فلا W | رأس الثعلب...طائر] رأس الثعلب اذا جعل في برج الحمام خرب وهرب منه الحمام G

(c) واذهب] واذهبت C

13.17	Fox right testicle: if it is dried, ground and given to the man suffering from kidney coldness and bladder complaint to drink with dates water, then he will recover.	*om.*	Fox right testicle: if it is dried, ground and given to the man suffering from liver complaint to drink, together with the water in which some dates have boiled, then this will be useful against kidney coldness and urine dripping, and it will also increases the sexual potency.
13.18	*om.*	Fox lung: if it is dried, ground and one *miṯqāl* is given to the man suffering from asthma to drink, with one cup of low quality dates water, this will increase the sexual desire and warm the kidneys.	*om.*
13.19	Fox gall: if it is mixed with green nut peel water and beet water—both of them boiled—and this is used to wash the dirt that is on the body, then this will go away.	If one dirham of fox gall is taken, with fresh nut peel water and blackberry water boiled and purified—one part of each one—the gall is mixed with it and spattered on the area of the abominable leprosy, this will change its colour.	Fox gall: if it is mixed with boiled green nut peel water and beet water, rubbed on the plain leprosy—that is the white vitiligo or leprosy—then this will cease.
13.20	Fox excrement: if it is ground, liquefied with rose oil and rubbed on the outer opening of the urethra at the moment of coitus, then this will strengthen the sexual desire.	Fox excrement: if it is mixed with rose oil and rubbed on the outer opening of urethra at the moment of coitus, then this will increase the sexual desire, and will help conceiving.	Fox excrement: if it is mixed with rose oil and rubbed on the outer opening of the urethra at the moment of coitus, this will strengthen the sexual desire.
13.21	If you want that a pigeon house is led to ruin and that the pigeons flee from that, hang on it the head of a fox, and then not a single bird will remain there.	If you want that a pigeon house is led to ruin and that the pigeons flee from that, then place there the head of a fox, and not a single bird will remain there.	If the head of a fox is placed on the pigeon house, then this will destroy it, and the birds will go away.

13.22

مرارة الثعلب يكتحل بها من في عينيه بد والماء والغشاوة ابرأه سريعا

مرارة الثعلب يكتحل بها من به دوء الماء في عينه ويخلط معه الاشياف النافع لهذا الشان ينفعه باذن الله تعالى

مرارة الثعلب يكتحل به من له في عينيه ماء اصفر فانه يذهب عنه والله اعلم

12.22: (a) This recipe is attested only in B
(b) يكتحل] اذا كحّل G | دوء] *om* W | ويخلط] *om*. G | معه الاشياف النافع لهذا الماء فينفعه] مع اشياف النافع لهذا الشان ينفعه G مع اشياف نفعه ;W
(c) مرارة الثعلب...سريعا] واذا اكتحل بمرارة الثعلب من بدا بعينيه ما او غشاوة ابرأها C | In L another recipe is added, with ground crab to reduce the salivation of babies; in C the same recipe is at the end of Ch. 14, see also 14.7

13.22	If a man who has yellow water in his eyes rubs some fox gall on them, then this will heal, and God knows best.	Fox gall: if it is applied on the eyes of the man affected by water in his eyes—and you mix it with the medicaments useful against this—then it will be useful to him.	Fox gall: if it is rubbed on the eyes affected by water and cataract, this will instantly cure them.

١٤. التمساح

	a	b	c
	ذكر منافع اعضاء التمساح	التمساح	باب منافع التمساح
14.1	مرارة التمساح يكتحل بها من في عينه البياض فيذهب عنه باذن الله تعالى	مرارة التمساح للبياض في العين يدهن به	مرارة التمساح اذا اكتحل بها صاحب البياض في العين ابرأه
14.2	كبد التمساح تبخر بها المجنون فيذهب عنه جنونه باذن الله تعالى	كبده يبخّر بها المجنون فيذهب عنه الجنون	كبد التمساح اذا بخر به المجنون اذهب جنونه
14.3	يؤخذ سن التمساح من الجانب الايمن فيبخر المحموم فتزول عنه الحمى النافض باذن الله تعالى	من أخذ شيئا من جانب حنك التمسح الأيسر ويعلق على من به الحمى النافض تركه	سن التمسح من الجانب الايسر اذا علق على المحموم ابرأه لوقته
14.4	شحم التمساح يدهن به عضة التمساح فيسكن عنه المه باذن الله تعالى	شحم التمساح اذا أخذ ووضع على موضع عضة التمساح سكن وجعه	*om.*

14.1: (a) البياض] بياض B | فيذهب عنه] يذهب B
(b) مرارة...به] يكتحل بها للبياض في العين فيبرئه W; مرارته اذا كحّل بها البياض في العين اذهبه G
(c) صاحب البياض في العين] من بعينه بياض من الجدري C | ابرأه] ابرأها C | In C two recipes are added, the first one with crocodile liver against leprosy, كبد التمساح اذا احرق وصار رمادا واذيب بالخل الخمر العتيق وطلى به البرص ابرأه وغير لونه; the second with black cow horn against scabies, وكذلك يفعل في الجرب وقرن البقرة السوداء يفعل ذلك.
14.2: (a) تبخر بها] يبخر به B | فيذهب عنه] يذهب B
(b) *om.* W | يبخّر] اذا بخّر G | فيذهب] ذهب G | الجنون] *om.* G
(c) كبد التمساح...جنونه] واذا بخر المجنون بكبد التمساح اذهب الجنون C
14.3: (a) من الجانب الايمن] من اليسار B | فيبخر] يبخر بها B | فتزول] يزول B
(b) من أخذ] ويؤخذ W | حنك التمساح] حنكه W | الأسير] الايمن والاسير G | ويعلق] فيعلق W; وعلقه G | تركه] فتتركه من ساعته W; ابرأه G
(c) المحموم] من به الحمى C | لوقته] *om.* C
14.4: (a) المه] الالم B
(b) شحم التمساح...وجعه] شحمه يبرأ عن عضته من ساعته W | شحم التمساح] شحمه G | اخذ] *om.* G | وجعه] وبرئ وجعه *add.* G

14. Crocodile

	a	b	c
	Exposition of the useful properties of the parts of the crocodile	**The crocodile**	**Chapter on the useful properties of the crocodile**
14.1	Crocodile gall: if it is rubbed on the eye affected by glaucoma, this will cure it, with the permission of God, may He be exalted.	Crocodile gall: [it is useful] against the glaucoma in the eye, if it is rubbed on it.	Crocodile gall: if it is rubbed on the eye affected by glaucoma, then this will cure it.
14.2	If the insane man is fumigated with crocodile liver, then his insanity will leave him, with the permission of God, may He be exalted.	Its liver: if the insane man is fumigated with it, then the insanity will leave him.	If the insane man is fumigated with the liver of crocodile, then its insanity will go away.
14.3	Tooth taken from the right side of a crocodile's mouth: if it is used to fumigate a feverish man, then will make the fever with shivers cease, with the permission of God, may He be exalted.	If a man takes the teeth from the left side of the crocodile's palate, hangs them on a man suffering from fever with shivers, then God will heal this.	Tooth from the left side [of its mouth]: if it is hung on a feverish man, then this will instantly cure him.
14.4	If the bite of a crocodile is rubbed with its fat, then this will make the pain cease, with the permission of God, may He be exalted.	Crocodile fat: if it is taken and applied on the part bitten by a crocodile, than its pain will cease.	*om.*

14.5	اذا اردت ان تتخذ كبشا للنطاح فأخذ من شحم التمساح ويدهن به قرنه وبين عينيه فلا يقدر كبش به ابدا ولا يقوي به وهذا مليح عجيب	واذا دهن به جبين كبش النطاح ففرّ منه ولا يقربه	شحم التمساح اذا ذوب ودهن به قرن كبش المنطاح لا يقدر عليه كبش ولا يقف له ابدا
14.6	*om.*	واذا طرح في الخليج اصول العيدول وهو دار شَيشعان اصعد التمساح من الماء	*om.*
14.7	من أخذ سن التمساح من جنبه الايمن فعلقه عليك فيحرّ الجماع كثيرا والله اعلم	يؤخذ من اسنان من التمساح من الجانب الايمن فيعلقه الرجل على عضده الايمن فانه يحرك الجماع حركة قوية	سن التمساح من الجانب الايمن اذا علق على الرجل قوي شهوة الجما[ع]

14.5: (a) اذا اردت ان تتخذ كبشا للنطاح] *om.* B | ويدهن] اذا دهن B | قرنه] قرن الكبش النطاح B | فلا يقدر...عجيب] ولا يقدر عليه ولا يقهره والله اعلم B

(b) واذا...ولا يقربه] شحمه اذا طلى به جبهة الكبش النطاح مع جبينه قهر W; وهذا الشحم يدهن به جنب الكبش النطاح فينفر من الكبش الذي يناطحه غريمة الذي يناطحه G

(c) ذوب] *om.* C | كبش المنطاح] من كباش النطاح C

14.6: (b) دار شَيشعان] داسَيسَقان T | واذا طرح] ويطرح W; وان طرح G | في الخليج] في الخليج الذي فيه التمساح *add.* W | العيدول وهو دار شَيشعان] الدار سَيْشان W | اصعد] ظهر W; طلع G

14.7: (a) *om.* B

(b) يؤخذ...قوية] ويقويه فيحرك الجماع *om.* | الرجل] G | وعلق] فيعلقه G | يؤخذ] اذا اخذ G | ويؤخذ من اسنانه من الجانب الايمن فيعلق على عضد الايمن فيحرك الجماع W | فانه يحرك الجماع] تحرك للجماع G | قوية] شديدة G

(c) علق على الرجل] اذا علقه احد عليه C | الجما[ع]] قوى شهوة الجماع C | كانت له قوة عظيمة في الجماع C | In C another recipe is added, with ground crab to reduce the salivation of babies, whereas in L this recipe is at the end of Ch. 13: السرطان اذا سحق بزيت وطلى به ليت الصبيان قطع اللعاب L; السرطان اذا سحق بزيت وطلى لثة الصبيان قطع اللعاب السائل اي الريق المندفق من الفم على صدور الاطفال C.

14.5	If you want to take a ram for butting, take the fat of the crocodile, rub it on its horns and the area between the eyes, then no other ram will never be able to defeat him and will ever be stronger than him, and this is witty and amazing.	If it is rubbed on the forehead of a butting ram, then [its adversary] will flee from him and will not approach him.	Crocodile fat: if it is liquefied and rubbed on the horns of a butting ram, then no other ram will be able to defeat him, nor will dare to go against him.
14.6	*om.*	If the roots of spiny broom—that is the *dār al-šayšʿān*— is thrown in the bay, then this will make the crocodile emerge from the water.	*om.*
14.7	The man who takes the tooth of the crocodile from the right side [of its mouth] and hangs it on you, will warm up the coitus, and God knows best.	If the teeth of the crocodile are taken from the right side of the mouth and hung on the right arm, then this will incredibly excite the coitus.	Crocodile tooth from the right side of the mouth: if it is hung on a man, then this will strengthen the desire of coitus.

١٥. البقر

	a	b	c
	ذكر منافع اعضاء البقر	البقرة	باب منافع البقر
15.1	يؤخذ قرن البقر فيحرق ويسحق فيؤخذ منه جزء ومن دم الاخوين جزء وملح اندراني جزء ويسحق الجميع ويذر على الظهر الدابة وتركب من ساعتها	يؤخذ عظم بقرة السوداء فيحرق حتى يصير رمادا ثم يؤخذ منه جزء ويخلط مع دم الاخوين وملح اندراني من كل واحد جزء وبالسوية ويدر على دبر في ظهر الدواب وتركبها من ساعتك فانه ينفع	*om.*
15.2	يؤخذ قرن البقرة السوداء يحرق حتى يصير رمادا ويذاف بالخل واطلِ به البرص فيزول باذن الله تعالى	قرن البقرة يحرق حتى تصير رمادا ويذاف بالخل ويطلي به البرص ويستقبل الشمس ينصبغ	قرن البقر السود اذا احرق وصار رماد واذيب بالخل الخمر الحادق وطلى به البرص الوضح ابرأه وغير لونه وكذا الجرب
15.3	لبن بقرة سوداء ويخلط معه دقيق السعتر ويجعل على البواسير فيذهب باذن الله تعالى	يؤخذ لبن البقرة ويخلط معه دقيق شعير ويضمد به البواسير يسكن الضربان	لبن البقرة السوداء اذا خلط معه دقيق الشعر وضمد به البواسر سكن وجعه

15: (b) البقرة] البقر G; البقرة السوداء W

15.1: (a) يؤخذ قرن البقر] قرن البقرة السوداء B | الاخوين] الاخين B

(b) يؤخذ...ساعتك] عظم البقرة السودا اذا احرق حتى يصير مثل الرماد يؤخذ منه جزء ومن دم الاخوين جزء وملح اندراني جزء ويدق ويخلط ويذر عقر الدواب G; عظمها يحرق يؤخذ من رماد جزء ويخلط معه دم الاخوين جزء وملح اندراني اجزاء بالسوية ويدر على دبرة ظهر الدابةويدركه ساعة يوضع عليه W | فانه ينفع] *om.* G; فلا يضره صاحبه W

15.2: (a) يؤخذ] *om.* B | يحرق] تحرق B | واطلِ] ويطلي B

(b) قرن البقرة] قرنها G; قرون بقرة W | يحرق] اذا احرق G | حتى تصير رمادا] *om.* G | ويذاف بالخل] واذيف بخل G; يضاف الرمد بخل W | ويطلي] وطلى G; فيبرأ W | ينصبغ] اذهبه G; ويستقبل به الشمس W | ويستقبل الشمس] في الشمس G; موضع *add.* W

(c) وصار...الجرب] احرق الى ان يصير رمادا ويذوّب بخل خمر حادق بكرور ودهن به من فيه برص الوضح أبرأه وغير لونه وكذا الجرب C

15.3: (a) *om.* B

(b) يؤخذ لبن البقرة ويخلط معه] لبن البقر اذا اخلط بدقيق G; لبن بقر سوداء اذا خلط معه W | ويضمد] وضمد G W | البواسير] الناصور والبواسير *add.* W | يسكن الضربان] سكن ضربانها G; سكن ضربان W

(c) وجعه] وجعها C

15. Cow

	a	b	c
	Exposition of the useful properties of the parts of the cow	**The cow**	**Chapter on the useful properties of the cow**
15.1	Cow horn: if it is burnt, ground, one part of it is taken, one part of dragon's blood, and one part of rock salt, everything ground together and applied on the back of the beast, and then you can immediately ride it.	Bone of the black cow: if it is burnt until it becomes ash, then one part of it is mixed with dragon's blood and rock salt—one part of each one, in the same quantity—and poured on the back of the beast, then you can ride it immediately, in fact this is useful.	*om.*
15.2	Horn of the black cow: if it taken, burnt until it becomes ash, mixed with vinegar, and rubbed on the leprosy, then this will cease, with the permission of God, may He be exalted.	Cow horn: if it is burnt, mixed with vinegar, and rubbed on the leprosy, and this is exposed to the sun light, then this will change colour.	Horn of the black cow: if it is burnt, turned into ash, then it is mixed with acid wine vinegar, and rubbed on the leprosy, then this will cure it and will change its colour, and the same happens with scabies.
15.3	Milk of the black cow: if it is melted with wild thyme powder, and applied on the haemorrhoids, then these will go away, with the permission of God, may He be exalted.	Milk of the cow: if it is taken, melted with barley flour, and the haemorrhoids are bandaged with it, then their acute pains will cease.	Milk of the black cow: if it is melted with barley flour, and the haemorrhoids are bandaged with it, then their pain will cease.

15.4

مرارة البقرة السوداء اذا ضرب بالخطمية وغسل بها من في راسه حزازة ابرأه

مرارة البقرة يضرب بها الخطمي ويغسل بها الرأس من الحرارة

مرارة البقر يخلط معها شيء من دقيق الخطمي واطل به الرأس نفع من القرع والحرارة ويربي الشعر ويحسنه

15.5

مرارة البقر السوداء وشيء يشبه الحجر وتسمى بالفارسية جاورد اذا أخذ منها مقدار عدسة واذيفت بماء الاصول وماء الشاهترج وسعط به صاحب اللقوة ومن بصره خفيف صلح حاله

ويكون في مرارة البقرة شيء يشبه بالحناء يسمى بالفارسيّة حاورة يؤخذ منه قدر عدسة ويذاف بماء اصول الرطبة والشهدانج ويسعط للقوة وضعف البصر ينفع

يؤخذ في مرارة البقرة شيء يشبه الحجر وهو يسمى بالفارسية الخاوز تأخذ منه مقدار عدسه ويذاب بماء الاصول السوس وبماء الشاهترج ويسعّط به صاحب اللقوة وضعف البصر ويوجد في مرارة البقرة ذلك

15.6

وكذا اذا سعط من هذا الدواء بماء السلق المصفى اعان على نفعه

ويسعّط به الصداع مقدار عدسة مذوبا بماء السلق الطري مصفى غير مغلى او ماء اصول السلق نافع باذن الله تعالى

om.

15.7

شحم البقرة ومخ الغطام منه يذاف ويدهن به العروق المشنجة فانها تلين العروق والعصب ويلقي في المراهم المنبتة للحم وينفع الجميع الاورام ويصحها

شحم البقر او مخه اذا طلى به الاورام التي في العصب حلله

يؤخذ شحم البقرة وامخاخ الافخاذ فيذاب على النار ويدهن به العروق المشنجة فيمدّها وكان الحكماء المتقدمون يتحدون منه مراهم فينبت بها اللحم الميت

15.4: (a) مرارة البقر] يؤخذ لبن بقر سوداء B | وأطل] ويحشا B | نفع] ينفع B
(b) مرارة البقرة] مرارة البقر G W | يضرب بها] اذا خلطت G; يخلط مع W | ويغسل بها] وبعسل وغسل بها G; ويغسل به W | من الحرارة] نقّي الحزازة منه G; فينقي الحرارة من الرأس W
(c) This recipe is attested only in C

15.5: (a) *om.* B
(b) ويكون في مرارة البقرة شيء يشبه بالحناء] اذا أخذ من مرارة البقر شيء يتحنبه المحصي G; ويؤخذ في مرارة البقرة شيء يشبه بالحجر W | حاورة] جاوازن G; حارّبأن W | يؤخذ منه] *om.* G | ويذاف بماء اصول الرطبة والشهدانج] تذاف بماء اصول الرطبة او بماء الشهدانج G; فتضاف بماء اصول الرطبة او بماء اصول الرطب وبماء الشهبانج W | ويسعط...ينفع] وسعّط بصاحب اللقوة برئ G; ويسعط به للقوة ويضعف البصر فينفع نفعا بينا W
(c) وتسمى] التي يسمى C | واذيفت] واذيب C | وماء الشاهنزج] وهو الشارطوج وهو الشاطراج بماء الاصول C | بصره خفيف] يبصره ضعف C | صلح حاله] نفع نفعا جيدا C

15.6: (b) به الصداع] منه صاحب الصرع G; منه ايضا من به الصرع W | مذوبا] يذاف G; يضاف W | غير مغلى] *om.* G | او ماء اصول السلق] *om.* G W | نافع] نفعه G; فينفع نفعا بينا W
(c) *om.* C

15.7: (a) يؤخذ] *om.* B | فيذاب] يذاب B | به] *om.* B | وكان...الميت] *om.* B
(b) This recipe is attested only in G and W | شحم البقر...حلّله] شحوم البقر ومحاخها تحلل الاورام ويلين الميليه من اللحم W
(c) الغطام منه يذاف] غطامه اذا اذيب C | ويدهن] واندهنت C | العروق...للحم] العروق المشنجة لينها C

15.4	Cow gall: if it is melted with a bit of marshmallow powder and rubbed on the head, then this will be useful against the ringworm and the stinging, will make the hair grow, and will make it nicer.	Cow gall: if it is whipped with marshmallow, then this will wash away the impetigo from the head.	Gall of the black cow: if it is whipped with marshmallow, and the man affected by impetigo washes his head with it, then this will cure him.
15.5	In the gall of cow there is something similar to a stone—called in *ḫāwz* [?] in Persian—if the amount of a lentil of it is taken, mixed with liquorice roots water and fumitory water, and inhaled by the man suffering from facial paralysis and weakness of the eyesight [it will be useful]; this is found in the gall of the cow.	Black gall of the cow: there is something resembling a stone—called *ḥāwra* [?] in Persian—if the quantity of a lentil is taken, mixed with fresh roots water and Indian hemp, inhaled against facial paralysis and weakness of the eyesight, then this will be useful.	Gall of the cow and something similar to a stone—called *ḫāwrad* [?] in Persian—if they are taken in the amount of a lentil, mixed with roots water and fumitory water, then inhaled by the man suffering from facial paralysis and weakness of the eyesight, then this will cure him.
15.6	*om.*	If the man suffering from epilepsy inhales the quantity of one lentil with purified—but not boiled—water of fresh beet or water of beet root, then this will be useful, with the permission of God, may He be exalted.	In the same way, if this remedy is inhaled with purified beet water, then this will enhance its usefulness.
15.7	Cow fat and the marrows of the legs: if it is melted on the fire, and rubbed on the contracted nerves, then this will relax them. The ancient wise men used to make ointments to make the dead flesh grows again.	Cow fat and its marrow: if they are rubbed on the swellings of the nerves, then this will make them subside.	Cow fat and the marrow of its bones: if they are mixed, and rubbed on the contracted veins, then this will loosen the veins and the nerves; and if it is added to the ointments for the growth of the flesh, then this will be useful against all the swellings, and will cure them.

15.8	*om.*	*om.*	دماغ البقرة الوحشية يؤخذ منها مثقال ومن مرارتها نصف مثقال ويطعم للمتحاربين تقع بينها العداوة والبغضة القاطعة
15.9	*om.*	*om.*	الثور اذا نزل عن البقرة ثم بال بعده خذ من ذلك الطين وطلى به الاحليل فانه يهيج الباه
15.10	*om.*	*om.*	شانته اذا جففت وسحقت تنفع لمن يبول في الفراش
15.11	للدوى في الاذن يؤخذ بول الثور يغمس فيه قطنة وتقطّر في الاذن فتبرأ باذن الله تعالى	بول العجل يقطّر منه في اذن من يسمع في اذنه مثل الدوى يذهب به	*om.*
15.12	دم البقر اذا صبّ على الجرح الذي يسيل منه الدم انقطع باذن الله تعالى	دم البقر اذا صبّ منه على الجرح الذي يسيل منه الدم وحبسه	*om.*
15.13	للاسهال يؤخذ مرارة البقر يخلط معها بورق احمر وشحم الحنظل وشيء من عسل فيطلي به المقعدة فينسهل الجوف باذن الله تعالى	مرارة البقر اذا اخلطت مع نطرون وشحم الحنظل وشيء من عسل ويطلي به الموضع المقعد سهّل البطن	مرارة البقرة اذا اذيفت بنطرون احمر وشحم حنظل وقليل عسل وطلى به حول المقعدة اسهل الجوف ويؤخذ منه فتائل تنفع القولنج
15.14	*om.*	واذا قطر منها قطرتين في الاذن الذي يسمع فيها الدوى نفع	*om.*

15.8: (c) يؤخذ] اذا أخذ C | مرارتها] المرارة البقرية C | ويطعم للمتحاربين] ودوب وأكل عليهما متحاربان C | تقع] وقعت C
15.9: (c) الثور اذا...بعده خذ] اذا بال الثور عقيب نزول عن البقرة وأخذ C | الباة] الباة ويقوي الانعاض *add.* C
15.10: (c) شانته...الفراش] [. . .] الثور اذا جففت وشربها من يبول في الفراش بخل وماء بارد نفعه C | In C another recipe is added, with the penis of the bull to give power to the coitus: ذكر الثور اذا جفف وشرب منه اخذ قدر مثقالين بيض برشت كانت له قوة في الجماع وجامع ما شاء
15.11: (a) للدواء في الاذن يؤخذ] *om.* B | فتبرأ] فيزول الدوي B
(b) بول العجل] بول العجول W | اذن...به] الاذن الذي يكون فيها الدوى اذهبه G
15.12: (b) وحبسه] قطعه G; قطع الدم وحبسه W
15.13: (a) معها] فيها B | وشيء من] *om.* B | فيطلي به] ويطلي بها B | فينسهل] فتسهل B
(b) اخلطت مع] اخلط معها G | ويطلي] وطلي G | موضع] *om.* G | *om.* W
(c) اذيفت] اذيبت C | وقليل] وشيء من C | ويؤخذ] واذا اتخذت C
15.14: (b) واذا...نفع] المرارة ايضا اذا قطر منها في الاذن ثلاث قطرات نفع من الدوى الذي فيها G; مرارة البقر اذا اخلط قطر منها في الاذن قطرات في اليمنى نفع من الدوى والطنين W

15.8	*om.*	*om.*	Cow brain: if one *miṯqāl* of it is taken with half *miṯqāl* of its gall, and this is fed to the enemies, then their enmity and hatred will cease.
15.9	*om.*	*om.*	When the bull stops to mount the cow, then he urinates: after this, take this earth and rub it on the outer opening of urethra, then this will excite the sexual desire.
15.10	*om.*	*om.*	Its skull [?]: if it is dried and ground, this will be useful to the man who wets the bed.
15.11	Against the buzzing in the ear, bull urine: if it is taken, a cotton cloth is soaked in it, and the urine is applied in drops inside the ear, then this will be cured, with the permission of God, may He be exalted.	Calf urine: if it is applied in drops inside the ear of the man who hears something like a buzz inside it, then this will cease.	*om.*
15.12	Cow blood: if it is poured on the wound from which blood flows, then this will stop, with the permission of God, may He be exalted.	Cow blood: if it is poured on a wound from which blood flows, then this will staunch it.	*om.*
15.13	To relieve [the bowels], cow gall: if it is taken, mixed with red natron, colocynth grease, and some honey, then the stomach is rubbed with it, the abdomen will be relieved, with the permission of God, may He be exalted.	Cow gall: if it is mixed with natron, colocynth grease, and a bit of honey, and the area of the stomach is rubbed with it, then this will ease the abdomen.	Cow gall: if it is mixed with red natron, colocynth grease, and a bit of honey, and rubbed around the stomach, then this will purge the abdomen, and will be useful against colic.
15.14	*om.*	And if two drops are applied in the ears in which a buzz is heard, then this will be useful.	*om.*

15.15	مرارة البقر اذا يخلط معها دهن ورد وقطران يقطر منها في الاذن الموجوعة يسكن وجعها	واذا خلط معها دهن ورد وشيء من قطران وقطر في الاذن سكن وجعها	مرارة البقر يخلط معها دهن ورد وقطران ويقطّر في الاذن الوجعة فتبرأ باذن الله
15.16	خصى العجل اذا ملحت وجففت وسحقت وشرب منها انسان قواة على النكاح وزاد في الباه	خصى العجاجيل اذا جففت ودقت وشرب منها انسان انعظ و قوى عليه الباه	خصى العجل تشرح وتملح وتبزر وتجفف وتسحق فاذا شرب منها انسان مقدار درهم بقليل لبن حليب ويكون لبن بقره فانه يقوي على الجماع ويزيد في شهوة النكاح
15.17	خثى البقر الرطب يخلط معه رماد وزيت ويضمد به النقرس يسكن المه	خثى البقر الرطب يضمد به النقرس بعد ان يخلط معه شيء من رماد وزيت [فينفع]	*om.*
15.18	*om.*	واذا أخذ منه واحرق نفخ منه في الانف قطع الرعاف	للرعاف يؤخذ حثى البقر اليابس يحرق ويذر في الانف فينقطع الرعاف
15.19	واذا اذيف بالخل وشمه من به الرعاف الدائم قطعت عنه	واذا أخذ منه وذيب بالخل وسعط نفع الرعاف	وكذلك اذيب بالخل كان ابلغ
15.20	قرن البقر يحرق ويسحق وينفخ منه في انف المرتعف يقطع عنه	قرن الثور يسحق ويسقي بالماء ويسعط للرعاف	قرن البقر اذا احرق وصار رمادا يسعط به صاحب الرعاف فينقطع باذن الله تعالى
15.21	واذا شربه من به اختلاف ارياح السدد برئ باذن الله	غظام فخذ الثور اذا احرقت وسعط منه المرعوف ايضا نفعه واذا سقى منه ايضا من به اختلاف نفعه	عظام افخاذ البقر يحرق حتى يصير رمادا ويسقي منها صاحب الارياح في الجوف فيبرأ باذن الله

15.15: (a) فتبرأ] يبرأ B
(b) واذا...وجعها] المرارة ايضا اذا خلطت بدهن ورد وقطران وقطر منه في الاذن نفع ايضا G | *om.* W
(c) مرارة البقر] *om.* C | اذا يخلط] اذا اخلط C | وقطران] *om.* C | يقطر] وقطر C | يسكن وجعها] سكن المها C
15.16: (a) وتبزر] *om.* B | شهوة النكاح] شهوته B
(b) العجاجيل] العجل G | ودقت] *om.* G
15.17: (b) In W this recipe is after 15.19 | احشاء] حثا T | احشاء...فينفع] احشاء البقر اذا خلط مع شيء من رماد وزيت وضمّد به النقرس نفعه G
(c) النقرس] من به النقرس C | يسكن المه] ابرأه C
15.18: (b) واذا أخذ منه واحرق نفخ منه] اخثى البقر اليابس اذا احرق ونفخ منه G; واحشاء البقرة اليابسة اذا احرقت ونفخ منها W
15.19: (b) واذا...الرعاف] وان اذيف بخل وسعّط منه صاحب الرعاف نفعه G; وان ضيفت المحرقة بخل ويسعط بها قطعه ايضا W
15.20: (a) قرن] ولذلك قرن *add.* B
(b) يسحق ويسقي] اذا سحق بمسك G | ويسعط للرعاف] وسعّط به من به الرعاف نفعه G
(c) يحرق ويسحق] اذا احرق وسحق C | عنه] عنه الرعاف C
15.21: (a) فيبرأ] فتزول B
(b) This recipe is attested only in G and W | غظام...نفعه] *om.* W | واذا...نفعه] ويسقي من به اختلاف ينفعهما W
(c) السدد برئ] او بريح الشدد ابرأه C

15.15	Cow gall: if it is mixed with rose oil and tar, and applied in drops inside the aching ear, then this will cure it, with the permission of God.	If some rose oil and some tar are mixed with it, and it is applied in drops inside the ears, then this will calm their pain.	Cow gall: if it is mixed with rose oil and tar, applied in drops inside the aching ears, then this will calm their pain.
15.16	Calf testicles, split, salted, spiced, dried: if a man drinks one dirham of this with a bit of cow milk, then this will give power to the coitus, and increase the desire of sexual intercourse.	Calf testicles: if they are dried, crushed, and a man drinks them, then this will excite him, and strengthen his sexual desire.	Calf testicle: if they are salted, dried, ground, and a man drinks them, then this will give him power in the sexual intercourse, and will increase the sexual desire.
15.17	*om.*	Cow fresh dung: if it is used to bandaged the gout, after that they have mixed with a bit of ash and oil, then this will be useful.	Cow fresh dung: if ash and oil are mixed with it, and they are used to bandage the gout, then this will calm its pain.
15.18	Against the nosebleed, cow dung: if it is taken, burnt, poured in the nose, then this will stop the nosebleed.	Cow dung: if some of it is taken, burnt, and blown inside the nose, then the nosebleed will stop.	*om.*
15.19	Likewise, if it is mixed with vinegar, this will be even more effective.	Likewise, if it is mixed with vinegar, this will be even more effective.	If it is mixed with vinegar and smelled by the man who has a constant nosebleed, then this will stop.
15.20	Bull horn: if it is burnt until it becomes ash, then the man who has a nosebleed sniffs it, then this will stop.	Bull horn: ground, given with water to drink, and sniffed, this will be against the nosebleed.	Bull horn: if it is burnt, ground and blown in the nose of the man with a nosebleed, then this will stop it.
15.21	Bone of cow legs: if it is burnt until it becomes ash, and given to the man affected by the winds in the abdomen to drink, then he will heal, with the permission of God.	Bone from a bull leg: if it is burnt, and the man with a nosebleed sniffs it, then it will be useful to him; and if it is also given to the man affected by a difference [?], then this will be useful to him.	And if the man affected by a variety of obstructing winds drinks it, then he will heal, with the permission of God.

15.22	كعب البقر اذا احرق وسحق وخلط معه سذاب وشربه من معه دود المسمى محب القرع فانه يخرجه من جوفه	كعب البقر اذا احرق وسقى مخلوط مع شراب وطلى على الاسنان نفع وجعها	كعب البقر اذا احرق وسحق ودلك به الاسنان فيزول وجعها
15.23	*om.*	واذا شرب منه مع العسل خرج حب القرع من البطن	*om.*
15.24	واذا شربه بسكتجبيل نفع من الطحال ووجع الكبد	واذا شرب بسكنجبين نفع من ورم الطحال وهيّج الباه ايضا	واذا شرب بسكنجبين نفع من وجع الطحال
15.25	دم البقر من شربه وجمد في مقعدته وشرب شراب السكنجبيل اذابه عنه	من شرب من دم الثور جمد في بطنه وقتله من اصابته هذه العلة وجمد دم الثور في بطنه يسقي سكنجبين وخل صرف حاذق يبرأ ان شاء الله تعالى	*om.*
15.26	اخثاء البقر اليابس يحرق ويسقي لمن به الاستسقاء او من يكون جوفه كبيرا يبرأ باذن الله	اخثاء البقر اليابس اذا احرق وشرب منه من به استسقاء نفعه	[اخثاء] البقر اليابس يحرق ويسحق ويسقي منه صاحب علة الاستسقاء بخل الخمر نفعه

15.22: (a) فيزول وجعها] نفعها B

(b) وسقى مخلوط مع شراب] وسحق وخلط بشراب G | نفع وجعها] نفع من وجعها G | كعب...وجعها] رماد كعب الثور يضاف بشراب ويلطخ على الاسنان ينفع من وجعها W

(c) دود المسمى مجب القرع] دود القرع C | جوفه] الذي في الجوف C | See also 15.23

15.23: (b) شرب] شرب ايضا *add.* G | العسل] عسل G W | خرج] نفع من G; اخرج W | القرع] القرع الذي يكون G; حب القرع W | من البطن] بالبطن واخرجه G; *om.* W

(c) المسمى...جوفه] القرع فانه يخرجه من الذي في الجوف C

15.24: (a) This recipe is attested only in B

(b) بسكنجبين] بسكنجبين ايضا *add.* G; سكنجبين W | ايضا] *om.* G W

(c) *om.* C

15.25: (b) من شرب...يبرأ] واذا شرب انسان من دم ثور جمد في معدته وقتله فاذا اردت خلاصه فاسقي سكنجبين مع خل G; ودم الثور حار اتعيل واذا خمد في المغرة نفعه الخل والسكنجبين W

(c) عنه] عنه وطبعة يحبس الدم *add.* C

15.26: (a) This recipe is attested only in B

(b) This recipe is attested only in G

(c) يبرأ] فانه يبرئه C

15.22	Cow anklebone: if it is burnt, ground, and rubbed on the teeth, then this will be useful for them.	Cow anklebone: if it is burnt, and given mixed with wine to drink, and rubbed on the teeth, then this will be useful against their pain.	Cow anklebone: if it is burnt, ground, melted with rue, and the man suffering from the worms called 'grains of ringworm', then these will come out from his abdomen.
15.23	*om.*	If it is drunk with honey, then the grain of ringworm will come out from the abdomen.	*om.*
15.24	And if it is drunk with oxymel, it will be useful against spleen complaint.	If it is drunk with oxymel will be useful against the swelling of the spleen, and will also excite the sexual desire.	If it is drunk with oxymel, this will be useful against liver complaint.
15.25	*om.*	If a man drinks the blood of the bull, this will coagulate in his abdomen, and will kill him; the one who is affected by this disease, and the blood of the bull has coagulated in his abdomen, should be given some oxymel and pure sour vinegar, then he will heal, God, may He be exalted, willing.	If a man drinks the blood of the cow, this will coagulate in his stomach; but if he drinks some oxymel, then this will dissolve it.
15.26	Cow dry droppings: if they are burnt, ground, and given to the man suffering from dropsy to drink with wine vinegar, this will be useful to him.	Cow dry droppings: if they are burnt and drunk by the man who suffers from dropsy, then this will be useful to him.	Cow dry droppings: if they are burnt, and given to the man suffering from dropsy or from abdomen swelling to drink, then this will heal, with the permission of God.

15.27	*om.*	خشى البقرة اليابس اذا شرب منه واحتقن به نفع من اسهال العارض من قروح الامعاء	لقروح الامعاء يؤخذ خشى البقر اليابس فيسحق ويحتفن به من في جوفه اسهال فيذهب باذن الله تعالى
15.28	اذا تحرقت البشيمة على المرأة وبخرت بشىء خشى البقر وشىء من المرارة وضعت الولد	لسقوط المشيمة تبخر المرأة بخشى البقر ومرارة البقر	اذا مسكت الحامل البشيمة في جوفها فبخرها باخثاء البقر فانها ترميها وكذلك اذا بخّرها بمرارة البقر فترميها
15.29	دم البقر يحبس الدم السائل الذي لم يكف اذا صب حارا	*om.*	*om.*
15.30	مرارة البقر مع العسل والشحم والنطرون يسهل البطن طلى على المقعدة	*om.*	*om.*
15.31	واذا قطر منها في الاذن يسكن الوجع	*om.*	*om.*
15.32	واذا شئت ان تجمع الذباب والفأر في بيت فرش ذلك البيت بمرارة عجل اصفر	واذا اردت ان تجمع الفأر والذباب في بيت فرشه بمرارة عَجل البقر اصفر فانهن يجتمعن	اذا [اردت] ان تجعل الذباب والفأر في البيت فرش فيه مرارة عجل اصفر فيمتلي منهم البيت
15.33	اذا أخذ اخثاء البقر وهو رطب وجعل في قدر فخار جديد وطين رأس القدر وجعل في زبل سبعة ايام واخرجت ما فيها واضفت اليه سذابا يابسا واسقيت منه	يؤخذ خشى ثور فيجعل في قدر ويدفن في الزبل سبعة ايام ثم يخرج ثم يؤخذ شراب ويجعل فيه شىء من السذاب مدقوق ويؤخذ من الاخثاء جزء يسحق	[يؤخذ] اخثاء ثور وهو رطب يجعل في قدرة جديدة ويدفن في زبل سبعة ايام ويخرج فيذاب بشراب عتيق ويذرّ عليه

15.27: (a) *om.* B

(b) خشى البقرة] الاخثاء ايضا G; ورماد احثاء W | منه واحتقن] او احتقن G | من] *om.* W

15.28: (b) لسقوط...البقر] المَشِيمة اسقطتها معها بقيت الذي الامرأة به بخّر اذا البقر اخثاء G; البشيمة اسقط البقر من والمرارة بالاخثاء بخر واذا W | البقر] كذلك مرارة البقر ايضا اذا بخرت بها *add.* G

(c) اذا تحرقت...الولد] واذا تعسرت البشيمة اي الخلاص من الولادة وتبخر بشىء من اخثاء البقر وشىء من المرارة C

15.29: (c) *om.* C

15.30: (c) *om.* C

15.31: (c) *om.* C

15.32: (a) This recipe is attested only in B

(b) فرشه] فرش البيت *add.* G | فانهن يجتمعن] فانهم يجتمعون W

15.33:(a) This recipe is attested only in B

(b) يؤخذ...الشراب] إخثاء ثور رطب اذا جعل في قدر حديد ويطبق ويدفن في زبل سبعة ايام ثم يخرج ويؤخذ شراب فيجعل في شىء من سذاب يابس مدقوق ويؤخذ من الزبل المدفون جزء ويسحق ويخلط بشراب ويسقي منه صاحب الاستسقاء يبرأ G; ولاستسقاء يؤخذ اخثاء ثور رطب فجعل في قدر جديد ويطين و يدفن في زبل سبعة ايام يجمع وقد صار لبنه ويؤخذ شراب ويجعل فيه سذاب يابس مدقوق ويؤخذ من الاخثاء جزء ويسحق ويضاف بهذا الشراب W

(c) البقر] الثور C | وجعل] وترك C | واضفت اليه] وجعل عليه C | واسقيت منه] وشربه C

15.27	Against the ulcers of the intestine: if they are taken, dried, ground, and subministrated with an enema to the one who has diarrhoea in his abdomen, then this will go away, with the permission of God, may He be exalted.	Cow droppings: if they are drunk and administrated with an enema, then these will be useful against the evident diarrhoea due to the ulcers in the intestine.	*om.*
15.28	If a pregnant woman retains the nausea in her womb, fumigated her with the droppings of the cow, then she will expel it. Likewise, if she is fumigated with the gall of the cow, she will expel it.	For the expulsion of the placenta, fumigate the woman with the droppings and the bile of the cow	If the placenta is burnt towards the woman, together with some droppings of the cow and a bit of its gall, then she will deliver the baby.
15.29	*om.*	*om.*	The blood of the cow staunches the bleeding that does not stop otherwise, if it is poured warm on this.
15.30	*om.*	*om.*	The gall of the cow, with honey, fat and soda, purges the abdomen, if rubbed on the posterior.
15.31	*om.*	*om.*	If it is applied in drops inside the ear, then this will stop its pain.
15.32	If you want to put flies and mice in the house, spatter the gall of a yellow calf inside it, then the house will fill up with them.	If you want to gather the flies and the mice in a house, then spatter it whit the gall of a yellow calf, and then they will gather there.	If you want to gather the flies and the mice in the house, spatter this house with the gall of a yellow calf.
15.33	Bull droppings, when they are moist: if they are taken, put in a new cooking pot, buried in the manure for seven days, taken out, mixed with old wine, abundant dry rue is added to this, and it is given	Bull droppings: if they are taken, put in a cooking pot, buried in the manure for seven days, then taken out, a bit of ground rue is added to it, one part of the droppings is	If the excrement of the cow is taken when it is moist, put in a new clay cooking pot, whose opening has to be covered with clay and put in the manure for seven days; than what is inside it should be taken out, added

صاحب الاستسقاء ومن في جوفه كبر ابرأه وازال ذلك عنه

ويذاف بهذا الشراب ويسقي منه صاحب الاستسقاء يبرأ

السذاب يابس ويسقي لصاحب الاستسقاء فيبرأ باذن الله تعالى

15.34

مرارة الثور اذا اذيفت بمقل ازرق محلول بخل وجعلت في حرقة وجعلت على الناسور ابرأته

مرارة الثور قيخلط مع خل خمر ويؤخذ مقل ازرق فيحل بالماء حتى يدوب

[يؤخذ] مرارة ثور يخلط معها شحم يجعل معها مقل ازرق محلول ويجعل على النسور فيبرأ

15.35

مرارة الثور اذا جعل عليها شحم حنظل والرازيانج واذيب الجميع ولطخ به صاحب القولنج اسهله وابرأه

ويخلط معها من شحم الخنظل وقليل رازيانج مدقوق ويدهن به صورة من به القولنج واحتباس الطبيعة يسهل البطن نافع

للقولنج يؤخذ مرارة الثور ويخلط معها شحم الحنظل وماء رازيانج اخضر ويلطخ به جوف صاحب القولنج احتبس الطبع فينسهل طبعه باذن الله تعالى

15.36

مخ الثور اذا اذيب على النار بدهن الغار ودهن الجوز والقى عليه ملح ومسح به اطراف اليدين والرجلين نفع من اليبس الشقاق

مخ الثور يذوب ويلقي معه دهن الجوز نصف جزء والمخ جزئين ويخلطا ويمسح به اليدين والرجلين التي تقرقعت ويبست بالغداة والعشى فانه ينحل التشبّك ويلين الاطراف

يؤخذ مخ الثور يداف بدهن الغار او بدهن الجوز ويلقي على ملح الطعام ويدهن به الاطراف اليدين والرجلين والركب فينحلوا باذن الله تعالى

15.37

اذا أخذ من الحنظل وزن درهم وعجن بمرارة ثور وجعل على صوفة وحملته من تعسر ولادتها ولدت سريعا

يؤخذ من ماء الخنظل الرطب وزن ثلاث قراريط فيخلط مع مرارة الثور ويصب على قطنة او صوفة وتحمله المرأة التي عسر عليها ولادتها فانها تلد سريعا

اذا عسر على المرأة الولادة يؤخذ مرارة ثور فتحل في ماء الحنظل الاخضر ويجعل في صوفة وتتحمل بها المرأة تلد سريعا باذن الله تعالى

15.34: (a) This recipe is attested only in B
(b) مرارة...يدوب] مرارة الثور اذا خلط مع خل ويؤخذ مقل ازرق فيحل بماء ويخلط مع المرارة ويصيّر على خرقة وتجعل على الناصور يبرأ G; يؤخذ مرارة ثور فتضاف بخل خمر ويؤخذ خل خمر ومقل ازرق ويخلط بماء ويخلط مع المرارة ويصير في خرقة على نصور W
(c) اذا اذيفت] اذا جعل عليه C | وجعلت] ووضعت C
15.35: (a) به جوف] *om.* B | طبعه] *om.* B
(b) ويخلط] مرارة ثور اذا خلط *add.* G | وقليل] *om.* G | ويدهن] ولطخ G | صورة من به] صاحب G | يسهل] نفع وسهل G | نافع] *add.* G | ويخلط...نافع] ولطخ معه على صاحب القولنج واحتباس الطبيعة اسهل W
(c) مرارة الثور] *om.* C | والرازيانج] والزيامج L, الرازابينج C | واذيب] ثم اذيب C | صاحب] جوف من به C | اسهله وابرأه] ابرأه وحلّه C
15.36: (a) يؤخذ] *om.* B | يداف] يداب B | بدهن الغار او] *om.* B | على] *om.* B | الاطراف] اطراف B | اليدين والرجلين] يديه ورجليه B
(b) مخ الثور يذوب] *om.* W | ويلقي...ويخلطا] يخلط الجميع جزئين على النار ويلقي عليه نصف جزء من دهن الغار ونصف جزء من دهن الجوز G; ولخفاف اليدين والرجلين وشهبها ويلقي عليه من نصف جزء من دهن الفار ودهن الجوز بصف جزء وملح جزئين يخلط الجميع W | التي تقرقعت ويبست] *om.* G | ينحل التشبّك ويلين الاطراف] يحل البرد والتشبّك ويلين ذلك G; ذلك التشبيك ولين الاطراف W
15.37: (a) اذا...سريعا] الطلق على المرأة يؤخذ مرارة ثور فتحبلها فتلده سريعا B
(b) يؤخذ...سريعا] مرارة ثور مع ثلاث قراريط من ماء الحنظل الرطب يعجن به ويجعل ذلك في صوفة وتتحمل به المرأة فانها يسهل عليها الولادة G; ولعسر الولادة يؤخذ الحنظل الرطب وزن قراط فتعجن بمرارة ثور بخل ويصير في صوفة وتحمل المرأة تلد من ساعته W
(c) وجعل] وجعلت C | ولادتها] عليها الولادة C

to the man suffering from dropsy to drink, then he will recover, with the permission of God, may He be exalted.

taken, ground, mixed with wine, and given to the man suffering from dropsy to drink, then he will heal.

to dry rue, and given to the man suffering from dropsy and large abdomen to drink, then this will cure him, and make this stop.

15.34 Bull gall: if it is taken, mixed with fat, some liquefied blue bdellium is added to it, and this is applied on the fistula, then this will heal.

Bull gall: mixed with wine vinegar, blue bdellium has to be taken and mixed with water.

Bull gall: if it is mixed with liquefied blue bdellium and vinegar, wrapped in a piece of cloth, and apply on the fistula, then this will cure it.

15.35 Against colic, cow gall: if it is taken melted with a bit of colocynth grease and green fennel water, spattered on the man suffering from colic and constipation, then will purge his him, with the permission of God, may He be exalted.

If it is mixed with colocynth grease and a bit of ground fennel, rubbed on the figure of the one suffering from colic and constipation, then this will purge his abdomen and cure him.

Bull gall: if the grease of colocynth and fennel are added to it, mixed and spattered on the man suffering from colic, then this will purge and cure him.

15.36 Bull marrow: if it is taken, mixed with laurel oil and nut oil together with cooking salt, rubbed on the extremities of hands, feet, and knees, then this will relax them, with the permission of God, may he be exalted.

Bull marrow: if it is mixed and nut oil—half part of oil and two parts of marrow—then they are mixed, the hands and the feet that have cracked are wiped with it—in the morning and in the evening—then this will loosen the contraction and relax the extremities.

Cow marrow: if it is mixed on the fire with laurel oil and nut oil, salt is added to it, and wiped on the extremities of hands and feet, then this will be useful against the dry lacerations.

15.37 When the a woman has difficulties in giving birth, bull gall: if it is taken, dissolved in green colocynth water, put in a piece of cloth, and the woman carries it, then she will quickly give birth, with the permission of God, may He be exalted.

If three carats of fresh colocynth are taken, mixed with bull gall, poured on a cotton or woollen cloth, and the woman who has difficulties in giving birth carries it, then she will quickly deliver.

If one dirham of colocynth is taken, kneaded with bull gall, then put in a woollen of cloth, and the woman who has difficulties in giving birth carries it, then she will quickly deliver.

15.38	ذكر الثور اذا جفف وسحق ناعما وحشى في بيضه واستعمل فانه يقوي الجماع ويعين على النكاح	يؤخذ ذكر الثور يجفف ويؤخذ منه شيء يسير فيسحق ويجعل في بيضة يتم رشت ويحسرها الانسان يزيد في الباه والجماع زيادة بينة	ما يقوي ويزيد في شهوة الجماع يؤخذ ذكور الثور فتجفّف وتسحق ناعما ويجعل منه في بيضه برشت ويتحساه الرجل فيقويه على ذلك
15.39	وينفع لضربان المفاصل	دماغ الثور يذاب بدهن ينفع من ضربان المفاصل	لضربان المفاصل يؤخذ دماغ الثور يداف بدهن ورد وتمسح به المفاصل فيسكن الضربان باذن الله تعالى
15.40	قضيب الثور الاحمر يخفف ويسحق ويسقي منه المرأة مثقال في شراب عتيق يسكن عنها غلمة النكاح	قضيبة الثور الاحمر يجفف ويسحق ويسقي المرأة منه وزن مثقال بنبيذ صرف يقطع عنها شهوة الجماع	يؤخذ قضيبة الثور يجفف ويسحق ويسقي منه المرأة وزن مثقال فتزول عنها علة النكاح
15.41	خصى العجل الاصفر اذا جففت وسحقت استغر اعان اعانة عجيبة	*om.*	*om.*
15.42	بول الثور اذا خلط بعسل نحل بلا نار وتكحل به من في عينيه غشاوة خلاها عنه ويحد البصر ويزيل الظلمة	بول الثور يخلط معه عسل ويكتحل به من الغشاوة وظلمة البصر فانه يحد البصر ويقوي النظر	لتقوية البصر يؤخذ بول ثور احمر ويخلط بعسل ويكتحل به فانه يقوي البصر ويزيل الغشاوة
15.43	خصوة الثور الاحمر تملح بملح وزاج اصفر وتجفف وتسحق ناعما وتذاب	خصية الثور الاحمر اذا ملّحت بملح وزاج اصفر يؤخذ منها جزء يذاف بدهن	خصى الثور الاحمر يشق ويجفف ويملح ويسحق والقى عليها زاج اصفر

15.38: (a) ما يقوي ويزيد في شهوة الجماع يؤخذ] *om.* B | برشت] ينمرشت B | على ذلك] على الجماع ويزيد في شهوته B
(b) يؤخذ] *om.* G W | الثور المستفحل] الثور المستفحل يجفف ويسحق ويؤخذ منه شيء يسير يلقي على بيضة برشت وتشرب فانها *add.* G W | ويؤخذ…بينة] تريد في الباه عجبا G; يجفف ويؤخذ منه شيء يسير فيسحق ويلقي على بين مرشت وويحشاها فتريد في الجماع حتى تريد العجب W
(c) واستعمل] واكلها C | فانه يقوي] قوى C | ويعين على النكاح] *om.* C
15.39: (a) يداف] يذاب B
(b) ذاب…المفاصل] ينفعه الوجعة به المفاصل يذاف وتدهن G | *om.* W
(c) This recipe is attested only in C
15.40: (a) This recipe is attested only in B
(b) قضيبة] دماغ W | ويسقي المرأة منه] ويسقي منه المرأة G; ثم يسقى منه المرأة W | مثقال بنبيذ صرف] مثقالين بنبيذ خالص G; مثقال نبيذ صلب W | يقطع] تنقطع G; فينقطع W
(c) يخفف ويسحق ويسقي] اذا خفف وسحق وشربت C | شراب] خمر C | يسكن] سكن C
15.41: (c) *om.* C
15.42: (a) البصر] النظر B | فانه يقوي] فيقوي B
(b) به] منه G W | فانه يحد البصر] *om.* G W | ويقوي النظر] *om.* G
(c) بول الثور] بول الثور الاحمر C | ويحد البصر ويزيل الظلمة] *om.* C
15.43: (a) والقى] والورم الاحمر B | ويجفف ويملح ويسحق] وتملح وتجفف وتسحق ويلقي B
(b) يؤخذ منها جزء] *om.* G | يذاف] وأذيفت G | ويطلي] موضع G | ينفع] نفع من G | اذا طلى به] *om.* G | W
(c) تملح بملح] اذا جعل فيها ملح C | وتجفف وتسحق] وجففت وسحقت C | وتذاب] واذيبت C | ويطلي] وطلى C | يحلل] حلله C | واذا طلى…وجعها] وسكن وجع المفاصل عنه C

15.38	What gives power and increases the desire of coitus, bull penis: if it is taken, dried, finely ground, put inside an egg to drink, and a man should licks it up, then this will give power to the coitus, and will increase the desire.	Bull penis: if it is taken, dried, a bit of it is taken, ground, put in an egg, and the man removes it, then this will improve the desire and the coitus in a tangible way.	Bull penis: if it is finely ground, stuffed into an egg and eaten, then this will give power to the coitus, and will help the sexual intercourse.
15.39	For the sharp pains in the joints, bull brain: if it is taken, liquefied with rose oil, and wiped on the joints, then their pangs will calm.	Bull brain: if it is mixed with oil, it will be useful against the sharp pains of the joints.	And this will be useful against the pangs of the joints.
15.40	Bull penis: if it is taken, dried, ground, given to the woman in the quantity of one *miṯqāl* to drink, will make cease for her the disease of the sexual intercourse.	Penis of the red bull: if it is dried, ground, given to the woman to drink, in the quantity of one *miṯqāl* with pure wine, then this will cut off her sexual desire.	Penis of the red bull: if it is dried, ground, and one *miṯqāl* of it is given to the woman to drink in some old wine, then her lust for the sexual intercourse will be calmed.
15.41	*om.*	*om.*	Testicles of the yellow calf: if they are dried and ground, then this will give a surprising and amazing help [to the coitus?].
15.42	To strengthen the eyesight, urine of the red bull: if it is taken and applied on the eyes, then this will strengthen the eyesight and make the cataract cease.	Urine bull: if it is mixed with honey, applied on the eye of the man affected by cataract and obscuration of the eyesight, then this will sharpen and strengthen the eyesight.	Bull urine: if it is mixed with honey—without fire—and rubbed on the eyes of the man affected by cataract, then this will make it cease, it will sharpen the eyesight and cure the obscuration.
15.43	Red bull testicles: if they are split, dried, salted, ground, yellow vitriol is poured on them, and this is	Red bull testicle: if it is seasoned with salt and yellow vitriol, one part of it is taken, mixed with henna oil,	Red bull testicle: if it is seasoned with salt and yellow vitriol, dried, finely ground, liquefied with henna berry oil and rubbed on the moist

بدهن تمر حناء ويطلي به الحاشى يحلل واذا طلى به من به وجع المفاصل سكن وجعها

الحناء ويطلي موضع الضربان والورم في الجسد ينفع

ويدهن به المفاصل والورم في الجسد فيذهب باذن الله تعالى

15.44

دم الثور الاحمر اذا خلط معه الدقيق وجعل في الشمس الى ان ييبس وسحق بعسل ودهن زنبق وشرب منها صاحب وجع الكبد مثقال بماء حار في الحمام برئ

دم الثور يخلط معه دقيق الارز ويخبز ويشرب منه وزن مثقال بماء حار لوجع الكبد الشديد

لوجع الكبد يؤخذ دم ثور احمر ويخلط معه دقيق ارز ويجعل في الشمس حتى يجف ويلتّ بعسل ودهن زنبق ويشرب منه وزن مثقال واحد فيسكن باذن الله

15.45

دماغ الثور اذا اذيف وهو طري بدهن كادي وقطر منه في الاذن الموجوعة الشديدة الضربان سكن ضربها وازال المها

دماغ الثور الطري يذاف بدهن كادي ويقطر في الاذن الوجعة يسكن الوجع باذن الله تعالى

لوجع الاذن الشديد يؤخذ دماغ لثور الطري ويداف بدهن الكادي ويقطر في الاذن فيسكن باذن الله تعالى

15.46

رية البقر اذا أخذتها المرأة معها حال جماعها فانها تحبل

واذا كانت المرأة لا تحبل فخذ من ورق الغبيراء جزء ويدق ويعجن بمرارة بقرة وتمسكه المرأة معها ويجامعها الرجل فتحبل باذن الله تعالى

[اذا] كانت المرأة لا تحبل فيؤخذ ورق الغبيراء يدق مع رية البقر وتمسكه المرأة ويجامها وزوجها فانها تحبل

15.47

مرارة البقر الاسود اذا اكتحل بها من لا يقدر على قرأة فص الخاتم فانه يقوي على ذلك يحد النظر

مرارة بقرة سوداء يكتحل بها من لا يقرأ فص خاتم من ضعف بصره فيحدّ بصره ويقويه

اذا اردت ان تقرأ فص اي خاتم اردت فخذ مرارة بقر سوداء فاكتحل بها ساعة ما تذبح فانك تقرأ فص اي خاتم شئت

15.44: (a) دقيق ارز] ازرق S | يجف] يسخن B | واحد] بماء حار B
(b) دم الثور] دمه ايضا G; وخصية الثور الاحمر W | يخلط معه] يخلط معها W | ويخبز] ويجعل في الشمس حتى يجفّ ويسحق ويلتّ يعسل وزنبق add. G
الوجع] ينفع من وجع G | W
(c) دم الثور الاحمر] om. C | وجعل] وترك C | وشرب منها] وشرب منه C | صاحب] من به C | برئ] ابرأه C
15.45: (a) om. B
(b) الطري] الكبير G | يذاف] يضاف W | ويقطر] ويقطر منه G | الوجعة] om. W | يسكن الوجع] تسكن G; فيسكن الوجع W
(c) اذيف] اذيب C | وهو طري] طريا C | المها] وازال وجعها add. C
15.46: (a) This recipe is attested only in B
(b) واذا...فتحبل] تحبل مرارة بقرة تعجن بورق غبيراء مدقوق وتحمله المرأة يجامعها الرجل G | om. W
(c) رية البقر...تحبل] رية البقر اذا حملت منها المرأة حال جماع حبلت باذن الله عز وجل C
15.47: (a) om. B
(b) فص] نقش G | من...ويقويه] حدّ بصره وقوى G | من لا يقرأ فص خاتم] om. W
(c) لا يقدر...النظر] حد حدت النظره C

rubbed on the joints and the swelling on the body, then these will go away, with the permission of God, may He be exalted.

and rubbed on the area of the acute pains and the swelling on the body, then this will be useful.

swelling, then this will subside; and if it is rubbed on the man suffering from joints pain, then their pain will be calmed.

15.44 Against liver complaint, blood of the red bull: if it is mixed with rice flour, left in the sunlight until it dries, then it is mixed with honey and lily oil, one *miṯqāl* of it is drunk with warm water, then the pain will calm, with the permission of God, may He be exalted.

Bull blood: if it is mixed with rice flour, baked, and one *miṯqāl* is given to drink with warm water, this will be against the intense pain of the liver.

Blood of the red bull: if it is mixed with flour, left in the sunlight until it dries up, ground with honey and lily oil, and drunk by the man suffering from liver complaint—one *miṯqāl* with warm water in the bath—then he will recover.

15.45 Against the intense pain of the ears, young bull brain: if it is taken, mixed with pandang oil, and it is applied in drops inside the ear, then the pain will calm, with the permission of God, may He be exalted.

Young bull brain: if it is mixed with pandang oil, and applied in drops inside the aching ears, then the pain will calm, with the permission of God, may He be exalted.

Bull brain: if it is mixed with pandang oil when it is still fresh, and applied in drops inside the severely aching ear, then this will calm its pangs, and will make his ache cease.

15.46 If a woman does not get pregnant, some rowan leaves have to be taken, ground with the lung of the cow, and the woman should keep it in her hand and have sexual intercourse, then she will get pregnant.

If the woman does not get pregnant, take one part of rowan leaves, grind them, knead it with cow gall, the woman should carry it, the man should take her, and then she will get pregnant, with the permission of God, may He be exalted.

Cow lung: if the woman carries it with her at the moment of the sexual intercourse, then she will get pregnant.

15.47 If you want to read the stone of any seal you want, take the gall of the black cow, apply it on the eyes when it is slaughtered, and then you will read the stone of any seal you want.

Gall of the black cow: if it is applied on the eyes of the man who cannot read the stone of a seal because of the weakness of his eyesight, then this will sharpen and strengthen his eyesight.

Gall of the black cow: if it is applied on the eyes of the man who cannot read the stone of a seal, then this will strengthen and sharpen the eyesight.

15.48	يؤخذ سمن بقر عتيق تذاف بدهن سوسن خالص ويجعل في مغرفة جديدة ويجعل على نار لينة فاذا اذاب فخذ منه ربع مثقال وسعط به صاحب اللقوة وادهن به وجهه فتزول اللقوة باذن الله	يؤخذ من سمن بقر عتيق جزء ودهن سوسن جزء ويخلطان جميعا ويصيران في مغرفة جديد على نار لينة ثم يصير في قارورة ويختم عليه فاذا اردت ان تعالج به فخذ منه وسعط به للقوة واطلى الجانب المسترخى فانه نافع	واذا أخذ بسمن البقر العتيق ودهن السوسن اذا خلطا وجعلا في مغلفة جديد وغلى النار وصار في اناء اذا سعط منه صاحب اللوقة بربع مثقال واذا دهن به صاحب العصب المسترخى نفعه
15.49	اذا اردت ان تقوي على الجماع فتأخذ سمن بقري خالص وبزر كرفس ووزن الجميع سكر ويسحق الجميع ويلقي على السمن فانه يقوي على الجماع ويزيد في الباه	يؤخذ من بزر الكرفس جزء ويدق وينخل ويخلط معه سكر ابيض مثله ومثل سمن بقر ويشرب منه ثلاثة ايام فانك تجامع مع ما شئت	واذا خلط ببزر الكرفس المنخول ومثله سكر ابيض واستعمل منه قوى الجماع وزاد الباه
15.50	*om.*	*om.*	مرارة البقر اذا خلط ببزر قطوناء مدقوقة وتحملت بها المرأة في صوفة نفع من ورم الارحام
15.51	للبهق يؤخذ روث البقر اليابس فيدق ويعجن بخل خمر ويدلك به البهق فيذهب باذن الله تعالى	خثى البقر اليابس يسحق ويعجن بخل حاذق ويطلي على موضع البهق ينفع	زبل البقر الخيس يدق ويعجن بالخل ويطلي به البهق ويجلس في الحمام ساعة فانه يدهب

15.48: (a) *om.* B
(b) يؤخذ...عليه] سمن البقر العتيق يؤخذ منه جزء وسوس جزء ويخلطا جميعا ويجعل في مغرفة حديد على النار لين ويصير في قارورة وتختم G; واللوقة
فاذا اردت ان [فخذ...نافع | W بسمن بقر عتيق جزء ودهن سوسا جزء ويخلطان جميعا ويصيران في مغرفة على النار لينة ثم يصير في قارورة وتختم عليه
W ويطلي منه الجانب المسترخى [فاذا...نافع | G تعالج به صاحب اللقوة فاطلى منه الجانب المسترخى وسعّط منه يبرأ
(c) واذا أخذ بسمن البقر العتيق] سمن البقر C | وجعلا] وتركا C | وصار] وجعل C | اذا سعط منه صاحب اللوقة] لوقت الحاجة C | دهن به] اندهن C
15.49: (a) فتأخذ] فخذ B | كرفس] ومن البورق من كل واحد جزء *add.* B | الجميع] الحراج B | فانه] فانه يقوي عند الحاجة *add.* B
(b) يؤخذ] سمن البقر يخلط معه جزء G | ويدق وينخل] المدقوق المنخول G | معه سكر ابيض] ومن السكر الابيض G | ومثل سمن بقر] مثله G W | ويشرب] *om.* W | فانك] فانه G W | شئت] ما شاء G W
(c) قوى الجماع وزاد الباه] من اراد قوة الجماع نفعه جدا وزاد في الباه قوة عظيمة C
15.50: (c) مرارة البقر] *om.* C | مدقوقة] *om.* C | وتحملت] وحملتها C
15.51: (b) يسحق...ينفع] نفعه البهق به وطلى بخل عجن اذا G | على موضع] مواضع اليمن W | ينفع] فيقلعه W | In G another recipe is added, one with cow dung to treat the stings of the hornet: الاخثاء ايضا الرطب واليابس بالخل ايضا يسكن وجع لسعة الزنبور G
(c) يدق ويعجن] دق وعجن C | ويجلس] وجلس C | فانه يدهب] ادهبه C

15.48 Cow old fat: if it is mixed with pure iris oil, put in a new ladle on a light fire; once it has liquefied, take a quarter *miṯqāl* of it, and the man suffering from facial paralysis inhales it and rubs his face with it, then the paralysis will cease, with the permission of God, may He be exalted.

Cow old fat: if one part of it is taken with one part with iris oil, these are mixed together, put in a new iron ladle on a light fire, then put in a long-necked flask and sealed; then, when you want to cure it, take it, use it for inhalation against facial paralysis, and rub it on the flaccid side, and then this will be useful.

If some old fat of the cow and iris oil are melted, put in a new ladle, boiled on the fire, and poured in a vessel, when the man suffering from facial paralysis inhales a quarter *miṯqāl* of it, and when the man with flaccid nerves applies it, then this will be useful to him.

15.49 If you want to increase the power of coitus, take some pure cow grease, celery seeds, and sugar in the same quantity of the rest, everything has to be ground and added to the grease, then this will increase the power of coitus and the sexual desire.

If one part of celery seeds is taken, ground and sieved, mixed with the same quantity of white sugar, and the same quantity of cow fat, then it has to be drunk for three days, and then you will have all the sexual intercourse you want.

If celery seeds, ground and sieved, are mixed with the same quantity of white sugar, and taken, then the coitus will be empowered, and the sexual desire will increase.

15.50 *om.*

om.

Cow gall: if it is mixed with ground dark psyllium, and the woman carries it in a woollen cloth, then this will be useful against the pain of the womb.

15.51 Against vitiligo, dry cow excrement: if it is taken, ground, kneaded with wine vinegar, and rubbed on the vitiligo, then this will heal, with the permission of God, may He be exalted.

Cow dry excrement: if it is kneaded with vinegar, and rubbed on the vitiligo, then this will be useful.

Cow dry excrement: if it is ground, kneaded with vinegar, and rubbed on the vitiligo while sitting in the bath for one hour, then this will cease.

15.52	اذا اصاب المرأة وجع في الاحشاء وورم في الرحم فيؤخذ مرارة بقري سوداء والقى عليها بزر قطوناء مسحوقه وتتحمل به المرأة فتبرأ باذن الله تعالى	يؤخذ مرارة البقرة ويخلط معها بزر قطوناء وتجعل منه المرأة يسكن الورم العارض في الرحم	مرارة البقر اذا خلطت ببزر قطوناء مدقوقة وتحملت بها المرأة في صوفة نفع من ورم الارحام
15.53	*om.*	وان طليت إناء بشحم بقر اجتمعت عليه البراغيث	*om.*
15.54	للصفار في الوجه والجسد يؤخذ لبن البقرة وهو حار فيشرب على الريق فيزول الصفار والابهار باذن الله تعالى والحيض منه ينفع للبواسير ووجع المقعدة	لبن البقر نافع لمن به صفار وهزال يشربه حارا على الريق اياما متولية	لبن البقر اذا شرب وهو حار على الريق نفع من البواسير ووجع المقعدة
15.55	*om.*	والحيض منه ينفع للبواسير ووجع المقعدة	*om.*
15.56	يؤخذ اخثاء البقر رطبا او يابسا ويطلي به لسعة الزنبور والهوام تبرأ باذن الله تعالى	خثى البقر اليابس او الرطب يخلط مع خل ويطلي على موضع لسع الزنبور فيسكن الوجع من ساعته	اخثاء البقر اذا اذيف بالخل سكن لسعة الزنبور العقرب
15.57	لليرقان والربو على الفؤاد يؤخذ سمن بقري فيذاف ويلقي عليه مر وكثيراء وكندر ويستعمل فيبرأ باذن الله تعالى	وسمن البقر يخلط مع شيء من مر وكندر وكثيراء ويسقي للربو وللسعال ويذهب اليرقان	سمن البقر مع مر بطارخ وكثيرة وكندر اذا شرب منه صاحب اليرقان والربو والسعال العتيق ابرأه

15.52: (a) In S and B this recipe is after 15.49 | فيؤخذ] فخذ B | بقري] بقرة B | مسحوقة] مسحوق B | وتتحمّل] وحمّل B
(b) وتجعل منه المرأة] *om.* G | يسكن] ينفعها من G | العارض] *om.* G | يؤخذ... الرحم] يؤخذ للورم العارض في الارحام add. G وتتحمل به المرأة في صوفة W مرارة بقرة يخلط معها بزر قطوناء فتحمله المرأة في صوفة فيسكن الورم
15.53: (b) طليت] طلى G | اجتمعت] اجتمع G W
15.54: (a) البقرة] بقرة B | فيشرب] يشرب B | والابهار] *om.* B | والخيض] والخيض والالبنها B | ينفع] يصلح B
(b) نافع...متولية] ولبن البقر نافع لمن به صفرة اللون وبهز وهزال يشربه حار G; لبن البقر اذا شرب حارا على الريق اياما متوالية نفع من صفار الوجع والهزال W على الريق اياما متوالية ويشرب يمخيض وللبواسر وضعف المعدة
15.55: (b) والحيض] والحيض والالبنها *add.* B | ينفع] يصلح B
15.56: (a) البقر] الثور B
(b) خثى البقر] *om.* G | اخثاء بقرة W | يابسة او رطبة] اليابس او الرطب W | مع خل] مع شيء من خل *add.* W
15.57: (a) فيذاف] يداف B | فيبرأ] *om.* B
(b) يخلط] اذا خلط G | مع شيء] بشيء G | ويسقي] واسقى منه صاحب *add.* G | للربو وللسعال] الربو والسعال G; للربو او للسعال W | اليرقان] اليرقان نفعهم *add.* G W
(c) وكندر] وكندر وهو الحصالبان الذكر *add.* C | صاحب] من به C | العتيق] المقرح C

15.52	If a woman happens to have bowel complaint and womb swelling, the gall of a black cow has to be taken, some ground black psyllium is added to it, and the woman carries it, then she will heal, with the permission of God, may He be exalted.	Cow gall: if it is mixed with dark psyllium, and a woman carries it, then this will be useful against the evident swelling of the womb.	Cow gall: if it is mixed with ground dark psyllium, and a woman carries with her it in a woollen cloth, then this will be useful against the swelling of the womb.
15.53	*om.*	If the fat of the cow is rubbed on a vessel, then the fleas will gather there.	*om.*
15.54	Against the yellow complexion of the face and the body, cow milk: if it is taken when it is warm, drunk it on an empty stomach, then the yellow complexion and breathlessness will cease, with the permission of God, may He be exalted.	Cow milk: it is useful to the one affected by paleness and consumption, if it is drunk warm on an empty stomach for some days in the same quantity.	Cow milk: if it is drunk when it is warm on an empty stomach, then this will be useful against haemorrhoids and pain of the posterior.
15.55	*om.*	Its menstrual blood is useful against haemorrhoids and pain of the backside.	*om.*
15.56	Cow droppings: if they are taken—either moist or dry—rubbed on the sting of the hornet and of other obnoxious insects, then these will heal, with the permission of God mat He be exalted.	Cow dung, moist or dry: if it is mixed with vinegar, and rubbed on the place of the hornet sting, then the pain will immediately calm.	Cow droppings: if they are mixed with vinegar, this will calm the pain of hornet and scorpion stings.
15.57	Against jaundice and asthma of the heart, cow fat: if it is taken, mixed, some myrrh, goat's horn and incense are added to it, and used, then these will heal, with the permission of God, may He be exalted.	Cow fat: mixed with a bit of myrrh, incense and goat's thorn, and given to drink against asthma and cough, also jaundice will go away.	Cow fat, with *baṭāriḫ* [?] myrrh, goat's thorn and incense: if it is drunk by the man suffering from jaundice, asthma and chronic cough, then this will cure him.

15.58 يؤخذ حجر يقال له الحاوور وهو يؤخذ في مرارة البقرة ويسحق ويخلط معه مسك خالص ويجعل في صوفة وتتحمل به المرأة فتزول عنها البروكة في الرحم والماء الاصفر فيبرأ باذن الله تعالى

واذا كان في رحم المرأة الماء الاصفر يؤخذ من الحروان الذي يكون في مرارة الثور جزء ويخلط معه شيء من مسك واشق واجعله على [صوفة] لون السماء وتمسكه المرأة فيذهب الماء الاصفر من رحمها

واذا أخذ حجر الحادود الذي يكون في مرارة البقر سحق ناعما بمسك عراقي ويسحظ ويجعل في صوفة وتحتمل به المرأة التي في رحمها الماء الاصفر يزول

15.58: (a) الحاوور] الحاوزن B | البقرة] *om.* B | البرودة] البرد B
(b) يؤخذ] فيؤخذ W | الحروان] الحلفاء G; الجوان W | الذي يكون في مرارة الثور] *om.* G W | ويخلط...ويخلط] في المرأة به وتتحمل واشق مسك من وشيء
W ويخلط معه شيء من مسك واشق ويجعل في صوفة لون السماء فتمسكة المرأة فيذهب الماء الاصفر G; صوفة بلون السماء يذهب
(c) ويسحق] *om.* C | ويجعل] وجعل C | وتحتمل] وحملته C | يزول] ازال ذلك عنها C

15.58 The stone called *ḥāwūr* [?], and it can be found in the gall of cow: if it is taken, ground, mixed with pure musk, wrapped in a woollen cloth, and the woman carries it, then the accumulation of liquid and yellow water in her womb will cease, with the permission of God, may He be exalted.

If there is yellow water inside the womb of the woman, one part of the *ḥarūn* [?]—that is in the bile of the bull—has to be taken, mixed with some musk and gum ammoniac, wrapped in a woollen cloth of the colour of the sky, and the woman should carry it, then the yellow water will go away from her womb.

If he stone called *ḥadūd* [?], that is in the gall of the cow, is taken, finely ground with Iraqi musk, wrapped in a woollen cloth, and the woman who has yellow water in her womb carries it with her, then this will cease.

١٦. الفرس

	a	b	c
	ذكر منافع اعضاء الفرس	الفرس	باب منافع الفرس
16.1	يؤخذ حافر الفرس فيحرق ويسحق ناعما ويخلط بطلاء خالص ويجعل منه في صوفة وتحمّل به المرأة فان الجنين سريعا ان كان حيا وان كان ميتا	يؤخذ حافر الفرس تحرقه حتى يصير رمادا ثم تذيف منه شيء بطلاء فتحمّله المرأة بصوفة فانه يخرج الولد من الرحم وان كان ميتا	حافر الفرس اذا احرق وسحق ناعما وخلط بطلاء خالص وجعل منه على الصوفة وحملت به من يعسر ولدها يخرج حيا كان او ميتا
16.2	يؤخذ خصى الفرس فيشرح ويملح ويجفف ويسحق ناعما ويذاف بمني الرجل الحار ويلطخ النقرس فيزول باذن الله تعالى	وخصية الفرس العتيق يشق ويملح بملح وصبر ويجفف ويؤخذ منها في وقت الحاجة فيسحق ويذاف بماء حار ويلطخ به النقرس [يذهب]	خصوة الفرس اذا سحقت بملح وأخذ منها شيء يسير واذيبت بماء حار وطلى به النقرس اذهب المه
16.3	*om.*	واذا بخّر بها النجل لم يقربها الزنابير	واذا بخر بهذا الدواء النحل لم يقربه الزنابير
16.4	يؤخذ لبن جحرة سوداء وبزر بنج يسحق ويعجن به اللبن ويعمل مثل حى البندق ويحرز عليه في جلد الايّل فكلما علق على المرأة حامل فيسقط ولدها والله أعلم	لبن الفرس يعجن به [بنج] ويؤخذ منه جزء ويصير في جلد ايل ويعلق المرأة عليها يسقط ولدها	لبن الفرس السوداء يدق ببنج ويعجن به ويعمل مثل الجوز واذا علق به على المرأة القت جنينها

16: (b) الفرس] الخيل G
16.1: (b) يؤخذ...ميتا] حافر الفرس اذا احرق وسحق واذيف يطلي وحمّلت منه المرأة في صوفة اسقطت الولد سريعا G; يأخذ حافر الفرس ثم يضاف من رماده ويطلي وتحمّله المرأة بصوفة فيخرج الولد وان كان ميت W
(c) بطلاء خالص] بطلاء وهو الخمر الخالص C | وحملت به] وحملته C | ولدها] الولادة عليها C | يخرج حيا كان او ميتا] اسرع نزول الولد حيا كان او ميتا C
16.2: وخصية الفرس] خصيته G | بملح] *om.* W | ويؤخذ منها في وقت الحاجة] *om.* G | ويذاف] وتذاف G; ويضاف W | به النقرس] يذهب به ارجل المنقرس G; على النقرس W
(c) بملح] بالملح C | بماء حار] بالماء الحار C | به النقرس] به وجع النقرس ابرأه C
16.3: (b) بها] منه G | النجل] النحل ايضا *add* G | يقربها الزنابير] لم يقربه الزنبور G
(c) الزنابير] الدبور C
16.4: (b) الفرس] *add.* الفرس السوداء G; *add.* الفرس الاسود W | يعجن] اذا عجن G; اذا يعجن W | ايل] اريل T | ويؤخذ منه جزء] *om.* G W | ويصير] واخرز G; ويعمل منه جوره ويخرز W | ويعلق...ولدها] وعلقت على المراة اسقطت الولد سريعا G; وتعلقه المرأة عليها فتسقط ولدها W
(c) يدق] اذا اذيب C | ويعمل] ويعمل منه C | علق به] *om.* C | القت] ارمت C

16. Horse

	a	b	c
	Exposition of the useful properties of the parts of the horse	**The horse**	**Chapter on the useful properties of the horse**
16.1	Horse hoof: if it is taken, burnt, ground, melted with pure liquid pitch, put it in a woollen cloth, and a woman carries it, then she will quickly give birth, no matter if her foetus is alive or dead.	Horse hoof: if it is taken, burnt until it becomes ash, pounded and mixed with some pitch, and a woman carries it in a woollen cloth, then the baby will come out of the womb, even if it is dead.	Horse hoof: if it is burnt, finely ground, mixed with pure liquid pitch, put it in a woollen cloth, and carried by a woman who has difficulties with her baby, then this will come out, alive or dead.
16.2	Horse testicles: if they are cut in slices, salted, dried, finely ground, mixed with warm human sperm, and spattered on the gout, then this will cease, with the permission of God, may He be exalted.	Horse testicle: if it is split, seasoned with salt and aloe, dried, taken at the moment of need, then ground, mixed with warm water and spattered on the gout, then this will go away.	Horse testicle: if it is ground with salt, a little bit of it is taken, mixed with warm water, and rubbed on the gout, then its pain will go away.
16.3	*om.*	If the bees are fumigated with it, then the hornets will not approach them.	If the bees are fumigated with this remedy, then the hornets will not approach them.
16.4	Black mare milk: if it is taken with the seeds of white henbane, made in a sort of pill, kept in the skin of a deer, and hung on the pregnant woman, then she will lose her baby, and God knows best.	Horse milk: if it is kneaded with white henbane, one part of it is taken, wrapped in the skin of a deer, and hung on a woman, then she will lose her baby.	Black horse milk: if it is ground with white henbane, and kneaded with it, then given the shape of a nut; and if this is hung on a woman, then she will expel her foetus.

16.5	اذا اردت ان تقتل الفرس فاسقيها زرنيخ اصفر مسحوق فتموت سريعا وكذلك جميع الدواب اذا سقى الزرنيخ	واعلم ان الخيل اذا سقيت الزرنيخ الاحمر قتلها وكذلك غيرها من الدواب	واذا سقيت الخيل الزرنيخ الاحمر قتلها وكذلك غيرها من الدواب اذا سقى الزرنيخ الاحمر قتله
16.6	قلله لطرد البعوض من البيت فلا يقربه بعوضة	واذا أخذ شعرة من ذنب فرس وجعلتها ممدودة على باب بيت لم يدخل ذلك البيت بغوض ما دامت عليه	واذا اردت ان تطرد البعوض من البيت ولا يقربه ابدا خذ شعرة من ذنب الفرس ومرها على الباب بكمالة فلا يقربه البعوض ابدا
16.7	اذا اردت ان تخرج للصغير اسنان بلا وجع ولا الم فتعلّق عليه سن الفرس فتخرج اسنانه بلا وجع ولا الم	وان أخذت شيئا من اسنان الفرس تريد اسنانه خرجت بلا الم ولا وجع ولا اذي	سن الفرس اذا علق على الطفل عند الطلوع اسنانه لا يتالم ولا يلحقه نكد
16.8	يؤخذ كبد الفرس تشوي وتشمّم لصاحب وجع الكبد واليرقان فيبرأ باذن الله تعالى	زيادة كبد الفرس ينفع من اليرقان الظاهر تشوي وتشقق صاحب اليرقان رايحته	كبد الفرس اذا اشويت وشقت في وجه صاحب اليرقان وشم رايحتها برئ وزيادة كبد الفرس ابلغ
16.9	للسعال والربو على القلب يؤخذ لبن جخرة حمراء او دمها فيسقي لصاحب العلّة فيبرأ باذن الله تعالى	لبن الفرس يسقي من به الربو والسعال العتيق	[لبن] الفرس اذا شربه صاحب السعال والربو الذي على القلب ابرأه
16.10	اذا اردت تسمّ النشاب فاحميها واسقيها عرق الخيل فاوفع في شيء الا هلك وهو من السموم القاتلة	عرق الخيل يسم به نصول النشاب بعد ان يحمي وتسقي به فلا تصيب انسانا الا قتله	*om.*

16.5: شرب [سقيت G; اسقيت W
C اذا شربه [اذا سقى الزرنيخ الاحمر قتله | C وقتل غيرها [وكذلك غيرها | C الزدنيخ [الزرنيخ (c)
16.6: (b) أخذ [أخذت G | وجعلت [وجعلتها G | يدخله [يدخل ذلك البيت G | عليه] *om.* G | *om.* W
C لم [فلا | C ومررت بها [ومرها | C ذنب الفرس اذا اخذ شعرة من ذيل [خذ شعرة من ذنب | *om.* C [واذا اردت ان تطرد البعوض من البيت ولا يقربه ابدا (c)
16.7: (b) سن فلو فرس اذا علق على صبي خرجت اسنانه بلا وجع [وان...اذي G | *om.* W | *om.* W
16.8: اذا شويت وتنشق منها صاحب اليرقان نفعه [ينفع...رايحته G | *om.* W
C ابراه [برئ | C من به [صاحب (c)
16.9: (b) اذا شرب منه صاحب الربو والسعال العتيق نفعه [يسقي...العتيق G | *om.* W
16.10: (b) In T this recipe is after 16.11 | يسم [سنّ اذا G | النشاب [السهام G | يحمي...قتله [تحمي فلا تمرّ بشيء الا قتله G | *om.* W

16.5	If you want to kill a horse, give it ground orpiment (yellow arsenic) to drink, then it will quickly die; likewise with all the beasts, when they are given arsenic to drink.	Know that the horse, when it is given realgar (red arsenic) to drink, then this will kill it; likewise with the other beasts.	If the horses are given realgar (red arsenic) to drink, this will kill them; likewise with the other beasts, when they are given realgar (red arsenic) to drink, this will kill them.
16.6	Take a smaller quantity to chase the mosquitos away from the house, and not a single mosquito will approach it.	Hair from the tail of the horse: if it is taken, stretched over the door of the house, then the mosquitos will not enter it as long as it remains there.	If you want to chase mosquitos away from the house, and that they never approach it again, take a hair from the tail of the horse, stretch it precisely over the door, and then the mosquitos will never approach it again.
16.7	If you want that the teeth of a child comes out without any pain or ache, hang on him a tooth of the horse, and then his teeth will come out without any pain or ache.	If the tooth of a foal is hung on a child, then his teeth will come out without any pain.	Horse tooth: if it is hung on the child at the moment in which his teeth come out, then this will not be painful, and will not give any trouble.
16.8	Horse liver: if it is taken, roasted, inhaled by the man suffering from liver complaint and jaundice, then he will heal, with the permission of God, may He be exalted.	Appendance of the horse liver: it will be useful against evident jaundice, if it is roasted, and the man affected by jaundice splits and smells it.	Horse liver: if it is roasted, and split in front of the man suffering from jaundice, and he sniffs its smell, then he will heal; and the appendance of horse liver is even more effective.
16.9	Against cough and asthma due to the heart, milk of a red mare or her blood: if it is taken, given to the man suffering from these diseases to drink, then he will recover, with the permission of God, may He be exalted.	Horse milk: it has to be given to drink against asthma and chronic cough.	Horse milk: if the man suffering from cough and asthma due to the heart drinks it, then this will cure him.
16.10	If you want to poison the arrowheads, make them red-hot and quench them with horse sweat, then these will not touch anything without destroying it, and this is one of the deadly poisons.	Horse sweat: to poison the arrowheads after that they have been made red-hot and quenched with it, and then they will not touch a man without killing him.	*om.*

16.11	عرق الفرس اذا شربته الحبلي اسقط ولدها	عرق الفرس ان أخذ منه ومزج بنبيذ وسقيت منه امرأة حامل اسقطت في الحين	اذا اردت ان تسقط المرأة الجنين من جوفها فاسقيتها عرق الخيل فانها سقط سريعا
16.12	مرارة الفرس اذا خلط معها مر ولبان ذكر وسنبل طيب من كل واحد جزء وشرب بماء الكمون ربع في الحمام لمن يبول الدم يبرأ	مرارة الفرس يخلط معها من كذا وسنبل ولبان وسعد ويشرب منه ثلاث قراريط بماء الكمون لمن يبول الدم	يؤخذ مرارة الفرس ويلقي عليها مر ولبان ووسنبل الطيب وسعد كوفي من كل شيء جزء وويسحق الجميع ويذاب بماء الكمون ويسقي منه لمن يبول دم فيبرأ باذن الله تعالى
16.13	اذا اردت ان تصلب الزجاج حتى يصير كالحديد يؤخذ من حوافر الفرس وصعدها بالقرع والانبيق واستقطر ماؤها كالورد واطل به الزجاج حتى يصير كالحديد فانه يتصلب ويقوم مقام النحاس وهو من الغرائب	اذا اردت ان تصلّب الزجاج حتى يكون اشد الحديد فخذ حوافر الخيل النقية الصافية فتصعد بماء في جرة خضراء ثم خذ ما قطر منها فاطلى على الزجاج الشامي من داخله ومن خارجه ثم اتركه حتى يجف ثم اطله ثانية وجففه وثالثة وجففه ثم ادنه من النار قليلا حتى يحمي فانه يصلب ولا يكسر	اذا اردت ان تصلّب الزجاج فيصير مثل الحديد فخذ خوافر الخيل فيصعّد ماؤها في الانبيق حتى يقطّر مثل الماء ورد فيؤخذ ذلك الماء ويطلي به الزجاج فانه يتصلب ويبقي مثل الحديد ولا يكاد ينكسر وهو عجيب مليح
16.14	*om.*	وادر فيه الذهب والفضة واطبخ فيه منهما اردت فانه يقوم مقام قدر النحاس	*om.*
16.15	اذا اردت ان تزيل الغطيط عن النائم ضع اسنان الفرس تحت رأسه	اسنان الفرس الفحل يصير تحت رأس من يغطّ في منامه فيذهب ذلك عنه	*om.*

16.11: (b) عرق...الحين] العرق ايضا ان مزج بنبيذ وشربت منه امرأة حامل اسقطت ولدها G | *om.* W
(c) اسقط] ارمت C
16.12: (b) مرارة...الدم] مرارتها اذا خلط مع مر ولبان وسعد وسنبل وشرب منه من يبول الدم وزن ثلاث قراريط بماء الكمون نفعه G | *om.* W
(c) مر] مر بطارخ وحصى *add.* C | ربع] ربع مثقال C | يبرأ] يبرأ فائدة C
16.13: (b) اشد] مثل G | النقية الصافية] *om.* G | فتصعد] فصاعدها G | بماء] *om.* G | جرة] خرقة T | خضراء] خضراء او انبيق *add.* G | على] به G | داخله] داخل G | خارجه] خارج G | وثالثة] واطله مرة ثالثة G | يصلب] يتصلب G | ولا يكسر] عجبا G | *om.* W
(c) يؤخذ] فخذ C | وصعدها بالقرع والابليق] كما في الكركرة استعطرها C | ماؤها كالورد] ماء الوردة C | الزجاج] الزجاج الصوري وغيره *add.* C | حتى يصير] *om.* C | كالحديد] *om.* C | من الغرائب] فائدة غريبة C
16.14: (b) واطبخ فيه] *om* G | قدر] *om.* G | *om.* W
16.15: (b) يصير] اذا جعلت G | من يغط] انسان ينغط G | منامه] نومه G | فيذهب ذلك عنه] اذهب عنه ذلك G | *om.* W
(c) اذ اردت...رأسه] اسنان الفرس اذا وضعت تحت رأس نائم لم يبق يغط في نومه C

16.11	If you want that a woman loses the foetus in her womb, give her the sweat of a horse to drink, then she will immediately lose it.	Horse sweat: if it is taken, diluted with wine, and drunk by a pregnant woman, then she will have a miscarriage on the spot.	Horse sweat: if it is drunk by a pregnant woman, then she will lose her baby.
16.12	Horse gall: if it is taken, mixed with myrrh, olibanum, nardus and Kufic sedge—one part of each one—everything ground and liquefied with cumin water, and given to the man who urinates blood to drink, then he will recover, with the permission of God, may He be exalted.	Horse gall: if some nardus, olibanum, and sedge are mixed with it, three carats of it have to be drunk with cumin water by the man who urinates blood.	Horse gall: if it is mixed with myrrh, olibanum and nardus—one part of each one—drunk with one quarter of cumin water in the bath by the man who urinates blood, then he will heal.
16.13	If you want to harden the glass and make it like iron, take the hooves of the horse, make their water evaporate in an alembic until it precipitate like rose water; take this water, and rub it on the glass, then this will harden, it will be as resistant as iron, and it will not be possible to break it, and this is amazing and witty.	If you want to harden the glass to the point that it becomes harder than iron, take the clean and pure hooves of the horse, let them evaporate in a green flask, then take what precipitates from it, and rub it on the Syrian glass—from the inside and the outside—then leave it there until has dried, then rub it a second time and let it dry, then a third time and let it dry; then bring it close to the fire until it becomes red-hot, then this will harden and will not break.	If you want to harden the glass to the point that it becomes like iron, take the hooves of the horse, make evaporate their water in the cucurbit and the alembic, let its water precipitate as it is done with the rose, rub it on the glass until it becomes like iron, then this will harden, and will become similar to copper, and this is one of the curious marvels.
16.14	*om.*	If it is poured on gold and silver, and one of them is cooked in it, then this will become like copper.	*om.*
16.15	*om.*	Stallion teeth: if they are put under the head of a man who snores in his sleep, then this will cease.	If you want that the snoring of a sleeping man ceases, put the teeth of the horse under his head.

16.16	اذا اردت تداوي عقر الدابة اغلى بول الفرس على النار والقى عليه نطرون احمر وضفار بيض وفلفل ووشق واطبخ الجميع واجعله على عقر الدابة يبرأ	بول الفرس اذا [غلى] على النار والقى عليه نطرون وصفار بيضة وقرفة وفلفل فهو اجود ما يكون لدبر الدواب تبلّ به قطنة ويحشي	يؤخذ بول الفرس يغلي على النار يضاف اليه صفارة البيض ونطرون احمر فيه وفلفل ويسحق الجميع ويعجن وهو دواء مليح لقلع الزنابير من الدابة
16.17	ان القى على ذلك شيء من العسل ووضع على الجرح أكل اللحم الميت وربي اللحم الحي	وان احتجت الى ذلك لجراحة أخذت منه قليلا وادقه بشيء من عسل وقطر على الجرح فانه يقطع اللحم الميت وينبت اللحم في الموضع سريعا	وينفع ايضا للجرح اذا تنسر نزل على الدواء قليل عسل نحل ويلصق على الجرح مثل المرهم فيأكل اللحم الميت ويربي غيره باذن الله تعالى
16.18	*om.*	الفرس الانثى اذا كان عنوفا ووطئتْ على اثر وطئة ذئب او دقت فجر عوقها يذهب الوداق	*om.*
16.19	الفرس العقوق اذا تودقت خذ من عرقها واجعله ذلك فانها تنصلح وكد	*om.*	للفرس اذا ودقت فخذ عرقها واجعله في صوفة وحمّلها به فانها تسكن باذن الله تعالى
16.20	اذا اردت ان توثب علها حمارا فاذا اجرى عرقها دلت وخضعت	وكذلك اذا اردت ان [لا] تنفروا عليها حمارا فانها اذا جر عرقها خضعت للحمار	*om.*

16.16: (b) والقى عليه] مع G | وصفار بيضة] وصفرة البيض G | وقرفة] وقنّه G | فهو اجود ما يكون] فانه نافع G | تبلّ به] يبلّ بقطنة G | *om.* W
(c) اذا اردت تداوي عقر الدابة] *om.* C | اغلى بول الفرس] بول الفرس غلى C | وضفار بيض] وضفار وبيض C | واطبخ] وطبخ C | واجعله] وجعل C
16.17: (b) وان...سريعا] وان جعل وشقه على جرح مع شيء من عسل فانه يقطع اللحم الميت ويبرأ سريعا G | *om.* W
(c) ان القى] واذا القيت C | العسل] العسل نحل *add.* C | ووضع] ووضعت منه C
16.18: (b) الفرس...الوداق] الفرس الانثى اذا وطيت على اثر ذيب ازلقت G; الفرس الانثى اذا كان عقر ماء وطئتْ على ابر وظنه رنت ادرقت W
16.19: (c) العقوق] العقور C | ذلك] في صوفة C | فانها تنصلح وكد] وحملها لها فايها تنصلح C
16.20: (b) وكذلك...للحمار] والفرس اذا ودقت ويرسن الحمر فجر عرقها سكن منها G; والفرس الانثى اذا ودقت فحزرت فجر عرفها فضع له W
(c) اذا اردت] وكذا اذا اردت C | اجرى] جرى C

16.16	Horse urine: if it is boiled on the fire, with egg yolk, red soda, and pepper—everything ground and kneaded—this will be a good remedy for the sting that the hornets give to the beasts.	Horse urine: if it is boiled on the fire with soda, egg yolk, cinnamon and pepper, then this will be the best that there is against the ulcers of the animals, if a cotton cloth is moistened with it and stuffed [inside the ulcer].	If you want to cure the bubos of a beast, boil the urine of the horse on the fire, add to it some red soda, yolk, pepper and gum ammoniac, cook everything, and apply these on the bubos of an animal, and this will heal.
16.17	This is also useful for the wounds, if you add a bit of honey to this remedy, applying it on the wound as an ointment, then this will remove the dead flesh, and will make the rest of the flesh grow, with the permission of God, may He be exalted.	And if you need this for a wound, take a bit of it, grind it with some honey, and apply it in drops on the wound; then this will remove the dead flesh, and will make the flesh grow quickly in that area.	And if some honey is added to this, and applied on the area of the wound, this will eat the dead flesh, and will make the living flesh grow.
16.18	*om.*	If some fiery mares walk over the tracks of the wolf, or bump against the first part of the obstacle, then the hot temperament will go away.	*om.*
16.19	For horses, when they stamp: take their sweat, moisten a woollen cloth with it, and let the horses carry it, then they will calm down, with the permission of God, may He be exalted.	*om.*	If the recalcitrant horse is restless, take its sweat and apply this to on it, and then its behaviour will be corrected, and it will work hard.
16.20	*om.*	Likewise, if you want that they do not flee from donkeys, then, when their sweat flows, will submit to the donkey.	If you want that a donkey mounts a mare, make her sweat flow, then she will submit to him.

16.21	للطحال يؤخذ طحال فرس عربي فانقعه في الخل يوما وليلة وجففه واذا جف فاسحقه فاذا اردت ان تعالج به المريض فخذ منه وزن مثقال وخلّا صاحب الطحال يجري كرتين ثلاثة حتى ينتفخ الطحال واسقه الطحال بشراب عتيق ثلاثة ايام فيزول الطحال باذن الله تعالى	يؤخذ طحال فرس عربي ينقع في خل خمر عتيق ابيض يوما وليلة ثم يخرجه وتعلقه في الشمس حتى يجف فاذا تعالج به فخذ منه وزن مثقال فدقه حتى يصير مثل الكحل وامر صاحب الطحال يعدوا حتى ينقتح طحاله ويربوا في بطنه وامره فليستف طحال الفرس مدقوقا ويشرب به رطلا من طلاء عتيق يفعل ذلك على الريق ثلاث مرات يوما ويوما فانه يبرأ	طحال الفرس ينقع في الخل يوما وليلة ثم يخرج يجفف في الشمس ويسحق ناعما ثم يومر صاحب الطحال يجري حتي يتعب ويربو الطحال في جوفه فيسف من ذلك الطحال المسحق ويشرب بعده رطلا من الخل الخالص يفعل ذلك ثلاثه ايا[م] متوالية يبرأ
16.22	يؤخذ دماغ الفرس فيذاب على النار ويلقي عليه شيء من الصبر والمر والبورق والعسل ويعمل منه مرهم ويلقي على الجرح فيأكل اللحم الميت ويربي اللحم الحى يلتحم الجرح	دماغ الفرس الانثى اذا القى عليه الصبر والبورق والمر والعسل ثم اغلى على النار حتى يصير ويخلط فهو اجود ما يكون من المراهم للجراحات	[اذا القى] على صبر وبورق احمر وعسلا وطبخ الجميع على النار حتى يصير مرهما اذا وضع منه على اي جرح كان ختم به
16.23	اذا كانت المرأة لا تحبل فيسقي لبن الفرس من حيث لا تعلم ويجامعها الرجل في ان ذلك فانها تحبل باذن الله تعالى	واذا كانت المرأة لا تحبل تسقي لبن فرس وهي لا تدري ويواقعها الرجل على المكان فتحبل	*om.*
16.24	للتخمة يؤخذ سن فرس النهر وهو من السباع موجودة في النهر ويعلق على من هلك من التخمة فانه يبرأ باذن الله تعالى	فرس النهر وهو من السباع الموجودة في النيل يخذ سنه فيعلق على من اشرف على الموت من وجع المِعدة من التخمة والامتلاء	*om.*

16.21: (b) يؤخذ طحال…به] ولوجع الطحال طحال فرس عربي اذا نقع في خل خمر عتيق ابيض يوما وليلة ثم يخرج ويعلّق في الشمس حتى يجف ثم خذ منه وزن مثقال فدقه حتى يصير مثل الكحل ثم أمر صاحب الطحال حتى يعدّ وحتى ينتفخ طحاله ويربو في بطنه خله يستفّ ذلك المدقوق ويشرب بعده رطلا من رطلا عتيق يفعل ذلك على الريق ثلاث مرات يوم بين يومين فانه يبرأ G; خذ…يبرأ] والورم العارض فيه يؤخذ طحال فرس عربي فينقع في خل خمر عتيق ابيض يوم وليلة ثم يعلق في الشمس حتى يجف فاذا اردت ان تعالج فخذ منه مثقال واسقه وقُلْ لصاحب الطحال حتى يعدُوا وينتفخ طحاله ويربوا في بطنه فاذا فعل ذلك مرة يستفّ ما دقة له ويشرب بعده بطل W | Here the text of W ends, followed by two pages filled with various *muğarrabāt* recipes

(c) ينقع] نقع C | يوما] يوما كاملا C | حتى يجري] ان يجري الى ان C | فيسف] فيستف C | يبرأ] فانه يبرأ C | يبرأ] *add.* C اذا أخذ عسل نحل ووضع فيه ملح ووضع منه على جرح الانسان اسكن وجعه وسكن سريعا

16.22: (b) والبورق والمر] والمر والبورق G | اغلى] يغلي G | حتى يصير ويخلط] *om.* G

(c) على صبر] عليه شيء من الصبر الاسقطري C | حتى] الى ان C | اذا] فاذا C | ختم به] ختم C | ختم به] *add.* C لوجع السن ضرس الفرس اذا سحق ودر منه قليلا على السن الوجع ابرأه لوقته وساعته

16.23: (b) واذا…فتحبل] لبن الفرس اذا اسقي للمرأة حتى يصير [...] التي لا تحتبل وهي لا تعلم وواقعها الرجل في الحال حبلت تحتبلها عاجلا G

16.24: (b) وهو من السباع الموجودة] التي تؤخذ G | يخذ] اذا أخذ G | فيعلق] وعلق G | من اشرف] من قد اشرف *add.* G | والامتلاء] والامتلاء من الطعام والشراب برئ *add.* G

16.21	For the spleen, spleen of an Arabian horse: if it is taken, macerated in vinegar for one day and one night, it will dry, once it has dried, grind it; when you want to cure a sick person, take one *miṯqāl* of it, then the man suffering from spleen complaint has to empty it three times until the spleen blows up, then give it to drink to the man together with old wine for three days, then the spleen [pain] will cease, with the permission of God, may He be exalted.	Arabian horse spleen: if it is macerated in old white wine vinegar for one day and one night, then taken out and hung in the sun until it dries; one *miṯqāl* of it is taken, ground until it becomes like an eye salve, then it is given to the man suffering from spleen until his spleen blows up and grows in his abdomen; then he has to eat the ground horse spleen, and drink with it one *raṭl* of old pitch, on an empty stomach for three times, day after day, and he will heal.	Horse spleen: if it is macerated in vinegar for one day and one night, taken out and dried in the sunlight, then given to the man suffering from spleen until he absorbs it all and the spleen grows in his abdomen, then he should swallow this spleen once it has been ground, drinking one *raṭl* of pure vinegar after this—this should be done for three days in the same quantity—and then he will recover.
16.22	Horse brain: if it is mixed on the fire, with the addition of some aloe, myrrh, natron and honey, an ointment is made from it, and it is applied on the wound, then this will eat the dead flesh, while the living flesh will cicatrize the wound.	Female horse brain: if some aloe, natron, myrrh and honey are added to it, then it is boiled on the fire, then this will be the best ointment that there is for the wounds.	If it is added to aloe, red natron and honey, cooked on the fire until it becomes an ointment, and it is applied on any kind of wound, then this will seal it.
16.23	If a woman does not get pregnant, give her the milk of the horse to drink—when she is not aware of it—the man should have sexual intercourse with her in that very moment, and then she will get pregnant, with the permission of God, may He be exalted.	If a woman does not get pregnant, give her horse milk to drink—when she does not know—the man has to take her on the spot, and then she will conceive.	*om.*
16.24	For indigestion, take the hippopotamus tooth—that is one of the wild animals that can be found in the river—hang it on the man who is dying for indigestion, and then he will heal, with the permission of God, may He be exalted.	The tooth of the hippopotamus—that is a wild beast that can be found in the Nile—taken and hung on the man who is close to death for the stomach ache due to indigestion and fullness [it will be useful].	*om.*

16.25	اذا اردت ان تطرد الفأر من البيت او حانوت فبخر البيت بحافر فرس وكبريت خفتاني فان الفار يهربون من المكان	حافره وكبريث القصّارين يبخّر به البيت فيهرب منه الفأر	*om.*
16.26	لعقد المرأة يؤخذ خيط نيرة ويعقد على قضيب فرس ميت سبع عقد على اسم الشخص واسم امه فيعقد ولا ينحل حتى تحله انتَ فتأتئ الى الفرس فتحل العقد فينحل وهو للمراة وللرجل وهو مليح وعجيب	*om.*	*om.*
16.27	*om.*	اعفاجه تبرأ من الجنون الذي يأخذ الانسان في رأس الشهر اذا سعط به ويعلق عليه	*om.*
16.28	*om.*	مرارته يسعط منها للفالج والقوة والصداع وكل علة من برد في الدماغ	*om.*

16.25: (b) حافره [حافر الفرس G | وكبريث [والكبريث G | القَصّارين [الذي يستعمله القصّار G | يبخّر [اذا بخّر G | فيهرب [هرب G

16.27: (b) اعفاجه...عليه [اعفاج الفرس النهري اذا أخذ في الهلال وسعط به المجنون وعلّق عليه برئ G

16.28: (b) مرارته [مرارة الفرس النهري G | يسعط [اذا سعط G | للفالج [صاحب الفالج G | من [تكون من *add.* G | الدماغ [نفعه الدماغ *add.* G

16.25	If you want to chase mice away from the house or from a shop, fumigate the house with the hoof of the horse and some *Ḫiftānī* sulphur, and then the mice will flee from the place.	Its hoof and sulphur of the washers: if the house is fumigated with it, then the mice will flee from the house.	*om.*
16.26	To tie a woman, a thread from the cane-roll of a loom has to be taken, tied on the penis of a dead horse with seven knots, in the name of that person and of her mother, tie it and it should not be untied until you untie it yourself; then give it to the horse, and untie the knot, this is suitable for women and men, and this is witty and amazing.	*om.*	*om.*
16.27	*om.*	Duodenum of the hippopotamus: the man who takes it at the beginning of the month will heal from insanity, if he inhales it and hangs it on himself.	*om.*
16.28	*om.*	Its gall: it has to be inhaled against paralysis, facial paralysis and epilepsy, and every disease that derives from the coldness in the brain.	*om.*

١٧. البغال

	a	b	c
	ذكر منفع اعضاء البغل	البغال	باب منافع البغل
17.1	يؤخذ وسخ اذن بغله ويجعله في قطعة جلد بغل ويعلّق على المرأة فلا تحبل ابدا	اذا أخذ جلد بغل فجعل فيه وسخ اذن بغلة وعلق على امرأة لم تحبل ما دام معلقا عليها	*om.*
17.2	يؤخذ عرق بغلة فتغمس فيه قطعة وتتحمّل به المرأة فلا تحبل ابدا	واذا أخذ من عرق في قطنة واحتملته المرأة لم تحبل ابدا	*om.*
17.3	اذا اردت ان لا يسكر احد من شرب النبيذ فخذ وسخ اذن بغل او بغلة وخلّه في قرّابة النبيذ فكل من شرب منه فلا يسكر ابدا	وسخ اذن البغلة او البغل اذا اذيف بنبيذ وسقيته رجلا لم يسكر سكرا	شرب انسان من وسخ اذنه في خمر سكر لوقته
17.4	اذا اردت ان تقطع البواسير فتأخذ الزنابير التي تكون في دبر البغلة أو الدابة فتجفف وتسحق وتبخر من به البواسير والارواح الظاهرة والباطنة فتذهب باذن الله	اذا جففت الزنابير التي تكون في دبر البغل وبخر بها من به البواسير ذهبت	*om.*

17.1: (b) فجعل] وجعل G | اذن] اذني G | لم تحبل] لم تحبل G | معلقا] *om.* G
17.2: (b) واذا أخذ...المرأة] وان تحمّلت المرأة بعرق بغل في قطنة G
17.3: (a) In S this recipe is after 17.4
(b) اذن] اذني G | وسقيته رجلا] وشرب منه انسان G | سكرا] سكرا مفرطا G
(c) شرب...لوقته] وسخ اذن البغل اذا وضع في الخمر سكر لوقته سكرا جيدا C
17.4: (b) الزنابي...ويذهب بها] اذا جففت الزنابير التي تكون في دبر البغل وبخر بها من به البواسير ذهبت G

17. Mule

	a	b	c
	Exposition of the useful properties of the parts of the mule	**The mule**	**Chapter on the useful properties of the mule**
17.1	Dirt from the ear of a mule: if it is put in a piece of mule skin and hung on the woman, then she will never get pregnant.	If the skin of the mule is taken, some dirt from the ear of a mule is put inside it, and this is hung on a woman, then she will never get pregnant as long as this remains on her.	*om.*
17.2	If a piece of cloth is soaked in the sweat of a mule and the woman carries it, then she will never get pregnant.	If its sweat is collected with a piece of cotton and a woman carries it, then she will never get pregnant.	*om.*
17.3	If you want that nobody gets drunk by drinking wine, take the dirt from the ear of a male or a female mule, marinate it in a demijohn of wine, and then no one who drinks from it will ever get drunk.	Dirt from the ear of a female or of a male mule: if it is mixed with wine and it is given to a man to drink, then he will get very drunk.	If a man drinks the dirt from the ear of a mule with somimmediatelye wine, then he will immediately get drunk.
17.4	If you want to cure the haemorrhoids, take the hornets that can be found on the back of a female mule or on any other animal, dry them, grind them and fumigate the man suffering from haemorrhoids and manifest or inner winds with them, and then the haemorrhoids will cease, with the permission of God, may He be exalted.	Hornets which can be found on the back of the mule: if they are dried and used to fumigate the man suffering from haemorrhoids, then this will make them disappear.	*om.*

17.5	*om.*	وسخ اذن البغلة اذا ذوب امرأة في نبيذ او وسقيت منه غيره لم تحبل ابدا	اذا اردت المرأة لا تحبل ابدا فخذ وسخ اذن بغلة فاذيبه واسقيه لامراة وهي لا تعلم فلا تحبل ابدا
17.6	*om.*	وان أخذ رحم بغلة وطبخته مع لحم حمار وغيره من اللحوم واطمعت منه امرأة وهي لا تعلم لم تحبل ابدا	*om.*
17.7	*om.*	*om.*	حافر البغلة الايسر اذا حملته المرأة معها فانها لا تحبل ابدا
17.8	وان بخر به هرب الفأر منه والهوام	واذا بخرت البيت بحافر البغل هرب منه الفأر	وتبخر به البيوت فلا يقربها فأر
17.9	*om.*	مخ البغل اذا خلط بالزيت فهو نافع لكل ورم حاسّ في البدن من شحمة وغير ذلك	*om.*
17.10	*om.*	واعلم ان البغل اذا اكثر من شمّ البغلة هرم سريعا	*om.*
17.11	بوله اذا شربته مرأة لم تحبل	بول البغل اذا شربت امرأة لم تحبل ويخلط مع ثلاث سكرجات في الماء الذي يطفي به الحديد وتشربه المرأة ثلاث ايام	*om.*
17.12	حافره اذا احرق وعجن بدهن آس انبت شعر الرأس وغيره من كل موضع	*om.*	*om.*

17.5: (b) وسخ] شحم G | وسقيت منه] وشربت G | ابدا] *om.* G

17.6: (b) وطبخته] وان أخذ رحم بغلة اذا طبخ رحم البغلة G | من اللحوم] *om.* G | واطمعت منه] واكلت G | ابدا] *om.* G

17.8: (b) واذا بخرت...الفأر] حافر البغل الاسير من الرجل اذا بخّر به البيت هرب منه الفار ومات G
(c) وان بخر] واذا بخر C | به] به في مكان *add.* C | الفأر منه والهوام] منه الفأر والحشرات C

17.9: (b) حاسّ] *om.* G | من شحمة وغير ذلك] *om.* G

17.10: (b) شمّ البغلة] شمّ بول الانثى G | هرم] كبر وهرم G

17.11: (b) شربت] شرب G | ويخلط] ان تخلطه G | ثلاث] ثلثة G | في الماء الذي يطفي به] من ماء الحدّاد الذي يطفي فيه G | المرأة] *om.* G | ثلاث] ثلثة G
(c) شربته] شربت C

17.12: (c) وغيره من كل موضع] وغيرها من الدقن وكل شعر يزيد انباته C

17.5	If you want that a woman will never get pregnant, take the dirt from the ear of a female mule, liquefy it and give it to drink to the woman—but she should not be aware of it—and then she will never get pregnant.	Dirt from the ear of a female mule: if it is liquefied and drunk by a woman in some wine or with something else, then she will never get pregnant.	*om.*
17.6	*om.*	Womb of a female mule: if it is taken, cooked with the meat of a donkey or with other meat and a woman eats it—but she should not be aware of this—then she will never get pregnant.	*om.*
17.7	If a woman carries with her the left hoof of a mule, then she will never get pregnant.	*om.*	*om.*
17.8	If a house is fumigated with it, then not a single mouse will approach it.	If the house is fumigated with the hoof of a mule, then the mice will flee from it.	And if it is fumigated [with its hoof], then the mice and the obnoxious insects will flee.
17.9	*om.*	Mule marrow: if it is mixed with oil, then this will be useful against every kind of painful swelling on the body, due to a piece of fat or something else.	*om.*
17.10	*om.*	Know that the mule, when he sniffs the smell of a female, quickly becomes decrepit.	*om.*
17.11	*om.*	Mule urine: if a woman drinks it, then she will not get pregnant; it has also to be mixed with three bowls of the water used by a blacksmith to quench iron, for three days.	If a woman drinks its urine, then she will not get pregnant.
17.12	*om.*	*om.*	If its hoof is burnt and kneaded with myrtle oil, then this will make the hair grow on the head and on other parts as well.

17.13	*om.*	*om.*	واذا دفن حافر بغلة السوداء او برذون ادهم تحت سكنة باب لم تقربه فأرة
17.14	*om.*	*om.*	ومن كان عاشقا فليتمرع في مراغة بغل ذكر لذكر وانثى لانثى فانه سلوه سلوا حقيقا
17.15	*om.*	حافر البغلة ان مسكته المرأة معها لم تحبل ابدا	*om.*
17.16	وايضا اذا اردت انها لا تحبل فخذ من قلب بغلة قطعة فجفّفها واسحقها واسقيها للمرأة في نبيذ فانها لا تحبل ابدا وهو عجيب مليح	قلب البغل اذا جفف وسحق وشرب منه المرأة في نبيذ لم تحبل ابدا مجرب	قلب البغلة اذا جفف وسحق وشرب منه احد مقدار حبة في شراب فانها البعضة القاطعة

17.13: (c) واذا دفن حافر بغلة السوداء] حافر البغلة C
17.14: (c) ومن كان عاشقا فليتمرع في مراغة] ومن تمرغ في مراغة C | ذكر لذكر وانثى لانثى] ذكر او انثى C
17.15: (b) ان مسكته] اذا حملته G | ابدا] *om.* G
17.16: (b) This recipe is attested only in G
(c) مقدار] قدر C | فانها] كانت هي C

17.13	*om.*	*om.*	If the hoof of a black female mule—or of a deep-black work horse—is buried under the door of the house, then not a single mouse will approach it.
17.14	*om.*	*om.*	The person who is sexually excited should rub the grease of a mule on his person —a male for the man and a female for the woman—then this will relieve him.
17.15	*om.*	Mule hoof: if a woman holds it, then she will never get pregnant.	*om.*
17.16	And also, if you want that a woman does not get pregnant, take one piece from the ear of a female mule, dry it, grind it, give it to drink to the woman in some wine, and then she will never get pregnant, and this is amazing and witty.	Mule heart: if it is dried, ground and drunk by a woman with some wine, then she will never get pregnant: this has been tried out.	If the heart of a female mule is dried, ground and one grain of it is drunk in some wine, then this will be the final hatred.

١٨. الحمار

	a	b	c
	ذكر منافع اعضاء الحمار	الحمير	باب منافع الحمار
18.1	يؤخذ طحال حمار فيجفّف في الظل فدق ويجعل في قطعة من جلد غزال وعلّقه على نفسك وادخل على اي مكان شئتَ فلا يراك احد من الناس الا اهابك وحبك	يؤخذ طحال حمار مجفّف في الظل ويدق ويصير في جلد غزال وعلّقه عليك وادخل حيث شئتَ فلا يراك الاّ اهابك واحبك	طحال الحمار يجفف في الظل ويجعل في جلد الغزال فاذا علق على احد احبه كان من يراه وان دخل في سلطان او كبار به
18.2	اذا اردت ان تجامع فلا تمل فخذ شعرة من ذنب حمار وهو فوق الحمارة وعلّقها على نفسك وقت الجماع فانه يقوي ويشتهي نفسك الجماع	ان أخذ انسان شعرة من ذنب الحمار وهو يقفز على اتانه فعلّقه عليك تنغط	اذا أخذ شعرة من ذنب الحمارة وعلقها عليه قوى شهوة الجماع
18.3	*om.*	يؤخذ حافر حمار يحرق يذاف بطلاء ويؤخذ منه في صوفة وتحتمله المرأة فيخرج الولد عاجلا	*om.*
18.4	بول الحمار يغمس فيه صوفة وتعّق على جنب المركب قريبا من الماء فانه السمك يجتمعون اليها فتصطادهم وهو عجيب مليح	بول الحمار اذا يؤخذ ويبل به اسفنجة وتعمل على وجه الماء فيجتمع اليها السمك	واذا غمست في بول الحمار صوفة وعلقها في جنب مركب قريبا الماء اجتمع السمك اليه من كل جانب
18.5	*om.*	*om.*	من أخذ من وسخ اذنه وسقى انسانا في شراب وغيره نام ولم يفعل شيئا

18.1: (a) فيجفف في الظل فدق] *om.* B | على نفسك] وعلقه عليك B | على اي مكان] الى مكان شئتَ B
(b) يؤخذ] *om.* G | حمار] الحمار الاهلي G | مجفّف] اذا جفف G | ويدق ويصير] وسحق وجعل G | غزال] الغزال G | وعلقه] وحمل G | وادخل...واحبك] لم يدخل على احد الا هابه واحبه G
(c) يجفف] اذا جفف C | ويجعل] وترك C | الغزال] غزال C | فاذا علق...كبار به] هو المحبة العكمي عند كل من يراى وان دخل على سلطان او كبير كان مهابا عند كل واحد C
18.2: (a) فلا] ولا B | وتشهي نفسك الجماع] ويزيد النكاح B
(b) ان] اذا G | شعرة] *om.* G | يقفز] ينزوا G | اتانه] اتان G | فعلّقه] وعلقه G | عليك تنغط] عليه انعظّ للجماع G
(c) الحمارة] الحمار C | عليه] عليه حال الجماع *add.* C
18.4: (a) من الماء] من المركب B | فتصطادهم] فتصيدهم B | مليح] عجيب B
(b) In G this recipe is after 18.6

18. Donkey

	a	b	c
	Exposition of the useful properties of the parts of the donkey	**The donkey**	**Chapter on the useful properties of the donkey**
18.1	Donkey spleen: if it is dried it in the shade, ground, put in a piece of gazelle skin and hung on your body, then you will be able to enter any place you want and no one will see you, but the one who desires and loves you.	Donkey spleen: if itis taken, dried in the shade, ground, put in some gazelle skin and hung on your person, then no one will see you, but the one who desires and loves you.	Donkey spleen: if it is dried in the shade, put in the skin of a gazelle, and hung on somebody, then anybody who sees him will love him; [this works] also if he enters in the presence of the sultan or of the mighty ones around him.
18.2	If you want to have sexual intercourse without getting tired, take a hair from a donkey's tail, while he is covering a donkey mare, hang it on your body at the moment of coitus, and this will give you power and excite you in the coitus.	If someone takes a hair from the tail of a donkey while he is mounting a donkey mare and hangs it on you, then you will get excited	Hair from the tail of a donkey mare: if it is taken and hung on the body, then this will increase the desire of coitus.
18.3	*om.*	Donkey hoof: if it is taken, burnt and mixed with liquid pitch, put in a woollen cloth, and a woman carries it, then the baby will quickly come out.	*om.*
18.4	If a woollen cloth is soaked in the urine of the donkey and hung on the broadside of the ship close to the water surface, then the fish will gather there and will be easy to catch them, this is amazing and witty.	If a sponge is moistened with its urine and suspended in the water, then the fish will gather there.	If a woollen cloth is soaked in the urine of the donkey and is hung on the broadside of a ship close to the water surface, then the fish will gather there from every direction.
18.5	*om.*	*om.*	If someone takes the dirt of its ear and gives it to another man in some wine or in another drink, then this will sleep and will not do anything.

18.6	*om.*	لحم الحمار وشحمه اذا طبخ بزيت عتيق ومسح به المفاصل المشبّكة اذهبه	*om.*
18.7	روث الحمار الطري يعصر ويسعط به صاحب الرعاف فينقطع باذن الله تعالى	روث الحمار الرطب يعصر ماؤه ويسعط به من به الرعاف اذهبه	وعصارة روثه اذا خلطت بالخل تقطع الدم السائل من جميع البدن والرعاف
18.8	*om.*	جلده ايضا اذا عمل منه خاتم وعلق على المجنون نفعه	وان حمل من حافر الايمن خاتما ولبسه المصروع ابرأه
18.9	مثله روث الحمار اليابس يسحق ويذاب بالخل ويطلي به الانف فينقطع الرعاف	والروث اليابس يسحق ويذاف بالخل ويطلي به الانف من الجانبين ينقطع الرعاف	روث الحمار اليابس اذا سحق واذيف بالخل وطلى به انف صاحب الرعاف قطعه
18.10	*om.*	وكذلك منقول على الجرح الذي يسيل منه الدم فيلحم الجرح وينقطع الدم منه	*om.*
18.11	لوجع الوركين والصلب يؤخذ مخ الحمار ويذاب بدهن الغار ويدهن به في الحمام فيذهب باذن الله تعالى	مخه اذا اذيف بدهن الغار وادهن به لوجع الوركين ووجع القلب في الحمام نفعه	مخ الحمار اذا اذيف بدهن الغار وطلى به الصلب والوركين في الحمام نفع من اوجاع ذلك
18.12	اذا اردت ان ينقطع دم الجرح ويمنع من القيح يؤخذ روث الحمار يابسا ويحرق جزء ومن عرق القبّار جزء ومن سواد القدر جزء ومن ملح الطعام جزء ويسحق الجميع سحقا ناعما ويتخذ منه درورا فيدر على الجرح فينقطع الدم منه ولا يقيح ابدا	روث الحمار يحرق ويؤخذ منه جزء ومن خرقة الكتان جزء ومن سواد القدر جزء ملح جزء ويدق ويخلط الجميع ويذر على جرح طري يقطع الدم منه ويجففه	روث الحمار اذا أخذ منه جزء ومن القبار جزء ومن سواد القدر جزء ومن ملح الطعام جزء ودرع على الجرح قطع دمه ولا يقيح

18.8: (c) *om.* C

18.9: (a) This recipe is attested only in B, see also 19.8.

18.11: (a) الصلب والوركين] الوركين والصلب B

(c) وطلى] ودلك C | الصلب والوركين في الحمام] الصلب في الحمام والوركين C | اوجاع] جميع اوجاع C

18.12: (a) ويمنع من القيح] *om.* B | يؤخذ] فخذ B | ويحرق] *om.* B | ومن سواد القدر جزء] *om.* B | سحقا] *om.* B | ولا يقيح] ولا ينقتح B

(c) ولا يقيح] ومنعه ان يقيح C

18.6	*om.*	Donkey meat and fat: if they are cooked with oil and this oil is wiped on the contracted joints, then the stiffness will go away.	*om.*
18.7	Donkey fresh excrement: if it is squeezed and inhaled by the man suffering from nosebleed, then this will stop, with the permission of God, may He be exalted.	Donkey fresh excrement: if it is squeezed and its water is inhaled by the man afflicted by nosebleed, then this will make it go away.	Juice of its excrement: if it is mixed with vinegar, this will stop every kind of bleeding from the body, and the nosebleed too.
18.8	*om.*	If a seal is made from its skin and is hung on an insane man, then this will be useful to him.	Its right hoof: if it is used to make a seal and an epileptic man wears it, then this will cure him.
18.9	Likewise, donkey dry excrement: if it is ground, mixed with vinegar, and rubbed on the nose, then the bleeding will cease.	Its dry excrement: if it is ground, mixed with vinegar and rubbed on the nose, then its bleeding will stop.	Donkey dry excrement: if it is pounded, mixed with vinegar and rubbed on the nose of a man suffering from nosebleed, then this will stop.
18.10	*om.*	Likewise, if it is applied on a bleeding wound, then the wound will cicatrize, and the bleeding will stop.	*om.*
18.11	For the pain in the legs the and in the spine, take the marrow of a donkey, liquefy it with laurel oil and anoint the body with it in the bath, and then the pain will cease, with the permission of God, may He be exalted.	If its marrow is mixed with laurel oil, anointed in the bath against the pain in the legs and in the loins, this will be useful against these.	Donkey marrow: if it is mixed with laurel oil and rubbed on the spine and the legs in the bath, then this will be useful against their pains.
18.12	If you want to stop the bleeding from a wound and prevent this from becoming infected, take the dry excrements of a donkey, burn one part of it, one part of capers root, one part of cooking pot's soot and one part of cooking salt, ground it into a fine powder, take an abundant portion of it, apply it on the wound, then the bleeding will stop and the wound will never become infected.	Donkey excrement: if it is burnt, one part of it is taken, with one part of linen cloth, one part of the soot from a cooking pot and one part of salt, everything mixed together and poured on the bleeding wound, then this will stop the bleeding and dry the wound.	If one part of donkey excrement, one part of capers, one part of soot from a cooking pot and one part of cooking salt are applied on a wound, then this will staunch the blood and the festering matter coming out from it.

18.13	*om.*	روثه الرطب يعصر ويصفي ماؤه ويسقي لصاحب الريح الذكر يذهبه	روث الحمار اذا عصر ماؤه وسعط به المرعوف ابرأه
18.14	للريح في الجوف يسقي روث الحمار اليابس يسقي لصاحب الريح بماء الرمان الحلو فيذهب باذن الله تعالى	ويؤخذ من روثه يابس يسقي من به الريح بماء الرمان الحلو ينفعه	روث الحمار اليابس اذا اذيف بماء الرمان الحلو وسقى منه صاحب الريح في الجوف برئ
18.15	يؤخذ قطعة من جلد حمار ميت وتعلق على المصروع فانه يفيق باذن الله تعالى	اذا أخذ من جلد جبهة حمار وعلق على المصروع افاق والله اعلم	جلد الحمار الميت اذا علق على المصروع افاق من ساعته
18.16	لطرد البراغيث من البيت يؤخذ لبن الحمارة فيطلي به عود واطرحه في وسط البيت فانّ البغاريث يجنمعون عليه بفعل ذلك مرتين او ثلاث فلا يبقي في البيت براغيث وهو مليح عجيب	وان طليت شيئا بلبن حمار وجعلته في البيت اجتمع عليه البراغيث	اذا اردت ان تطرد البراغيث من البيت اطل عود بلبن حمارة واجعله في البيت تجتمع اليه البراغيث
18.17	لوجع الاسنان يؤخذ لبن حمارة فيسحق على نار لينة ويتمضمض به فيسكن الوجع	اللبن ايضا اذا سخّن على النار وتمضمض به نفع من وجع الاسنان	لبن الحمار اذا سخن على النار وتمضمض صاحب وجع الاسنان سكن الوجع
18.18	*om.*	لبن الحمارة اذا شرب نفع من الادواء العاملة وقروح الامعاء وقروح الرحم	*om.*
18.19	اذا هاج بالصغير السعال والربو على فواد واوجاع الصدر فيسقي لبن حمارة حارا كما حلبوا يكون فيه رب السوس ربع مثقال مثقال كثيراء بيضاء مسحوقان	اذا هاج بالصبي سعال ووجع الصدر يسقي لبن الحمارة حارا كما يحلب ويذاف فيه كثيراء ورب السوس من كل واحد وزن دانقين مسحوقا ومنخولا مسح	اذا هاج على الطفل السعال والريق واوجاع الصدر خذ لبن الحماره كما حلب والق عليه رب السوس وكثيرة

18.13: (c) ابرأه] الرعاف C | الرعاف] ويفعل في ذلك فعل الكفور فانه اذا نشق منه المرتعف قطع الرعاف *add.* C
18.14: (a) للريح...فيذهب] للريح في الجوف يسقي روث الحمار فيزول عنه B
(c) الحمار] *om.* C | الحلو] *om.* C | وسقى] وشرب C | في الجوف] *om.* C | برئ] ابرأه C
18.15: (c) ساعته] وقته C
18.16: (a) البراغيث] البرغوث B | بفعل ذلك...عجيب] *om.* B
(c) تطرد] طرد C | اطل] طلى C | حمارة] الحمارة C
18.17: (c) صاحب] من تشتكي C | الوجع] الالم وازال الوجع C
18.19: (c) خذ لبن] خذ من لبن C | كما حلب] اذا حلب C | رب السوس] من الربّ سوس C | الطفل] الطفل منه C | يبرأ] فانه يبرأ C

18.13	*om.*	Its moist excrement, if its juice is extracted and purified, and its water is given to the man suffering from the wind, then this will go away.	Donkey excrement: if its water is extracted and the one affected by nosebleed inhales it, then he will heal.
18.14	Against the wind in the abdomen: give its dry excrement to drink to the man suffering from winds, with sweet pomegranate water, then this will heal, with the permission of God, may He be exalted.	Its dry excrement: if it is given to the man suffering from air with sweet pomegranate water to drink, then this will be useful to him.	Donkey dry excrements: if it is mixed with sweet pomegranate water and given to the man suffering from air in the abdomen to drink, then he will recover.
18.15	A piece of dead donkey skin: if it is taken, hung on an epileptic man, then he will recover, with the permission of God, may He be exalted.	If the skin from the donkey forehead is hung on the epileptic man, then he will recover, and God knows best.	If the skin of a dead donkey is hung on the epileptic, then he will instantly recover.
18.16	To chase the fleas away from the house, take the milk of a donkey mare, rub it on a branch and place it in the middle of the house, then the fleas will gather there. Do this two or three times, and then no flea will remain in the house, this is witty and amazing.	If some milk of donkey mare is rubbed on something, and this is placed in the house, then the fleas will gather there.	If you want to chase the fleas away from the house, rub a branch with the milk of a donkey mare, place it in the house, and then the fleas will gather there.
18.17	For the tooth pain: take the milk of a donkey mare, warm it over a low fire and make a mouthwash with it, and then the pain will be relieved.	If its milk is warmed on the fire and used to do mouthwashes, then this will be useful against the toothache.	Donkey milk: if it is warmed on the fire and used to do mouthwashes by the man suffering from tooth pain, then the pain will be relieved.
18.18	*om.*	Donkey mare milk: if it is drunk, it will be useful against the 'active' diseases, and against the ulcers in the intestine and in the uterus.	*om.*
18.19	If cough, asthma of heart and chest pains trouble a child, give him the milk of a donkey mare to drink—as warm as it is when it is milked—and in it there should be one-quarter *miṯqāl* of liquorice jelly and one *miṯqāl* of astragale—both of them ground—then wipe the chest with	If cough and chest pain trouble a child, give him the milk of a mare donkey to drink—as warm as when it is milked—mix it with astragale and liquorice jelly, two *dāniq* of each one, pound it and sieve it, then rub the child's chest with wax and sweet violet oil for some days,	If cough, asthma and chest pains trouble a child, take the milk of a donkey mare—just like it is when it is milked—add liquorice jelly and astragale to it, give it to the child to drink and anoint his chest with

	ويمسح الصدر بشيء او دهن بنفسج وشمع فانه يبرأ باذن الله	صدره بموم ودهن بنفسج اياما نافع باذن الله تعالى	بيضاء واسق الطفل وادهن صدره بدهن بنفسج يبرأ ان شاء الله تعالى
18.20	لبن الحمارة يسقي لصاحب وجع السل على هذه الصفة في أيام الربيع فينفعه باذن الله تعالى	وان سقى من به السل على هذه الصفة في الربيع نفعه ان شاء الله تعالى	*om.*

	some of it or with sweet violet oil and wax, and then the child will recover, with the permission of God, may He be exalted.	and then this will be useful, with the permission of God, may He be exalted.	sweet violet oil, and then he will recover, God, may He be exalted willing.
18.20	Donkey mare milk: if it is given during the Spring to the man suffering from consumption pain to drink—following this preparation—then this will be useful for him, with the permission of God, may He be exalted.	If the man suffering from consumption drinks it during the Spring, then this will be useful to him.	*om.*

١٩. حمار الوحش

	a	b	c
	ذكر منافع اعضاء حمار الوحش	*om.*	باب منافع حمار الوحش
19.1	مخ حمار الوحش يسقي بماء الخَسّ لمن [يجنب كثيرا] يبول في كثيرا فانه يقلله	مخ حمار الوحش لمن يبول في الفراش ولمن تصيبه الجنابة كثيرا يذاف بماء الخس ويسقي عند النوم	مخ حمار الوحش يذاف بماء الجبن ويسقي لمن يبول كثيرا فانه يقل بوله
19.2	شحم حمار الوحش يداف بدهن زنبق خالص ويدلك به الكلف فيقلعه باذن الله تعالى	شحمه يذاف بدهن الزنبق خالص ويطلي على الوجه الذي فيه الكلف فيقلعه باذن اللع تعالى	شحم الحمار الاهلي يذاب على النار ويدلك منه الكلف يبرأ والق عليه دهن زنبق فانه انفع المكلف والبهق الذي يكون على الوجه يقلعه
19.3	*om.*	واذا كان الصبي كثير البكاء يؤخذ من اذن الحمار اليسرى ومن شحم اي حمار كان فيسقي الصبي اياما بلبن امه فيبرأ وينام ويهدي باذن الله تعالى	*om.*
19.4	بول حمار الوحش يخلط بدهن كادي وشيء من نشاء القمح ويسقي لصاحب الضربان في الجسد والمفاصل فيذهب باذن الله تعالى	بوله ودهن كادي يغلي على النار ويذاف فيه قلب الحنطة ويشرب منه في الحمام ويدهن به المفاصل ينفع لظلمة البصر ولغشاوة العين	بول حمار الوحش اذا القى عليه دهن وغلى على النار والقى عليه نشاء وشرب منه صاحب وجع المفاصل في الحمام ودهن به البدن والمفاصل ابرأه

19.1: (a) يقلله] يقل البول B
(b) مخ حمار...النوم] مخ حمار الوحش اذا شرب بماء الخَسّ عند النوم لمن يجنب كثيرا ويبول في الفراش فانه مجرب G
(c) يذاف] اذا اذيف C | ويسقي لمن] وشربة من C | يقل] اقل C
19.2: (a) يداف] يذاب B | ويدلك] ويدهن B | فيقلعه] فينفعه B
(b) الزنبق] زيبق T | شحمه...فيقلعه] شحمه ايضا اذا اذيف بدهن الزنبق وطلى به الكلف الذي في الوجه اذهبه G | In G another recipe is added, to prepare a seal with wild donkey skin for the treatment of insanity, see also 18.8: جلده ايضا اذا عمل منه خاتم وعلق على المجنون نفعه.
(c) الحمار الاهلي] الحمار الوحش والاهلي C | ويدلك منه] ودلك به C | يبرأ] ابرأه C | والق] واذا القى C | فانه انفع] نفع C | يقلعه] فيقلعه C
19.3: (b) واذا كان...ويهدي] اذنه ايضا اليسرى مع شحم اي حمار كان واسقي للصبي الذي لا ينام في لبن امه فانه ينام G
19.4: (a) وشيء من نشاء القمح] *om.* B | فيذهب] وشيء من نشا القمح المغص الشديد بقليل عسل نحل B
(b) بوله...العين] بوله ايضا اذا أخذ مع دهن كادني واغلي على النار مع لباب الحنطة واسقى لصاحب الضربان في الحمام وادهّن به نفعه G
(c) دهن] دهن الزنبق C

19. Wild Donkey

	a	b	c
	Mention of the useful properties of the parts of the wild donkey	*om.*	**Chapter on the useful properties of the wild donkey**
19.1	Wild donkey marrow: if it is given with lettuce water to the man who is affected by a severe pleurisy and wets the bed to drink, then this will reduce it.	Wild donkey marrow: for the one who urinates in bed and for the one who is severely affected by pleurisy, mixed with lettuce water, and given to drink at the moment of sleeping.	Wild donkey marrow: if it is mixed with cheese water and given to the man who urinates copiously to drink, then this will reduce his urination.
19.2	Wild donkey fat: if it is mixed with pure lily oil and rubbed on the freckles, then this will remove them, with the permission of God, may He be exalted.	Its fat: if it is mixed with lily oil and rubbed on the face spotted with freckles, then this will remove them, with the permission of God, may He be exalted.	Domestic donkey fat: if it is liquefied on the fire and rubbed on the freckles, this will cure them. Add to it some lily oil, then this will be useful to the man with freckles and vitiligo on his face, and will remove them.
19.3	*om.*	If a baby cries a lot, take a part of the left ear of a donkey and some fat of any donkey, give it to the baby with his mother's milk for some days, then he will heal, sleep, and behave, with the permission of God, may He be exalted.	*om.*
19.4	Wild donkey urine: if it is mixed with pandang oil and some corn starch, given to the man suffering from pangs in the body and in the joints to drink, then these will cease, with the permission of God, may He be exalted.	Its urine: if it is boiled with pandang oil on the fire with kernels of wheat starch, drunk in the bath and rubbed on the joints, then this will be useful against the obscuration of the eyesight and the cataract.	If some oil is added to the urine of wild donkey, boiled on the fire with the addition of starch, then drunk in the bath by the man suffering from joints pain and rubbed on the body and on the joints, then this will cure him.

19.5	خصيته تشق وتملح وتسحق وتسقي لصاحب المغص الشديد ووجع الجوف بقليل عسل فيذهب باذن الله تعالى	خصى حمار وحشا يشقّ ويملح بملح وورس ويجفف ويسقي منه من به مغص ووجع الجوف بعسل وماء حار نفعه	خصوة حمار الوحش شرح وتملح ويشرب منها صاحب المغص بالعسل وزن درهم يبرا باذن الله تعالى
19.6	حافر حمار الوحش يحرق ويسحق ناعما اسقي ويكتحل به من في عينيه الغشاوة وضعف النظرة فيذهب باذن الله تعالى	حافره اذا احرق واسقى وكحل به العين نفع من الظلمة والغشاوة	حافر حمار الوحش اذا احرق وسحق ناعما واكتحل به صاحب غشاوة العين ابرأه
19.7	مرارة حمار الوحش يخلط بها خولنجان وبورق ويسقي منها صاحب برد الكلي ورخو المثانة بماء الكرفس فهو يفت الحصاة باذن الله تعالى وتكون الهر به وزن درهم اول النهار ووزن درهم بالعشاء	مرارته اذا خلط معها خولنجان وبورق وشرب منها من به الحصاة وزن اربعة قراريط بماء بزر الكرفس المغلى المصفى نفعه	مرارة حمار الوحش اذا القى عليها خولنجان مكي وبورق احمر وخولنجان وشرب منه صاحب الحصاة ورخو المثانة وبرد الكلي اربعة دوانق بماء الكرفس مغلى مصفى تنفعه
19.8	روث حمار الوحش يسحق ويذوّب بمخ بيضة ويلطخ به جنبين صاحب الرعاف فينقطع باذن الله تعالى	*om.*	*om.*

19.5: (a) *om.* B

(b) خصي حمار...ويسقي منه] خصيته اذا شقت وملحت بملح وورس وجففت وشرب منها G

(c) شرح وتملح ويشرب] شرحت وملحت وجفف وشرب C | المغص] المغص وزن درهم *add.* C | يبرأ] ابرأه C

19.6: (a) In B this recipe is after 19.5 | اسقى] *om.* B | وضعف] وضعف النظرة *add.* B

(b) *om.* T | In G this recipe is after 19.5

19.7: (a) بها] معها B | ويسقي...الحصاء] ويخلط معها كثيراء بيضاء وعسل ويسقي لصاحب الحمى والسعال وغشاوة البصر فيبرأ B | الحصاء] وتكون شربه درهم بالغداة ودرهم بالعشاء *add.* B, see also 19.15

(b) *om.* T

(c) صاحب] من به C | اربعة] قدر اربعة C | الكرفس مغلى مصفى] الافسنتين الرومي C | تنفعه] وشربه صاحب وجع الكلى في الحمام ابرأه C

19.8: (a) *om.* B, see also 18.9

(b) *om.* G

19.5	Its testicles: if they are split, salted, ground, given with honey to the man suffering from acute gripes and abdomen pain to drink, then this will cease, with the permission of God, may He be exalted.	Its testicles and bowels: if they are split, seasoned with salt and curcuma, dried and drunk with honey and warm water by the man suffering from colic and abdomen pain with honey and warm water, then this will be useful to him.	Wild donkey testicle: if it is salted and taken with honey by the man who suffers from colic—in the amount of one dirham—then he will heal, with the permission of God, may He be exalted.
19.6	Wild donkey hoof: if it is burnt, ground into a fine powder, given to drink and rubbed on the eyes of the man affected by the cataract and weakness of the eyesight, then these will cease, with the permission of God, may He be exalted.	Its hoof: if it is burnt, given to drink and rubbed on the eyes, this will be useful against the obscuration of the eyes and the cataract.	Wild donkey hoof: if it is burnt, ground into a fine powder and rubbed on the eyes of a man with the cataract in the eye, then this will disappear.
19.7	Wild donkey gall: if it is mixed with galangal and natron, given to the man suffering from kidney coldness and bladder loosening to drink, together with celery water, then this will crumble the stones, with the permission of God, may He be exalted. The correct amount is of one dirham at the beginning of the day and one in the evening.	Its gall: if it is mixed with galangal and natron, drunk by a man suffering from stones, in the amount of four carats with boiled and purified celery water, then this will be useful to him.	Wild donkey gall: if it is added to Meccan galangal, red natron and galangal, drunk by a man suffering from stones, bladder loosening and kidneys coldness—four *dāniq* with boiled and purified celery water—then this will be useful to him.
19.8	Wild donkey excrement: if it is ground, liquefied with the yolk of an egg and spattered on the temples of a man suffering from nosebleed, then this will stop it, with the permission of God, may He be exalted.	*om.*	*om.*

19.9	*om.*	وكذلك يسحق ويخلط معه مرارة البقرة ويطلي على الشعر يجعّده ويحسّنه	روث حمار الوحش يسحق ويخلط معه مرارة البقر ويضمخ به الشعر فانه يحسنه ويطوله ويلينه ويكون بعيد الشيب
19.10	*om.*	لبن حمارة الوحش ينفع اذا شرب من وجع الظهر والوركين	لحم حمار الوحش يشوي ويطعم لصاحب وجع الظهر والكلى فينفعه باذن الله تعالى
19.11	*om.*	مخ حمار وحشا ينفع من النقرس اذا طلى عله مع دهن ورد	مخ حمار الوحش يذاف بدهن ورد ويطلي به النقرس فيزول باذن الله تعالى
19.12	زبل حمار الوحش اذا اذيف بماء الافسنتين الرومي وشرب منه صاحب الكلى في الحمام برئ	ودم حمار الوحش جيد لوجع الكلى والتقطير يشرب منه جزء بماء الافسنتين مغلى مصفى في الحمام على الريق	دم حمار الوحش يذاب بماء الافسنتين الرومي ويسقي لصاحب وجع الكلى في الحمام فيذهب عنه باذن الله تعالى
19.13	لحم حمار الوحش وشحمه وكبده يدق ناعما ويلقي في قدر ويجعل عليه سمن البقر والعسل ويطبخ ويجعل في اخر الطخ حلبة ودار فلفل وخولنجان من كل واحد جزء ويزيد في شهوة الجماع ويقويه	لحم حمار الوحش وكبده تدق دقا ناعما وهو طري ثم يطبخ بعسل وسمن بقرة ويغلي فيه حلبة وورس ودار فلفل وخولنجان من كل واحد جزء ويدق وينحل ويخلط معه ويشرب منه ينفع للحصاة في المثانة والكلى والتقطير وبرد الكلى ويزيد في الباه	لحم حمار الوحش وشحمه وكبده يدقه الجميع يطبخ بسمن بقري وعسل ويلقي عليه حلبة وورس وخولنجان ودار فلفل من كل واحد جزء وسقى لصاحب الحصاة في القضيب الذي يبول الدم ولتقطير البول فانه ينفعه وهو ايضا يزيد في الباه

19.9: (a) *om.* B
(b) وكذلك...ويحسّنه] زبله اذا سحق وخلط معه مرارة البقر وطلى به الشعر جعّده وحسّنه G
19.10: (a) *om.* B
(b) ينفع اذا شرب] اذا شرب نفع G
19.11: (a) *om.* B
(b) مخ حمار...ورد] مخ حمار الوحش اذا طلى على النقرس مع دهن ورد نفعها G
19.12: (a) *om.* B | الافسنتين] الافسيتين S
(b) الافسنتين] الافستيين T | *om.* G
(c) om. C | الافسنتين] الافسيتين L
19.13: (a) *om.* B
(b) لحم حمار...لحصاة] لحمه وشحمه وكبده يدق الجميع ناعما يطبخ بعسل وسمن بقر ويلقي فيه حلبة وورس ودار فلفل وخولنجان من كل واحد جزء مدقوق ومنخول ويشرب منه ينفع من الحصاة G
(c) ويزيد في شهوة الجماع ويقويه] فانه في يقوي شهوت C | ويجعل في اخر الطخ حلبة] ويلقي عليه شيء من الحلبة C | ويجعل] ويلقي C | ويلقي] ويجعل C الجماع

19.9	Wild donkey excrement: if it is ground, mixed with cow gall and rubbed on the hair, than this will make it longer, softer, and will prevent it from becoming white.	Likewise, if it is ground, mixed with cow gall and rubbed on the hair, this will make it curly and nicer.	*om.*
19.10	Mare donkey meat: if it is roasted and fed to a man suffering from kidney and back pain, then this will be useful against these pains, with the permission of God, may He be exalted.	Milk of a donkey mare: if it is drunk, it will be useful against the pain of the back and of the legs.	*om.*
19.11	Wild donkey marrow: if it is mixed with rose oil and rubbed on the gout, then this will cease.	Wild donkey marrow: it is useful against the gout, if it is rubbed on it with rose oil.	*om.*
19.12	Wild donkey blood: if it is mixed with absinth water, given in the bath to the man suffering from kidney complaint to drink, then this will cease, with the permission of God, may He be exalted.	Wild donkey blood: it is good for the pain of the kidney and urine dripping, if one part of it is drunk with boiled and purified absinth water, in the bath on an empty stomach.	Wild donkey excrement: if it is mixed with absinth water and drunk in the bath by a man suffering from kidney complaint, then he will recover.
19.13	Wild donkey meat, its fat and its liver: if they are minced together, cooked with cow fat and honey, with the addition of fenugreek, curcuma, galangal and long pepper—one part of each one—and given to drink to a man suffering from stones in the penis, and who urinates blood and against urine dripping, then this will be useful against this, and it will also increase the sexual desire.	Wild donkey meat and its liver: if they are finely minced when they are fresh, cooked with honey and cow fat; then fenugreek, curcuma, long pepper and galangal are boiled with it—one part of each one—ground, sieved, and then drunk, this will be useful against bladder stones, kidneys and urine dripping, and it will also increase the sexual desire.	Wild donkey meat, its fat and its liver: if they are finely minced , put in a cooking pot with the addition of cow fat and honey, cooked with the final addition of fenugreek, long pepper and galangal—one part of each one—then these will increase the desire of coitus and will improve it.

19.14	رية حمار الوحش تجفف وتدق ويخلط معها كثيراء بيضاء وعسل ويسقي لصاحب الحمى والسعال والغشاوة البصر فيبرأ باذن الله تعالى وتكون الهر به وزن درهم اول النهار ووزن درهم بالعشاء	ريته تجفف وتدق ويخلط معه كثيراء ويعجن بعسل ويلعق منه صاحب الربو والسعال وعسر النفس في كل يوم مرتين بالغداة والعشاء جيد مجرب	رية حمار الوحش اذا جففت ودقت ناعما وخلط معها كثيرة بيضاء وعسل وعجن الجميع بعسل واستعمله صاحب الحمى والسعال والغشاوة البصر كل يوم بالغداء والعشاء ابرأه
19.15	مخ حمار الوحش يذاب بماء الكرفس والعسل ويسقي لمن به السل في الحمام ثلاثة ايام فيبرأ	دماغه يذاف بماء الكرفس والعسل وتغليه على النار غلية وويسقي لمن به السل اياما متوالية في الحمام على الريق جيد نافع	دماغ حمار الوحش يداف بماء الكرفس وشرب منه صاحب علة السل والحمى العتيقة في الحمام ينفع نفعا جيدا
19.16	مخ حمار الوحش يداف بدهن سوسان ويطلي به الركب والمقعدة تحلل باذن الله تعالى	*om.*	*om.*

19.14: (a) *om.* B

(b) صاحب...جيد] على الريق في العشاء فانه ينفع من الربو والسعال وعسر النفس G

(c) بعسل] بعسل نحل C | واستعمله] واستعمل منه C | صاحب] من به C | ابرأه] راى من ذلك عجبا C

19.15: (a) This recipe is attested only in B

(b) يذاف...نافع] اذا اذيف بماء الكرفس والعسل وغلى على النار وشرب منه صاحب السل اياما من اليه في الحمام على الريق نفعه G

(c) يداف] اذا اذيب C | صاحب علة] من به مرض C | والحمى العتيقة] والحمى الربع C | ينفع] نفع C

19.16: (a) يداف] يذاب B | سوسان] سوس B | تحلل] *om.* B

19.14 Wild donkey lung: if it is ground, mixed with astragale and honey, given to a man suffering from fever, cough and cataract to drink, then he will heal, with the permission of God, may He be exalted. The correct amount is of one dirham at the beginning of the day and one dirham in the evening.

Its lung: if it is dried, pounded, mixed with astragale and kneaded with honey, then the man affected by asthma, cough and breath difficulties should lick it twice every day in the morning and in the evening, then this will be good. This has been tried out.

Wild donkey lung: if it is dried, ground into a fine powder, mixed with astragale, then everything is kneaded with honey and given to a man affected by fever and cataract—every day once in the morning and once in the evening—then this will cure him.

19.15 Wild donkey marrow: if it is liquefied with celery water and honey, given to a man suffering from consumption to drink in the bath for three days, then he will recover.

Its brain: if it is mixed with celery water and honey, boiled on the fire and given to a man suffering from consumption to drink, for some days in a row, in the bath on an empty stomach, this will be useful to him.

Wild donkey brain: if it is mixed with celery water and drunk in the bath by a man suffering from consumption and chronic fever, then this will be very useful to him.

19.16 Wild donkey marrow: if it is mixed with iris oil and rubbed on the knees and on the back, then this will relax these parts, with the permission of God, may He be exalted.

om.

om.

٢٠. الجمل

	(a)	b	c
	ذكر منافع اعضاء الجمل	الجمل	باب منافع الجمل
20.1	عظم ساق الجمل يحرق ويدق ويذاف بماء السماء ويصب في جحرة الفار فانه يموت باذن الله تعالى	يؤخذ عظم ساق البعير البختي فيدق ويذاف بالماء ويصبّ في جحرة الفار فانه يقتله	عظم ساق الجمل المنخور والعتيق منهم حديقة العظم واحرقه واسحقه واعجنه بالماء والقه في جحر الفيران فلا يبقي في الجحر شيء حي
20.2	بول الجمل يجعل في وعاء ويلقي عليه ورق الاراك وزيت خالص ويغلي الجميع حتى يذهب البول ويبقي الزيت فيرفع في اناء فاذا احتاج اليه صاحب وجع السرطان والشقاق ويندهن به ويغسله بخمر عتيق فيزول باذن الله تعالى	للسعلة والسرطان وكل ورم حاس يكون في الجسد يؤخذ ابوال ابل الرعي وورق الأراك يجمع ذلك مدقوقا يلقي عليه من الزيت ما يعمّر ويجعل في قدر ثم يطبخ حتى لا يبقي غير الزيت ثم يصفي ويصير في قارورة فاذا اردت ان تعالج به فخذ منه بصوفة وصيّره على المواضع واغسله بعد ذلك بخمر عتيق	بول الجمل ووبعر الوبر وورق الاراك يغلي الجميع بالبول ويغسل منه الشقاق والسرطان وكل وجع حاس فانه يبرأ واذا نطل الموضع بعد ذلك بخمر عتيق كان ابلغ
20.3	بول الجمل الحار كما يبوله فيفقد ويحشي به البواسير فتزول	مما ينفع الناسور ابوال الابل المعقودة	واذا حشى النسور ببول الابل برئ
20.4	رية الجمل يجفف ويسحق سحقا ناعما	واذا كانت وجه الانسان متغيرا او اصفر من مرض او علة فخذ رية الجمل ساعة	اذا كان الوجه مصفرا من مرض خذ رية

20.1: (a) عظم ساق الجمل] ساق الجمل النخر B | ويذاف] ويذاب B | فانه يموت] فيموت B

(b) يؤخذ عظم] *om.* G | البعير] *om.* G | فيدق ويذاف] اذا دق ناعما واذيف G | ويصبّ] وصبّ G | فانه يقتله] قتلهن G

(c) عظم ساق...شيء حي] بعد الدق عظم ساق الجمل الدائر اذا دق ناعما واذيب بالماء وصب في بيت الفأر اذهبه من الدار واذا عجن عظم الجمل بالماء والقى منه في جحر الفأر قتله C

20.2: (a) وعاء] أناء B | الجميع] *om.* B | فيرفع] ويرفع B | اليه] عليه B | والشقاق] والنسعا B

(b) للسعلة...واغسله] ثم ابوال الابل غير معقودة وورق الضاك يدق ويلقي عليه الزيت ويوضع الجميع في قدر ويطبخ حتى يذهب البول ويبقي الزيت يصفي ويصير في قارورة فاذا اردت ان تعالج السلعة التي في الجسد والسرطان وكل ورم يكون في الجسد فخذ من الدواء بصوفة وامسح به الوجع ثم اغسله G

(c) وكل وجع حاس] *om.* C

20.3: (a) This recipe is attested only in B

(b) مما...المعقودة] ابوال الابل المعقودة اذا مسحت في الناصور نفعه G

(c) برئ] ابرأه C

20.4: (a) يجفف] *om.* B | سحقا ناعما] *om.* B | منها] *om.* B | بلا] ملا B

(b) واذا...لونه] ريته الجمل اذا نزعت من جوفة ساعة نزعها تلقي على وجع الانسان فانه يزول ما به من الصفرة والتغبيب من مرض او علة G

(c) اذا كان الوجه مصفرا من مرض خذ] *om.* C | والصقها على وجهه يرد اليه لونه] اذا لصقها وجه من به صفار من الم عاد الوجه الى لونه وازال الصفار منه C

20. Camel

	a	b	c
	Exposition of the useful properties of the parts of the camel	**The camel**	**Chapter on the useful properties of the camel**
20.1	Bone from a camel leg: if it is burnt, ground, mixed with rain water, and poured in the mice hole, then the mice will die, with the permission of God, may He be exalted.	Bone from the leg of a female camel: if it is taken, ground, mixed with water, and poured in the mice hole, then this will kill the mice.	Old and eaten bone of a camel leg: if it is burnt, ground, kneaded with water, and poured in the mice hole, then not a single mouse will remain alive.
20.2	Camel urine: if it is poured in a vase, with arak leaves and pure oil, everything boiled until the urine has evaporated while the oil remains, then this has to be preserved inside a vessel; when the man suffering from cancer and splitting pain needs it, rub him with this, and wash him with old wine, and then the pain will cease, with the permission of God, may He be exalted.	Against cough, cancer and every moist swelling on the body, urine of different camels from the herd and arak leaves, pounded with the addition of enough oil to cover it, placed in a cooking pot; then cooked until the urine has evaporated while the oil remains, then purified and poured in a long-necked flask; when you wish to cure with this, take it with a woollen cloth, and wipe it on the areas, after this wash him [the man] old wine.	If the urine of the camel, the droppings of the hyrax and anise leaves are boiled together, and used to wash splitting [pain] and the cancer, and every acute pain, then this will heal;and if the part is washed with old wine after this, then this will be even more effective.
20.3	Camel urine, as warm as it comes out: if it is stuffed in the haemorrhoids, then these will cease.	Among the things that are useful against the fistula: thickened urine of different camels.	If the fistula is stuffed with camel urine, then this will heal.
20.4	Camel lung: if it is dried, finely ground, and applied on the face	If the face of a man has changed its colour or it is yellow for a disease or an illness, take the lung of the	If the face is yellow for a disease, take the lung of camel, warm as

	الجمل ساعة تخرج من جوفه حارة والصقها على وجهه يرد اليه لونه	ان تنزع من جوفه والصقها على وجهه وهي حارة فانها ترده لونه	ويجعل منها على الوجه الاصفر بلا مرض فيزول الصفرة
20.5	دماغ الجمل اذا اذيف بماء الكراث النبطي وتمسح به عند النوم يبرأ	دماغ الجمل للزحير يخلط بماء الكراث النبطي ويمسح به السفل وقت المنام نفعه	دماغ الجمل يخلط بماء الكراث النبطي يمسح به فم الصفرة فينفع من الزحير ورمى الدم باذن الله وينفع ايضا من البواسير
20.6	شعر الجمل اذا حرق قطع الدم السائل لوقته والرعاف درورا	*om.*	*om.*
20.7	الجوز أكله على الريق يقطع السموم ونماده في المصرة يمنع المغص	*om.*	*om.*
20.8	سنام الجمل يذاف بدهن المشمش ويلقي عليه ما الكراث النبطي ويدهن به النسور الذي يكون في فم الجرح يسكن المه	سنام الجمل يذوّب ويخلط بدهن المشمش وشيء من ماء الكراث النبطي ويمسح به من به البواسير في السفلة فيذهب	*om.*
20.9	لعاب الجمل الهائج اذا شرب منه انسان وزن نصف درهم تغير عقله واختل	وكذلك سنام الجمل يذاف في لغام الجمل العائج ويسقي منه انسان في رأس الهلال بشراب الجرز يخبط مثل الجمل الهائج المجنون	لعاب الجمل الهائج يسقي منه الانسان يختل عقله

20.5: (c) ويمسح [وتمسح C | يبرأ] ازال ذلك ايضا C
(b) اذا خلط بماء الكرفس النبطي ومسح به ما يقعد عليه صاحب الزحير للقيام [للزحير...المنام G
(c) الكرات [الكراث L C
20.6: (c) In C this recipe after 20.1
20.7: (c) *om.* C | In L another recipe is added, with an onyx tied to the hair of a woman to ease the birth: الجزع اذا الف به شعر المطلقة اسرع الولد
20.8: (a) This recipe is attested only in B
(b) This recipe is attested only in G; In T the ingredient is mentioned in the following recipe
(c) المشمش] نواء قلب المشمش C | ويدهن] ودهن C | يسكن الجرح] سكن المجرح C
20.9: (a) This recipe is attested only in B
(b) وكذلك...المجنون] من أخذ من لعاب الجمل الهائج فسقي لانسان في رأس الهلال جن G
(c) واختل] واحتبل C

	with a yellow complexion that is not due to any disease, then this will cease.	camel, in the moment in which it is taken out from its abdomen, and apply it on his face while it is still warm, and then this will revert to its [normal] colour.	when it is taken out from the abdomen, apply it on the face, and then it will return to its own colour.
20.5	Camel brain: if it is mixed with wild leek water, and wiped on the anus, then this will be useful against the dysentery and the expulsion of blood, with the permission of God, may He be exalted; it is useful against haemorrhoids too.	Camel brain, against dysentery: if it is melted with celery water and rubbed on the bottom the man suffering from dysentery, then this will be useful to him.	Camel brain: if it is melted with wild leek water, and rubbed on a man during his sleep, then he will recover.
20.6	*om.*	*om.*	Camel hair: if it is burnt, this will instantly stop the bleeding and the nosebleed.
20.7	*om.*	*om.*	If the heart is eaten on an empty stomach, then this will stop the poisons; and if it is applied on the belly, then this will prevent the colic.
20.8	*om.*	Camel hump: if it is melted, mixed with apricot oil and some wild leek water, then rubbed on the man suffering from haemorrhoids in his bottom, then these will cease.	Camel hump: if it is mixed with apricot oil, with the addition of wild leek, and rubbed on the fistula that has formed on the wound, then this will calm its pain.
20.9	Saliva of the excited camel: if it is given to a man to drink, then his mind will become disordered.	The hump likewise, if it is mixed with the foam of the excited camel, given to a man at the new moon to drink with wine from the barrel, then he will stamp and stumble like a crazy excited camel.	Saliva of the excited camel: if a man drinks half dirham of it, this will affect his mind and will put it in disorder.

20.10	*om.*	*om.*	فاذا اردت خلاصه المعمة الهعمة سمنا بقريا وخلا حادقا
20.11	مخ الجمل يذاب بماء المر ويسقي لصاحب وجع الظهر فينفعه باذن الله تعالى	مخ الجمل لوجع الصلب يذاف بماء المر المطبوخ ثم يشربه في الحمام على الريق ثلاثة ايام متوالية	مخ الجمل يذاب بماء المر ويطبخ على النار ويسقي لصاحب وجع الظهر في الحمام ثلاث ليال متواليات فانه يبرأ
20.12	بعر الجمل البرية يجفف ويسحق معه دقيق الدرمك ويعجن بحمر خالص ويدهن به الحلق الوارم ويزول ورمه	بعر الابل البرية يسحق يابسا ويخلط معه دقيق ورمل ويعجن بطلاء عتيق ويضمّد به من كان به ورم في حلقة من داخل او خارج ويذهبه ان شاء الله تعالى	بعر الابل البرية يسحق ويخلط بماء الدرمك ويعجن يخمر عتيق ويضمد به صاحب الحناق وورم الحلقوم يبرئه
20.13	*om.*	ابوال الابل البرية يؤخذ فتعقد على النار ويلقي عليه شيئا من المر الورس ويجفف في الشمس فاذا جفّ يكتحل به من الرطوبة في العين والدمعة والحمرة والجرب والغشاوة	*om.*
20.14	*om.*	ومن كان به شيء من صفار او مليلة في ظاهره او باطنه فليدق منه بماء وزن مثقال ويشربه بلبن البقر ثلاثة ايام على الريق وربما شربت ابوال الابل مع البانها لاوجاع الكبد والاورام العارضة فيها	*om.*

20.10: (a) This recipe is attested only in B
(c) خلاصة المعمة الهعمة] والخلاص منه اطعمه C
20.11: (a) This recipe is attested only in B
(b) لوجع الصلب] *om.* G | الم] التمر G | الحمام] الحمام صاحب وجع الصلب *add.* G
(c) يذاب] اذيب C
20.12: (a) This recipe is attested only in B
(b) يسحق] *om.* G | بطلاء عتيق] يطلي G | او خارج] وخارج G | ويذهبه] فيذهبه G
(c) بماء الدرمك] بدقيق الفريك C | به صاحب] به حلق صاحب C | يبرئه] برأ C
20.13: (b) يؤخذ] *om.* G | فتعقد] تعقّد G | عليه شيئا من المر والورس] فيه مر وورس G | ويجفف] وتجفف G
20.14: (b) شيء من] *om.* G | او مليلة] ومليلة G | في ظاهره او باطنه] ظاهرة او باطنة G | فليدق] فيدق G | بماء] *om.* G | ويشربه] ويشرب G | فيها] *om.* G

20.10	*om.*	*om.*	If you want to bring this to an end, take cow fat and sour vinegar.
20.11	Camel marrow: if it is melted with myrrh water, and given to the man suffering from back pain to drink, then this will be useful to him, with the permission of God, may He be exalted.	Camel marrow, against the pain of the spine: if it is mixed with cooked myrrh water, then drunk in the bath by the man suffering from spine pain—on an empty stomach for three days in the same quantity [it will be useful].	Camel marrow: if it is melted with myrrh water, cooked on the fire, and given to the man suffering from back pain to drink—the same quantity for three nights—then he will recover.
20.12	Wild camel droppings: if they are dried, ground with first quality flour, kneaded with pure vinegar, and rubbed on the swollen throat, then its swelling will subside.	Wild camel droppings: if they are ground dry, mixed with flour and sand, kneaded with old pitch, and the man who has a swelling in his throat is bandaged with it—from inside or outside—then this will go away, God willing.	Wild camel droppings: if they are ground with first quality flour water, kneaded with old wine, and the man suffering from throat swelling is bandaged with it, then this will subside.
20.13	*om.*	Urine of different wild camels: these have to be thickened on the fire, with the addition of a bit of myrrh and curcuma and dried in the sunlight; then once it has dried, it has to be applied in the eyes affected by moistness, lachrymation, irritation, scabies and the cataract.	*om.*
20.14	*om.*	The man who is affected by yellow bile and feverish heat outside or inside, should crush one *miṯqāl* of it, drink it with cow milk for three days on an empty stomach; the urine of different camels may be drunk with different milks against the liver complaint and the occasional swellings.	*om.*

20.15	رية الجمل البكر الذي ليس به علة تشرح رقيقا ويدر عليها كاشم مسحوق منخول وكثيرة وباقلا مسحوقان ويخلط الجميع ويشرب منه من ضيف النفس في كل يوم خمسه دراهم على الريق ويشرب بعده حليب الضان خمسه ايام متولية ينفع نفعا جيدا	من السدد والربو وعسر النفس يؤخذ رية جمل ليس به علة فتشرّح تشريحا رقيقا ثم يذر عليها كاشم مسحوق منخول ويخلط معه من ماء الكسبرة المنخولة جزء ومن الباقلا المقشور جزء مسحوقا منخولا ويسقي منه لصاحب هذه العلة في كل يوم على الريق وزن خمس دراهم ومثلها بالعشى ويسقي بعده لبن ضأن حليبا كما يحتلب	رية الجمل تشرح ويذر عليها كاشم مسحوق منخول وبقلا مسحوق وكثيرة بيضاء مسحوقة من كل واحد جزء ويخلط الجميع ويسقي لصاحب ضيق النفس والربو على الفواد كل يوم خمس دراهم باذن الله ويسقي بعده كذلك لبن حليب الضان ينفعه
20.16	دماغ الجمل يعجن بخل ويسقي منه المصروع في الشهر ثلاثه ايام في كل عشرة ايام مرة واحدة يبرأ	دماغه اذا جفّف واذيف بخل وسقى منه من يصرع من المرّة السوداء في رأس كل هلال او وسطه	دماغ الجمل يجفف ويعجن بخل خمر ويسقي منه المصروع من السوداء في رأس كل هلال مرة فيبرأ باذن الله
20.17	اذا كانت الدابة تنفر من الجمال خذ مخلاة واملاها بعر الجمل وعلقها في رأس الدابة من الغداء الى العشاء فانها يسكن نقورها وتانس بالجمال باذن الله سحبانه وتعالى	اذا كانت الدابة تنفر من الجمال فخذ مقدار نصف مخلاة من بعر الجمال وعلقه على الدابة المخلاة بما فيها من البعر من غدوة الى نصف النهار حتى تشم ريح البعر ثم ينزع فاذا علقتَ الشعير فرد عليه مخلاة البعر فانه يذهب نفاره	للدابة يؤخذ بعر الجمل وتملا منه مخلاة ويعلق في رأسها نهارا كاملا فلا تقود تنقر ثم يلبس بالجمل وغيرها والله تعالى اعلم
20.18	*om.*	يؤخذ من قردان الجمل واحدة على اسم من تريد محبه واسم امّه فتعلقه على كمّ العاشق من حيث لا يعلم يذهب الحب من قلبه	*om.*

20.15: (a) This recipe is attested only in B

(b) من السدد...حليبا] رية الجمل الذي ليس به علة تشرّح ثم يذر عليها كاشم مسحوق منخول وتجفّف في الشمس فاذا جفّت يؤخذ منها جزأ مسحوقا منخولا ويخلط معه كثيرا مسحوق منخول جزء ومن الباقلي المقشّر المسحوق المنخول جزين ويسقي منه صاحب الربو وعسر النفس وزن خمس دراهم كل يوم على ريق ومثلها بالعشى يسقي بعده لبن ضان حليبا مقدار ربع رطل حار G

(c) وباقلا] وهو الفول *add.* C | الجميع] جميعا C | من] من به C | جيدا] جيدا انتهي C

20.16: (a) This recipe is attested only in B

(b) دماغه] دماغ البعير G | من يصرع من] منه من يصرع من به لمن G | في] عند G | او وسطه] وفي وسط شهر نفعه G

(c) دماغ الجمل] دماغ البعير C

20.17: (a) This recipe is attested only in B

(b) In T this recipe is after 20.19 | مقدار] قدر G | وعلقه] وعلقها G | المخلاة بما فيها من البعر] *om.* G | غدوة] اول النهار G | نصف النهار] وسطه G | البعر] الجمال G | ثم ينزع...نفاره] ثم انزعها عنه وافعل ذلك مرارا فانه يذهب G

(c) وعلقها] وتعلقها C | بالجمال] بالجمال فائدة C | In C another recipe is added, to calm an animal with a Qur'anic verse (3:83): اذا كانت الدابة شموصة فاقرا في اذنها قول تعالى ﴿أفغير دين الله يبغون وله أسلم من في السماوات والأرض طوعا وكرها وإليه يرجعون﴾

20.18: (b) يؤخذ...يذهب] اذا أخذ قرادة من ناقة باسم من يحب واسم امّه ثم عُلقت في كمّ العاسق وهو لا يعلم ذهب G

20.15	Camel lung: if it is cut in slices, with the addition of ground and sieved Mediterranean moon carrot, pounded broad beans and ground astragale—one part of each one—everything melted and given to drink to the man suffering from breath weakness and asthma, five dirhams every day [this will be useful], with the permission of God; after this, he should be given to some sheep milk to drink, and this will be useful to him.	Against obstruction, asthma, breath difficulties, lung of a camel without any disease: if it is finely cut in slices, then some ground and sieved Mediterranean moon carrot is poured on it, mixed with one part of ground and sieved coriander water, one part of ground and sieved peeled broad beans, and given to drink to the man suffering from this disease—five dirhams every day on an empty stomach, and the same quantity in the evening—after this he has to be given sheep milk to drink as it comes out when milked.	Lung of a young camel without any disease: if it is cut in fine slices, with the addition of some ground and sieved Mediterranean moon carrot, goat's thorn and broad beans—both ground and sieved—everything melted and given to the man suffering from breath weakness to drink—five dirhams every day on an empty stomach—drinking after this the milk of a sheep, the same quantity for five days, then this will be very useful to him.
20.16	Camel brain: if it is dried, kneaded with wine vinegar, and given to drink at the new moon to the man affected by epilepsy due to black gall, then this will heal, with the permission of God.	Its brain: it has to be dried, mixed with vinegar, and given to the man who has epilepsy due to black gall, at the beginning of the lunar month or in its middle.	Camel brain: if it is kneaded with vinegar, and given to the epileptic man to drink—three days per month, once every ten days—then this will heal.
20.17	For the domestic beasts, take some camel droppings, fill the nosebag with them, and hang it on its head for a whole month, but do not let it rip, then let it wear to the camel or to another animal, and God knows best.	If a domestic beast has an aversion for the camel, take half nosebag of camel droppings, hang it on the beast with what is in it, from the morning until half of the day, so that it can sniff the smell of the droppings, then remove it; and when you give it barley again, then this will echo the camel droppings and the aversion will cease.	If a domestic beast has an aversion for the camel, take a nosebag and fill it with camel droppings, hang it on the head of the beast from the morning until the evening, then its aversion will be appeased, and it will like the company of camels, with the permission of God, may He be exalted.
20.18	*om.*	If one tick from the camel is taken in the name of the one whose love you want [to take away], and the name of his mother, then hung on the sleeve of the lover when he is not aware of it, then the love will leave his heart.	*om.*

٢١. الضأن

	a	b	c
	ذكر منافع اعضاء الحروف	الضأن	باب منافع الضأن
21.1	دماغ الخروف يكتحل به من في عينيه الماء المكمد فيزول باذن الله تعالى	دماغ الضأن اذا اكتحل به الماء في العين نفعه	دماغ الضأن اذا اكتحل به من في عينيه الماء المكمد ابرأه
21.2	مخ الخروف اذا يذاب بدهن على النار ويلقي عليه سكر ودهن زنبق ويسقي لصاحب بول الدم ورمى الحصاة فيزول باذن الله تعالى	مخ الخروف اذا اذيف بدهن الجوز على النار وخلط معه سكر طبرزذ وقطّع عليه زنبق خالص وشربه من به الخصاة فتّته	مخ الخروف اللطيف يدهن بدهن الجوز علي النار ويلقي عليه جلاب السكر ويقطر عليه دهن الزنبق ويسقي لمن به الحصاة وبول الدم يبرأ
21.3	وينفع ايضا المحرقات في الاحليل ووجع الخاصرة	وكذلك ينفع ايضا لمن يبول الدم ويجد حرقة في الاحليل وينفع من وجع الكلى ومن وجع الخاصرة اذا اذيف بشراب وشرب في الحمام	ينفع للحرقات في الاحليل ووجع الخاصرة
21.4	دم النعجة حار كما يذبح يدلك به الوضح فيغير لونه	دم الشاة الحار كما تذبح اذا لطخ به مواضع الوضح [بماء السذاب] غيّر لونه وقلعه	واذا شرب بماء السذاب ودم الانثى من الضأن وهو حار كما وتجت وطلى به موضع الوضح ابراها وصيرها بلون الجسد ويقلع الآكلة من البدن
21.5	*om.*	دم الشاة حار كما تذبح يلطخ على مواضع فيها شعر حلقه ونثره	*om.*

21.1: (b) يكتحل] اذا اكتحل G | من به] *om.* G | الماء ينفعه] الماء في العين نفعه G
21.2: (a) بدهن] بدهن الجوز *add.* B | فيزول] فيزول عنه B
(b) وقطّع...فتّته] *om.* T
(c) يدهن] اذا اذيف C | ويقطر] وقطر C | دهن] شيء من دهن C | ويسقي لمن] وشربه من C | وبول الدم] ورمى الدم C
21.3: (a) *om.* B
(b) This recipe is attested only in B
(c) ينفع...الخاصرة] نفع ايضا واذا شرب بماء السذاب وينفع وجع الخاصرة C
21.4: (a) *om.* B
(b) This recipe is attested only in B
(c) ويقلع الآكلة من البدن] يمنع الآكلة C
21.5: (b) دم الشاة...ونثره] وكذلك دم الشاة اذا طلى به الشعر حلقه G

21. Sheep

	a	b	c
	Exposition of the useful properties of the parts of the lamb	**The sheep**	**Chapter on the useful properties of the sheep**
21.1	Lamb brain: if it is applied on the eyes of the man affected by dark water, then this will cease, with the permission of God, may He be exalted.	Sheep brain: if it is applied on the water in the eye, then will be useful against it.	Sheep brain: if it is applied on the eyes of the man affected by dark water, then this will cure him.
21.2	Lamb marrow: if it is liquefied with oil on the fire, with the addition of sugar and lily oil, and given to drink to the man who urinates blood and expels stones, then this will cease, with the permission of God, may He be exalted.	Lamb marrow: if it is mixed with nut oil on the fire, melted with rock sugar, with the addition of pure lily [oil] in drops, and drunk by the man suffering from stones, then this will crumble them.	Brain of a tender lamb: if it is mixed with nut oil on the fire, with the addition of some sugar julep and of lily oil in drops, and given to drink to the men suffering from stones and blood in the urine, then he will recover.
21.3	It is also useful against the burnings in the outer opening of urethra, and against the pain of the hips.	Likewise, it is also useful to the man who urinates blood, and has a burning in the outer opening of urethra; it is useful against the pain of the kidneys and of the hips, if it is mixed with wine and drunk in the bath.	It is also useful against the burnings in the outer opening of urethra and the pain of the hips.
21.4	Ewe blood, as warm as at the moment of the slaughtering: if it is rubbed on the leprosy, then this will change its colour.	Blood of female sheep, as warm as when it is slaughtered: if it is spattered on the areas affected by leprosy with rue water, then this will change its colour, and will eradicate it.	If some rue water and the blood of female sheep—as warm as when it comes out—are rubbed on the areas affected by leprosy, then this will cure it, will change the colour of the body, and will eradicate the gangrene from the body.
21.5	*om.*	Ewe blood, as warm as when it is slaughtered: if it is spattered on the areas with hair, then this will remove and disperse it.	*om.*

21.6	*om.*	لحم الضأن يؤكل فيورث صاحب الحفض حتى يحفظ حتى يحفظ كلما يسمعه	*om.*
21.7	مرارة الخروف يطلي به الآكلة التي في الجسد فيذهب باذن الله تعالى	مرارة الضأن اذا طلى بها مواضع الآكلة نفعه نفعا بينا	*om.*
21.8	للاستسقاء يؤخذ رأس النعجة تضف جيدا وشرحه ثلثة اجزاء ثم جعل في كل جزء منه ورق الجوز البري ويحشي منه المنخرين والاذنين ويجعل في التنور ليلة فاذا كان من الغداء تخرجه وتستخرج ذلك الورق ثم تطعم لصاحب الاستسقاء ثلثة ايام فيزول باذن الله تعالى	يؤخذ رأس الشاة وينقي ويجود تنظيفه كما يهيأ للاكل ويشرّح كل حد ثلاث تشريحات وتحشي ورق الجوز البري او تحشي منخره واذناة وغلصمته واجعله في تنور الرواس وفرغ ما فيها ويطعم صاحب الاستسقاء ثلاثة ايام يبرأ باذن الله تعالى	رأس الشاة الضان يشرح ويحشي اذناه وحلقومه بورق الزيتون او الجوز البري ويجعل في تنور الذى للمرواسين من الغشاء الى بكرة يأكل منها صاحب الاستسقاء بعدان تخرج من التنور ويرمي ما فيه من الورق ثلاث مرات يبرأ
21.9	للطحال لحم بشتمازك التي يكون للخروف تشرح ارقّ ما يكون وتكبّ على الجمر فاذا سال ماؤها وكادت ان تنضج يؤخذ ويجعل في خل خمر حاذق ثم يأخذ صاحب الطحال ذلك اللحم فيمصه ويشرب ذلك الخل يذهب عنه الطحال وحمى الكبد	للطحال يؤخذ لحم ضأن من البشتمازك فيشرّحه ارقّ ما يكون ثم يكب على النار فاذا سال ماء اللحم فكاد ان ينضج يصير في الخل ثقيف يومر صاحب تلك العلة ان يمضغ اللحم ويحسى ذلك الخل الذي كان فيه منقعا ويرمي الثقل ولا يبلعه فانه يبرأ باذن الله تعالى	لحم الخروف يشرح رقيقا ويجعل على الفحم فاذا سال ماؤه يجعل في كل خل حادق ويعطى لصاحب الاستسقاء والطحال يزول عنه

21.6: (b) يؤكل فيورث] اذا أكل اورث G

21.7: (b) بها مواضع الآكلة] به المواضع الذي قد وقعت فيه الآكلة *add.* G | نفعا بينا] *om.* G

21.8: (a) تضف] ينصف B | وشرحه] او يقسم B | ورق الجوز البري] ورق البرنوق وهي الجوز البري ويجعل فيه سافات B | ويحشي] وتحشي B | المنخرين والاذنين] المناخير والاذان B | من الغداة] بالغداة B | فيزول] فينفعه ذلك B
(b) يؤخذ...يهيأ] اذا اردت ان تعالج الاستسقاء فخذ رأس شاة وجوّد تنظيفه كما يجوّد G | ورق الجوز البري] بورق ودنوا رطب وهو الجوز البري السرد G | واجعله] ويجعل G | واجعله] بذلك ويجعل G | في تنور الرواس] اتون الرواسين G | وفرغ...يبرأ] فاذا كان من الغد أخذت الرأس ونزعت ما فيه من البورق واطعمته صاحب الاستسقاء ثلاثة ايام فانه يبرأ G | وتسميه العامة خلال المامون *add.* G
(c) ويحشي] حشيت C | تنور] التنور C | بكرة] بكرة النهار C | صاحب] من به C | تخرج] يخرج C | ويرمي] ورمي C | ثلاث مرات يبرأ] *om.* C

21.9: (a) بستمازك التي يكون للخروف] بستمازكة الخروف B | وتكبّ] وتترك B | تنصبح] تقيج B | حاذق] عتيق B | صاحب الطحال] *om.* B | يأخذ] تأخذ B | فيمصه] فيمضغه B | ويشرب] وشرب B | يذهب] فيذهب B
(b) البشتمازك] المبشمار T; البشتمارج G | الطحال...فيشرّحه] وكذلك اذا اردت علاج الطحال فخذ لحم البشتمازك وشرّحه G | يكب] يكبّب ويجعل G | فكاد] وكاد G | يصير] أخذت الكباب وجعل في G | يومر...الثقل] ثم يأخذ صاحب ذلك الوجع الكباب ويمضغها ويرمي ثقلها G
(c) يشرح رقيقا] اذا شرح C | ويجعل] وجعل C | يجعل في كل خل حادق] جعل في نصف حادق C | ويعطى لصاحب] واستعمله صاحب C | يزول] ازول ذلك C

21.6	*om.*	Sheep meat: if it is eaten, by a man, this will expand the memory to the point that he will remember everything he hears.	*om.*
21.7	Lamb gall: if it is rubbed on the gangrene that affects the body, then this will go away, with the permission of God, may He be exalted.	Sheep gall: if it rubbed on the areas affected by the gangrene, then this will be clearly useful.	*om.*
21.8	Against dropsy, ewe head: if it is cleaned well, cut in three pieces, then a leaf of wild nut is placed inside each piece, stuffed in the nostrils and in the ears, then it is put inside a baking oven for one night; when the morning comes, take it out and remove the leaves, then feed these for three days to the man affected by dropsy, then this will cease, with the permission of God, may He be exalted.	Ewe head: if it is taken, cleaned well as if it were meant for eating, then each side cut in three, stuffed with wild nut inside the nostrils, the ears and the throat, then put it in the oven of the heads seller; when the morning comes, remove what is inside it, and give it to the man suffering from dropsy for three days to eat, then he will heal, with the permission of God, may He be exalted.	Ewe head: if it is cut, the ears and the throat are stuffed with olive or wild nut leaves, put inside a backing oven that is used by the sellers of sheep heads, from the evening until the morning, then fed to the man suffering from dropsy—taken out from the backing oven with a branch and the leaves removed from inside it—for three days, then he will heal.
21.9	For the spleen, meat that is at the extremity of the ribs of the lamb: if it is minced very finely, made soft, and roasted as a roll on the live coal; when its water has gone and it is well cooked, take it and put it in sour wine vinegar; then the man suffering from spleen complaint should take this meat, chew it, and drink the vinegar, then the spleen complaint and the fever of the liver will leave him.	For the spleen, meat from the extremity of the ribs of the sheep: if it is cut very finely, softened, and roasted on the fire as a roll; once the water of the meat has gone and it is well cooked, it has to be put in good vinegar; then the man suffering from this disease has to be told to chew the meat and sip this vinegar in which there is some usefulness, throwing the solid part away without swallowing, and then he will heal.	Lamb meat: if it is finely cut, and put on the live coal, once the water has gone, put in any kind of vinegar, and offered to the man suffering from dropsy and spleen, then these will cease.

21.10

واذا اردت ان ينضج التين في شجرة قبل اوانه خذ قرن كبش وادفنه تحت الشجرة فانها تننضج سريعا

واذا اردت ان ينضج التين سريعا فادفن في اصل الشجرة قرن كبش

اذا اردت ان تنضج التين في غير وقته فخذ قرن كبش فادفنه في اصل الشجرة تنضج سريعا

21.11

اذا اردت ان يذهب داء الغنم خذ جوف كبش واطبخه بشراب وماء ثمر صبه في الحوض الذي شرب منه الغنم التي بها فان ديها يذهب

بطن الكبش اذا طبخ بشراب وماء وخلط ماء وسقى للغنم ذهب عنها دواء والفناء

اذا اردت ان تذهب الدواء الذي تسلط على الغنم فيقتلها فخذ كبشا كبيرا واطبخه بشراب وقليل ماء وصبّه في الماء الذي تشرب منه الغنم فيذهب الداء باذن الله تعالى

21.12

اذا أكل من به البرص كل يوم بالغداة شرائح الضأن وشرب فوقها رطل شراب عتيق وقف عنه

يطعم من به البرص كبابا من البشتمازك الضان مع شيء من السذاب فانه يبرأ

يؤخذ لحم الخروف الذي يكون انثى فيشرح ويكب على الجمر بلا ملح ولا ازار ويسقي المرض بعد ان اكله ثلاثة ايام بشراب صرف فيزول عنه باذن الله تعالى

21.13

اذا كان المرأة استرخاء الرحم خذ رأس شاة الغنم الضأن منعها على النار بعد ان تنصب لها عيدان الطرفاء وتجعلها عليهم حتى يتصعد الدخان وتقف المرأة على ذلك الدخان حيث يدخل جوفها فانها تبرأ

لاستداد الرحم يؤخذ دود من رأس شاة فيضع على جمر ويصير عليه طرفاء وتنفخ المرأة عليه حتى يطلع اليها الدخان

اذا كان بالمرأة برودة في فم الرحم يؤخذ رأس نعجة يعمل على عيدان طرفاء ويجعل على الجمر ثم تنفح عليه المرأة حتى يصعد اليها الدخان فتنري باذن الله تعالى

21.10: (a) التين] الشيء B | فادفنه] وادفنه B
(b) This recipe is attested only in G
(c) واذا اردت ان ينصج التين في شحره قبل او انه] *om.* C | خذ قرن كبش وادفنه] اذا ادفن قرن الكبش C | الشحرة] التين شجرة C | تنضبح سريعا] ينضبح عاجلا C
21.11: (a) *om.* B
(b) This recipe is attested only in G
(c) بها
فان ديها يذهب] فانه يذهب الدا عنها C
21.12: (a) *om.* B
(b) يطعم...يبرأ] بشتمازج الضأن يجعل كباب مع شيء من سذاب ويأكله صاحب البرص مع الخبز اربعين يوما لا يذوق غيره فانه يبرأ G
(c) اذا أكل...وقف عنه] كل يوم بالغداة شرائح الضان وشرب فوقها عتيق وقف عنه الوضح C
21.13: (a) رأس] *om.* B | على الجمر] على النار B | على المرأة] تنفح عليه ويوقد عليها B | فتنري] فتنري B *add.* حتى يصعد اليها من ذلك الدخان
(b) لاستداد...الدخان] رأس الشاة اذا وضع على الجمر وجعل عليه ظرف ونفخ عليه تفجّجت عليه المرأه التي بها انشداد الرحم حتى يدخل فيها نفعها G
(c) اذا كان...فانها تبرأ] اذا دخل الدخان الى رحم امرأة حصل لها مرض استرخاء الرحم فاذا دخل الدخان [...] على النار وضع عليها عيد [...] حتى يتصعد الدخان الى جوفها ابرأها C

21.10	If you want that the figs ripen outside their season, take the horn of ram and bury it under the roots of the tree, then this will quickly give fruit.	If you want that the figs become ripe quickly, bury the horn of a ram among the roots of the tree.	If you want that the figs become ripe before their time, take the horn of a ram and bury it under the tree, then this will quickly give fruit.
21.11	If you want to cure the disease that affects the sheep and kills them, take a big ram, cook it with wine and a bit of water, then pour this in the water that is drunk by the sheep, and the disease will cease, with the permission of God, may He be exalted.	Ram abdomen: if it is cooked with wine and water, the water is mixed and given to drink to the sheep, then the disease and the ruin will leave them.	If you want that the disease of the sheep goes away, take the abdomen of a ram, cook it with wine and dates water, pour it in the basin from which sheep affected by the disease drinks, then this will cease.
21.12	Meat of a female lamb: if it is cut and roasted like a roll on the live coal—without salt or any dressing—give it to the sick man after he has eaten it for three days with pure wine, and then this will cease, with the permission of God, may He be exalted.	If the man affected by leprosy eats a roll of the meat that is at the extremity of the ribs of the sheep with some rue, then he will heal.	If the man affected by leprosy eats every morning a ram stew, drinking one *raṭl* of old wine with it, then [the leprosy] will leave him.
21.13	If a woman has the coldness in the neck of the womb, ewe head: if it is taken, pierced with a branch of tamarisk, and put on the live coal, then the woman should blow until the smoke reaches her, and then she will heal, with the permission of God, may He be exalted.	Against the obstruction of the uterus: the worm from the head of the ewe has to be taken, placed on the live coal, tamarisk has to be placed on top of it, and the woman blows on it so that the smoke rises towards her.	If the woman is affected by the flaccidity of the uterus, take the head of a sheep, place it on to the fire after having laid some tamerisk branches on top of it, until the smoke rises while the woman stands over it, so that it can enter in her abdomen, then she will recover.

21.14

خصوة الكبش اذا ملحت وجففت وأخذ زرواند مطاول ونطرون احمر وكمون كرماني من كل واحد جزء ودق الجميع ويحل وشرب منه صاحب البرص البهق اوقف عنه

للبرص والبهق ووجع الكبد يؤخذ خصية كبش يملّح ويذرّ عليها زراوند طويل وكمون كرماني ونطرون من كل واحد جزء مدقوق ويخفّفت ويسحق منها وزن مثقال وينخل ويشرب بماء حار

للبرص والبهق يؤخذ مخصى الكبش الكبير فتشرح وتملح بملح ونطرون وكمون كرماني ويجفف ويسحق ويسقي منها صاحب البرص علي الريق وزن مثقال بماء حار نفعه

21.15

اذا أخذ دم الضأن وشحمه وزيادة الكبد ودق الجميع والقى عليه نطرون احمر واذيب الجميع بماء القراط واكتحل به من به العمش والجهر ابرأه

للعمش وكثرة القذاة في البصر لحم الضأن وشحمه وكبده فيدق ويخلط بماء القرط ويخلط مع نطرون ويكتحل به لهذه العلة نافع

ان كان الانسان اغمسا او اجهرا يؤخذ لحم الخروف وشحمه وكبده يداف الجميع ويخلط بماء القرط ويلقا عليه نطرون فانه يزول باذن الله تعالى

21.16

مراره الكبش السمين اذا طلى بها الاحليل عند الجماع هيج المرأة هيجا عظيما وزاد في القوة

من أخذ مرارة كبش سمين يطلي به احليله في وقت الجماع احبت حبا شديدا

اذا اردت ان تقوي على الجماع فخذ مرارة كبش سمين واطلى بها الاحليل عند الجماع فانه يهيج ذلك كثيرا وهو عجيب

21.17

دماغ الخروف اذا جعل على النار ودرن عليه دقيق الكرسنه والورس والحلبة وضرب الجميع حتى تصير كالمرهم وجعل على خرقة وشد علي مواضع الكسر في الانسان ابرأه وجيده

دماغ الخروف يصير على النار ويصير معه دقيق حُوّاري وورس وحلبة ويضرب حتى يصير مثل الضماد ويضمّد موضع الكسر والوثي ويشد فيبرأ باذن الله تعالى

اذا اردت ان تجبر الكسر في اليدين او الرجلين يؤخذ دماغ الخروف طريا فيجعل في وعاء وتلقي عليه دقيقا ابيضا حواري وورسا وحلبة ويضرب الجميع ويشال على النار فاذا صار مثل المرهم يشد على الكسر فتجبره

21.14: (a) مخصى] خصى B | فتشرح] تشرح B | ونطرون] ونطرون احمر B | ويسحق] om. B | منها] منه B | نفعه] نافع B
(b) للبرص...حار] خصية الكبش اذا ملّحت وذرّ عليها زراوند طويل ونطرون وكمون كرماني من كل واحد جزء ومدقوق منخول وخفّفت وسقى منها صاحب الربو والبهر ووجع الكبد وزن مثقال نفعه G
(c) وتحل] ويحل C | اوقف عنه] ازال ذلك عنه C
21.15: (a) اغمسا او اجهرا] اغمس او اجهر B | يداف] يدق B | القرط] القراط B | نطرون] نطرون احمر B | فانه يزول] فتذهب به العلل ويكتحل B
(b) للعمش وكثرة القذاة في البصر] واذا اردت ان تصنع كحلا ينفع للعمش والجهر وكثرة الاذي في البصر فخذ G | فيدق...نافع] ودق الجميع واطبخه بماء القرط واخلط مع نطرون واستعمله هذه العلل G
(c) اذا أخذ] om. C | نطرون احمر] النطرون الاحمر C | القراط] القرط C | به الغمش والجهر ابرأه] بعينيه غمش وجهر فانه يبرأه C
21.16: (a) وهو عجيب] om. B
(b) من أخذ] om. G | سمين] الكبير G | يطلي به] طلى بها الرجل G | في] om. G | احبت] احبت المرأة G | شديدا] ابدا G
(c) هيجا] تهييجا C | في القوة] في القوة الاعاض C
21.17: (a) om. B
(b) In G this recipe is after 21.15 | يصير على النار ويصير] اذا خلط G | الضماد] المرهم على النار G | ويضمّد] وضمّد G | ويشد فيبرأ] نفعه G
(c) وضرب] وخلط C | حتى] الى ان C | الانسان] عظم الانسان C

21.14 Against leprosy and vitiligo, testicles of the big ram: if they are seasoned with salt, soda and cumin, dried, ground and one *miṯqāl* of it is given to the man suffering from leprosy to drink on an empty stomach with warm water, then this will be useful to him.

Against leprosy and vitiligo: salted, seasoned with long aristolochia, soda and cumin—one part of each one, crushed and sieved— one *miṯqāl* of this dried, ground, sieved and given to drink with warm water.

Ram testicle: if it is salted, with long aristolochia, red soda and cumin—one part of each one—everything ground and dissolved; and if the man suffering from leprosy and vitiligo drinks it, then this will make them cease.

21.15 If a man is bleary-eyed and affected by nyctalopia, lamb meat: if it is taken with its fat and its liver, everything mixed and melted with alfalfa water, with the addition of some soda, then this will cease, with the permission of God, may He be exalted.

Against the disease of the eye and the abundance of fine particles in the eye, sheep meat, its fat and its liver: if they are minced and melted with alfalfa water, mixed with red soda, and applied on the eyes affected by this disease, then this will be useful.

If the blood of the sheep, its fat and the outgrowth of its liver are taken with the addition of red soda, everything liquefied with alfalfa water, and applied on the eyes of the man who is bleary-eyed and affected by nyctalopia, then this will cure him.

21.16 If you want to give power to the coitus, take the gall of a fat ram, rub it on the outer opening of urethra at the moment of coitus, then this will excite it very much, and this is amazing.

The man who takes the gall of a fat ram, rubs it on the outer opening of the urethra at the moment of coitus, then [the woman] will love him intensely.

Gall of fat ram: if it is rubbed on the outer opening of urethra at the moment of coitus, then this will extremely excite the woman, and will increase the sexual power.

21.17 If you want to set a broken bone in the hands or in the feet, lamb brain: if it is taken fresh, put in a vessel, some white gypsum powder, curcuma and fenugreek are added to it, everything is beaten, placed on the fire and, once it has become like an ointment, fixed on the fracture, then this will set.

Lamb brain: if it is melted with crushed gypsum, curcuma, and fenugreek, beaten until it becomes like a cream, and used to bandage the fracture, then this will be useful to it.

Lamb brain: if it is placed on the fire, with the addition of vetches flour, curcuma and fenugreek, everything beaten until it becomes like a cream, put in a piece of cloth, and fixed on the area of the fracture, then this will cure it, and this will be good for it.

21.18	اذا اردت ان تكثر الشعر في الجانبين فخذ مرارة نعجة سوداء فاحرقها اسحقها واخلط معها زيت شامي واطلى به الحواجب بريشة فانه يربي الشعر ويسوده	لكثرة الشعر في حاجب ينتف الانسان منه ما اراد وتأخذ مرارة شاة فتحرقها وتخلطها بزفت شامي ويطلي الموضع بريشة ويتبع موضع النتف	مرارة الشاة السوداء من الضأن اذا احرقت وسحقت وخلط معها ذرور شامي واطلى به الحاجبين بريشة فانه يربي الشعر ويسوده ويغزره ويكثره ويحسنه والله سبحانه وتعالى اعلم
21.19	اذا اردت ان تشد رحم امراة تاخذ صوفة فتحرقها وتحمّل بها المراة فهو جيّد مليح	*om.*	*om.*
21.20	*om.*	مخ الضأن يطلي به موضع لثة الصبي الذي يريد ان تخرج اسنانه فتخرج بلا وجع ولا اذية وكذلك يفعل شعر الغنم	*om.*
21.21	اذا كان الانسان به ذبول وضعف وهزال وصفار في اللون يؤخذ لبن حليب فيجعل في قدر ويلقي عليه دقيق سميد وعسل ويغلي على النار ويلقي عليه سنبل وقرنفل وزعفران من كل واحد جزء ويطبخ ويفرغ في اناء ويستعمل منه صاحب هذه العلات كل يوم اوفيه على الريق عند النوم فيبرا باذن الله تعالى	السل والهزال والصفار يؤخذ لبن حليب حار بسميد وشيء من عسل ويلقي فيه سنبل وقرنفل من كل واحد جزء حتى يصير مشوى وياكلهن به السعلة يبرأ باذن الله تعالى	*om.*

21.18: (b) الكثرة...النتف] اذا اردت ان تنتف الشعر الذي في الحاجب وغيره ولم فخذ مرارة شاة سوداء فأحرقها وخلطها بزيت شامي وطلى به المواضع التي تريد نتفها بريشة وانتفه G
(c) ذرور] ورد C | ويحسنه] ويسوده ويغزره ويكثره ويحسنه ويغزره ويكثره C
21.19: (a) فتحرقها] تحرقها B | المرأة] *om.* B | مليح] *om.* B
(c) For this recipe, see also 22.27
20.20: (b) يطلي] اذا طلى G | موضع لثة] *om.* G | ان تخرج] خروج G | فتخرج] خرج G
21.21: (a) وهزال] *om.* B | لبن حليب] لبن حليب حار B | فيجعل] يجعل B | قدر] قدرة B | سميد وعسل] نحل وعسل سمند B | ويفرغ] ويرفع B | العلات] العلل B | فيبرأ] فانه يبرأ B
(b) السل...يبرأ] لبن الحليب الحار الغنم اذا طبخ بسميد وشيء من عسل والقى فيه سنبل وقرنفل من كل واحد جزء مدقوق منخول مع شيء من جوف الكبش وطبخ حتى يستوي واكله صاحب السل والدبول والهزال والصفار برئ G
(c) For this recipe, see also 22.28

21.18	If you want to increase the hair on the temples, take the gall of a black ewe, burn it, grind it, melt it with Syrian oil, and rub it on the eyebrows with a feather, then this will increase the hair and make them black.	For the removal of the hair from the eyebrows and for shaving the man from what he wants to shave, take the gall of a black sheep, burn it, melt it with Syrian pitch, and rub it on the area with a feather, then the area will get shaved.	Gall of the black sheep: if it is burnt, ground and mixed with Syrian powder, rubbed on the temples with a feather, then this will increase the hair, make it black and abundant, multiply it and make it nicer, and God, may He be praised and exalted, knows beast.
21.19	If you want to strengthen the uterus of a woman, take a woollen piece of cloth and the woman should carry it, and this is good and witty.	*om.*	*om.*
21.20	*om.*	Sheep marrow: if it is rubbed on the gums of the baby whose teeth you wish to come out, then these will come out without any pain or ache; and the hair of the sheep does the same.	*om.*
21.21	If a man is affected by weakness, impairment and paleness of the complexion, its milk: if it is taken, put in a cooking pot, some semolina and honey are added to it, boiled, again with the addition of hyacinth, cloves and saffron—one part of each one—then it is cooked, poured in a vessel, and given to the man suffering from these diseases—one ounce everyday on an empty stomach at the moment of sleeping—then he will heal, with the permission of God, may He be exalted.	Consumption, weakness, and paleness, warm milk cooked with semolina and some honey, with the addition of hyacinth and cloves—one part of each one—until it becomes a poultice, eaten against the cough, then this will be cured, with the permission of God, may He be exalted.	*om.*

21.22

om.

دم الضأن يخلط بدقيق شعير ويحفف ثم يسحق ويلتّ بزيت ويشرب للسعال بعسل وماء حار نافع انفحة الخروف جيد اذا سحقت بعسل وشيء من صبر ينفع لكل وجع يعرض لثدي المرأة والقدم يطلي عليه فيحلل الورم ويسكن الوجع ان شاء الله تعالى

يؤخذ دم الخروف يلت بدقيق شعير ويجفف ويسحق ويربب بزيت ويسقي لصاحب السعال بعس منزوع الرغوة وماء حار فيذهب عنه السعال باذن الله تعالى

21.23

من أخذ مخة الخروف اذا جففت وسحقت ولتت بعسل وصبر وطلى بها البدن الذي قد ورم ذهب المه وزال ورمه

انفحة الخروف جيد اذا سحقت بعسل وشيء من صبر ينفع لكل وجع يعرض لثدى المرأة والقدم يطلي عليه فيحلل الورم ويسكن الوجع ان شاء الله تعالى

يؤخذ منفحة الخروف تجفف وتسقي وتضرب بعسل وصبر ويطلي بها اليدين والرجلين فيسكن وجههم باذن الله تعالى

21.24

ساق الخروف اذا كسر وجد فيه شيء بكسر المدة واذيف بلبن شاة سوداء ودهن بنفسج واستعط به صاحب النمش واندهن ببقية الدهن فانه يزول

واذا سمطت الخروف فخذ ساقه واخرج المخ الذي في فذوبه في مسعط بلبن جارية ودهن بنفسج واسعط به من في وجهه النمش ويلطخ من في وجهه النمش يذهب ويحسّن لون الوجه

للنمش يؤخذ ساق خروف فيكسر ويؤخذ المخ الذي يكون في فاجعله في مسعط والق عليه لبن جارية سوداء ودهن بنفسج ويسعّط به صاحب النمش الذي يكون في الوجه وادهن به وجهه وموضع النمش فيزول باذن الله تعالى

21.22: (a) ويسحق] ويسقي B | بعسل] بعسل منزوع B | عنه السعال] *om.* B
(b) يخلط…للسعال] دم الضان اذا خلط دقيق الشعير وحفف ثم سحق ولتّ بزيت وشربه صاحب السعال G
(c) For this recipe, see also 22.29
21.23: (a) تجفف وتسقي وتضرب] يجفف ويسقي ويضرب B | وجههم] *om.* B
(b) جيد] *om.* G | الثدى] في ثدى G | والقدم] وقدمها G | يطلي…الوجع] يلطخ به G
21.24: (a) *om.* B
(b) واذا سمطت] اذا سمط G | واخرج…مسعط] فاكسره تجد فيه مخ شبه الغدد فخذ ذلك ودقه G | ودهن] مع دهن G | واسعّط به ويلطخ من] نمش وطلى به الوجه بعد ذلك فانه G
(c) For this recipe, see also 22.30

21.22	Lamb blood: if it is taken, mixed with barley flour, dried, ground, melted with oil, and given to the man suffering from cough to drink, with honey without foam and warm water, then the cough will leave him, with the permission of God, may He be exalted.	Sheep blood: if it is mixed with barley flour, dried, then ground, mixed with oil, and drunk against the cough, with honey and warm water, then this will be useful, with the permission of God, may He be exalted.	*om.*
21.23	Lamb rennet: if it is taken, dried, ground, beaten with honey and aloe, rubbed on the hands and on the feet, then their pain will be calmed, with the permission of God, may He be exalted.	Lamb rennet: if it is ground with honey and some aloe, this will be useful against every pain that affects the breast of the woman; and if the feet are rubbed with it, then the swelling will subside and the pain will cease.	If one who takes lamb marrow, dries it, pounds it, mixes it with honey and aloe, and rubs it on the swollen body, then its pain and its swelling will cease.
21.24	Against the freckles, lamb leg: if it is broken and the marrow that is inside it is taken, then it is put in a snuff box, and the milk of a black maiden and sweet violet oil are added to it; then it is given to sniff to the man who has freckles on his face, and the face and the areas with freckles are rubbed with it, then these will disappear, with the permission of God, may He be exalted.	If the lamb is prepared, then take its leg, extract the marrow inside it, pour it in a snuff box with the milk of a maiden and violet oil, then let it sniff to the man who has freckles on his face—spatter it on the face with freckles as well—then these will disappear, and the colour of the face will become nicer.	Lamb leg: if it is broken, inside it there is something, then if this is mixed with the milk of a black sheep and violet oil, inhaled by the man who has freckles, and he is rubbed with the rest of the oil, then these will cease.

٢٢. الماعز

	a	b	c
	ذكر منافع اعضاء الماعز	الماعز	باب منافع المعز
22.1	يؤخذ قرن تيس ويجعل في يد المطلقة فتلد سريعا باذن الله تعالى	اذا تعسّر على المرأة الولادة فخذ قطعة من قرن عنز فاجعلها في فمها وتمسكه المرأة معها او تضعه على فخذها فانها تلد سريعا	قرن الماعز اذا حكته من تعسر ولدها وجعله تحت اقدامها وضعته سريعا
22.2	*om.*	ظلف عنز وتيس يحرق ويسحق ويسقي منه من يبول في الفراش وزن مثقال بخل عسل يبرأ باذن الله تعالى	*om.*
22.3	لوجع القلب والريّة يؤخذ دم الماعز يجفّف ويسحق ويخلط معه دقيق الباقلا ويسقي به صاحب المرض بماء حار فيبرأ باذن الله تعالى	مرارة العنز اذا اذيفت بسمن بقر وشربها من به عسر النفس بماء حار نفعه	دم المعز اذا جفف وسحق وخلط بدقيق الباقلة ويسعط من به وجع القلب والرية بماء حار برئ
22.4	*om.*	*om.*	كبد المعز اذا شويى وأكل بسماق وكزبرة نفع من القيام المفرط
22.5	اذا اردت ان تقوي على الجماع تاخذ شحم خصى التيس وبزر عواطيس	*om.*	

22.1: (a) تيس] ماعز كبير B
(b) تعسّر] عسر G | الولادة] ولادتها G | فاجعلها...فخذها] وتمسكه في فمها او تحمله او تضع على فخذها G | سريعا] سريعا فاذا ولدت نحّته *add.* G
(c) حكته] مسكت C | تعسر ولدها] عسرت عليها الولادة C | وضعته] وضع C
22.2: (b) ظلف] ضلف T | عنز وتيس] العنز والتيس G | يحرق ويسحق ويسقي] اذا احرق وسقى G | من] لمن G | وزن مثقال بخل عسل] *om.* G | يبرأ] ذهب عنه G
22.3: (a) المرض] الوجع B | فيبرأ] ينفعه B
(b) *om.* G
(c) الباقلة] الباقلا C | ويسعط] وسعط C | برئ] ابرأه C
22.4: (b) In G another recipe is added, with goat blood against the pain of the waist: دم الماعز اذا جفف وخلط مع من دقيق الباقلى وسحق وسقي منه صاحب وجع الخاصرة بماء حار نفعه G
(c) C places this recipe after 22.5
22.5: (a) عواطيس] عرطسا S | تاخذ] فخذ B | عرطسا] قطر B | واذب] وذيّب B | وألق] والقى B | واطل] واطلى B | فانه عجيب] *om.* C
(c) In L this recipe is after 22.26

22. Goat

	a	b	c
	Exposition of the useful properties of the parts of the goat	**The goat**	**Chapter on the useful properties of the goat**
22.1	Billy goat horn: if it is taken, put it in the hand of a woman who is giving birth, then she will deliver quickly, with the permission of God, may He be exalted.	If a woman has some difficulties in giving birth, take a piece of فاث billy goat's right horn, put it in her mouth—or let her carry it or place it on her leg—then she will deliver quickly.	Goat horn: If the woman who has some difficulties in giving birth scrapes it, then she will deliver; and if it is placed under her feet, then she will deliver quickly.
22.2	*om.*	Billy goat hoof: if it is burnt, ground, and given to drink to the man who wets the bed—one *miṯqāl* with honey vinegar [oxymel?] then he will heal, with the permission of God, may He be exalted.	*om.*
22.3	For the pain of the heart and خب the lung, goat blood: if it is dried, ground, melted with broad beans flour, and inhaled by the sick man with warm water, then he will heal, with the permission of God, may He be exalted.	Goat gall: if it is mixed with cow fat, and drunk with warm water by the man suffering from breath difficulties, then this will be useful to him.	Goat blood: if it is dried, ground, melted with broad beans flour, and inhaled with warm water by the man suffering from heart and lung pain, then he will recover.
22.4	*om.*	*om.*	Goat liver: if it is roasted and eaten with sumach and coriander, then this will be useful against the insurgence of the excess [?].
22.5	If you want to give power to the coitus, take the fat from the testicles of a billy goat and finely ground	*om.*	Billy goattesticles: if they are mixed with sneezewort seeds, and rubbed

	مسحوقا ناعما واذب الشحم والق عليه البزر واطل به الاحليل عند الجماع فانه عجيب		خصى التيس اذا اذيف والقي عليه بزر عواطيس وطلى به الاحليل عند الجماع اعان على ذلك
22.6	لورم الطحال يؤخذ خصى الجدى الصغير وتملحه بملح وصعتر وبورق ودقيق شعير ويجفف ويسحق ويسقي لصاحب الطحال بخل عنصل فيذهب الطحال باذن الله	خصية الماعز اليمنى اذا ملّحت بملح وبورق وتنكار وصعتر وجففت وسحقت وشرب منها صاحب الطحال وزن مثقال بخل العنصل نفعه	خصوة الجدى اذا ملحت وأخذ البورق ودقيق الشعير وسحقا ودقا معار شرب من ذلك صاحب الطحال وزن درهم بخل عنصل ابرأه
22.7	اذا اردت ان يذهب الشعر من الجسد فتاخذ كلى التيس الكبير فتشرح وتيجفف في الشمس ويسحق ناعما والقى عليه زفتا شاميا وادلك به الجسد في الحمام وقبل الحمام فيزول الشعر باذن الله تعالى	واذا اردت ان لا ينبت في جسدك شعر فخذ كلوتي تيس بمعالقها فصير في الشمس حتى تجف فاذا جف فدقها واخلطها مع الزيت وادهن به الموضع الذي تريد ان لا ينبت فيه الشعر	اذا اردت ان لا ينبت الشعر فخذ قطعة قطعا [كلى التيس] وجفف في الشمس واسحقه ناعما وخلط معه زفت شامي واطلى به ذلك الموضع فلا ينبت فيه شعرا
22.8	*om.*	واذا بخرت الكرم الذي فيه الدود بظلف شاة لم فيه شيء منه وكذلك تفعل عروق السوس	*om.*
22.9	*om.*	واذا كان البق في الاسرة فخذ مرارة التيس ويخلط بزيت وتضرب ضربا ويطلي به الحائط والسرير فيذهب باذن الله تعالى	*om.*

22.6: (a) الصغير] صغير يشق *add.* B | وتملحه] ويملح B | وصعتر وبورق] ونطرون وذعز B | ويسحق] *om.* B
(b) This recipe is attested only in G
(c) In L and C this recipe is after 22.26 | وأخذ] مع ودق C | وسحقا ودقا] دقا ناعما C | شرب من ذلك صاحب] به من ذلك واستعمل C | وزن] زنة C
22.7: (b) واذا...الشعر] لم ينبت فيه الشعر ان نبت يريد لا الذي الموضع دهن او رفيقا معها وخلط وسحقت الشمس في جففت اذا بمعاليقها التيس كلوة G
(c) In L and C this recipe is after 22.30 | اذا اردت ان لا ينبت الشعر] *om.* C | فخذ قطعه قطعا] اذا قطع التيس كلى C | واطلى به ذلك الموضع] واذا طليت به مكانا C
22.8: (b) بظلف] بضلف T | *om.* G
22.9: (b) واذا كان البق في الاسرة فخذ] *om.* G | ويخلط] اذا خلطت G | وتضرب ضربا] جيدا ضربا به وضرب G | ويطلي] وطلى G | والسرير] او السرير G | فيذهب] البَق منه ذهب G

	seeds of sneezewort, liquefy the fat, pour it on the seeds, and rub it on the outer opening of urethra at the moment of coitus, then this will be amazing.		on the outer opening of urethra at the moment of coitus, then this will help it.
22.6	Against spleen complaint, testicles of a young billy goat: if they are taken, seasoned with wild thyme, natron and wheat flour, dried, ground, and given to the man suffering from spleen complaint to drink with red squill vinegar, then this will make it cease, with the permission of God, may He be exalted.	Right testicle of the goat: if it is seasoned with salt, natron, tin and wild thyme, then dried and ground, one *miṯqāl* of it is drunk by the man suffering from spleen complaint, with red squill vinegar, then this will be useful to him.	Young billy goat testicle: if it is salted, natron and wild thyme finely ground are taken along with it, then this is drunk by the man suffering from spleen complaint—one *miṯqāl*, with red squill water—then this will cure him.
22.7	If you want to remove the hair from the body, take the kidneys of a big billy goat, cut them in slices, dry them in the sunlight, grind it finely, pour some Syrian pitch, rub the body with it in the bath before bathing, then the hair will be removed, with the permission of God, may He be exalted.	If you want that the hair do not grow on your body, take both the kidneys of a billy goat, place them in the sun until they dry; once they have dried, grind them, mix this with oil, and rub with it this the zones in which you do not want that the hair grow.	If you want that the hair do not grow, take one piece [of billy goat kidney], dry it in the sun, grind it finely with Syrian pitch, and rub a zone with it, then the hair will not grow there.
22.8	*om.*	If the vine on which there are worms is fumigated with the hoof of the billy goat, then none of them will remain there; and liquorice roots have the same effect.	*om.*
22.9	*om.*	If there are bedbugs in the beds, take the gall of the billy goat, mix it with oil, whip it well, and rub the wall and the bed with it, then these will go away, with the permission of God, may He be exalted.	*om.*

22.10	*om.*	دماغ الجدى يطبخ بعسل ويلقي عليه مُر وسكر وكمون كرماني ويخلط ناعما ويشرب فيه وزن متقال بماء حار لوجع الصلب والرية نافع	*om.*
22.11	*om.*	دم المعز يطلي به موضع الدوّالي وهى المعروق المجتمعة في الساقين المعقدة فينفعها	اذا أخذت الدوالي التي تكون في الساقين وهي العروق المجتمة في كراع المعز ودقت ونقعت قي الخل الحادق وسلقت في قدر واطعمت لمن به وجع الرية والقلب ابرأه
22.12	*om.*	مخ الماعز يطلي به العصب المنتقض المشبّك اليابس فيليّنه	*om.*
22.13	*om.*	لغثى النفس مرارة العنز تذاف بسمن بقر وتشرب بماء حار لوجع الخاصرة والمثانة	*om.*
22.14	*om.*	دم الماعز يجفف ويخلط معه دقيق الباقلا جزء يسحق ويغلي بماء حار	*om.*
22.15	*om.*	شحم حصى التيس وبزرعرطنيثا وشيء من عرطنيثا يسحق سحقا ناعما ويطلي به الاحليل فتجد له لذة عظيمة	*om.*
22.16	*om.*	لورم الطحال يؤخذ خصية الماعز القتي فتملح بملح وبورق وشعير وتجفف ويسحق ويسقي وزن مثقال بخل العنصل يبرأ باذن الله تعالى	*om.*

22.10: (b) يطبخ] اذا طبخ G | ويلقي] ورمى G | وسكر] *om.* G | ويخلط...فيه] وخلط وشرب منه G | لوجع الصلب والرية نافع] نفع من وجع القلب والرية G
22.11: (b) يطلي] اذا طلى G | الدوّالي] الروّابي G | المعقدة] *om.* G | فينفعها] فانه يلينها G
(c) In L and C this recipe is after 22.30 | أخذت] *om.* C | ونقعت] *om.* C | ونقعت] *om.* C | الريه والقلب] القلب والرية C
22.12: (b) يطلي] اذا طلى G | المنتقض] *om.* G | المشبّك] المتشبك G | اليابس] *om.* G | فيليّنه] ليّنه G| In G another recipe is added, with goat milk (the best after human milk) against the cough: لبن المعز ارقّ الالبان بعد البان النساء الاتُنّ والبان الخيل وهو نافع سعال اليابس G

22.10	*om.*	Young billy goat brain: if it is cooked with honey, myrrh, cumin and sugar are poured on it, then it is mixed well, and one *miṯqāl* of it is drunk with warm water against the pain of the back and the lung, this will be useful.	*om.*
22.11	*om.*	Goat blood: if it is rubbed on the areas of the varicose veins—that are the veins entangled together in the leg—then this will be useful against them.	If you take the varicose veins that are in the legs—they are the veins entangled in the legs of the goats—crush them, soak them in sour vinegar, boil them in a pot, and give them to the man suffering from pain in the lung and in the heart, then this will cure him.
22.12	*om.*	Goat marrow: if it is rubbed on the contracted and dry nerve, then this will relax it.	*om.*
22.13	*om.*	Against the indisposition of the breath, goat gall: mixed with cow fat, given to drink with warm water against the pain of the waist and the bladder.	*om.*
22.14	*om.*	Goat blood: dried, mixed with one part of broad beans flour, ground, and boiled with warm water [?].	*om.*
22.15	*om.*	Billy goat testicle fat and cyclamen seeds, and some cyclamen, finely ground, and rubbed on the outer opening of the urethra, then you will find a great pleasure in this.	*om.*
22.16	*om.*	Against the swelling of the spleen, goat testicle: if it is taken, seasoned with salt, natron and barley, dried, ground, and one *miṯqāl* of it is given to drink with red squill vinegar, then this will cure it, with the permission of God, may He be exalted.	*om.*

22.17	*om.*	زيادة كبد الماعز اذا شرّحت وذر عليها دار فلفل مسحوق وشيء من بورق ارمني والقي على جمر لين الحرارة وكحل منها من به الغشاوه في عينيه نفعه	*om.*
22.18	*om.*	وباقي الكبد تشقّ شقا وتجعل في قدر حديد ويجعل عليها ماء غمرها ويغطي رأس القدر ويوقد تحتها وقودا ليّنا حتى تتهرّأ ثم تنزل القدر وتدني من صاحب الغشاوة وتجعل هذا وجهه ويلقي رأسه فيها ويوضع على رأسه ثوبا حتى بخارة الى عينيه فان ذلك يذهب	*om.*
22.19	اذا اردت ان تحسن الياقوت ويقوي حمرته خذ دم التيس حال دبخه وخذ من مخه واخلط الجميع والطخ به الياقوت واعبر به النار ساعة واخرجه واغسله فانه يزيد في لونه ويحسنه	دم التيس وزنجفر يخلطان جميعا ويلطخ به حجر الياقوت ويدخل في النار ويترك حتى يحمي ويجفّف ثم يخرج ويغسل فانه ذلك يزيد في لونه وحسنه	اذا اردتَ ان تحمّر الياقوت وتحسنه فالطخه بشيء من دم التيس وشيء من مخه فادخله النار وخليه حتى ينسف واخرجه واغسله فانه يخرج اجود ما كان ويزيد في ثمنه
22.20	واذا اردت ان يطول الشعر خذ دم تيس واوقية لاذن واعجنه بماء الآس الاخضر	من أخذ دم تيس فجففه ثم خلطه بلاذن وسحقه سحقا ناعما وعجنه بماء	اذا اردت ان تطول الشعر تأخذ دم تيس فيجفف ويسحق ويلقي عليه لاذنا عنبريا وماء الآس الاخضر واعلف به الشعر

22.17: (b) الكبد] كبد الماعز G | وذر عليها] ويدر فيها G | فلفل] فلفل مسحوق add. G | والقي على] ويلقي فيه G | لبن الحرارة] لبن add. G | وكحل] ويكتحل به منها G | الغشاوة] الغشاوه في عينيه add. G | ولا يبصر بالليل] om. G

(c) In L and C this recipe is after 22.30

22.18: (b) وتصير...ويؤخذ] وتجعل شقا وتشقّ الكبد وباقي G | ويصير] ويجعل G | من] om. G | يغمره] غمرها G | فاذا...بصره] صاحب من وتدني القدر تنزل ثم G الغشاوة وتجعل هذا وجهه ويلقي رأسه فيها ويوضع على رأسه ثوبا حتى نجارة الى عينيه فان ذلك يذهب

(c) In L and C this recipe is after 22.30

22.19: (a) بشيء من دم التيس] بدم تيس B

(b) يخلطان وزنجفر] اذا خلط بزنجفر G | جميعا] om. G | ويلطخ] ولطخ G | ويدخل] وادخل G | في] om. G | يحمي] om. G | ويجفّف] يجفّ G | ذلك] om. G | لونه وحسنه] حمرته ولونه G

(c) In L this recipe is after 22.30| *om.* C

22.20: (a) الشيب...اذا اردت] بعيد الشيب ويكون ويطوّله يحسنه فانه التيس بدم الحمام في اغسله الشعر تطول ان اردت اذا B

(b) خلطه...من] وخلط جفف اذا ايضا ودم G | وعجنه...وسحقه] وعجن ناعما وسحقا G | وعلف] وطلي G | شعرا] شعر الامرأة add. G | خلاف بلا وقواه] *om.* G

(c) In L and C this recipe is after 22.30 | يطول الشعر] واذا اردت ان *om.* C | شيبه...خذ دم] الآس بماء لادن به وعجنت اوقية منه أخذت اذا التيس دم الاخضر وعلقت به الشعر طوله وغزره وسوده وابطاء بشيبه C

22.17	*om.*	Goat liver appendance: if it is cut in slices, with the addition of ground long pepper and some Armenian natron, put on the live coal, then this will mitigate the hotness; and if it is rubbed on the eye affected by cataract, then this will be useful against it.	*om.*
22.18	*om.*	What remains of the liver: if it is split, put it in an iron cooking pot, abundant water is poured over it, then covered, cooked on a light fire until it is well done, then removed from the fire, and brought close to the man affected by the cataract, it is applied on his face and his head goes inside the pot, with a piece of cloth placed over it so that the fumigation goes to his eyes, then this will go away.	*om.*
22.19	If you want to make the ruby more red and beautiful, spatter it with some billy goat blood and some of its marrow, place it in the fire, and leave it there until the blood is pulverized, then you will take it out nicer than it was, and its value will increase.	Billy goat blood and cinnabar: if they are mixed, and spattered on the ruby, then this is placed in the fire, and left there until it becomes hot and dries, then it is taken out and washed, its colour and its beauty will improve.	If you want to make a ruby more beautiful and intensify its red colour, take the blood of the billy goat when you slaughter it, take its marrow, melt everything up, and spatter it on the ruby, leave it in the fire for one hour, then take it out and wash it, then its colour will be intensified, and it will become nicer.
22.20	If you want that the hair becomes longer, take the blood of the billy goat, dry it, grind it, and add some amber, laudanum and green myrtle water, apply it on the hair, and	The one who takes the blood of a billy goat, dries it, then mixes it with laudanum, grinds it well, kneads it with green myrtle water, and applies it on the air, then this	If you want to make the hair stronger, take the blood of a billy goat, one ounce of laudanum and green myrtle water, apply it on the

	واغسله في الحمام فانه يحسنه ويطوّله ويكون بعيد الشيْب	الآس وعلف به شعرا طوله وغلظه وقواه بلا خلاف	واعلف به الشعر فانه يطوله ويحسنه ويسوده وبطى شيبه
22.21	اذا اردت ان تطول الشعر ونوم الانسان فخذ قرن تيس ولفّه في خرقة واجعله تحت رأس من شئت فلا ينتب حتى تشيل من تحت رأسه	ومن أخذ قرن تيس في منديل وجعله تحت رأس انسان وهو لا يعلم نام ما دام تحت رأسه	قرن الماعز اذا لف خرقة وجعل تحت رأس النائم فلا ينتب حتى ينزع من تحت رأسه
22.22	اذا اردت ا[ن] لا ينبت الشعر على الجسد فاطل الجسد بمرارة شاة وقليل نوشاذر فلا يطلع فيه الشعر ابدا	يؤخذ مرارة عنز وشيء من نوشادر ويخلطان جميعا ويطلي به الموضع الذي ينتف منه الشعر فلا ينبت ابدا	مرارة المعز اذا خلطت بالنوشاذر وطلى به المواضع المنتوفة لم يطلع فيها شعر
22.23	*om.*	[بعر الماعز] واذا طلى على لسع الهوام ونهش السباع نفع باذن الله تعالى	*om.*
22.24	اذا اردت ان تطرد جميع الذبيب فخذ بعر المعز فبخر به البيت فانه يطرد جميع الذبيب	بعر الماعز اذا بخر الموضع به طرد الذبيب والهوام	بعر المعز اذا بخر به لم يبق ذبيب
22.25	بعر المعز يعجن بالماء ويطلي به لسعة العقرب او الزنبور فانها تسكن باذن الله تعالى	*om.*	*om.*

22.21: (a) ونوم] نوم B | ولفّه] واجعله B | رأس من شئت] رأسه B | تشيل] تقلعته B
(b) *om.*G
(c) In L and C this recipe is after 22.30 | الماعز] الغزال L | وجعل] وترك C | فلا ينتب] *om.* C
22.22: (a) فاطل] فاطلى B | نوشاذر] نشادر B
(b) يؤخذ] *om.* G | عنز] الماعز G | وشيء] مع شيء G | نوشادر] نوشاذر G | ويخلطان جميعا ويطلي به] على منها ويطلي ويخلط G | ينتف منه] يخلط G | فيه] ينبت G | ابدا] *om.* G
(c) المعز] الماعز C | المواضع المنتوفة] الموضع المنتوف C | لم يطلع فيها شعر] منع انبات الشعر C
22.23: (b) In T this recipe is after 22.31
22.24: (a) اذا اردت ان تطرد جميع الذبيب] *om.* B | فخذ بعر المعز فبخر] اذا بخرت بعر الماعز B | فانه يطرد] طرد B
(b) In T this recipe is after 22.31 | الموضع به] به الموضع G
(c) به] البيت به *add.* C | ذبيب] شيء من الذبيب *add.* C
22.25: (a) بعر المعز...تسكن] نعر الماعز اذا طلى به لسعة العقرب بعد ان يكون عجنته بماء او سمن بقر فانه يسكن وجهه وكذلك لسعة الزنبور C

	wash it in the bath, then the hair will become nicer and longer, and it will not turn white.	will—no doubt—make it longer, thicker and stronger.	hair and then it will become longer, nicer and black, and it will not turn white.
22.21	If you want to make the hair and the sleep of the man longer, take the horn of billy goat, wrap it in a piece of cloth, put it under the head of the man you want, and then he will not get up as long as this remains under his head.	The one who takes the horn of a billy goat in a handkerchief, and places it under the head of a man—but he should not be aware of it—then this one will sleep as long as the horn remains under his head.	Goat horn: if it is wrapped in a piece of cloth, and placed under the head of a sleeping man, then he will not get up until this is removed from under his head.
22.22	If you want that the hair will not grow on the body, rub it with the gall of a sheep and a bit of ammonia, then the hair will never grow again.	Goat gall: if it is melted with some ammonia, and rubbed on the area where the hair grows, then this will never grow again.	Goat gall: if it is melted with ammonia, and rubbed on the areas where the hair grows, then it will not grow there.
22.23	*om.*	Goat droppings: if they are rubbed on the sting of obnoxious insects and the bite of the beats of prey, then this will be useful, with the permission of God, may He be exalted.	*om.*
22.24	If you want to chase all the flies away, take the droppings of the goat, fumigate the house with them, and then this will chase all the flies away.	Goat droppings: if the place is fumigated with them, then this will chase flies and obnoxious insects away.	Goat droppings: if they are used for fumigation, then the flies will not remain in that place.
22.25	Goat droppings: if they are kneaded with water, and rubbed on the sting of a scorpion or of a hornet, then [the pain] will calm down, with the permission of God, may He be exalted.	*om.*	*om.*

22.26	وايضا اذا سحق وعجن بالعسل وطلى به القدمين من فوق اليدين نفع وجع المفاصل	واذا سحق وعجن بالعسل وطلى به القدمين واليدين نفع من وجع المفاصل	وبر المعز يعجن بالخل ويطلي به اليدين والرجلين ينفع للضربان
22.27	واذا كانت امرة تشتكي النتة يخرج من تحتها شيء يشبه الماء الاصفر ولا يقدر الرجل ان ينالها تحرق صوف الغنم ويحمل منه فانه يسكن الوجع وضيق المكان	*om.*	*om.*
22.28	لبن الماعز اذا القي على النار مع شيء من سمن وعسل والقى عليه سنبل وقرنفل من كل واحد جزء و[غلى] على النار حتى يعقد واستعمله من به الصفار والهزال ابرأه	*om.*	*om.*
22.29	من أخذ مخة الخروف اذا جففت وسحقت ولتت بعسل وصبر وطلى بها البدن الذي قد ورم ذهب المه وزال ورمه	*om.*	*om.*
22.30	ساق الخروف اذا كسر وجد فيه شيء بكسر المدة واذيف بلبن شاة سوداء ودهن بنفسج واستعط به صاحب النمش واندهن ببقية الدهن فانه يزول	*om.*	*om.*

22.26: (a) *om.* B
(b) In T this recipe is after 22.31 | وكذلك] *om.* G | اذا سقى] واذا سحق G
(c) ايضا] *om.* C | بالعسل] بعسل النحل C | وطلى] وطليت C | من فوق اليدين] واليدين C | المفاصل] والضربان *add.* C
22.27: (a) For this recipe, see also 21.19
(c) واذا كانت...المكان] صوف الغنم اذا احرقت وتحمل منه المرأة التي تشتكي نتنة الفرج ويخرج منها شيء يشبه الما الاصفر ولا يقدر الرجل ينالها سكن ذلك الوجع وضيق المسلك وطيب الرايحة وفي نفع كبير C
22.28: (a) For this recipe, see also 21.21
(b) For this recipe, see also 21.21
(c) لبن الماعز] الحار *add.* C | القى] رفع C | حتى يعقد] الى ان ينعقد C
22.29: (a) For this recipe, see also 21.22
(b) For this recipe, see also 21.22
(c) من أخذ مخهمنن] فحة C | وصبر] استعطري بروصببير *add.* C | بها] به C | قد ورم] اعتراه الورم C | ذهب المه وزال ورمه] فشه واذهب الورم وزاله C
22.30: (a) For this recipe, see also 21.24
(b) For this recipe, see also 21.24
(c) وجد فيه] خرج منه C | بكسريش] به C | واستعط] وتسعط C | صاحب] من به C | واندهن ببقية الدهن فانه يزول] ثم اندهن منه ببقيته ازال النمش C

22.26	Goat droppings: if they are kneaded with vinegar, and rubbed on the hands and on the feet, then this will be useful against the pangs.	If they are ground, kneaded with honey, and rubbed on the feet and on the hands, then this will be useful against the pain of the joints.	Also, if it is ground, kneaded with honey, and rubbed on the feet from the back of the hands, then this will be useful against the pain of the joints.
22.27	*om.*	*om.*	If a woman suffers from womb pain, and something similar to yellow water comes out from her lower parts, and the man cannot take her, burn the wool of the goat and the woman should carry it, then the pain will be calmed, and the lower parts will heal.
22.28	*om.*	*om.*	Goat milk: if it is put on the fire, with some grease and honey, with the addition of hyacinth and clover—one part of each one—boiled on the fire until it thickens, and it is given to the man suffering from yellow complexion and emaciation, then this will cure him.
22.29	*om.*	*om.*	If one takes the marrow of the ram, and if this is dried, ground, mixed with honey and aloe, and rubbed on the body that suffers from a swelling, then this will make its pain go away, and its swelling will cease.
22.30	*om.*	*om.*	Ram leg: if it is broken, one finds something inside it, then if this is mixed with the milk of a black sheep and violet oil, inhaled by the man with freckles—and he is rubbed with the rest of the oil—then these will disappear.

	(a)	(b)	(c)
22.31	*om.*	دم التيس يفتّت الحجر الماس	*om.*
22.32	*om.*	لبن الماعز اذا شرب نفع من قروح الامعاء	بعر المعز اذا شرب وهو حار نفع من قروح الامعاء
22.33	*om.*	*om.*	واذا اسحق واذيب بالخل وطلى به البدن والرجلين سكن ما بذلك من الضربان
22.34	يؤخذ لبن المعز ويجعل في قدرة ويلقا عليها نشاء وقلت وحنطة وورس خالص ويلقي عليه بوزن الجميع سكر خالص ويستعمله صاحب علة السل والدق والحمى العقبة فتزول باذن الله تعالى	لبن الماعز الحار الحليب فيؤخذ ويطبخ ويخلط معه لبّ القمح وورس مكان الزعفران وسكر طبرزذ بقدر الحاجة ويقطّر عليه دهن اللوز مكان سمن البقر فهو اجود ما يكون لنفى الاوجاع الحادة في الصدر والرية ولمن به حمّى الربع	لبن المعز اذا جعل في قدر مع نشاء القمح وورس وسكر طبرزد ويطبخ طبخا جيدا والقي عليه دهن اللوز واستعمل نفع من مرض السل والوجع الحار وحمى الدق
22.35	لبن الماعز اذا اخلط معه بول الثور وتحمي الاسنّة وتسقيها به فانها تصير قاطعة	لبن الماعز حامضا ويخلط معه بدم ماعز وبول تيس ويحمي الاسنّة ونصول النشاب وتغمس فيه وهي حارة ويتردد فيه ثم تخلا فان الحديد يصير مسموما اذا خالط الدم قتل	لبن المعز اذا حميت الاسنة ونصول النشاب وسقيت به كان مسا فاتلا لا يقع في شيء الا قتله وكانت الملوك تدخر ذلك في خزائنهم
22.36	*om.*	للدوى وللصمم يؤخذ بول غنز جزء ومن الاذريون جزء يدق وينخل ويذاف بالبول ويقطر منه في الأذن نافع باذن الله تعالى	اذا أخذ من دم الماعز جزء ومن الادريون جزء ودق الجميع ويعجن بالبول وقطر في الاذن الصماء نفعها

22.32: (B) This recipe is attested only in G

22.33: (c) ما بذلك من الضربان] الم الضربان C

22.34: (a) This recipe is attested only in B

(b) فيؤخذ ويطبخ ويخلط] اذا طبخ وخلط G | القمح] الفيج G | ويقطّر] وقطّر G | يكون لنفى الاوجاع] يسقي منه للاوجاع G | الربع] الدق G

(c) القمح] *om.* C | ويطبخ طبخا جيدا] وطبخ طبخا جيدا C | والقى] ثم القى C | نفع من] منه من به C | الدق] ابراه وازال ذلك عنه *add.* C

22.35: (a) This recipe is attested only in B

(b) حامضا] الحامض G | ويخلط] اذا خلط G | معه] *om.* G | ماعز] ماعز فجل *add.* G | تيس] ثور G | ويحمي] وسقيت به G | النشاب] النشاب والرماح *add.* G | وتغمس…قتل] فهو اجود ما يكون للعدوّ فانه اذا اصابه قليلا منه قتله G

(c) لبن المعز…خزائنهم] واذا أخذ المعز وبول ثور احمر واحميت الاسنّة ونصول النشاب وسقيت منه كان سما قاطلا لا يقع في شيء الاقتله وكانت الملوك تدخره في خزائن C

22.36: (b) للدوى…غنز] يؤخد منه بول الغنز G | بالبول] في البول G | نافع] الاذن الصمى وللدوى G

(c) اذا أخذ من دم الماعز] اذا أخذت منه دم المعز C | ودق] ودقت C | ويعجن] وعجنته C | وقطر] وقطرت C | الاذن المصما نفعها] الاصمّ فتق السمع وازال الصمم C

22.31	*om.*	The blood of the billy goat crumbles the diamond.	*om.*
22.32	*om.*	Goat milk: if it is drunk, this will be useful against the ulcers of the intestine.	Goat milk: if it is drunk when it is warm, then this will be useful against the ulcers of the intestine.
22.33	*om.*	*om.*	If it is ground, mixed with vinegar, and rubbed on the body and the legs, this will calm their pangs.
22.34	Goat milk: if it is taken, poured in a cooking pot, some starch, *qlt* [?], wheat, and pure curcuma are added to it, pure sugar is added in the same quantity, and given to the man suffering from consumption, phthisis and fever, then these will cease, with the permission of God, may He be exalted.	Warm goat milk: if it is taken, cooked with the wheat kernel, curcuma instead of saffron and rock sugar—as much as it is needed—with the addition of almond oil drops instead of cow grease, this is the best thing to drink against the acute pains in the chest and in the lungs, and for the man suffering from quartan fever.	Goat milk: if it is poured in a cooking pot with wheat starch, curcuma and rock sugar, cooked well with the addition of almond oil and applied, then this will be useful against consumption, acute pain and the quartan fever.
22.35	Goat milk: if it is mixed with the urine of the bull, thenthe spearheads are made red-hot and quenched in it, then these will become sharp.	Goat sour milk: if it is mixed with goat blood and billy goat urine, then spearheads and arrowheads are made red-hot, and quenched in it while they are still hot, then thrown back in it, and let rest, then the iron will become poisonous, and when it mixes with blood, it will kill.	Goat milk: if the spearheads and the arrowheads are made red-hot, and quenched in it, this will be a mortal poison, that will not touch anybody without killing him; the kings keep this in their treasures.
22.36	*om.*	Against the ear buzz and the deafness, goat urine: one part of it, one part of calendula, ground, sieved, and mixed with urine, and applied in drops in the ears, then this will be useful, with the permission of God, may He be exalted.	If a one part of goat blood is taken, and one part of calendula, then everything is ground, kneaded with urine, and applied in drops inside the deaf ears, then this will be useful for it.

22.37	*om.*	لعسر الولادة يعلق على قرن المرأة الايمن قرن المعز الايمن فانه يسهل الولادة	*om.*
22.38	قرن ماعز ابيض فتحرقه وتدقّه وتخله ويؤخذ رماده ويجعل في خرقة كتان جديد وتجعل تحت رأس النائم وهو لا يعلم فلا ينتبه حتى تنزعها وذلك يفعل بالمريض اذا لم ينام	يؤخذ قرن عنز ابيض فيحرق ويؤخذ رماده وفيصير في حرقة كتان وتصير تحت رأس المريض وهو لا يعلم فلا يزال نائما حتى ينبّه بشدة او تشال الخرقة من تحت رأسه	قرن الماعز يحرق ويدق وينخل ويجعل في خرقه كتان جديده وتجعل تحت رأس النائم المريض الذي يشتكي قله النوم فلا يزال نائما حتى ينزع من تحت رأسه
22.39	*om.*	واذا اردت ان يسلم الباز من الحصر [؟] فاطعمه في كل شهر ثلاث مرات او اربع من لحم التيس ولا تكثر	واذا اردت ان يسلم البازي من القرنصة خذ دم تيس اطعمه في اول الشهر كره ويكون الدم ثخينا فانه يخلص ذلك
22.40	*om.*	واذا اردت ان يسمن الباز فاطعمه دم تيس ملطوخا بالدم الذي يأكله فانه يسمن	واذا اردت ان تسلم البازي ويكون قليل المرض فالطخ له اللحم الذي يأكله بدم تيس
22.41	اذا اردت ان تقتل السبع فخذ لحم الماعز وتبله بماء وزيت فوق فان اكله مات لساعته	دواء يقتل السباع يؤخذ شحم ماعز ويخلط معه مُرّ مدقوقا ناعما ويعجن به ويلقي للسباع فلا ياكل منه سبع الا مات في وقته	واذا اردت ان تقتل السبع خذ لحم معز ودقه واخلطه بلوز مدقوق فانه ان اكله مات

22.37: (b) *om.* G

22.38: (b) يؤخذ] *om.* G | عنز ابيض] العنز الابيض G | فيحرق ويؤخذ] اذا احرق وأخذ من G | وفيصير] وجعل G | وتصير] وجعل G | المريض] مريض G | ينبّه] تنزع G | بشدة او تشال الخرقة] *om.* G

(c) قرن الماعز...رأسه] قرن المعز الابيض اذا حرق ودق ونحل وجعل في خرقة من كتان جديدة وتركت تحت رأس انسان نائم فلا ينتبه حتى تنزع من تحته C

22.39: (b) This recipe is attested only in G

(c) *om.* C

22.40: (b) بالدم] على لحم G | الذي ياكله فانه يسمن] *om.* G

(c) *om.* C

22.41: (b) دواء يقتل السباع يؤخذ] *om.* G | ماعز] الماعز G | ويخلط] اذا دق وخلط *add.* G | مرّ] لوز مرّ *add.* G | ويعجن] وعجن G | ويلقي] ويوضع G | في وقته] *om.* G

(c) واذا اردت ان تقتل السبع] *om.* C | خذ لحم...مات] لحم المعز اذا دق ناعما وخلط بلوز مدقوق وأكل منه بسع مان ذلك السبع C

22.37	*om.*	For the difficulties in giving birth: if the goat horn is hung on the horn of the woman [on top?], then this will ease the birth.	*om.*
22.38	Horn of the white goat: if it is ground, its ash is taken, put in a new cotton cloth, and placed under the head of a sleeping man—but he should not be aware of it—then he will not wake up until this is removed, this is done with the sick person who cannot sleep.	White goat horn: if it is burnt, its ash taken and put in a cotton cloth, placed under the head of the sick man—but he should not be aware of it—then he will not stop sleeping until this is removed from under his head.	Goat horn: if it is burnt, pounded, sieved, put into a new cotton cloth, this is placed under the head of a sleeping sick man, who suffers from lack of sleep, then he will keep sleeping until this is removed from under his head.
22.39	*om.*	If you want to cure the hawk from emaciation, feed it three or four times every month—but not more—with the meat of a billy goat, but do not do it more often.	If you want that the hawk recovers from the purchase, take the blood of billy goat, feed it to the hawk in the first month—and the blood should be thick—then the hawk will be fine.
22.40	*om.*	If you want that the hawk gets some weight, feed him with the blood of the billy goat mixed with the blood with which is fed, and then he will gain some weight.	If you want that the hawk recovers when it is a bit sick, spatter the meat that the hawk eats with the blood of the billy goat.
22.41	If you want to kill a beast of prey, take the meat of the goat, moisten it with water and oil on top, and if the animal eats it, then it will die immediately.	Remedy that kills the beasts of prey, goat fat: if it is taken, mixed with finely ground myrrh, kneaded with it, and poured on the beasts of prey, then no beast of prey will eat it without dying on the spot.	If you want to kill a beast of prey, take the meat of the goat, mince it, melt it with ground almonds, and if the wild animal eats it, then it will die.

22.42

om.

يؤخذ قطعة من كبد ماعز ويغرز فيها خمس عيدان دار فلفل ويملّح بملح اندراني مسحوق وتصير الكبد في عود وتلوّح على النار ويجمع ما يسيل منها من الماء في صدفة فاذا انقطع تنحّ النار ويخرج العيدان دار فلفل منه وتطعم صاحب العلة ذلك الكبد ثم تجفف تلك العيدان في الظل ويسحق منها جزء ومن ملح اندراني جزء فيسحق الجميع سحقا ناعما ويكتحل منه صاحب العلة الطرية عليه من العمى في وقته وساعته ساعة طريان العمى عليه في ذلك اليوم مرارا فانه يبرأ باذن الله تعالى

om.

22.43

om.

ظلف الماعز يحرق ويؤخذ رماده ويعجن بخل خمر حاذق ويطلي به الموضع الذي فيه القرع يبرأ

om.

22.44

للشقيقة والصداع خذ اول يوم ثلاث اكارع ماخر اول ما يدبح وهو حار كارعين من المقدم وكارع من الموخر وتأخذ في اليوم الثاني كارعين من الموخر وكارع من المقدم وتكسر الجميع وتخلط مخاخه وتجعل في مسعط وتأخذ وزن قيراط من ذلك يسعط به صاحب الشقيقة والصداع ثلاثة ايام متواليا يبرأ

للشقيقه يؤخذ في يوم ثلاثة اكراع ماعز طرية ساعة ان تذبح كان عين المقدّم وكراع من الموخر اليوم الثاني كراعين من الموخر وكراع من المقدم فتكسر ويؤخذ مخّها فيصير في مسعط ويخلط معه قدر سمسم ويذوب على نار او رماد حار ويسعط منه من اصابه الشقيقه من البرد ثلاثة ايام متوالية فانه يبرأ

للشقيقة والصداع تأخذ في يوم الاول ثلاثة كراع من كراع الماعز تذبح كارع من الموخر وكارعين من المقدم فتكسرهم وتأخذ مخاخها وتجعل في اناء وتأخذ منه مقدار دانق واخلط معه وزن حبّة عنبر خام ويسعط به صاحب الشقيقة فانه يزول باذن الله وهو يكون ٣ ايام

22.42: (b) [وتطعم صاحب | om. G [دار فلفل | G واخرج [ويخرج | add. G ما يسيل منها يختّها على [تنحّ | om. G [وتصير الكبد في عود | G الماعز [ماعز
الجميع | G واسحقها [حق | G ثم اسحقهم واأخذ منهفيس [ويسحق | G وجفف [ثم تجف | G الغشاوه وهو الذي لايبصر بالليل [العلة | G واطعمتها لصاحب
G فهو [فانه | om. G [الطرية عليه من العمى في وقته وساعته ساعة طريان العمى عليه | add. G هذا العلة [العلة | G وكحّل به [ويكتحل منه | om. G [سحقا

22.43: (b) G القرع في الرأس او في غيره اذهبه [الموضع...يبرأ | G وطلى [ويطلي | G خمر حار [حاذق | G وعجن [ويعجن | G اذا احرق واخذ [يحرق ويؤخذ

22.44: (a) This recipe is attested only in B

(b) ويؤخذ في اليوم الثاني كراع من المقدم [اليوم...من اصابه | G ومما يستعمل للشقيقه يؤخذ في اول يوم كراعين ماعز طرية ساعة الذبح [للشقيقه...عين وكراعين من الموخر ويؤخذ في اليوم الثالث كراعين من المقدم وكراع من الموخر يكسر الجميع ويؤخذ مخّها ويجعل في مسعط ويخلط معه قدر سمسمه عنبر ويذوب على النار او على رماد حار ويسعط منه صاحب G

(c) ما في العظام من [مخاخه | C وهو الايدي [المقدم | add. C اي الرجلين [الموخر | C ساعة [اول ما | C كوارع ماعز [اكارع ماخر | add. C يوم تريد عمله [يوم C فانه يبرأ [يبرأ | C وتسعط [يسعط | C وترفع في اناء [وتجعل في مسعط | C المخ

22.42	*om.*	Piece of goat liver: if it is taken, five branches of long pepper are stuck into it, it is salted with ground rock salt, then it is put on a stick and burnt, all the liquid that comes out of it is collected in a shell; when the fire stops to make sounds, the branches of long pepper have to be taken out, and fed to the man suffering from the disease of this liver; these branches have to be dried in the shade, then one part of it has to be ground with one part of rock salt, then everything is finely ground, and applied on the eyes of the man affected by this moist disease that immediately brings blindness with it, on that very day for some times, and then he will heal, with the permission of God, may He be exalted.	*om.*
22.43	*om.*	Goat hoof: if it is burnt, its ash is taken, kneaded with sour wine vinegar, and rubbed on the ringworm of the head or of another area, then this will heal.	*om.*
22.44	Against migraine and headache, on the first day take three legs of a slaughtered goat—one from the front and two from the back—break them and take their marrow, put it in a vessel and take one *dāniq* of it, mix it with one grain of fetid amber, and let it inhale to the man suffering from migraine, then this will go away, with the permission of God; and this has to be done for three days.	Against migraine: three legs have to be taken from a fresh goat—the best is when it is slaughtered—on the second day, two from the back and one from the front; they have to be broken, their marrow has to be taken, put in a snuff-box, mixed with a measure of sesame, melted on the fire or on the warm ash, and inhaled by the man affected by the migraine due to the cold, for three days in the same quantity, then he will heal.	Against migraine and headache, take on the first day three legs of a goat that has been slaughtered while it is still warm, two legs from the front and one from the back; on the second day, take two from the back and one from the front, break everything and melt their marrows, put this inside a snuff-box, take one carat of it, and let it sniff to the man suffering from migraine and headache, for three days in the same quantity, then he will heal.

٢٣. بقر الوحش

	a	b	c
	باب منافع اعضاء بقر الوحش	بقر الوحش	باب منافع بقر الوحش
23.1	يؤجد في مرارة بقر الوحش خرزة يؤخذ منها مقدار دانق ويسعط منها صاحب اللقوة والفالج يبرأ باذن الله تعالى	خرزة بقر الوحش تنفع من اللقوة اذا سُعّط بها وهي انجع من الجاوازن اي خرزة بقر الاهلي و الارمنية	يؤخذ فيها خرزة اذا أخذ وسعط بها صاحب اللقوة والفالج ابرأته
23.2	*om.*	مخ بقر الوحش يليّن الاوصال المنعقدة	مخ بقر الوحش يذاب على النار وتدهن به الاوجاع المتعقدة والمنكسرة تبرأ
23.3	منفحة بقر الوحش تذاف بماء الكمون الابيض ويسقي منها المبطون فانه يمسك الجوف باذن الله تعالى	انفحة عجاجيل بقر الوحش تسقي منها المبطون قدر مثقالين بماء الكمون المغلى المصفى يقطع الاسهال باذن الله تعالى	اذا أخذ عجل بقر الوحش وسقى منه المبطون وزن مثقال بماء الكمون المغلى ابرأه

23.1: (b) In T only part of the recipe is attested: وهي انجع واقوى فعلا من الكازور الذي يؤخذ في البقر الاهلي
(c): يؤخذ] توجد مرارة بقر الوحش C | أخذ] أخذت C | بها] منها C | ابرأته] ابرأه C
23.2: (b) المنعقدة] المتشبّكة G
(c) يذاب] اذيبته C | وتدهن] ودهنت C | الاوجاع المتعقدة] الاوجاع والاوصال المتعقدة C | والمنكسرة] برئت *add.* C | تبرأ] *om.* C
23.3: (b) عجاجيل] *om.* G | تسقي] اذا اسقى G | قدر] وزن G | يقطع] قطع G | الاسهال] عنه ذلك G | In G another recipe is added, with the worm that can be found in the head of the buffalo, see also 29.1: يري في رأس الجاموس ودماغه دود متشبك لا يدعه ينام ان أخذ انسان من ذلك الدود وهو حي وعلقه عليه لم ينم

23. Wild Cow

	a	b	c
	Exposition of the useful properties of the parts of the wild cow	**The wild cow**	**Chapter on useful properties of the wild cow**
23.1	Small stone that can be found in the gall bladder of the wild cow: if one *dāniq* is taken, inhaled by the man suffering from facial paralysis and paralysis, then this will cure him, with the permission of God, may He be exalted.	The small stone from wild cow is useful against facial paralysis, if a man inhales it; this is even more beneficial than the bead of the domestic and from the Armenian cow.	Take the small stone inside it, and let it inhale to the man suffering from facial paralysis and paralysis, then this will cure him.
23.2	*om.*	The marrow of the wild cow relaxes the contracted limbs.	Wild cow marrow: if it is melted on the fire, and rubbed on the pains of the joints and of the fractures, then this will cure them.
23.3	Wild cow rennet: if it is mixed with white cumin water, and given to the man suffering from an intestinal ailment to drink, then this will contain the abdomen, with the permission on God, may He be exalted.	Rennet of wild cow's calf: if two *miṯqāl* of it is given to the man suffering from an intestinal ailment with boiled and purified cumin water, then this will stop the diarrhoea, with the permission of God, may He be exalted.	If the calf of the wild cow is taken, given to drink to the man suffering from intestinal ailments with boiled cumin water, then this will cure him.

٢٤. اليحمور

	a	b	c
	ذكر منافع اعضاء اليحمور	اليحمور	باب منافع اليحمور
24.1	خصى اليحمور تملح بملح وحليب وسذاب يابس ويجفف وتسقي لصاحب الدمعة فانها تذهب	خصية اليحمور تملم بملح وحلتيت وسذاب يابس ويجفّف ويسحق ويسقي به من به الحمى ربع وزن مثقال بماء القرط المغلى المصفى ثلاثة ايام متوالية مجرب	خصوة اليحمور ويجعل فيها ملح وحلتيت خالص وسذاب يابس ويجفف ويسحق ويشرب منها صاحب حمى الربع وزن مثقال بماء القرط المغلى المصفى ثلالة ايام متوالية فان الحمى تذهب عنه
24.2	للبهر وضيق النفس يؤخذ مرارة اليحمور فيذاف بسمن بقري ويشرب على الريق في الحمام بماء حار فيبرأ	لبهق والنفس يؤخذ مرارة اليحمور فيذاف بسمن بقر ويشرب لهذه العلة في الحمام على الريق بماء حار بفعه	مرارة اليحمور اذا اذيفت بسمن البقر وشرب منها المنبهرا ومن به ضيق النفس في الحمام برئ
24.3	للمرو والبلغم وبرد المعدة وحمى الكبد يؤخذ لحم اليحمور يطبخ طبخا جيدا ويجعل في صلاية ويلقي عليه كمون كرماني ما في وشب يماني ويهرس ناعما منه يسقي منه صاحب هذه الامراض فيبرأ باذن الله	لغلبة البغلم في البدن وبرود المعدة والكبد يؤخذ لحم اليحمور وشحمه فيطبخ طبيخا ناعما ويدق في الهاون ويلقي عليه كمون الكرماني وشبّ يماني ويخلط خلطا جيدا ويسقي منه وزن مثقال بماء حار في الحمام ينفع من البغلم والبول	لحم اليحمور اذا طبخ طبخا جيد ودق على صلابة ويلقي عليه كمون كرماني وشب يماني وسقى منه في الحمام مثقال لمن كثيرة البلغ وبرد المعدة ووجع الكبد ابرأه

24.1: (a) This recipe is attested only in B
(b) خصية اليحمور] خصيته G | وحلتيت] وحليبت T | تملم] اذا ملحت G | يابس] om. G | ويجفّف ويسحق ويسقي به] وجفّفت وسحقت وسقى منها G | متوالية مجرب] لم تعاوده G
(c) اليحمور] بقر الوحش C | وحلتيت] وحنتيت L | ويجفف ويسحق] om. C | خالص وسداب يابس ويجفف ويسحق] om. C | ويشرب منها...تذهب عنه] وشرب منه وزن مثقال بماء القرط المغلى المصفى ثلالة ايام متوالية اذهب الحمى عنه وازالها C
24.2: (a) فيذاف] فتذاب B | بقري] بقر B
(b) البهر] لبهق T | يؤخذ مرارة...لهذه العلة] مرارته اذا اذيفت بسمن بقر وشرب منها صاحب البهر والنفس G
(c) المنبهرا] om. C
24.3: (a) للمرو...الكبد] لكثر البلغم وبرد المعدة وحمو الكبد B | ويلقي] ويجعل B | ما في] om. B | ويهرس ناعما] ويهرش B | فيبرأ] يبرأ B
(b) برود] يزود T | لغلبة البغلم في البدن وبرود المعدة والكبد] post. G | يؤخذ...ويلقي] لحمه وشحمه اذا طبخ ناعما ودق في الجرن والقى G | وشبّ يماني] وشبّ يماني ومور G | ويخلط...والبول] وخلط الجميع جيدا وسقي منه لغلبة البغلم في البدن البرودة في المعدة والكبد وزن مثقال بماء حار في الحمام نفعه G
(c) مثقال] زنة مثقال بماء حار add. C | كثره البلغ وبرد المعدة] وبردت معدته واعتراه C

24. Roe Deer

	a	b	c
	Exposition of the useful properties of the parts of the roe deer	**The roe deer**	**Chapter on the useful properties of the roe deer**
24.1	Roe deer testicles: if they are seasoned with salt, cow milk and dry rue, dried and given to the man suffering from lachrymation to drink, then this will cease.	Roe deer testicles: if they are seasoned with salt, asafoetida and dry rue, dried, pounded and given in the quantity of one *miṯqāl* to the man affected by quartan fever to drink with boiled and purified alfalfa water for three days, [it will be useful]: tried out.	Roe deer testicles: if they are seasoned with salt, pure asafoetida and dry rue, then dried, pounded and given in the quantity of one *miṯqāl* to the man affected by quartan fever to drink with boiled and purified alfalfa water—the same quantity for three days—then the fever will leave him.
24.2	Against breathlessness and weakness of the breath: if the gall of roe deer is taken, mixed with cow fat and drunk on an empty stomach in the bath with warm water, then this will cure it.	Against difficult respiration, roe deer gall: if it is taken, mixed with cow fat, and given against this disease to drink in the bath on an empty stomach, then this will be useful against it.	Roe deer gall: if it is mixed with cow fat, and drunk in the bath by the man affected by breathlessness and by the man with a weak breath, then this will heal.
24.3	Against stones, phlegm, stomach coldness and liver fever, roe deer meet: if it is taken, cooked very well, put in a mortar, with the addition of the available cumin and Yemeni alum, crushed finely, and given to the man suffering from this illnesses to drink, then he will recover, with the permission of God.	Against the phlegm in the body and the coldness in stomach and in the liver, roe deer meat and its fat: if they are taken, well cooked, minced in a mortar, with cumin, Yemeni alum, mixed well, and one *miṯqāl* of it is given to drink with warm water in the bath, then this will be useful against the phlegm and the urine.	Roe deer meat: if it is well cooked, ground in a mortar with cumin and Yemeni alum, one *miṯqāl* of it is given to the man who has phlegm, stomach coldness and liver complaint to drink in the bath, then this will cure him.

24.4	لوجع الخاصرة يؤخذ دماغ اليحمور يذاب بماء الجرجير يسحق على النار ويشرب صاحب وجع الخاصرة وايضا الجبين	دماغ اليحمور يذاف بماء الجرجير ويسخن على النار ويشرب منه لوجع الجبين والخاصرتين وزن مثقال بماء عسل	دماغ اليحمور اذا اذيف بماء الجرجير وفتر على النار وشرب منه في الحمام من يشتكي وجع الخاصر والجبنين ابرأه
24.5	يؤخذ مخ اليحمور فيذاب بماء السذاب وعسل نحل ويسحق على النار ويسقي لصاحب الفهاق فانه يزول باذن الله تعالى	للفواق مخ اليحمور بماء والعسل ويسخن على النار ويشرب على الريق جيد	مخ اليحمور يذاب بماء السذاب الاخضر والعسل يسحق على النار ويسقي لصاحب الفهاق فانه يبرأ باذن الله تعالى
24.6	زبل اليحمور يبخر به البيت فانه لا يقربه الذبيب والله اعلم	*om.*	*om.*

24.4: (a) This recipe is attested only in B
(b) *om.* G
(c) اليحمور] *om.* C | اذيف] ذوب C | وفتر على النار] *om.* C | الحمام] مثقال وزن حار بماء الحمام *add.* C | يشتكي] وجع C | والجبنين] وذات الجبن C | ابرأه] *om.* C
24.5: (a) فيذاب] يذاب B | ويسحق] وسحق B | الفهاق] البهق B
(b) للفواق...جيد] نفعه على الريق صاحب القولنج وشربه على النار والعسل بماء السذاب اذا اذيف مخه G
(c) يذاب] اذا اذيب C | يسحق] تسحق C | ويسقي لصاحب] به من ويشربه C | يبرأ] *om.* C
24.6: (a) فانه لا] فلا C

24.4	Against the pain of the waist, roe deer brain: if it is taken, liquefied with rocket water, ground on the fire, and given to the man suffering from waist pain to drink, [this will be useful] also against the pain of the forehead.	Roe deer brain: if it is mixed with rocket water, pounded on the fire, given to drink against the pain of the temples and the forehead—one *miṯqāl* with honey water—[it will be useful].	Roe deer brain: if it is mixed with rocket water, made lukewarm on the fire, and drunk by the man suffering from waist and temples pain, then this will cure him.
24.5	If the gall of roe deer is taken, mixed with rue water and honey, ground on the fire, and given to the man suffering from a lesion in the neck to drink, then this will cease, with the permission of God, may He be exalted.	Against irregular respiration, roe deer marrow, with water and honey, pounded on the fire, and drunk on an empty stomach, then this will be very useful.	Roe deer marrow: if it is liquefied with fresh rue water and honey, pounded on the fire, and given to the man suffering from a lesion of the neck to drink, then this will cure him, with the permission of God, may He be exalted.
24.6	Roe deer excrement: if it is fumigated inside the house, then the flies will not approach it, and God knows best.	*om.*	*om.*

٢٥. النمر

	a	b	c
	ذكر منافع اعضاء النمر	النمر	باب منافع النمر
25.1	يؤخذ خصى النمر تملح بملح ومر وزعفران ولبان وتجفف في الظل ويؤخذ منه مقدار حمصة يذاب بماء الكمون ويسقي لصاحب هذا المرض ويدهن به الجسد يبرأ	خصية النمر اذا تملح بملح ولبان ومُرّ وزعفران وتجفّف ويؤخذ بقدر حمصة منه ويشرب يطرد البرد ويسخن ويشربه الصبيان والنساء بماء الكمون	خصوة النمر اذا ملحت بملح ومر وشرب منها الصبيان والنساء ويتبخر بها وطلى الجسد نفعت نفعا جيدا
25.2	مرارة النمر تذاب بقطران ويسقي منها صاحب وجع الكبد والصفار وزن ثلاث قراريط بدهن زنبق خالص وماء حار نافع باذن الله تعال	مرارة النمر يذاف بقطران ويشرب منها لوجع الكبد والصفار وزن ثلاثة قراريط بزنبق وماء حار[نفعه]	مرارة النمر تذاف بقطرن خالص وتسقي لمن به وجع الكبد والصفار وزن مثقال بدهن زنبق وماء حار فانه ينفع
25.3	دم النمر يلطخ به العين فانه نافع من كل داء يكون في العين	دم النمر يلطخ على العين [نفع] لكل عاهة تكون في البصر	اذا الطخت العين بدم النمر نفعها من كل داء فيها
25.4	يؤخذ لحم النمر وشحمه يطبخ بماء الزيتون حتى يتهرا ويلطخ به الجسد فينفع من الشرى والحرارة	لحم النمر وشحمه يطبخ بماء الزيتون حتى يتهرّا وهو اجود ما يكون للشرى والقروح والحزاز	دم النمر ولحمه وشحمه اذا طبخ بماء الزيتون حتى تهري ثم لطخ به الجسد نفع من الشرية والحرارة

25.1: (a) This recipe is attested only in B
(b) خصية النمر] خصيته G | اذا تملح] اذا ملحت G | وتجفّف ويؤخذ بقدر] وخفّفت وسحقت وشرب منها وزن G | ويشرب…الكمون] وشرب منها وزن حمصة بماء الكمون وتبخّر بشيء منها ومسح جسده بشيء منها نفع من النظرة والسحر G
(c) ملحت] شننت C | ويتخر بها] *om.* C | نفعت نفعا جيدا] نفع البدن كله نفعا جيدا C
25.2: (a) نافع] فينفعه B
(b) مرارة النمر] *om.* G | يذاف] اذا اذيف G | ويشرب] وشرب G | وزن] *om.* G | ثلاثة] ثلثة G | بزنبق] بزيبق T | حار] نفعه *add.* G
(c) نافع] فينفعه C | تداف] اذيبت C | بقطرن خالص] بقطران برفي خالص C | وتسقي] وشرب C | لمن به] صاحب C | ينفع] نفع نفعا جيدا ازال ذلك عنه C
25.3: (a) *om.* B
(b) دم النمر] دمه G | يلطخ على] اذا طلى به G | العين] العين نفع add. G | عاهة] علة G | في البصر] فيها G
25.4: (a) ويلطخ…والحرارة] *om.* B
(b) لحم النمر] لحمه G | يطبخ] يطبخا G | والحزاز] اذا طلى به *add.* G

25. Cheetah

	a	b	c
	Exposition of the useful properties of the parts of the cheetah	**The cheetah**	**Chapter on the useful properties of the cheetah**
25.1	Cheetah testicles: these have to be taken, seasoned with salt, myrrh, saffron and olibanum, dried in the shade; the quantity of a chick-pea has to be taken, liquefied with cumin water and given to the man suffering from this illness to drink, and rubbed on his body, then he will recover.	Cheetah testicles: if they are seasoned with salt, olibanum, myrrh and saffron, and dried, and if the quantity of a chick-pea is taken and drunk, this will remove the cold; if it is ground, it can be drunk by children and women with cumin water.	Cheetah testicles: if they are seasoned with salt and myrrh, drunk by children and women, fumigated and rubbed on the body, then they will be really very useful.
25.2	Cheetah gall: if it is liquefied with tar, and three carats of it are given to the man suffering from liver complaint and yellow complexion to drink with pure lily oil and warm water, then this will be very useful to him, with the permission of God, may He be exalted.	Cheetah gall: if it is mixed with tar and drunk against the liver complaint and the yellow complexion, in the quantity of three carats with lily and warm water, then this will be useful against this.	Cheetah gall: if it is mixed with pure tar, given to the man suffering from liver complaint and yellow complexion to drink with lily oil and warm water, then it will be very useful.
25.3	Cheetah blood: if it is spattered on the eye, then this will be useful against all the diseases that affect it.	Cheetah blood: if it is spattered on the eye, this will be useful against all the diseases that affect the eyesight.	If the eye is spattered with the blood of the cheetah, then this will be useful against all the diseases that affect it.
25.4	Cheetah meat and its fat: if they are taken and cooked with olives water until they are well done, and then spattered on the body, this will be useful against the itching skin eruption and the hotness.	Cheetah meat and its fat: if these are cooked with olives water until they are well done, this will be the best remedy against the itching skin eruption, ulcers and the impetigo.	Cheetah blood, its meat and its fat: if they are cooked until they are well done, then spattered on the body, then this will be useful against the itching skin eruption and the hotness.

25.5

دماغ النمر اذا اذيب بماء الجرجير ودهن الزنبق ودهن به الرجل احليله نفعه وانشطه

دماغه اذا اذيف بماء الجرجير مع شيء من زنبق ودهن الرجل به احليله نشط للجماع

دماغ النمر يذاف بماء الجرجير ودهن زنبق ويدهن به الرجل احليله عند الجماع فانه يقوي شهوة النكاح ويقوي على الجماع

25.6

مخ النمر اذا اذيب بدهن زنبق وحملت به المرأة في صوفة نفعها من وجع الرحم ان شاء الله تعالى

مخه اذا ذوّب بزنبق وتحملت به المرأة في صوقة نفعها من وجع الارحام

مخ النمر يذاف بدهن الزنبق تحمله المرأة لوجع الرحم فانه اجود ما يكون والله أعلم

25.5: (a) دماغ النمر] *om.* B | ويقوي على] *om.* B
(b) This recipe is attested only in G
(c) نفعه وانشطه] نعضه انعاضا شديدا وحسّن له الجماع C
25.6: (a) يداف بدهن الزنبق] يذاب بزيت B | لوجع الرحم فانه اجود ما يكون] نافع لوجع الرحم B
(b) This recipe is attested only in G
(c) الرحم] الرحم نفعا جيدا *add.* C

25.5	Cheetah brain: if it is mixed with rocket water and lily oil, and a man rubs this on the outer opening of the urethra at the moment of coitus, then this will give power to the sexual desire and to the coitus itself.	Its brain: if it is mixed with rocket water with some lily, and the man rubs the outer opening of his own urethra with it, then this will have an invigorating effect on the coitus.	Cheetah brain: if it is liquefied with rocket water and lily oil, and rubbed on the outer opening the urethra, then this will be useful, and will invigorate it.
25.6	Cheetah marrow: if it is mixed with lily oil, and carried by a woman against the pain of the womb, then this will be the best against it, and God knows best.	Its marrow: if it is liquefied with lily and carried by the woman, then this will be useful to her against the pain of the womb.	Cheetah marrow: if it is liquefied with lily oil and carried by a woman, then this will be useful to her against the pain of the womb, God, may He be exalted, willing.

٢٦. الفيل

	a	b	c
	ذكر منافع اعضاء الفيل	الفيل	باب منافع الفيل
26.1	شحم الفيل يبخر به صاحب الصداع والشقيقة فتزول	شحم الفيل يدهن به صاحب الصداع يبرأ	شحم الفيل اذا بخر به صاحب الصداع ابرأه
26.2	ناب الفيل يدق ناعما ويسقي منه صاحب الجذام بماء الفودنج النهري فيقف عنه	يؤخذ من العاج وزن درهم ويعجن ويبرد بالمبرد ويشربه الانسان الذي قد بدأ به الجذام بوزن عشرة دراهم ماء الشعير والعدس والفوذنج فيقف الجذام باذن الله تعالى	ناب الفيل اذا برد وسحق وسقى منه صاحب الجذام وزن عشرة دراهم بماء العصفر وهو الفوذنج النهري وقف عنه
26.3	لحم الفيل يطبخ بالخل والكاشم حتى ينهرا وتسقي المرأة الحامل تسقط الجنين	[لحم الفيل] واذا طبخ بالخل والكاشم حتى ينهرا وحست وشربت امرأة حبلي من مرقته القت ما في بطنها	لحم الفيل اذا طبخ بالخل الكاشم وشربت مرقته المرأة الحامل وضعت الجنين لوقتها
26.4	للسعال العتيق والبهق على الجوف يؤخذ لحم الفيل يطبخ بالخل والكاشم حتى يتهرا ويسقي للمرأة الحامل فيسقط الجنين من جوفها باذن الله تعال	لحم الفيل يطبخ بماء وملح وكاشم حتى ينهرا ويحسي من مرقته من به السعال عتيق [نفعه]	*om.*

26.1: (a) فتزول] يزول عنه B
(b) شحم الفيل] شحمه G | يدهن] اذا دخن G | يبرأ] برئ G
(c) صاحب] من اصابه C | ابرأه] ابرأه وازال عنه الالم والشقيقة *add.* C
26.2: (a) الفودنج] الفوتينخ B
(b) يؤخذ] اذا أخذ G | ويعجن ويبرد] وسحق او برد G | ويشربه] وشربه G | بوزن] مع وزن G | والفوذنج] والفوذج T | ماء الشعير والعدس والفوذنج] من ماء السعتر G | فيقف الجذام] وقف الجذام G | العزلي وهو الفوذنج الجبلي
(c) وسقى منه] برد وسحق وشرب منها وسحقت برادته C | وزن] زنة C | وقف] اوقفه C
26.3: (a) This recipe is attested only in B
(b) In T the order of this recipe and of the following one is inverted | وشربت] *om.* G | حبلي] *om.* G
(c) وشربت] وشرب C
26.4: (a) *om.* B
(b) In T the order of this recipe and of the previous one is inverted | لحم الفيل] لحمه G | يطبخ] اذا طبخ G | السعال العتيق] السعال القديم والربو G

26. Elephant

	a	b	c
	Exposition of the useful properties of parts of the elephant	**The elephant**	**Chapter on the useful properties of the elephant**
26.1	Elephant fat: if man suffering from headache and migraine is fumigated with it, then these will cease.	Elephant fat: if it is rubbed on the man affected by headache, then he will heal.	Elephant fat: if a man suffering from headache is fumigated with it, then this will cure him.
26.2	Elephant tusk: if it is finely ground, and given with river sedge water to the man suffering from elephantiasis, then this will cease.	If one dirham of elephant's tusk is taken, ground, filed with a rasp, and the man who has already contracted the elephantiasis drinks it with ten dirhams of barley, lentils and pennyroyal, then the elephantiasis will cease.	Elephant tusk: if it is filed, ground, ten dirham of it with river sedge water are given to the man suffering from elephantiasis to drink, then this will cease.
26.3	Elephant meat: if it is cooked with vinegar and Mediterranean moon carrot until it is well done, and this is given to drink to a pregnant woman, then she will lose the baby.	Elephant meat: if it is cooked with vinegar and Mediterranean moon carrot until it is well done, and a pregnant woman sips and drinks its broth, then she will lose what is in her belly.	Elephant meat: if it is cooked with vinegar and Mediterranean moon carrot, and a pregnant woman sips its broth, then she will immediately lose the baby.
26.4	Against the chronic cough and the vitiligo on abdomen, elephant meat: if it is taken, cooked with vinegar and Mediterranean moon carrot until it is well done, and it is given to a pregnant woman to drink, then she will have a miscarriage, with the permission of God, may He be exalted.	Elephant meat: if it is cooked with water, salt, and Mediterranean moon carrot until it is well done, and the one affected by the chronic cough sips it, [it will be useful to him].	*om.*

26.5	يؤخذ مرارة الفيل يذاف بمسك خالص ويسعط بها المصروع فيبرأ باذن الله تعال	مرارة الفيل يسعط منها وزن قيراط مع مثله مسك لمن به وجع الكبد نفعه	مرارة الفيل تذاب بمسك ويسعط منها صاحب الصرع وزن مثقال فانه يبرأ
26.6	يؤخذ كبد الفيل يطبخ بماء وورق الريحان والسماق ويسقي منها صاحب وجع الكبد فيبرأ باذن الله	كما السماق مع ورق الريحان وهو البارز بحبوبه ينفع نفعا بينا	زيادة كبد الفيل اذا طبخت بورق الريحان والسماق وأكل منها صاحب وجع الكبد نفعه جيدا
26.7	*om.*	زبل الفيل ينفع للقمل اذا طلى به الجسد وترك حتى يجفّ عليه فانه اذا فعل ذلك لم يبق في بشرته ولا جلده قملة الا خرجت عند جفاف الزبل	*om.*
26.8	زبل الفيل يبخر به البيت فلا يقربه البروض	زبله اذا بخّر الموضع الذي فيه البعوض قتله وهرّبه	زبل الفيل اذا بخرت به البعوض قتله
26.9	اذا اردت المرأة لا تحبل ابدا فخذ زبل الفيل فاذيبه بماء واسقيه للمرأة فلا تحبل ابدا	واذا شرب من زبله امرأة بنبيذ وزن دانق لم تحبل ابدا	واذا شربت منه امرأة لم تحبل ابدا

26.5: (a) يذاف] تذاب B | ويسعط بها] ويسقي B
(b) مرارة الفيل] مرارته G | يسعط] اذا سعط G | قيراط] قراط G | وجع الكبد] الصرع G
26.6: (a) *om.* B
(b) كما...بينا] زيادة كبده اذا اكل منها من به وجع الكبد بماء السماق مع ورق الريحان نفعه G
(c) صاحب] من اصابه C | نفعه جيدا] نفعه نفعا جيدا C
26.7: (b) زبل الفيل] زبله G | ينفع للقمل] *om.* G | فانه...الزبل] قتل القمل ولم يعد تبقي عليه قملة G | In G a remark about the antipathies of the elephant is added: والفيل يخاف من الفأرة والخنزير
26.8: (b) This recipe is attested only in G
(c) بخرت] بخره C
26.9: (a) ابدا] *om.* B | واسقيه للمرأة] واسقى المرأة B | فلا] فانها لا B
(b) This recipe is attested only in G
(c) ابدا] *om.* C

26.5 Elephant gall: if it is taken, mixed with pure musk, and the epileptic man inhales it, then he will recover, with the permission of God, may He be exalted.

Elephant gall: if the epileptic man inhales one carat of it with the same quantity of musk, then this will be useful to him.

Elephant gall: if the epileptic man inhales one *miṯqāl* of it mixed with musk, then he will recover.

26.6 Elephant liver: if it is taken, cooked with basil leaves water, and given to the man suffering from liver complaint to drink, then he will recover.

In the same way the sumach with basil leaves—that is *al-bāriz*—with its seeds—this will be greatly useful.

Elephant liver appendage: if it is cooked with basil leaves and sumach, and the man suffering from liver complaint eats it, then this will be very useful to him.

26.7 *om.*

Elephant excrement: it is useful against lice, if it is rubbed on the body and left until it dries; and when this has been done, not a single louse will remain on the body or on the skin without coming out when the excrement dries.

om.

26.8 Elephant excrement: if the house is fumigated with it, then the mosquitos will not approach it.

Its excrement: if the place in which there are mosquitos is fumigated with it, then this will kill and destroy them.

Elephant excrement: if the mosquitos are fumigated with it, then this will kill them.

26.9 If you want that a woman will never get pregnant, take the excrement of the elephant, mix it with water and give it to the woman to drink, then she will never get pregnant.

If a woman drinks one *dāniq* of its excrement with wine, then she will never get pregnant.

If a woman drinks it, she will never get pregnant.

٢٧. النمس

	a	b	c
	ذكر منافع اعضاء النمس	النمس	باب منافع النمس
27.1	اذا اردت ان يفرّق الحمام من البرج فيبخره بذنب نمس فلا يبقي به شيء من الحمام	ذنبه اذا بخّر به برج الحمام هرب منه الحمام	ذنب النمس اذا بخر به برج الحمام لم يوي اليه الحمام ولم يبق به طير
27.2	مرارة النمس تذاف ببياض البيض ويضمد بها العين فلا يبقي فيها شيء من الالم والحمرة والورم ويقطع الدمعة باذن الله تعالى	مرارته اذا اذيف ببياض البيض وضمّد به العين لقط الحرارة وقطع الدمعة	مرارة النمس اذا اذيفت ببياض البيض وضمد بها العين لقطت الحمرة التي بها وجفت الدمعة
27.3	يبخر المجنون بوزن حبة من دم النمس فانه يفيق باذن الله تعالى	دمه اذا سعط منه المجنون وزن قراط بلبن امرأة وبخّر منه نفعه	دم النمس اذا سعط به المجنون قراط وبخر به نفع نفعا كثيرا
27.4	لتقطير البول ورخاء المثانة يؤخذ ذكر نمس فيقطع ويطبخ ويلقي عليه قرنفل وتحسي مرقته فانه نافع باذن الله تعالى	*om.*	ذكر النمس اذا طبخ مع شيء من القرنفل وشرب منه من به وجع المثانة ابرأه
27.5	اذا كان السذاب في موضع فلا يقربه النمس وهدا عجيب	السذاب اذا وضع في موضع مجمع الدجاج لم يقربهن نمس	المكان اذا كان فيه سذاب لا يقربه نمس

27.1: (a) يفرّق] يهرّب B
(c) يوي] ياوي C | طير] طاير ابدا C
27.2: (a) تذاف] تضاف B | الالم والحمرة] الم ولا حمرة B | والورم] *om.* B
(c) اذيفت] اذيبت C | وضمد بها] وضمدت به C | وجفت] وجففت C
27.3: (a) يبخر...يفيق] دم النمس اذا بخرت به المجنون وزن خمسة دراهم فانه يفيق B
(c) This recipe is attested only in C
27.4: (a) ورخاء] ورخو B | فيقطع] يقطع B
(c) من به] من اصابه C
27.5: (c) *om.* C

27. Ichneumon

	a	b	c
	Mention of the useful properties of the parts of the ichneumon	**The ichneumon**	**Chapter on the useful properties of the ichneumon**
27.1	If you want to scatter the pigeons from the pigeon house, fumigate it with the tail of the ichneumon, then no pigeon will remain there.	Its tail: if the pigeon house is fumigated with it, then the pigeons will flee from it	Ichneumon tail: if the pigeon house is fumigated with it, then the pigeons will not seek shelter there, nor a single bird will remain there.
27.2	Ichneumon gall: if it is mixed with egg white, used to bandage the eye, then no pain, inflammation or swelling will remain, and this will also stop the lachrymation, with the permission of God, may He be exalted.	Its gall: if it is mixed with egg white and applied with a bandage on the eye, then this will eliminate the inflammation and the lachrymation.	Ichneumon gall: if it is mixed with egg white, and used to bandage the eye, this will stop the inflammation that affects it, and will dry the lachrymation
27.3	If the insane man is fumigated with one grain of ichneumon's blood, then he will recover, with the permission of God, may He be exalted.	If the insane inhales one carat of its blood mixed with woman's milk, then this will be useful to him.	If the insane man inhales one carat of ichneumon's blood and uses it for fumigations, this will be very useful for him.
27.4	Against urine dripping and bladder prolapse, ichneumon penis: if it is taken, chopped up, cooked, some cloves are added to it, and its broth has to be sipped, with the permission of God, may He be exalted.	*om.*	Ichneumon penis: if it is cooked with some cloves and the man suffering from bladder complaint eats it, then this will cure him.
27.5	If there is some rue in a certain place, then no ichneumon will approach it, and this is amazing.	If some rue is put in the place where the hens gather, then no ichneumon will approach them.	No ichneumon will ever approach the place in which there is some rue.

٢٨. الضب

	a	b	c
	ذكر منافع اعضاء الضب	الضب	باب منافع الضب
28.1	شحم الضب ولحمه يطبخ ويؤخذ دسمه فيخلط مع دهن زنبق ويطلي به الرجل احليله عند الجماع فانه يقوي شهوة الجماع	لحمه وشحمه اذا طبخ وأخذ دسمه فخلط معه زنبق وطلى به الاحليل عند الجماع كثُر جماعة	لحم الضب وشحمه اذا طبخ وأخذ دسمه فخلط مع زنبق ودهن به الرجل احليله كثر الجماع
28.2	للبياض في العين خرؤ الضب يسحق ناعما ويخلط به الاثمد ويكتحل به من في عينه بياض فيزول باذن الله تعالى	خرؤه الابيض اذا خلط مع الاثمد واكتحل به من في عينه البياض او الرطوبة او الحمرة نفعه	بعر الضب الابيض اذا سحق واكتحل به صاحب البياض الذي في العين ابرأه
28.3	اذا اردت ان تسمن الدابة فخذ لحم الضب واطبخ بحنطة واطعم منه [...] الدابة الهزيلة فانها تسمن حتى تكاد تنفلك وان اكل منه ابن ادم فانه جيدا	لحمه اذا طبخ بحنطة واوجرت منه الدابة المهزولة سمّنها	وان خلط بالاثمد كان انفع
28.4	*om.*	خرؤه اذا اذيف بعسل واكتحل به من بعينه بياض نفعه	اذا اردت ان تسمن الدابة
28.5	لداء الثعلب يؤخذ مرارة الضب يذاف بماء السلق وتسعطها فمن في رأسه داء الثعلب فينبت فيها الشعر باذن الله تعالى	مرارته اذا سعّط منها بماء اصول السلق نفع من داء الثعلب	*om.* مرارة الضب اذا سعط بها من به وجع داء الثعلب ابرأه

28.1: (a) شهوة الجماع] السيميا B
(c) فخلط] وخلط C | كثر الجماع] اعانه اي كثرت الجماع وانعضه C
28.2: (a) *om.* B
28.3: (a) *om.* B
28.4: (a) *om.* B
28.5: (a) *om.* B
(c) من به] من اصابه C | داء الثعلب ابرأه] داء الثعلب والرحري لشعر ازال زبك منه وابرأه وابرأ الشعر وانبت الشعر باذن الله تعالى C

28. Stellion

	a	b	c
	Mention of the useful properties of the parts of the stellion	**The stellion**	**Chapter on the useful properties of the stellion**
28.1	Stellion fat and its meat: if they are cooked, their grease is taken apart, mixed with lily oil, and a man rubs the outer opening of his urethra with it at the moment of coitus, then this will increase the desire of coitus.	Its meat and its fat: if they are cooked, their grease is taken, mixed with lily and rubbed on the outer opening of the urethra at the moment of coitus, then this will multiply the copulations.	Stellion meat and its fat: if they are cooked, their grease is taken apart, mixed with lily oil, and a man rubs the outer opening of the urethra with it, then this will multiply copulations.
28.2	Against the glaucoma of the eye: excrement of the stellion pounded into a fine powder, mixed with antimony and applied on the eye affected by glaucoma, then this will disappear, with the permission of God, may He be exalted.	Its white excrement: if it is melted with antimony and applied on the eye, this will be useful to against glaucoma, the moistness and the inflammation of the eye.	White droppings of the stellion: if they are pounded and applied on the eye of a man affected by glaucoma, then this will cure it. And if you melt them with antimony, it will be even more effective.
28.3	If you want that a beast gains some weight, take the meat of a stellion, cook it with wheat and feed it to the skinny animal, then this will gain weight until it becomes nicely plump; it is also good if a man eats it.	Its meat: if it is cooked with wheat and ruminated by a skinny beast, then it will put on weight.	If you want that the a beast puts on weight [...].
28.4	*om.*	Its excrement: if it is mixed with honey and applied on the eyes of the man affected by glaucoma, then this will be useful to him.	*om.*
28.5	Against alopecia: if the gall of the stellion is taken, mixed with beet water and inhaled, then the man affected by alopecia on his head will see his hair growing again, with the permission of God, may He be exalted.	Its gall: if it is inhaled with beet's root water, then this will be useful against the alopecia.	Stellion gall: if it is inhaled by the man suffering from the pain of alopecia, then this will cure him.

٢٩. الجاموس

	a	b	c
	ذكر منافع اعضاء الجاموس	—	باب منافع الجاموس
29.1	يؤخذ في رأس الجاموس دودة تشتكي في دماغه فلا تدعه ينام لكثرة حركتها فان أخذ الانسان ذلك الدودة وجعلها في عرقة وعلقها عليه فانه لا ينام ابدا مما كانت عليه فاذا رميها عنه نام وكل من علق عليه فانه لا ينام وهذا عجيب	—	رأس الجاموس اذا أخذ منه الدود الذي لا يدعه ينام لكثره حركته وهو حي وعلقه انسان عليه فانه لا ينام ما دام ذلك عليه ولو دودة لو اقامت شهرا
29.2	خرؤ الجاموس ينعرك به في الحمام يزيل الطبوع من البدن	—	*om.*
29.3	زبل الجاموس من يبخر به البيت فانه يطرد منه الحيوان باذن الله تعالى	—	*om.*

29.1: (b) In G a similar recipe is added at the end of the chapter on the wild cow, see also 23.3

(c) الذي] التي C | وهو] وهي C | وعلقه] وعلقت ذلك الدود C | عليه] *om.* C | لا ينام] لا يكاد ان ينام C | ذلك عليه ولوروده] ذلك الدود معلقا عليه C

29. Buffalo

	a	b	c
	Mention of the useful properties of the parts of the buffalo	–	**Chapter on the useful properties of the buffalo**
29.1	Take the worm that is inside the head of the buffalo, the worm that does not let it sleep with all its movements; if a man takes this worm, wraps it in a piece of cloth and hangs it on his person, then he will not sleep as long as this remains on him; and if he throws it away, he will sleep again, but everyone that carries the worm on himself will not be able to sleep, and this is amazing.	–	Buffalo head: if the worms that do not let it sleep for all their movements are taken—while they are still alive—and someone hangs them on his body, then he will not sleep as long as this remains on him; and if it were just one worm, he would not sleep for one month.
29.2	Buffalo excrement: if it is rubbed on the body in the bath, then all the marks on the body will disappear.	–	*om.*
29.3	Buffalo manure: if someone fumigates the house with it, then this will chase all the animals away, with the permission of God, may He be exalted.	–	*om.*

٣٠. السنور

	a	b	c
	ذكر منافع اعضاء السنور	السنور	باب منافع السنور
30.1	مخ السنور يذاف بماء الجرجير ويسحن على النار ويسقي لصاحب قطار البول وبرد الكلى	مخه اذا اذيف بماء الجرجير وسحق على النار وشرب منه من به وجع الكلى وتقطير البول في الحمام على الريق وهو حار نفعه	مخ السنور اذا اذيب بماء الجرجير على النار وشرب منه من به قطار البول في الحمام بماء حار نفعه ونفع برد الكلى
30.2	يؤخذ جوف السنور الاسود يجعل على الجمر وسخر به امرأة في جوفها جنين ميت وكذلك القطران اذا حملته المرأة في صوفة وضعت الجنين	جوف السنور الاسود اذا دخّن به تحت المرأة الحاملة رمت الولد الميت. ثم بعد ذلك يؤخذ [من ماء] الحنظل البري وزن ثلاثة قراريط ويخلط معه مرارة ثور فحل وتبلّ فيه صوفة وتتحمل به المرأة	اذا أخذ جوف السنور الاسود ويغلي على النار ورقت عليه المرأة الحامل التي تتوهم ان جنينها ميت قطعه والقاه وكذلك اذا حملت القطران القت من ساعتها
30.3	اذا اردت ان تنظر الى الجانّ وتعرف طرايق السحر تأخذ مرارة سنور اسود ومرارة دجاجة سوداء فيخلط الجميع بالاثمد ويكتحل به قليلا يبي الجانّ ويخبرك بما تريد	ومن اراد ان ينظر الجن فلياخذ مرارة سنور اسود ومرارة دجاجة سوداء يسحقا جميعا مع الاثمد يكتحل بهم فانه يرى الجن ويخبرونه بماء يريد	مرارة السنور الاسود ومرارة الدجاجة السوداء اذا أخذ من كل واحد جزء بالسوية وخلطا جميعان على الاثمد واكتحل بذلك انسان فانه يرى الجان
30.4	ويؤخذ زبل السنور ويذاف بدهن الأس وهو موجود في بمارستان ويدهن به صاحب الحمى النافض فتزول باذن الله تعالى	زبل السنور اذا اذيف بدهن الاس وادهن به انسان وقت الحمى نفعه	زبل السنور اذا اذيب بدهن الاس واندهن به صاحب الحمى زالت عنه ساعتها
30.5	يؤخذ لحم السنور يدق ويطبخ ويضمد به النقرس فيزول باذن الله تعالى	لحمه اذا طبخ ودق وضمّد به النقرس نفعه	*om.*

30.1: (c) اذيب] اذيبته C | اذيب] اذيبته C | من به] من اصابه C | نفعه] نفعه نفعا جيدا *add.* C | ونفع برد] وينفع من اعتراه برد C
30.2: (c) اذا أخذ] *om.* C | ويغلي] اذا جعل C | تتوهم] توهمت C | جنينها ميت] ولدها مات C | والقاه] القت *add.* C | القت] القته C
30.3: (c) اذا أخذ...بالسوية] اجزاء مساويه C | جميعان] جميعا C | الاثمد] الاثمد وهو الكحل *add.* C | بذلك انسان] به احد اعانه على زوجه C | يرى] ورويه C
30.4: (c) زالت] ازالها C | ساعتها] من وقته وساعته C

30. Cat

	a	b	c
	Exposition of the useful properties of the parts of the cat	**The cat**	**Chapter on the useful properties of the cat**
30.1	Cat marrow: if it is mixed with rocket water, ground on the fire and given to the man suffering from urine dripping and coldness of the kidneys to drink, [it will be useful].	Its marrow: if it is mixed with rocket water, ground on the fire and drunk by the man suffering from kidneys complaint and urine dripping, in the bath on an empty stomach while it is warm, then this will be useful to him.	Cat marrow: if it is liquefied with rocket water on the fire and drunk by the man suffering from urine dripping, in the bath with warm water, this will be useful against it; and it is also useful against the coldness of the kidneys.
30.2	Abdomen of a black cat: if it is taken, placed on the embers, and a woman who has a dead foetus in her womb uses it, [then she will expel it]. Likewise, with the tar, if a woman carries it in a woollen cloth, she will deliver the foetus.	Abdomen of a black cat: if it is fumigated under a pregnant woman, then she will expel the dead foetus. After this, take three carats of wild colocynth and mix the gall of a bull with it, moisten a woollen cloth with it and give it to the woman to carry.	If the abdomen of a black cat is taken, boiled on the fire and a pregnant woman, who is believed to have a dead foetus in her womb, sits on it, then she will abort and expel the foetus. Likewise, if she carries some tar, she will instantly expel it.
30.3	If you want to see the jinns and know the ways of magic, take the gall of a black cat and of a black hen, mix everything with antimony and apply a bit of this on your eyes, then you will see the jinns, and they will tell you everything you want to know.	If someone wants to see the jinns, he should take the gall of a black cat and of a black hen, ground everything with antimony and smear it on his eyes, then he will see the jinns and they will tell him everything he wants to know.	Gall of black cat and gall of black hen: if one part of each one is taken in the same quantity, mixed together with antimony and applied on the eyes of a man, then he will see the jinns.
30.4	Cat excrement: if it is mixed with myrtle oil—and this can be found in a hospital—rubbed on the man affected by fever with shivers, then this will cease, with the permission of God, may He be exalted.	Cat excrement: if it is mixed with myrtle oil and rubbed on a man while he is feverish, then this will be useful to him.	Cat excrement: if it is liquefied with myrtle oil and rubbed on a feverish man, then the fever will instantly cease.
30.5	Cat meat: if it is taken, minced, cooked, and applied with a bandage on the gout, then this will cease, with the permission of God, may He be exalted.	Its meat: if it is cooked, minced and used to bandage the gout, then this will be useful against it.	*om.*

30.6	*om.*	وان دهن انف سنور بدهن ورد مات	*om.*
30.7	*om.*	وان طلى رأسه بماء السذاب جنّ	اذا اردت ان يحسن القط فاطل رأسه بماء السذاب وشحمة السنبل الطيب
30.8	*om.*	مرارة السنور الاسود اذا أخذ منها نصف درهم واذيف بريق وسعّط به صاحب اللقوة نفعه	مرارة القط الرطبة اذا اذيبت ببورق وسعط بها صاحب القوة ابرأه
30.9	*om.*	اذا اردت ان يحبك انسان حبا شديدا فخذ سنور شديد النمرة فشق اذنه وخذ من دمها خمس قطرات واجعله في سويق او نبيذ او طعام او حلو واطعمه لمن تريد فانه يجن من حبّك ثم احبس السنور عندك واحسن اليه فانه ان هرب السنور او مات مات الذي اطعمته	اذا اردت ان يذهب بعقل الرجل والمرأة من المحبة خذ من دم اذن القط ثلاث قراط واجعلها في الطعام او نبيذ او سويق او حلو واطعمها ذلك للرجل تريد محبته فانه ابلغ في المحبة احبس السنور عندك واحسن اليه فان مات السنور مات الشخص
30.10	*om.*	واذا اردت حله فاطعمه لحم قنفذ مطبوخا او مشويا فاذا ذهب عنه فحلّ عن السنور	وان اردت ان تخلص الشخص مما حملت به افراط المحبة فاطعمه لحم قنفد مطبوح فانه يتخلص واطلق السنور الى حال سبيله
30.11	اذا اردت ان تطرد الشياطين فخذ خصى سنور اسود شقّها وملحها بملح وكندر ومر وبخر بها البيت والدار فلا يقرب الشيطان ولا جان ولا شيء من الهوام	خصية السنور الاسود اذا دقت وملحت بملح وكندر ومُر وتبخّر بها طردت الرياح الردية من الشياطين وغيرهم	اذا ان اردت ان تطرد الشياطين من البيت خذ خصية سنور اسود ودق مع ملح وبخر بها الموضع فان الشياطين يهرب من ذلك والارواح الردية

30.7: (c) السذاب] بماء الفيحول وهو السذاب C

30.8: (c) القط] القط اي السنور *add.* C | الرطبة] اذا أخذتها طرية C | اذا اذيبت] واذبتها C | ببورق] ببورق مسحوق *add.* C | بها] به C

30.9: (c) اذا اردت ان يذهب بعقل الرجل والمرأة من المحبه] *om.* C | خذ من دم اذن القط] اذا أخذ منه دم اذن القط C | وسويق واحلو] شيء حلو C | في] [واحسن] اذا حبست ذلك السنور C | احبس السنور] لاحد على ان يحبك ان اكلها افرط في محبتك ولا يستطيع عندك صبرا C | او اطعمها ذلك...المحبة] واحسنه اليه كان ابلغ *add.* C | فان] واذا C | الشخص] الشخص المحبة *add.* C

30.10: (c) وان اردت ان تخلص الشخص مما حملت به افراط المحبة] *om.* C | فاطعمه] واذا اطعمته شيئا من C | واطلق] فانه يتخلص واطلق] تخلص مما عملته C

30.11: (c) اذا ان اردت ان تطرد الشياطين من البيت] *om.* C | اذا دقت] خذ...ودق C | خصوة السنور الاسود] مع ملح C | بملح والمرا البطارخ *add.* C | من ذلك] وكذلك تهرب الارواح الردية C | والارواح الردية] من ذلك الموضع *add.* C

30.6	*om.*	If the nose of the cat is anointed with rose oil, then it will die.	*om.*
30.7	*om.*	And if its head is rubbed with rue water, it will become insane.	If you want to make a cat nicer, rub its head with rue water and nardus grease.
30.8	*om.*	Black cat gall: if half dirham of it is taken, mixed with saliva and a man affected by facial paralysis inhales it, then this will be useful to him.	Fresh cat gall: if it is liquefied with natron and inhaled by the man affected by facial paralysis, then this will cure him.
30.9	*om.*	If you want that a man loves you passionately, take a cat that is as strong as a cheetah, split its ear and take five carats of its blood and put it in some *sawīq* [mush made of wheat or barley, also with sugar and dates], or wine, or food or into something sweet, feed it to anyone you want, then he will go out of its mind for his love for you. Then keep the cat with you and take care of it, because, if the cat flees or dies, the man who has eaten it will die too.	If you want that either a man or a woman goes crazy for love, take three carats of the blood from its ear, put it in the food, or in the wine, or in the *sawīq* [mush made of wheat or barley, also with sugar and dates] or in something sweet, and feed it to the man whose love you want, then he will love you with great intensity. Then keep the cat with you and take care of it: if the cat dies, the person will die too.
30.10	*om.*	And when you want to set him free, feed him the meat of a hedgehog—stewed or roasted—and once [the love] has left him, release the cat too.	And if you want to free the person from the excess of love you have imposed on him, feed him with stewed hedgehog meat, and he will be set free; then let the cat go its way.
30.11	If you want to chase the devils away, take the testicles of a black cat, season them with salt, incense and myrrh, fumigate the house with this, then neither a devil, nor a jinn or any other pest will approach it.	Black cat testicle: if it is minced and seasoned with salt, incense and myrrh and fumigated, then the evil winds derived from devils and other creatures will be chased away.	If you want to chase the devils away from the house, take the testicle of a black cat, ground it with salt and fumigate the place with it, then the devils and the evil spirits will flee from it.

30.12	اذا اسقيت الساحر او الساحرة وسخ اذن سنور وهو لا يدري شيء كل سحر يعرفه	اذن السنور الاسود اذا سقيت منها الساحرة وهي لا تعلم نسيت السحر	*om.*
30.13	اذا عقلت على دراعك الايسر قلب سنور اسود في قطنة فانك تكفي شر كل انسان سيء ولم تخشش او لا شيئا ما دام معلقا عليك	قلبه ايضا اذا علق على انسان في قطن على ذراعه الايسر لم يخش بوسا ولا ضررا	اذا علقت قلب سنور اسود في قطنة على ذراعك الايسر لم تخف من شيء ابدا
30.14	دماغ السنور اذا اذيب بماء الريحان وقطره عليه دهن زنبق وشرب منه صاحب وجع الكبد ابرأه	دماغ السنور اذا اذيف بماء الريحان وقطر عليه قليل زنبق وسحق وشرب نفع لوجع الكبد والبهر	*om.*
30.15	قلب السنور الاسود اذا جعل في قطعة من جلد الذئب المدبوغ وعلق على عضد الانسان كان مخفيا عن الناس	اذا اردت ان لا يراك احد او رسولك فخذ قلب سنور اسود واجعله في قطعة من جلد دُب مدبوغ وعلّقه على العضد الايسر فلا يراك احد	اذا اردت ان لا يراك احد فخذ قلب سنور اسود جميعه فاجعله في جلد ذئب فاحرزه وعلّقه في عصدك الايسر فلا يراك احد وهو من علم السماء
30.16	اذا شربت الدابة واردت ان تردها على صاحبها بعيب خذ مخلاة واجعل فيها السنور وعلقها على الدابة فانه ينهشها فتفزع من ذلك المخلاة فردها بذلك العيب	واذا اردت ان تردّ الدابة على صاحبها بغير علة بها توجب الرد فخذ سنور واجعله في مخلاة وعلّقه على الدابة حتى ينهشه وينفزع فيصير اذا راى المخلاة هرب منها من فزعه فيصير عيبا تردّ به	اذا اردت ان تردّ الدابة على صاحبها من غير غيب فخذ سنورا اسودا فاجعله في مخلاة وعلقها علي رأس الفرس فانه ينهشها فنفر من المخلاة ولا تعود تقابلها ابدا فترمها على صاحبها والسلم
30.17	اذا شققت جوف السنور بالحياة وأخذت مرارته وشحم الدجاجة بيضاء كلها واذيب الشحم بالمرارة واكتحل به انسان	اذا اردت ان ترى ما يخفي عن الناس فخذ مرارة سنور ذكر وشحم دجاجة بيضاء ليس فيها سواد ودقها جميعا	يشق بطن السنور وهو بالحياة وتأخذ مرارته وشحم دجاجة بيضاء كلها فيذاف الشحم والمرارة ويكتحل بها فانك ترى ما يخفي من الناس فاذا

30.12: (c) *om.* C
30.13: (c) اذا عقلت...في قطنة] قلب السنورالاسود اذا جعل في قطنة وعلق على ذراعك الايسر C | تكفي] تكتفي C | ولم تخشش] ولا تخش C
30.14: (c) وقطره] وقطر C | صاحب] من اصابه C
30.15: (c) *om.* C
30.16: (c) *om.* C
30.17: (c) يخفي] خفى C

30.12	*om.*	Black cat ear: if it is given to drink to a sorceress—and she is not aware of it—this will make her forget magic.	If you give the dirt from a cat ear either to a sorcerer or to a sorceress to drink, then he or she will not remember anything of the magic he used to know.
30.13	If you hang the heart of a black cat in a piece of cotton on your left forearm, then you will not be afraid of anything anymore.	Its heart too: if it is hung on a man in a piece of cotton on his left forearm, then he will not be afraid of suffering, or of any harm.	If you hang on your left forearm the heart of a black cat inside a piece of cotton, then you will be protected from the malice of every evil man, and you will not be harmed as long as it remains on your body.
30.14	*om.*	Cat brain: if it is mixed with basil water, with some drops of lily, ground and drunk, it will be useful against liver complaint and breathlessness.	Cat brain: if it is liquefied with basil water, with the addition of some drops of lily oil, drunk by the man suffering from liver complaint, then this will cure him.
30.15	If you do not want to be seen by anybody, take the whole heart of a black cat, put it in a wolf's skin, pierce it and hang it on your left arm, then no one will see you, and this pertains to the 'science of heaven'.	If you want that no one can see you or your messenger, take the heart of a black cat, place it in a piece of tanned wolf skin and hang it on the left arm, then no one will be able to see you.	Black cat heart: if it is put in a tanned wolf skin and hung on the arm of a man, then he will be invisible to the other people.
30.16	If you want that an animal comes back to its master without hiding itself, take a black cat, put it inside a nosebag and hang it on the horse's head, then the cat will bite the horse, it will stampede away from the nosebag and will never approach it again, so it will go back to its master and to its safe place.	If you want that an animal comes back to its master safe and sound, and that it finds its way back, take a cat and put it inside a nosebag, hang it on the animal until the cat bites it and flounders inside the bag; then when the beast sees the nosebag, it will flee from it and its floundering, will be scared and it will come back.	When an animal has drunk, and you want that it comes back with shame to its master, take a nosebag and put a cat inside it, hang the bag on the animal, the cat will bite it and will flounder inside the bag, and this will make the animal return.
30.17	If the abdomen of a cat is ripped open while it is still alive, its gall and the fat of a completely white hen are taken, the fat and the gall are mixed and rubbed on the eyes, then you will see what is hidden to	If you want to see what is hidden from people, take the gall of a male cat and the fat of a white hen—without any black spot on her—mince everything and rub it on	If you split open the abdomen of a cat while it is alive, take its gall and the fat of a completely white hen, liquefy the fat with the gall and rub it on the eye of a man, then he will

فانه يرى ما يخفي على الناس اذا اردت ذهاب ذلك فاغسل عينيك بخمر عتيق	واكتحل بهما ترى ذلك واذا اردت ذهابة عنك فاغسل عينيك بخمر	اردتَ ان يزول عنك ذلك فاغسل عينيك بخمر عتيق وهو من علم السيميا	
مرارة سنور الاسود واخلط معها كمون كرماني وملح وطليت به الجراحات فانها تبرأ ونفع ايضا لمن في رأسه القرع	مرارة السنور الاسود اذا خلط معها ملح وكمون كرماني وطلى به على الجراحات والقرع برئ	يؤخذ مرارة سنور اسود واخلط معها ملح وكمون كرماني واخلط الجميع خلطا جيدا واطلِ به القرع في الرأس فتزول واطل به الجراحات تبرأ باذن الله	30.18
زبل السنور البري اذا سحق وعجن بالماء وطلى به صاحب النقرس رجليه فانه يبرأ	زبل السنور البري اذا سحق واذيف بالماء وطلى به النقرس نفعه	يؤخذ زبل سنور بري فيعجن بالماء واطلِ رجلي صاحب النقرس فيبرأ باذن الله تعالى والله اعلم	30.19

30.18: (c) واخلط] اذا خلط C | وطليت] وطرحت C | في رأسه القرع] برأسه السبخ والقرع الفاحش C
30.19: (c) فانه] *om.* C | يبرأ] اباه C

	people; and when you want to make this cease, wash your eyes with old wine, and this is part of the 'natural magic'.	the eyes, then you will see that; and when you want to make this cease, then wash your eyes with wine.	see what is hidden to people.; and when you want to make this cease, wash your eyes with old wine.
30.18	Black cat gall: if it is taken and mixed with salt and cumin, everything mixed up and rubbed on the ringworm on the head, then it will cease. Rub it also on the wounds and they will heal, with the permission of God, may He be exalted.	Black cat gall: if it is mixed with salt and cumin and rubbed on the wounds, then this will heal them.	Black cat gall: if it is mixed with cumin and salt, and rubbed on the wounds, then these will heal; and it is also useful to the man affected by the ringworm on the head.
30.19	Wild cat excrement: if it is taken and kneaded with water, rubbed on the feet of the man afflicted by gout, then he will recover, with the permission of God, may He be exalted, and God knows best.	Wild cat excrement: if it is ground, mixed with water and rubbed on the gout, this will be useful against it.	Wild cat excrement: if it is ground, kneaded with water and used to rub the man affected by gout, then this will cure him.

٣١. الفهد

c	b	a	
باب منافع الفهد	الفهد	ذكر منافع اعضاء الفهد	
مـرارة الفهـد اذا خلـطت بـعسل وملـح وجعلت على الجرح انقطع دمه ولا يعود يفتح	مرارتـه اذا اذيـف بـعسل وملـح وصـيّرت على جرح انقطع دمه ولم يفتّح	مرارة الفهد يخلط معها عسل القصب وملح ويجعل على الجراحات التي يسيل منها فينقطع الدم ولا يفتح ابدا	31.1
دم الفهد اذا اذيف بخل العنصل وطلى به صاحب النقرس رجليه سكن المـها سريعا ان شاء الله تعالى	دمـه اذا اذيـف بشـيء مـن خل عـنصل وطلى به النقرس نفعه	دم ابخل العنصل ويطلي به القدمي مـن صاحب النقرس فيسكن المـه باذن اللـه تعالى والله اعلم	31.2

31.1: (a) القصب] قصب B | ولا يفتح] ولا يسيل B
(c) ولا يعود يفتح] ولم يفتّح C
31.2: (a) يداف] يذاب B | القدمي] قدمي S | فيسكن المه] *om.* B
(c) اذيف] اذيب C | صاحب] من اصابه C | المها سريعا] الالم وازاله C

31. Lynx

	a	b	c
	Exposition of the useful properties of the parts of the lynx	**The lynx**	**Chapter on the useful properties of the lynx**
31.1	Lynx gall: if it is mixed with sugar cane, honey, and salt, applied on the bleeding wounds, then this will stop the bleeding, and the wounds will not open again.	Its gall: if it is mixed with honey and salt, and poured on a wound, then this will stop the bleeding, and will prevent the wound from opening again.	Lynx gall: if it is mixed with honey and salt, and applied on the wound, then this will stop the bleeding, and the wound will not open again.
31.2	Lynx blood: if it is mixed with red squill vinegar, rubbed on the feet of the man suffering from gout, then its pain will be relieved, with the permission of God, may He be exalted, and God knows best.	Its blood: if mixed with red squill vinegar and rubbed on the gout, then this will be useful against it.	Lynx blood: if it is mixed with red squill vinegar, and the man affected by gout rubs it on his feet, then the pain will quickly cease, God, may He be exalted, willing.

٣٢. الغرير

	a	b	c
	ذكر منافع اعضاء الغريري	*om.*	—
32.1	اذا اردت ان تطرد العقارب من الدار فبخرها بشعر الغريري فلا يبقي فيه شيء يؤذي باذن الله تعالى	شعر العزير اذا بخّر به البيت طرد منه كل عقرب وحية وجميع الذبيب	—
32.2	لحم الغريري اذا أكل مطبوخا نفع من علة الجذام	*om.*	—
32.3	*om.*	زبل الكاكسة اذا سحق واذيف بخل وطلى به موضع النملة نفعه	—
32.4	*om.*	وان عضّت انسانا وهي حبلي قتلته	—
32.5	*om.*	يقول ان هذه الدابة ابن عرس. ويقال ان غيرها	—

32.2: (a) نفع من] *om.* B

32. Badger

	a	b	c
	Exposition of the useful properties of the parts of the badger	*om.*	–
32.1	If you want to chase the scorpions away from the house, fumigate it with the hair of a badger, then nothing that can damage the house will remain there, with the permission of God, may He be exalted.	Badger hair: if the house is fumigated with it, then this will chase every scorpion, snake, and insect away from it.	–
32.2	Badger meat: if it is eaten cooked, it will be useful against elephantiasis.	*om.*	–
32.3	*om.*	*Kākasa* excrement: if it is mixed with vinegar and rubbed on the part affected by tingle, then this will be useful to it.	–
32.4	*om.*	If it bites someone while it is pregnant, then this will kill him.	–
32.5	*om.*	It is said that this beast is the weasel, but it is also said that it is something else.	–

٣٣. ابن عرس

	a	b	c
	ذكر منافع اعضاء ابن العرس	ابن عرس	باب منافع بنات عرس
33.1	يؤخذ شحم ابن العرس يدلك به باب البيت فلا يقربه العرس ابدا	ان أخذ ودلك به في باب بيت لم يدخله ابن عرس	شحم بنات عرس اذا ادهن به باب البيت لا يقربه عرس
33.2	زبل ابن العرس يبخر به صاحب النزف فينقطعه وان حملته فكان اجود	زبله اذا تبخّرت به المرأة انقطع عنها النزف	واذا بخر بزبله صاحب النزيف ابرأه
33.3	اذا اردت ان تقلع الضرس بلا حديد فخذ لحم ابن عرس جففه واجعله على الضرس الوجع فانه ينقلع بلا حديد	لحمه يؤخذ ويجفف ويسحق ويجعل منه على الضرس الوجع المأكول قلعه بغير شيء وهو الذي يعالجوا به الاضراس	ولحمه اذا جفف ودق ناعما وجعل على الضرس المسوس الوجع قلعه بلا اذى
33.4	يؤخذ زبل ابن عرس يداف بالنبيذ ويقطر على الجرح الذي يسيل منه الدم فانه ينقطع باذن الله تعالى	زبله اذا اذيف بماء وقطّر منه على جراحات الذي يسيل منها الدم حبس الدم من ساعته	زبل اذا اذيب ووضع على الجراحات التي يسيل منه الدم ابرأها
33.5	[جلد] بن العرس يدبغ ويكتب فيه حرز ويلقي على المصروع او الجنون فيبرأ	جلد ابن عرس الذكر اذا دبغ وكبت فيه وعلق على المجانين والمسحورين نفعهم	وجلد المذكر منه اذا دبغ وكتب فيه حرزا وعلق على المجنون افاق
33.6	*om.*	*om.*	دماغه اذا دلك به زجاج اجتمع البراغيت

33.1: (a) ابن العرس] العرس S | يدلك] واطلى B
(c) باب البيت] الباب البيت L | عرس] عرسة C
33.2: (a) ابن العرس] العرس S | يبخر] يتبخر B | فينقطعه] *om.* B
33.3: (a) اذا اردت ان تقلع الضرس بلا حديد فخذ] *om.* B | جففه واجعله] جففته وجعلته B | الوجع] *om.* B | فانه ينقلع] قلعه B
33.4: (a) منه الدم] دمه B | فانه ينقطع] فينقطع B
33.5: (a) This recipe is attested only in B

33. Weasel

	a	b	c
	Exposition of the useful properties of the parts of the weasel	**The weasel**	**Chapter on the useful properties of the weasel**
33.1	Weasel fat: if it is taken, and the door of the house is greased with it, then the weasels will never approach it.	If it is taken, and rubbed on the door of the house, then the weasels will not enter it.	Weasels fat: if it is rubbed on the door of the house, then the weasels will not approach it.
33.2	Weasel excrement: if the man suffering from loss of blood is fumigated with it, then this will cease; and if he carries it with him, it is even better.	Its excrement: if a woman is fumigated with it, then her bleeding will stop.	If the man suffering from loss of blood is fumigated with its excrement, then this will cure him.
33.3	If you want to extract a molar without using an iron instrument, take the meat of a weasel, dry it, apply it on the aching tooth, then it will be extracted without any iron instrument.	Its meat: if it is dried, minced, and applied on the eaten tooth that aches, then this will extract it without using anything else. This is the way in which the molars are cured.	Its meat: if it is dried, finely minced, and applied on the rotten tooth that aches, then this will extract the tooth without any pain.
33.4	Weasel excrement: if it is taken, mixed with wine and applied in drops on the bleeding wounds, then the bleeding will stop, with the permission of God, may He be exalted.	Its excrement: if it is applied in drops on the bleeding wounds, then this will instantly staunch the bleeding.	Excrement: if it is liquefied and applied on the bleeding wounds, then this will cure them.
33.5	Weasel skin: if it is tanned, an amulet is written on it, and applied on the epileptic or the insane man, then he will heal.	Male weasel skin: if it is tanned, inscribed, and hung on the insane men, or on those who have been bewitched, then this will be useful to them.	Skin of its male: if it is tanned, an amulet is written on it, and it is hung on the insane man, then he will recover.
33.6	*om.*	*om.*	Its brain: if it is rubbed on some glass, then the fleas will gather there.

33.7	*om.*	*om.*	زبله اذا اذيب بتراب وصرف ورد منه على الجرح الرطب جففه
33.8	*om.*	*om.*	خصيته اذا جعلت في جلد وعلقت على المرأة لم تحمل ما دامت عليها

33.7: (c) بتراب [بشراب C | ورد [وقطرت C
33.8: (c) دامت [ذلك معلقا C

33.7	*om.*	*om.*	Its excrement: if it is mixed with dust, prepared, and later applied on a moist wound, then this will dry up.
33.8	*om.*	*om.*	Its testicles: if they are placed in a skin and hung on a woman, then she will not get pregnant as long as these remain on her.

٣٤. ابن اوي والاروى

	a	b	c
	ذكر منافع اعضاء ابن اوي	—	باب منافع ابن اوي
34.1	*om.*	*om.*	قلبه اذا علق على العضداء من سائر السباع وعين الينمى اذا علقت منعت العين والنظرة
34.2	*om.*	*om.*	خصيته اذا شويت واكلها رجل وجامع امرأته حملت من وقتها
34.3	*om.*	*om.*	لسانه اذا اكل يمنع قطار البول
	—	الاروى	باب منافع الاروى
34.4	مرارة بن اوي يخلط معها كندر وزنجبيل ويسقي لصاحب الطحال في الحمام فيبرأ باذن الله تعالى	مرارته اذا خلط معها كندر وزنجبيل وشربت بماء حار في الحمام على الريق نفع من وجع الطحال	مرارته اذا خلط بالعسل وماء السذاب وسقى منها في الحمام صاحب وجع الكبد نفعه
34.5	دم ابن اوي يذاف بماء السذاب والعسل ويسقي لصاحب وجع الكبد فيبرأ باذن الله تعالى	دماغه اذا اذيف بعسل وماء السذاب وشرب منه صاحب وجع الكبد وزن مثقال على الريق وهو حار نفعه	*om.*

34:(c) باب منافع ابن اوي] باب منافع واوي اي ابن آوي C | الاروي] الازوي L; الازدي C
34.1: (c) قلبه] قلب ابن آوي C | وعين] عينه C | علقت] اذا علقت على انسان C
34.3: (c) اكل] اكله C | يمنع] منع من C
34.4: (a) مرارة...فيبرأ] يؤخذ مرارة بن اوي يخلط معها كندر وزنجبيل ويسقي لصاحب الطحال في الحمام فيبرأ B
(c) This recipe is attested only in C
34.5: (a) *om.* B
(c) مرارته] دمه C | وسقى منها] وشرب منه C | في الحمام] *om.* C | نفعه] ابرأه C

34. Jackal & Chamois

	a	b	c
	Exposition of the useful properties of the parts of the jackal	**–**	**Chapter of the useful properties of the jackal**
34.1	*om.*	*om.*	Its heart: if it is hung on the limbs of other wild animals—along with its right eye as well—then this will keep the evil eye away.
34.2	*om.*	*om.*	Its testicle: if it is roasted, a man eats it, and he has sexual intercourse with his woman, then she will immediately get pregnant.
34.3	*om.*	*om.*	Its tongue: if it is eaten, then this will stop the urine dripping.
	–	**The chamois**	**Chapter on the useful properties of the chamois**
34.4	Jackal gall: if it is melted with incense and ginger, given to the man suffering from spleen complaint to drink, then this will cure him, with the permission of God, may He be exalted.	Its gall: if it is melted with incense and ginger, and drunk with warm water in the bath on an empty stomach, this will be useful against spleen complaint.	Its gall: if it is melted with honey and rue water, given to the man suffering from liver complaint to drink in the bath, then this will be useful to him.
34.5	Jackal blood: if it is mixed with rue water and honey, given to the man suffering from liver complaint to drink, then this will cure him, with the permission of God, may He be exalted.	Its brain: if it is mixed with honey and rue water, and one *miṯqāl* of it is drunk warm on an empty stomach by a man suffering from liver complaint, then it will be useful to him.	*om.*

34.6	مخ ابن اوي يخلط معه ورس وبورق ويذاف الجميع بخل خمر ويطلي به البرص فانه يغير لونه ويبرأ باذن الله تعالى	مخه اذا خلط بورق وورس واذيف بخل وطلى به موضع البرص والحصف اذهبه	ومخه اذا خلط معه بورق وشق واذيب الجميع بخل ويطلي به البرص غير لونه ووقع عن صاحبه
34.7	*om.*	مصرانه اذا دلك به قدح او جلم وكبّة في بيت اجتمع البراغيث	*om.*

34.6: (a) ويذاف [ويذاب B | بخل خمر [بالخل الخمر B | ويبرأ [ويزول B
(c) ويطلي [وطلى C | ووقع [واوقعه وازاله C | صاحبه [صاحبه ونفع نفعا جيدا *add.* C

34.6	Jackal marrow: if it is mixed with curcuma and natron, everything is diluted with wine vinegar, and rubbed on the area affected by leprosy, then this will change its colour, and this will heal, with the permission of God, may He be exalted.	Its marrow: if it is melted with natron and curcuma, liquefied with vinegar and rubbed on the area affected by leprosy and dry scabies, then this will cure them.	Its marrow: if it is melted with natron, everything liquefied with vinegar, and rubbed on the area affected by leprosy, then this will change its colour and make it disappear.
34.7	*om.*	Its bowels: if they are rubbed on a drinking bowl, or also on some shears, or a hank of yarn that are in a house, then the fleas will gather there.	*om.*

٣٥. القرد

	a	b	c
	ذكر منافع اعضاء القرد	القرد	باب منافع القرد
35.1	يؤحذ قلب قرد يشوي ويجفف ويسحق ويسقي منه صاحب الرجيف والخفقان يذهب عنه ويكون بنبيذ عسلي عتيق وهو ايضا يقوي القلب وجيد لحدة النظر	قلبه اذا شوى وجفف وسحق وشرب منه وزن درهم بعسل عتيق ذهب بالخفقان وسقوط النفس ويشجّع الجبان ويزيد في الذهن	قلب القرد اذا شوى وجفف وسحق ناعما بنبيذ عسل نفع صاحب خفقان القلب والرجيف
35.2	اذا اردت ان يرى الرجل في منامه ما يهوله ويفزّعه فاجعل تحت رأسه شعر قرد وهو عجيب	اذا اردت ان يستوحش الرجل في منامه فاجعل تحت رأسه شعر قرد	اذا اردت ان يستوحش الرجل في منامه مما يهوله فاجعل فاجعل تحت رأسه شعر القرد فانه يرى في منامه ما يوحشه
35.3	دم القرد يلطخ على البهق والكلف فيبرأ باذن الله	*om.*	دم القرد اذا اذيف بدهن الزنبق وطلى به اماكن الشعر الذي على المعانة لا ينبت ابدا

35.1: (a) This recipe is attested only in B
(c) وجفف] *om.* C | بنبيذ] بنبيذ مرلب C | صاحب] من وجع C
35.2: (a) اذا اردت ان يرى الرجل] اذا أراد الرجل ان يرى B | يهوله ويفزّعه] ويعرجه B | وهو] فانه B
(c) *om.* C
35.3: (a) يلطخ] اذا طلى B | تذاف] تذاب B | فيبرأ] يذهب B
(c) In C other two recipes to prevent the growth of unwanted hair are added, one with monkey blood: وكذلك اذا لطخ بدهن الى ان يتقسح ودهن به المشاعر بعد التنظيف من الشعر منع من انبات جدا; the other with dried frogs, وكذا الضفدع المجفف اذا سحق بالخل وطلى به المشاعر لم ينبت بذلك الموضع شعرا ابدا باذن الله تعالى.

35. Monkey

	a	b	c
	Exposition of the useful properties of the parts of the monkey	**The monkey**	**Chapter on the useful properties of the monkey**
35.1	Monkey heart: if it is taken, roasted, dried, minced and fed to a man suffering from convulsions and palpitations, then these will go away; and if it is served with old honey wine, this will also strengthen the heart and sharpen the eyesight.	Its heart: if it is roasted, dried, one dirham of it is eaten with old honey, then this will cure palpitations and apnoea; and it will also embolden the coward and increase the intelligence	Monkey heart: if it is roasted, dried, finely minced with honey wine, this will be useful against heart palpitations and convulsions.
35.2	If you want that someone sees what scares him during his sleep—and also that he is struck by terror—then put the hair of a monkey under his head, and this is amazing.	If you want that a man is afraid during his sleep, then put the hair of a monkey under his head.	If you want that a man is frightened during his sleep by the things that usually scare him, then put under his head the hair of a monkey, and he will see in his sleep what scares him.
35.3	Monkey blood: if it is spattered on vitiligo and freckles, then they will heal, with the permission of God.	*om.*	Monkey blood: if it is mixed with lily oil, and rubbed on the hair around the eyes, then this will never grow again.

٣٦. الوبر

c	b	a	
—	الوبر	ذكر منافع اعضاء الوبر	
—	بوله اذا أخذ منه جزء وخلط معه فلفل واكتحل منه نفع من غشاوة في العين	يؤخذ بول الوبر فيخلط معه لحك اثمد ويكتحل به من في عينه غشاوة فتزول باذن الله تعالى	36.1
—	بوله اذا سعط منه بقدر عدسة بلبن جارية بدهن بنفسج نفع من الريح التي تكون في الرأس	ويسعط منه ايضا مقدار عدسة بلبن مرأة سوداء ودهن بنفسج وهو ايضا للبرود في الدماغ والله اعلم	36.2

36: (a) ذكر منافع اعضاء الوبر] *om.* B

36. Hyrax

	a	b	c
	Mention of the useful properties of the parts of the hyrax	**The hyrax**	–
36.1	Hyrax urine: if it is taken, then mixed with antimony glue, rubbed on the eye affected by cataract, then this will go away, with the permission of God, may He be exalted.	Its urine: if one part of it is taken, mixed with pepper, and rubbed on the eye, then this will be useful against the cataract.	–
36.2	And also, if it is inhaled in the quantity of a lentil, with the milk of a black woman and sweet violet oil, this will be useful against the coldness inside the brain, and God knows best.	Its urine: if it is inhaled in the quantity of a lentil with a maid's milk and sweet violet oil, this will be useful against the wind that is inside the head.	–

٣٧. القسطوريون

	a	b	c
	ذكر منافع اعضاء القسطريون	*om.*	—
	وهو الجرذ الكبير وهو الجندبادسير		
37.1	شحم هذا الحيوان يذاب مع الشمع ودهن زنبق ويدهن به مواضع القرع في الرأس فينبت الشعر وينفع ايضا لداء الثعلب	شحم القسطوريون ويعرف بالجارود وهو كلب الماء اذا اذيف مع شمع بزنبق ودهن به مواضع القرع في الرأس انبته	—
37.2	خصية هذا الدابة يسحق ويضرب بخمر عتيق ويسقي منها صاحب الخفقان والرجيف ووجع الكلى	خصيته اذا شرب منها نفع لكل برد يكون في الجسد وللخفقان ولضعف القلب بنبيذ او شراب	—
37.3	يسعّط ايضا من به لقوة فيبرأ باذن الله تعالى	ويسعّط منه للقوة وزن ثلاث حبات بماء اصول الرطوبة والشهدانج مع دهن الزنبق	—
37.4	*om.*	الجارود جندبادسير اذا جفف وسحق وشرب منه وزن دانقين بشراب ممزوج نفع من الكزاز والخفقان العارض من المرة السوداء	—
37.5	*om.*	ويسخّن الاعضاء الباردة وينفع من النسيان اذا سعط منه	—

37: (a) قسطوريون] القسطبون S; *om.* B | جندبادسير] الجنادسير S

37.1: (a) الشمع] شحم هذا B | ويدهن] وادهن B | وينفع ايضا لداء الثعلب] *om.* B

37.2: (a) *om.* B

37. Beaver

	a	b	c
	Exposition of the useful properties of the parts of the beaver that is the big rat, that is *al-ğundbāsīr.*	*om.*	–
37.1	Fat of this animal: if it is liquefied with wax and lily oil, rubbed on the parts of the head affected by ringworm, then the hair will grow again, and this is also useful against alopecia.	Fat of the beaver, also called *ğārūd*, that is the otter: if it is mixed with wax and lily, rubbed on the parts affected by ringworm, then this will make the hair grow again.	–
37.2	Testicle of this beast: if it is ground, whipped with old wine and given to drink to a man suffering from palpitations, convulsions and liver complaint [this will be useful to him].	Its testicles: if it is drunk, this will be useful against every coldness that can be found in the body; it is also useful against palpitations and heart weakness, with wine or another drink.	–
37.3	If it is inhaled by a man afflicted by facial paralysis, then he will heal, with the permission of God, may He be exalted.	If inhaled, it is useful against facial paralysis, three grains of it with fresh Indian hemp roots water and lily oil.	–
37.4	*om.*	Beaver: if it is dried, pounded, and two *dāniq* of it are drunk with mixed wine, then this will be useful against tetanus and the occasional palpitations due to the black gall.	–
37.5	*om.*	It will warm the cold organs and will be useful against forgetfulness, if it is inhaled	–

٣٨. القنفد

	a	b	c
	ذكر منافع اعضاء القنفد	القنفد	باب منافع القنفد
38.1	يؤخذ طحال القنفد يشوي ويطعم لصاحب وجع الطحال فيذهب فان اكل نصفه نفع نصفه وان اكل جميعه ابرأه جميعه وهو عجيب	طحاله اذا جفف في التنّور واخرج واطعم لمن به الطحال	طحال القنفد اذا شوى في التنور وأكل منه صاحب الكبد والطحال ان أكل كله نفع كله وانصفه نفع نصفه
38.2	يؤخذ قنفد فيحرق جميعه ويسحق ويحشي به الناسور فانه يبرأ باذن الله تعالى	[...]	اذا جفف القنفد وسحق ناعما وحشى به الناسور ابرأه
38.3	مرارة القنفد تذاف بالكافور القديم وتسعط به صاحب هذا الصداع فيذهب باذن الله تعالى	—	مرارة القنفد اذا خلطت بشيء من كافور القنصوري وتسعط به صاحب الصداع ابرأه
38.4	لحم القنفد وشحمه يخلط الجميع يطبخ بعسل ويلقي على سذاب يابس ومر من كل واحد جزء ويضربا حتي يستوي ويسقي منه صاحب البواسير والقولنج بماء الاقحوان فانه يبرأ باذن الله تعالى	—	لحم القنفد وشحمه اذا دق الجميع وخلط بعسل القى عليه شراب وملح الطعام وضرب بعضه ببعض وشرب منه صاحب القولنج والبواسير بماء الاقحوان على الريق ابرأه

38.1: (a) يشوي] *om.* B | فان...يشوي] *om.* B
(c) شوى] شويته C | في التنور] *om.* C | وانصفه] او نصفه C
38.2: (b) This chapter is attested only in G
(c) جفف] جففت C
38.3: (a) مرارة القنفد] *om.* B | تذاف] يذاب B | بالكافور] بماء كفور C | هذا] *om.* B
(c) كافور] الكافور C | القنصوري] *om.* C | In C another recipe is added, with hedgehog gall to expel the dead foetus from the womb: مرارة القنفد اذا عجن بها قليل من العنبر وتحملت بها المرأة في فتيلة القت الولد الميت من بطنها
38.4: (a) يخلط الجميع] *om.* B | ومر] *om.* B | من كل واحد] من واحد B | ويضربا حتى يستويا] *om.* B
(c) وشحمه] وشحمه وكبده *add.* C | ومن] *om.* C

38. Hedgehog

	a	b	c
	Exposition of the useful properties of the parts of the hedgehog	**The hedgehog**	**Chapter on the useful properties of the hedgehog**
38.1	Hedgehog spleen: if it is taken, roasted, and fed to a man suffering from spleen complaint, then this will disappear; and if he eats half of it, then this will be half-useful; if, instead, he eats the whole of it, then this will be fully useful.	Its spleen: if it is dried in a baking oven, and fed to a man suffering from bladder complaint, then this will cure him.	Hedgehog bladder: if it is roasted in a baking oven, and eaten by a man suffering from liver and bladder complaint, [it will be useful]. If he eats the whole of it, then this will be fully useful; if, instead, he splits it into two parts, then this will be half-useful.
38.2	If a hedgehog is taken, completely burnt, ground, and stuffed inside a fistula, then this will disappear, with the permission of God, may He be exalted.	[...]	If a hedgehog is dried, ground into a fine powder and stuffed inside the fistula, this will cure it.
38.3	Hedgehog gall: if it is mixed with old camphor, given to a man suffering from this headache to inhale, then it will go away, with the permission of God, may He be exalted.	—	Hedgehog gall: if it is mixed with a bit of *Qanṣūrī* camphor, inhaled by a man suffering from headache, then this will cure him.
38.4	Hedgehog meat and its fat: if they are mixed together, cooked with honey, with the addition of some dry rue and some myrrh—one part of each one—then whipped until they have a uniform consistence, given to the man suffering from haemorrhoids and colic to drink with camomile water, then he will recover, with the permission of God, may He be exalted.	—	Hedgehog meat and its fat: if they are mixed with honey, with the addition of wine and cooking salt, whipped, and drunk with camomile water by a man suffering from colic and haemorrhoids, then this will cure him.

38.5

اذا اردت ان تطرد البراغيت اذبح قنفد واسلخه واغله بزيت وماء حتى يذهب الماء ويبقي الزيت خذ ذلك الزيت وادهن به عودا والقي البيت يجتمع اليه البراغيث ولا يبقي منهم شيء اربح

—

يؤخذ قنفد يذبح ويسلخ جلده ويجعل في قدر ويجعل عليه غمرة ماء ويطبخ حتى يسيل دهنه ودسمه ويؤخذ ذلك الدهن ويدهن به عصاة وترمي في وسط البيت فيجتمعوا البراغيت عليها يفعل ذلك ثلاث او اربع كرات فلا يبقي في البيت برعوث

38.6

مرارة القنفد اذا اكتحل بها صاحب البياض في العين اذهبه

—

يؤخذ للبياض في العين مرارة القنفد يكتحل بها من في عينه بياض فيذهب

38.7

مرارة القنفد اذا اذيبت بدهن زنبق وشرب منها صاحب الزحير والجذام بلا دهن ابرأه

—

مرارة القنفد تذاب بلبن ويسقي لصاحب الجذام فيجفف عنه

38.8

اذا ذبح القنفد وشق جوفه وطبخ حتى يبلي جميعه ويصفي دهنه ويدهن به الظهر وياكل الباقي من به وجع الظهور والكلى والوركين يعافا

—

لوجع الظهر والركب يؤخذ قنفد فيذبح ويسلخ ويطبخ في قدر بالماءِ حتى يتهرا ويؤخذ دهنه فيدهن الظهر والركب فيذهب الالم باذن الله

38.9

كلى القنفد اذا جفـفت وشربها من به عسر البول وزن درهم بماء الحمص الاسود المغلى المصفى نفعه جيدا

—

لعسر البول يؤخذ كلى القنفد يجفف ويسحق ويسقي لصاحب عسر البول فيبرأ باذن الله وان شربها بماء الحمص الاسود كان انفع وابلغ

38.5: (a) يذبح] فيذبح B | جلده] *om.* B | قدر] قدرة B | ويجعل عليه غمره ما] *om.* B | ويؤخذ ذلك الدهن] *om.* B | وسط] *om.* B | فيجتمعوا...برعوث] فان البراغيت يجتمعون عليها B
(c) اذا...البراغيت] اذا اردت ذلك طرد البراغيث C | اذبح] ذبح C | حتى] الى ان C | والقي البيت] والقه في البيت C | In C other two recipes to chase fleas away are added: وكذلك اذا أخذت جوزة شقفتها نصفين ونزعت ما فيها وملأت فيها ورق دفلا ودفنت في البيت فلا يقربه برغوث ابدا; وكذلك قتأ الحمار اذا سلقتها الى ان يهري واخذت من ماية ورشيته في البيت مات كل برغوث في البيت
38.6: (a) يؤخذ للبياض في العين] *om.* B | من...فيذهب] تذهب البياض من العين B
(c) صاحب البياض في العين] من بعينيه بياض C
38.7: (a) فيجفف] فيقف B
(c) مرارة القنفد] *om.* C | صاحب] من اصابه مرض C | بلا دهن] وادهن منه C
38.8: (a) *om.* B
38.9: (a) العسر البول] *om.* B | فيبرأ] يزول عنه B | كان انفع وابلغ] كان اجود B
(c) كلى...وشربها] اذا شق جوف القنفد وجفف وسحق وشرب منها C

38.5 If a hedgehog is taken, slaughtered and flayed, put it in a cooking pot, with the addition of some Indian yellow water, cooked until its fat and grease become liquid; then this fat is taken and used to grease a stick, this is thrown in the middle of the house, then the fleas will gather on it: repeat this three or four times, and not a single flea will remain in the house.

—

If you want to chase fleas away, slaughter a hedgehog, flay it, boil it with oil and water until the water has gone while the oil remains, take this oil and rub it on a branch, throw it in the house, then the fleas will gather on it and none of them will remain.

38.6 Against the glaucoma of the eyes: take the gall of a hedgehog, rub it on the glaucoma, and then this will disappear.

—

Hedgehog gall: if it is rubbed on the eyes of a man affected by glaucoma, this will make it disappear.

38.7 Hedgehog gall: if it is mixed with milk, and given to a man affected by elephantiasis to drink, then this will dry up.

—

Hedgehog gall: if it is mixed with lily oil, and drunk by a man affected by dysentery and elephantiasis—without oil—then this will cure him.

38.8 Against the pain of the back and the knees: if a hedgehog is taken, slaughtered and flayed, cooked in a cooking pot until it is well done, its grease is taken and rubbed on the back and on the knees, then the pain will cease, with the permission of God, may He be exalted.

—

If a hedgehog is slaughtered, its abdomen split and cooked until it melts, then the grease is purified and rubbed on the back of a man suffering from back pain; then the one afflicted by legs, kidneys and knees pain should eat the rest and he will recover.

38.9 Against urine retention: if the kidneys of a hedgehog are taken, dried, ground and given to a man suffering from urine retention to drink, then he will heal, with the permission of God, may He be exalted; and if it is drunk with black chick-peas water, this will be even more useful and effective.

—

Hedgehog kidney: if it is dried and drunk in the quantity of one dirham with boiled and purified black chick-peas water, then it will be very useful for this.

عين القنفد اليسرى اذا غليت بزيت وجعلت في قارورة و[اذا] اردت ان تنوم انسانا اجعل في اذنه زنة ربع درهم فلا يستفيق حتى توقضه	—	للنوم يؤخذ عين القنفد اليسرى فتغلي بالزيت وتصير في اناء فاذا اردت ان تنوّم انسانا فخذ منه شيئا يسير وصبه في اذن النائم فلا يزال نائما حتى يذهبه أنت ولو تركبه شهرا النام	38.10
اظفار القنفد من اليد اليمنى اذا بخر بها المحموم اذهبت الحمى عنه	—	اظفار القنفد يبخر بها المحموم فيبرأ باذن الله تعالى	38.11
مرارة القنفد اذا عجنت بعنبر وجعلت فتيلة وحملتها المرأة القت الجنين الميت من جوفها	—	لخروج الجنين من الجوف يؤخذ مرارة القنفد فيعجن بشيء من عنبر حام وتعمل فتيلة وتحملها المرأة فتلقي الجنين الميت باذن الله تعالى	38.12
عين القنفد اليمنى اذا غليت بدهن وخل وتصير في اناء نحاس احمر واكتحل به من اراد ينظر في [الليل كما ينظر في] النهار فانه يفعل ذلك وهو عجيب	—	عين القنفد اليمنى تغلي بدهن ورد وخل خمر ويصيّر في اناء نحاس ويكتحل بها انسان فانه يرى بالليل مثل ما يرى بالنهار	38.13
خرقة لحم القنفد اذا خلطت بالعسل وتغرز به من في حلقه مخه نفعه ونفعت الصوت من الخشونة	—	لخرجة الصوت دم القنفد يخلط بعسل يتعر عسر به فيصفي الصوت ويحسّنه	38.14

38.10: (a) للنوم يؤخذ] *om.* B | اليسرى] اليسار B | في اذن النائم] في اذن انسان وهو نائم B
(c) اجعل] فاجعل C | حتى توقضه] الى ان قظه C
38.11: (c) بخر] بخرت C | المحموم] من اصابه الحمى C
36.12: (a) بشيء] مع شيء B | وتعمل] ويعمل B
(c) بعنبر] بالعنبر C | وجعلت فتيلة] وعملت في الفتيلة C
38.13: (a) مثل ما] كما B
(c) وتصير] وتركت C | احمر] *om.* C | فانه...عجيب] راى من ذلك امرا عجيب C

38.10	For the sleep: if the left eye of a hedgehog is taken, boiled with oil and poured into a vessel; then when you want to make a man sleep, take some of it and pour it inside the ear of a sleeping man, then he will not stop sleeping until you remove it; but if you left it there, he would keep sleeping.	—	If the left eye of a hedgehog is boiled with oil and put in a long-necked flask; then when you want that a man falls asleep, pour a quarter dirham of this inside his ear, and then he will not wake up until you decide for it.
38.11	Hedgehog nails: if they are taken and used to fumigate a feverish man, then he will heal, with the permission of God, may He be exalted.	—	Nails taken from the right forepaw of a hedgehog: if a feverish man is fumigated with them, then the fever will leave him.
38.12	To make the foetus come out of the womb: if hedgehog gall is taken, kneaded with some warm ambergris, a tampon is made out of it, and it is given to a woman to carry, then she will expel the dead foetus, with the permission of God, may He be exalted.	—	Hedgehog gall: if it is kneaded with ambergris, made into a tampon that a woman has to carry, then she will expel the dead foetus from her womb.
38.13	Hedgehog right eye: if it is boiled with rose oil and wine vinegar, poured into a copper vessel and rubbed on the eye of a man, then he will be able to see during the night as he can see during the day.	—	Hedgehog right eye: if it is boiled with oil and vinegar, poured in a vessel of red copper, then who wants to see during the night as he does during the day should rub it on the eyes, this will produce such an effect, and this is amazing.
38.14	For the emission of the voice, hedgehog blood; if it is mixed with honey, this will solve the difficulties with it, will clean the voice and make it nicer.	—	Shred of hedgehog meat: if it is mixed with honey, and is inserted inside a man who has his marrow in the back of the throat, this will be very useful to him; and it is also useful against the roughness of the voice.

38.15 دم القنفذ اذا أخذ من غير ذبح وخلط وعلق على من به عسر البول ابرأه

—

لعسر البول يؤخذ قنفذ فيذبح ويسلخ جلده ويخلع عظمه ويعلق على من عسر عليه بوله او الدابة اذا كان بها المغل فيدرّ البول باذن الله تعالى وان علق عليه عظامه كان ابلغ والله اعلم

38.16 واذا علق على الدابة المغولة ابرأه

—

om.

38.15: (a) العسر البول] *om.* B | من عسر عليه بوله] انسان عسر البول B | والدابة] او الدابة B | وان علق] وان كانت B
(c) وخلط وعلق] وخلط بدهن واستعمله دهنا C
38.16: (c) ابرأه] ازال عنها المغل وابرأها من ذلك C

38.15	Against urine retention: if a hedgehog is taken, slaughtered, flayed, one of its bones is taken out and hung on a man suffering from urine retention—or on an animal—then the urine will flow easily, with the permission of God, may He be exalted; and if more of its bones are hung on the man, then this will be even more effective, and God knows best.	—	Hedgehog blood: if it is taken without slaughtering it, melted and hung on a man suffering from urine retention, then this will cure him.
38.16	*om.*	—	And if it is hung on a beast suffering from an intestinal ailment, then this will cure it.

٣٩. القنفد الهندي

	a	b	c
	ذكر منافع اعضاء القنفد الهندي	—	باب منافع القنفد الهندي
	وهو يسمى باليناتية اسطرقس وزعموا اهل الهند انه يكون مثل الذئب		القنفد الهندي زعموا انه يشبه النمس
39.1	يؤخذ هذا الحيوان ويذبح ويؤخذ دمه فيطلي به عضة الكلب الكلب فتبرأ باذن الله تعالى	—	اذا أخذ هذا الحيوان وطليت به عضة الكلب الكلب بزيت [ابرأه]
39.2	يؤخذ كبد هذا الحيوان ايضا تشوي وتطعم لصاحب وجع الكبد فيبرأ باذن الله	—	واذا أخذ كبده وشوى وأكله صاحب وجع الكبد ابرأه
39.3	يؤخذ خصية هذا الحيوان تجفف وتسحق ويسحق حب بلسان ويخلط الجميع ويسقي منه المرأة وزن ربع مثقال فمنع عن الولد باذن الله وان شربتها بنبيذ كان ابلغ	—	خصية هذا الحيوان اذا جففت وسحقت واذيبت بدهن بلسان وشرب منها المرأة منعها من الحبل وان شربت بعسل كان ابلغ
39.4	*om.*	—	واذا أخذت خصيته اليمنى وجففت وسحقت وشرب منها وزن درهم مع عسل منزوع الرغوة فانه يزيد في الباه ويقوي الجماع

39. Indian Hedgehog

	a	b	c
	Exposition of the useful properties of the parts of the Indian hedgehog	–	**Chapter on the useful properties of the Indian hedgehog**
	In Greek it is called *isṭriqs*, the people from India maintain that it resembles the wolf.		It is maintained that the Indian hedgehog resembles the ichneumon.
39.1	If this animal is taken, slaughtered, its blood is taken and rubbed on the bite of a rabid dog, then this will heal, with the permission of God, may He be exalted.	–	When this animal is taken, and rubbed on the bite of the rabid dog, then this will cure this.
39.2	Again, liver of this animal: if it is taken, roasted, and fed to a man suffering from liver complaint, then this will heal, with the permission of God, may He be exalted.	–	Its liver: if it is taken, and a man suffering from liver complaint eats it, then this will cure him.
39.3	Testicle of this animal: if it is taken, dried, ground with a grain of balsam of Mecca, everything mixed together and a quarter *miṯqāl* of it is given to a woman to drink, then this will prevent her from getting pregnant, with the permission of God. And if she drinks it with wine, it will be even more effective.	–	Testicle of this animal: if it is died, ground, mixed with balsam of Mecca oil and a woman drinks it, then this will prevent her from getting pregnant. And if it is drunk with honey, it will be even more effective.
39.4	*om.*	–	If its right testicle is taken, dried, pounded, one dirham of it is drunk with honey without foam, then this will increase the sexual power and give power to the coitus.

٤٠. الكاشة

	a	b	c
	ذكر اعضاء الكاشة	—	—
	زعموا اقوام انها ابن عرس وزعم قوم انها وحش اخر		
40.1	زبل هذا الحيوان يسحق ويذاب بخل خمر ويطلي النملة التي يكون في الساق فيبرأ باذن الله	—	—
40.2	لحم هذا الحيوان اذا أكل مطبوخا فانه ينفع من داء الجنون والله اعلم	—	—

40. *Kāša*

	a	b	c
	Mention of the useful properties of the parts of the *kāša*	–	–
	Some people maintain that this is the weasel, while some other people maintain that this is another beast.		
40.1	Excrement of this animal: if it is mixed with wine vinegar and rubbed on the tingle which affects the leg, then this will heal, with the permission of God, may He be exalted.	–	–
40.2	Meat of this animal: if it is eaten cooked, then this will be useful for the insane man, and God knows best.	–	–

٤١. السمندل

	a	b	c
	ذكر منافع اعضاء السمندل	—	باب منافع السمندل
41.1	وهي دابة لا تخاف من النار وتلد بالنار كما يلذ ابن ادم بالماء ويتخذ من هذا الدابة الثياب والمناشف وتهدي للملوك وكل اتسخ غسله بالنار	—	وهي دابة لا تخاف من النار وتلذّ بها كما تلذ جميع الحيوانات بالهواء ويتخذ من جلده الثياب واذا توسخت غسلت بالنار
41.2	مرارة هذه الدابة يسقي للمحموم والمسموم فلا يعمل فيه السم ولو شرب من السم ما عسى ان شرب وان شربها بها بماء الحمص المغلى جيد وان لم يكون والا بلبن حليب	—	مرارة هذه الدابه اذا سقيت لمن شرب السم فيه [فلا يعمل] شيئا وقيل انها تذاف بماء الحمص بلبن الضان سداد حمصة
41.3	لذاء في العين [الماء] وضعف البصر يؤخذ دماغ هذه الدابة يخلط مع الاثمد ويكتحل به من في عينه الماء فيذهن باذن الله تعالى	—	دماغ هذه الدابة اذا خلطت مع الاثمد واكتحل به من بعينيه ماء وجفف بصره ابرأه
41.4	يؤخذ دم هذه الدابة فيطلي به الوضح وهو سحن فيغير لونه ويمنعه ان يزيد باذن الله تعالى	—	اذا أخذ دم هذه الدابة وهو حار وطلى به الوضح ابرأه وغير لونه

41.1: (a) بالنار] بها B | بالماء] *om.* B | وكل] فكلما B
41.2: (a) للمحموم والمسموم] للسموم B
41.3: (a) لذا في العين وضعف البصر] *om.* B | من في عينه الماء فيذهن] العين يذهن البياض من العين B
41.4: (a) فيطلي] اذا طلى B

41. Salamander

	a	b	c
	Exposition of the useful properties of the parts of the salamander	–	**Chapter on the useful properties of the salamander**
41.1	This beast is not afraid of fire, on the contrary, it is delighted by it in the way in which all the other living beings are delighted by fresh water; its skin is used to make cloths and towels, and it is offered as present to the kings; it can be cleaned with fire from everything that has soiled it.	–	This is a beast that is not afraid of fire, on the contrary it is delighted by it in the same way in which all the other living beings are delighted by air; its skin is used to make cloths and, when these get dirty, they should be cleaned with fire.
41.2	Gall of this wild animal: if it is given to a feverish man and to a poisoned man to drink, then the poison will have no effect, whatever poison he has drunk. It is also good if you drink it with boiled chick-peas water. If this is not available, it can be substituted with cow milk.	–	Gall of this beast: if it is given to a man who has drunk poison, then this will have no effect. It is said that is should be mixed with chick-peas water and sheep milk.
41.3	For a man who has water in his eye and a weak eyesight: if the brain of this beast is taken, mixed with antimony and rubbed on the eye with water in it, then this will heal, with the permission of God, may He be exalted.	–	Brain of this wild animal: if it is mixed with antimony, and rubbed on the eye with water, then this will dry it and cure the eyesight.
41.4	Blood of this animal: if it is taken, and rubbed on the leprosy while it is still warm, then this will change its colour and will prevent it from expanding.	–	If the blood of this animal is taken while it is still warm, and rubbed on the leprosy, then this will cure it and change its colour.

٤٢. كركدن

	a	b	c
	ذكر منافع اعضاء كركدن	—	باب منافع كركدن
42.1	هي دابة تطلع من البحر وهي بالسريانية ويما ولها بين عينيها قرن وهي تحمل به على الفيل فلا تجزع منه	—	وهي دابه تخرج من البحر تسمى بالسريانية ربما لهذه الدابة قرن بين عينيها يقال انها تحمل الفيل ولا تفزع منه وقتله وهذه الدابة دون المرائم
42.2	ويتخذون من قرن هذه نصب للسكاكين وهي يكون في بلاد النوبة والحبشة	—	*om.*
42.3	يؤخذ مرارة هذه الدابة فيبخر بها الدار فلا يحيك فيها السحر	—	مرارة هذه الدابة اذا بخر بها طردت كل سحر قديم ويتخذ منها ايضا مضارب للعيد ان تذخره الملوك امانا من السحر وما تصاد هذه الدابة الا لاجل قرنها
42.4	ونصاب السكين من قرن هذه الدابة يجعل في الطعام المسموم فتغرقه وهو عجيب	—	اتخذ من ذلك انصبة السكاكين تدخرها الملوك في خزينها وكثر ما يكون في بلاد النوبة والحبشة فاذا أخذت الملوك حادث من امر السم يؤخذ النصاب الذي من قرن هذه الدابة ويوضع في الطعام فان يمرق النصاب الذي من قرن هذه الدابة يكون الطعام سموما وان لم يغرق فيلبس فيه السم

42: كركدن] كرك S | كركند L

42.1: (a) وهي] وهي تسمى *add.* B | ويما] ديما B | In B a reference to the enmity between the rhinoceros and the elephant is added: وهذه الدابة كثر ما تحمل على الفيل فتغلبه وتقتله.

The transcriptions of the alleged Syriac name may be a corruption of the Syriac root *y-ʿ-l*. This originally means 'ibex, mountain goat', but its meaning might have been extended to the rhinoceros. However, another possible origin may be the Syriac word *raymā*, 'rhinoceros' (R. Payne Smith, *Thesaurus Syriacus*, Oxford, 1879-1901, p. 3807).

42.2: (a) ويتخذون] فيتخذ B | بلاد النوبة والحبشة] الحبشة والنوبة B

42.3: (a) فيبخر] يبخر B

(c) In L this recipe is after 42.4

42. Rhinoceros

	a	b	c
	Exposition of the useful properties of the parts of the rhinoceros	–	**Chapter on the useful properties of the rhinoceros**
42.1	This wild animal emerges from the sea, in Syriac it is called *w-y-m-ā*, it has a horn between its eyes with which it lifts the elephant, and it is not afraid of this.	–	This wild animal that comes out from the sea is called in Syriac *r-b-m-ā*; this wild animal has a horn between its eyes, it is said that it lifts the elephant with this, and that it is not afraid of it, on the contrary, it kills the elephant and this beast has no females.
42.2	Knives are made from the horn of this [animal], it dwells in the countries of Abyssinia and Nubia.	–	*om.*
42.3	Gall of this wild beast: if it is taken and the house is fumigated with it, then magic will not be woven there.	–	Gall of this animal: if it is fumigated, this will repel every ancient magic; from it also sticks for the feast [are made]; they store it away as a protection from magic and this animal is hunted for nothing but its horn.
42.4	If a knife handle made of its horn is put in some poisoned food, then it will sink into it, and this is amazing.	–	The kings take these knife handles and keep them in their treasures, there are many of them in the countries of Abyssinia and Nubia; and if an accident concerning poison occurs, then the handle made with the horn of this wild beast is taken and placed on the food: if the handle made of rhinoceros horn sinks into the food, then it is poisoned; whereas, if it does not sink, then the food is not poisoned.

٤٣. الفأر

	a	b	c
	ذكر منافع اعضاء الفأر	—	باب منافع الفأر
43.1	من أخذ فأرا كبيرا وذبحها واطعم من لحمه صاحب وجع الكبد الشديد ينفعه باذن الله تعالى	—	اذا أخذ فأر كبير وذبح وطبخ لحمه وأكل منه صاحب وجع الكبد ابرأه
43.2	واذا بخر البيت بلحم الفأر موضع فلا يبقي فيه فار	—	*om.*
43.3	واذا القي على حجرة الفار بصل الفار فيهربون من ذلك المكان	—	اذا عجن بصل الفأر وعمل منه بنادق وبخر به مكان الفار والجرذون فلا يبقي من ذلك هناك شيء وان أكل منه ساقتله
43.4	لنبات الشعر يؤخذ فأر ويحرق ويؤخذ رماده فيعجن بوسخ السراج ويطلي به الموضع الذي وقع منه الشعر فينبت باذن الله تعالى	—	الفأر اذا احرق وعجن رماده بوسخ السراج وطلى به الموضع القليل الشعر انبته وغزره وحسنه
43.5	يؤخذ رأس فأرة ميته ويشد في خرقة كتان قوارة جيب ويعلق بين عيني المصروع فيفيق	—	اذا أخذ فأر ميت وشد في ثوب كتان وجعل بين عيني المصروع افاق من وقته

43.1: (a) فأرا كبيرا] فأرة كبيرة B | لحمه صاحب] واطعم لحمها لصاحب B | الشديد] *om.* B | ينفعه] نفعه B
(c) *om.* C
43.2: (a) بلحم الفأر] بلحمه B | فيه] في البيت B
(c) *om.* C
43.3: (a) حجرة الفأر] حجر الفأر B | من ذلك المكان] ايضا B
(c) *om.* C
43.4: (a) لنبات الشعر] *om.* B | فيعجن] يعجن B | الذي وقع منه] *om.* B | فينبت] فانه ينبت B
(c) *om.* C
43.5: (a) فأرة ميتة] فأر ميت B | في خرقة كتان] في قوارة B | قوارة جيب] *om.* B
(c) *om.* C

43. Mouse

	a	b	c
	Exposition of the useful properties of the parts of the mice	–	**Chapter on the useful properties of the mice**
43.1	If a man takes some big mice, slaughters them, gives this to someone suffering from acute liver complaint to eat, then this will be useful to him, with the permission of God, may He be exalted.	–	If a big mouse is taken, slaughtered, cooked and given to a man suffering from liver complaint to eat, then this will cure him.
43.2	If a house is fumigated with mouse meat, then not a single mouse will remain there.	–	*om.*
43.3	If some sea onions [lit., mouse onion] are thrown in a mice hole, then the mice will flee from that place.	–	If some sea onions are kneaded, made in pills, and used to fumigate the hole of mice and rats, then they will not remain there; and if they eat it, then this will kill them.
43.4	For hair growth: if some mice are taken and burnt, their ash taken and kneaded with lantern soot, then rubbed on the part where the hair has fallen, then it will grow again, with the permission of God, may He be exalted.	–	If some mice are burnt, the ash is kneaded with lantern soot, and rubbed on the part where there is only a few hair, then this will make it grow, thicker and nicer.
43.5	Head of a dead mouse: if it is taken, wrapped in a linen cloth—like in a pocket—hung between the eyes of an epileptic man, then he will recover.	–	If a dead mouse is taken, wrapped in a linen cloth, and placed between the eyes of an epileptic man, then he will instantly recover.

اذا ذبحت فأر في نصف الشهر وجعلتها في اناء والقي عليها غمرها زيت واصابت انسان حمى الربع وأخذ من ذلك الزيت بريشة ودهن من رقيته الخاصرة واطراف اناء مثله قبل طلوع الشمس فانه يبرأ	—	يؤخذ فأرة تذبح في نصف الشهر فتجعلها في اناء القي عليها غمرها زيت طيب فاذا كان بالانسان حمى فخذ من ذلك الزيت فادهنه بريشة من رأسه الى متنه واطراف يديه ورجليه فتزول الحمى باذن الله تعالى	43.6
شحم الفأر اذا اذيف وطلى به الكلف الاسود الذي يكون على الوجع قلعه وغير لونه	—	يؤخذ شحم فأرة فيذاب على النار ويطلي به الكلف الاسود الذي يكون على الوجه فيزول باذن الله تعالى	43.7
زبل الفأر اذا عجن بعسل وجعل فتيلة وحمله المحقون سهل جوفه	—	يؤخذ زبل الفأر وبورق ويسحق سحقا ناعما ويسقي ويعجن بعسل ويتخذ منه فتيلة ويتحمل بها الانسان فيسهل طبعته	43.8
اذا اردت طرد الفأر من البيت خذ جرذونا واقطع ذنبه وخصيه واطلقه في البيت فلا يبقي هناك فأر الا هرب	—	اذا اردت ان تطرد الفأر من الحانوت او الدار فخذ جرذ كبير فتقطع ذنبه وخصيه وتسيبه في الموضع فلا يقربه الفأر ابدا وهو عجيب مليح	43.9
واذا اردت ان يخرج الفأر من الزرع خذ جرذونا كبيرا اقطعه [واقطع] ثلاث عيدان اجعل على كل عود قطعة واذا راوه الفيران لا يقربوا ذلك الزرع ابدا	—	واذا اردت ان تطرد الفأر من الزرع تأخذ جرذ تقطعه ثلاث قطع ويخط في الارض خطة مثل القوس ثم تأخذ ثلاث عيدان ويجعل على كل عود قطعة وتعرز في طرف الخطة عودا وفي وسطها عودا وفي طرفها عودا فاذا راوهم الفيران هربوا جميعهم	43.10

43.6: (a) *om.* B
(c) *om.* C
43.7: (a) ويطلي] ويدهن B | الذي يكون على الوجه] *om.* B | فيزول] يزول B
(c) *om.* C
43.8: (a) وبورق] وملح *add.* B | سحقا ناعما] الجميع B | فيسهل] فتسهل B
(c) وعمل منه] وجعل C | احد مكتوم] المحقون C
43.9: (a) من الحانوت او الدار] من الدار او الحافت B | فخذ جرد كبير] فتأخذه B | فتقطع] وتقطع B | وهو عجيب مليح] النبات ابدا *om.* B
(c) *om.* C
43.10: (c) واذا...الزرع ابدا] طرد الفأر اذا اردت طرده من الدار او الزرع فالحلمة انك جردودا كبيرا قطعه ثلاث قطع واجعل في الارض نصف دائرة مثل القوس وخذ ثلاث عيدان اجعل على كل عودة قطعة فاذا راوه الفيران فروا من ذلك المكان ولم يقربوا الزرع C

43.6	If a mouse is taken, slaughtered in the middle of the month, put it in a vessel, and abundant good oil is poured in it; then when someone is feverish, take this oil and apply this on him, from the head to half of the back, using a feather—and also the extremities of his hands and feet—then the fever will cease, with the permission of God, may He be exalted.	—	If some mice are slaughtered in the middle of the month, put in a vessel and abundant oil is poured on it; then, when a man contracts the quartan fever, this oil has to be taken with a feather and rubbed on the waist and the extremities of the vessel before sunrise, then he will recover.
43.7	Mouse fat: if it is taken, liquefied on the fire, rubbed on the black spots on the face, then they will disappear, with the permission of God, may He be exalted.	—	Mouse fat: if it is mixed, and rubbed on the black spots on the face, then this will make them disappear, and will change their colour.
43.8	Mice excrement: if it is taken with natron, ground into a fine powder, kneaded with honey, a compress is made with it and a man uses it, then his bowels will be relieved.	—	Mice excrement: if it is kneaded with honey, made into a compress and carried by a constipated man, then this will relieve his abdomen.
43.9	If you want to scare the mice away from a shop or a house, take a big rat, cut its tail and its testicles and leave this in that place, then the mice will never approach it again, and this is amazing and witty.	—	If you want to scare the mice away from a house, take a rat, cut its head and its testicles and release it inside the house, then the mice will not approach it, but only flee from it.
43.10	If you want to scare mice away from a field, take a rat, cut it in three pieces and trace on the ground a line similar to a bow, take three branches and place a rat's piece on each of them, then place one branch on one edge of the line, another in its middle and one on the other edge; then, when the mice see these, all of them will flee.	—	If you want to chase the mice away from a field, take a big rat, and cut it in pieces, cut three branches and place a rat's piece on each branch, and when the mice see it, they will never approach this field again.

43.11	*om.*	—	اذا أخذ من زبل الحمام جزئين ومن قثاء الحمار جزئين ومن الفودنج وهو المردقوش جزء وثلاث بيضات وجزء من دهن ودقت الادوية وضربه الدهن والبيض ضربا جيدا وطلى به البدن نفع من الكلف والبهق والعلة السوداء
43.12	[شعر] الجفون اذا كثر فاطل عليه دم الفأر فلا ينبت فيه شعر	—	دم الفأر اذا طلى به جفن العين لا ينبت في شعره
43.13	دم الجرد الكبير يعجن بدقيق الحمّص ويسقي منه صاحب القولنج بماء الصعتر الاخضر فيزول عنه باذن الله تعالى وينفع ايضا لصاحب وجع الجنب	—	دم الجرذون اذا عجن بدقيق الحمص وشرب منه على الريق نفع من القولنج وايضا لجميع امراض الجوف
43.14	بول الفأر اذا طلى به جبين المصروع فاق من ساعته باذن الله		*om.*

43.12: (a) This recipe is attested only in B
(c) العين] العين الذي فيه الشعرة بعد نتفها *add.* C | لا ينبت] لم ينبت C | في شعره] فيها شعر C
43.13 (a) الصعتر] السعتر S | الجرد] الجردون B | السعتر] الصعتر B | فيزول عنه] فتزول B | ايضا لصاحب] *om.* B
43.14: (a) *om.* B

43.11	*om.*	—	If two parts of pigeon excrement are taken, with two parts of squirting cucumber, one part of marjoram, three eggs and one part of oil; all the single ingredients are crushed, and the eggs well whipped, then the oil has to be taken and rubbed on the body, and this will be useful against the spots on the skin, vitiligo, and the black disease.
43.12	When the hair of eyelids becomes too much, rub some mouse blood on it, and then not a single hair will grow there.	—	Mouse blood: if it is rubbed on the eyelid, then not a single hair will grow there.
43.13	Blood of a big rat: if it is kneaded with chick-peas flour, and given to the man sufferings from colic to drink with fresh thyme, then the colic will cease, with the permission of God, may He be exalted. It is also useful to the one suffering from the pain caused by pleurisy.	—	Rat blood: if it is kneaded with chick-peas flour, and drunk on an empty stomach, then it will be useful against colic, and also against any disease of the abdomen.
43.14	Mice urine: if it is rubbed on the forehead of an epileptic man, then he will instantly recover, with the permission of God.	—	*om.*

٤٤. الخلد

	a	b	c
	ذكر منافع اعضاء الخلد	—	باب منافع الخلد
44.1	من أخذ قلب الخلد فينقع في لبن ماعز ويسقي منه الصغير الذي يكون قليل الفهم والذكاء فانه ينصلح ويصير كثير الذكاء والفهم	—	اذا أخذ قلب خلد ونقع في لبن ماعز وشرب منه غلام قليل الحفظ بليد الذهن اصلح فهمه وقوى ذكاؤه
44.2	*om.*	—	اذا اردت ان تصيد الخلد اجعل على باب وكره بصلة فانه اذا شم الرائحة ظهر وبصل العنصل اجود
44.3	دماغ الخلد يذاب بدهن ورد ويطلي البهق والبرص والحزازة والخنازير فيبرأ باذن الله تعالى	—	دماغ الخلد اذا اذيف بدهن الورد وطلى به البرص والبهق الابيض والاسود غيره واصلح لونه ويصلح ايضا للقوبة والخنازير التي يكون في الحلق وهو اجود ما يكون لهذه الامراض
44.4	رأس الخلد يحرق ويؤخذ رماده فيذاف بدهن ورد ويطلي به الرأس فيسكن الصداع باذن الله تعالى	—	اذا احرق رأس الخلد وأخذ رماده واذيف بدهن ورد ودهن به الرأس المصدع ابرأه

44.1: (a) من أخذ] يؤخذ B | ينصلح ويصير] يصلح ويكون B
(c) اذا أخذ] *om.* C | ماعز] الماعز C | اصلح] انصلح C
44.2: (c) تصيد] صيد C
44.3: (a) البهق والبرص] والبهق الابيض B | والحزازة والخنازير فيبرأ] يبرأ وكذلك للحزازة والخنازير B
(c) اذيف] اذيب C | واصلح] واخلص C
44.4: (a) فيذاف] فيذاب B | ويطلي] ويدهن B | فيسكن] يسكن B
(c) اذا احرق رأس الخلد] رأس الخلد اذا احرق C

44. Mole

	a	b	c
	Exposition of the useful properties of the parts of the mole	–	**Chapter on the useful properties of the mole**
44.1	The one who takes the heart of a mole, macerates it in goat milk, and gives it to the child who is not so clever or intelligent to drink, then this will be fine, and will become more intelligent and clever.	–	If the heart of the mole is taken, macerated in goat milk, this is drunk by the boy who has just little memory, this will enhance his intellect and improve his intelligence.
44.2	*om.*	–	If you want to hunt the mole, put an onion in front of the entrance of its hole, when this sniffs its smell, then it will come out; the onion of the red squill is even better.
44.3	Mole brain: if it is mixed with rose oil, and rubbed on vitiligo, leprosy, impetigo and the scrofula, then these will heal, with the permission of God, may He be exalted.	–	Mole brain: if it is mixed with rose oil, and rubbed on the leprosy and white or black vitiligo, these will change and improve their colour. It is also good against tetter and the scrofula that affects the back side of the throat: this is the best that there is against this illness.
44.4	Mole head: if it is burnt, its ash taken, mixed with rose oil, and rubbed on the head, then the headache will cease, with the permission of God, may He be exalted.	–	If the head of the mole is burnt, its ash is taken, mixed with rose oil, and rubbed on the aching head, then this will cure it.

44.5	للفزع في النوم يؤخذ اسنان الخلد العلية فتعلّق على من يفزع في النوم كبيرا او صغير فلا يخاف ابدا	—	اذا أخذت اسنان الخلد وعلقتها على من يفزع في نومه من كبير او صغير زال ذلك عنه
44.6	شفة الخلد العلية تعلّق على من به الحمى النافض فيذهب عنه باذن الله	—	شفة الخلد العلية اذا علقت على من به الحمى اذهب عنه
44.7	دم الخلد يجفف ويسحق ويخلط مع بياض البيض ويجعل على قطنة ويجعل على العين الرمدة فيبرأ باذن الله تعالى	—	دم الخلد اذا اذيف ببياض البيض وقطر في العين المرمدة ابرأه
44.8	دم الخلد يجفف ويحرق ويسحق ويكتحل به الرمد فيبرئ باذن الله وانه ايضا يحد النظر ويجلي البياض من العين	—	دم الخلد اذا جفف وسحق واكتحل به انسان حد نظره واجلا غشاوة العين
44.9	يؤخذ خلد فيشوي بجلده وياكله انسان قبل الطلوع الشمس فانه يكون عالما بالاشياء التي تحدث في العالمين	—	اذا أخذت الخلد بجلده وشق كما هو واكل قبل طلوع الشمس من اكله كان ذكيا فهيما عالما بالاشياء التي تحدث في العالم
44.10	مرارة الخلد يذاف بدهن الزنبق ويقطر في الاذن الثقيلة السمع فيبرأ باذن الله	—	مرارة الخلد اذا اذيفت بدهن زنبق وقطر في الاذن الثقيلة السمع انفتحت وازال المها ونفعها جدا

44.5: (a) *om.* B
(c) اذا...وعلقتها] اسنان الخلد اذا علقت C
44.6: (a) فيذهب] فانها تذهب B
(c) اذهب] اذهبها C
44.7: (a) يجفف ويسحق] *om.* B | ويجعل] يوضع B
(c) المرمدة ابرأه] الرمدة ابرأها C
44.8: (a) ويحرق] *om.* B | وانه ايضا] فانه B
(c) دم الخلد] *om.* C | العين] عينه C
44.9: (a) في العالمين] في العالم C
(c) اذا أخذت...هو] فائده اذا شق الجلد بجلده وطبخ C | ذكيا فهيما] ذكاء عظيما C | عالما] وكان عارفا C
44.10: (a) *om.* B

44.5	Against terror during the sleep, superior teeth of the mole: if these are taken, hung on the man who is taken afraid during the sleep—either an adult or a child—then he will never be afraid again.	—	If the teeth of the mole are taken, hung on the man who is taken by fear during the sleep—either an adult or a child—then this will cease.
44.6	Upper half of the mole: if it is hung the man who has fever and shivers, then these will cease, with the permission of God, may He be exalted.	—	Upper half of the mole: if it is hung on a feverish man, then this will make the fever cease.
44.7	Mole blood: if it is dried, ground, melted with egg white, put on a cotton piece of cloth to be applied on the eye affected by ophtalmia, then this will cure it, with the permission of God, may He be exalted.	—	Mole blood: if it is mixed with egg white, and applied in drops in the eye affected by ophtalmia, then this will cure it.
44.8	Mole blood: if it is dried, burnt, ground, and smeared on the eyes affected by an inflammation, then it will be cured, with the permission of God. This will also sharpen the eyesight and remove the glaucoma from the eye.	—	Mole blood: if it is dried, ground, and smeared on the eye of a man, then this will sharpen the eyesight and remove the cataract.
44.9	If the mole is taken, roasted with its skin, given to a man before sunrise to eat, then he will know everything that happens in the world.	—	If you take a mole with its skin, quarter it as it is, and it is eaten before sunrise, then the one who eats it will know and understand everything that happens in the world.
44.10	Mole gall: if it is mixed with lily oil, applied in drops into the ear that is hard of hearing, then this will cure it, with the permission of God, may He be exalted.	—	Mole gall: if it is mixed with lily oil, applied in drops into the ear that is hard of hearing, then this will open it, will make its pain cease, and will be very useful to it.

44.11	يؤخذ التراب الذي يبول عليه الخلد فتربط في جلد الخلد واعقد عليه عقد اسم من تريد واسم امه فما يبول ابدا ما دام معقودا فان اردت ان تحله فيحل ذلك التراب فان بخر بجلد الخلد فانه فينحل	—	اذا أخذ من تراب الخلد الذي يبول عليه وجعل في جلده على اسم من تريد ان تعقد بوله واسم امه فلا يبول ما دام معلقا عليه اذا اردت حله خذ من ذالك التراب من ذلك الجلد فانه ينحد
44.12	*om.*	—	بيضته اذا جففتا وسحقتا وشرب من ذلك من به عسر البول بشراب عتيق ادر بوله
44.13	*om.*	—	بول الفأر اذا مسح منه بصوفة حبين المصروع افاق من وقته ومعرفة
44.14	واذا أخذت البول الخلد فاجعله في مصيدة واريه السنور وهو القط فانه يبول من الفزع فخذ ذلك البول ثم اجعله في قرورة فاذا رأيت المجنون قد عرض به عارض فخذ من ذلك البول بصوفة وامسح بها على جبين المصاب فانه يفيق وكذلك الفار يفعل به كذلك فهة	—	أخذ بول الفاران تجعله في اناء زجاج ثم اره قطا فانه اذا اراه بال من الفزع فاعلم ذلك

44.11: (a) واعقد عليه] واعقده B | تحله فيحل] حله فحل B | بخر] بخرته B | من ذلك الجلد فانه ينحد] فانه ينحل ويبول C | تعقده عن البول] تعقد بوله C | (c) In C this recipe is after 44.12

44.14: (a) السنور وهو القط] القط B | ثم اجعله] واجعله B | في قرورة] فتينيه B | عرض به] *om.* B | به كذلك] في المعبني B (c) أخذ بول...ذلك] بول الفأران تجعله في اناء من زجاج ثم اره قطافا فاذا راه فزع منه وبال فخذ عند ذلك بوله وامسح به الجبين او سعطه منه فانه ينيق من الصرع لوقته ويبرأ منه باذن الله عز وجل وهذه حكمة عظيمة C

44.11	If the earth on which the mole has urinated is tied up inside the skin of a mole, then a knot is tied with it—in the name of any man you want and his mother—then he will not urinate until the earth remains tied. And if you want to free him, untie that earth. And also, if you fumigate him with mole skin, then he will be freed.	—	If the earth where the mole has urinated is taken, put inside its skin in the name of any man whose urine one wants to tie—and in the name of his mother—then he will not urinate until this remains hung on him.
44.12	*om.*	—	Its testicles: if they are dried, ground, and drunk by the man suffering from urine retention, then this will make his urine flow copiously.
44.13	*om.*	—	Mice urine: if it is wiped with a woollen cloth on the forehead of the man suffering from headache, then he will instantly recover, and his mind too.
44.14	If the urine of the mole is taken, put into a hunting net and the cat sees it, then it will urinate for the fear. Then take this urine, and put inside a long-necked flask; when you see an insane man who has a seizure, take this urine with a woollen piece of cloth and wipe his forehead with it, then he will recover. Likewise, the mouse and the dyer's madder have the same effect.	—	Mice urine: if it is taken, poured into a glass vessel, then shown to a cat, then this will urinate for the fear when it sees this, so you should know this!

٤٥. الحجل

	a	b	c
	ذكر منافع اعضاء الحجل وهو القبج	—	باب منافع الحجل
45.1	يؤخذ مرارة الحجل يسعط بها قليل الفهم في رأس كل شهر فانه يجود فهمه ويقوي ذكائه ويقل لسانه	—	مرارة الحجل اذا سعط منها من يكون قليل الفهم كثير النسيان في رأس كل شهر فانه يجود فهمه ويقل نسيانه
45.2	مرارة الحجل تجفف وتسحق ويؤخذ جزء حرذون ولؤلؤ غير مثقوب من كل واحد جزء وحبّة مسك يسحق الجميع ويكتحل به صاحب الغشاوة والظفرة البيضاء فيذهب باذن الله تعالى	—	مرارة الحجل اذا اذيفت بجوز وخرؤ الحرذون ولؤلؤ غير مثقوب من كل واحد جزء والقي بعد السحق مسك ويكتحل به صاحب البياض الذي في العين والغشاوة والحمرة والجرب ازاله وان اضفت اليه عسل بلا نار كان [ابلغ] في المنفعة
45.3	دم الحجل ينشّف ويسحق ناعما ويسحق معه زجاج فرعوني ودار فلفل من كل واحد جزء ويكتحل به من في عينيه البياض والجرب والحمرة وان خلط معه عسل نحل بلا نار وكان للمنعة	—	*om.*

45.1: (a) كل شهر] كل هلال B | ويقل لسانه] *om.* B
(c) رأس] *om.* C | فانه يجود] اجاد C | ويقل] وقلل C
45.2: (c) مرارة الحجل اذا اذيفت] واذا اذيفت المرارة C | غير] *om.* C | من كل...ازاله] وسحق والقي عليه المسك واكتحل به من بعينه بياض وغشاوة وحمرة وجرب ازال ذلك عنه وبرئ C
45.3: (a) ينشّف] يجفف B

45. Sandgrouse

	a	b	c
	Exposition of the useful properties of the parts of the sandgrouse	–	**Chapter on the useful properties of the sandgrouse**
	that is the perdrix.		
45.1	Sandgrouse gall: if it is taken, inhaled at the beginning of every month by a man who has little acumen in his head, then his acumen will be improved, its intelligence will be strengthen, while his tongue will become smaller.	–	Sandgrouse gall: if it is inhaled at the beginning of every month by a man who has little intellect and great forgetfulness in his head, then his intellect will be improved while his forgetfulness will become smaller.
45.2	Sandgrouse gall: if it is dried, ground, one part of it is taken with a rat and some non pierced pearls—one part of each one—and one grain of musk, everything is ground and rubbed on the eyes of a man affected by the cataract and the white nail, then these will go away, with the permission of God, may He be exalted.	–	Sandgrouse gall: if it is mixed with nut, rat excrement and unpierced pearls—one part of each one—and ground, then some musk is added to it, and it is rubbed on a man affected by glaucoma, cataracts, reddening, and scabies, then these will go away. And if it is mixed with honey that has not been heated on the fire, then it will be even more effective.
45.3	Sand grouse blood: if it is dried, ground into a fine powder with crystal and long pepper—one part of each one—rubbed on the eye of a man affected by glaucoma, scabies and reddening, [then these will go away]; if it is mixed with honey which has not be heated on the fire, then it will be good for the vigour.	–	*om.*

45.4	يؤخذ صدر الحجل وشحمه يدق ويخلط معه انيسون وميعة رطبة ويعجن بعسل ويسقي لصاحب وجع الجنب بماء الرازيانج مغلى مصفى ويذهن عنه	—	لحم صدر الحجل وشحمه يدق الرازيانج الشم المغلى ينفع صاحب وجع الجنب ويبرأه
45.5	يؤخذ بيض الحجل وينقع في خل خمر يأكله صاحب وجع الجوف والمغض فانه يبرأ باذن الله تعالى	—	بيض الحجل اذا سلق وينقع في الخل فانه ينفع لوجع الجوف والمغص
45.6	مرارة الحجل تخلط بلبن جارية ويكتحل بها من في عينيه الماء ويزول باذن الله تعالى	—	مرارة الحجل اذا اكتحل بها من به ابتداء الماء الذي في عينه نفعه جدا
45.7	دماغ الحجل يذاف بزعفران وقليل عنزروت وبياض بيضة ويقطر في العين الوارمة المحمرة فانها تبرأ باذن الله تعالى	—	دماغ الحجل اذا اذيف بزعفران وعنزوت مسحوق بياض بيضة قطر في العين الوارمة الحمر برئها باذن الله تعالى
45.8	يؤخذ شخم الدراج فيذاف بدهن كاذي ويقطر في الاذن الوجعة فتبرا باذن الله تعالى	—	*om.*

45.4: (a) انيسون] B انبسون | مصفى] B فيصفي
(c) ويبريه ...لحم صدر] وهو ماء الرازيانج وشرب بماء العسل النحل وشيء من سايلة وميعه اتيون وخلط معه الجميع اذا دق وشحمه الحجل صدر لحم
C الشومر الاخضر المغلى نفع من وجع ذات الجنب وابراه
45.5: (c) فانه...والمغص] C واكل منه من يشتكي من وجع الجوف والمغص ابراه وازال المه
45.6: (a) تخلط] B تذاف | الماء ويزول] B الما المكمن ينفعه
(c) نفعه جدا] C نفعه ومنع من الماء وازاله
45.7: (a) يذاف] B يذاب
(c) وعنزوت مسحوق] C والعنزروت المسحوق | بياض بيضة] C مع بياض البيض | قطر] C وقطر منه
45.8: (a) فيذاف] B يذاب | فتبرأ] B تبرأ
(c) For this recipe, see also 46.1

45.4	Sandgrouse breast and its fat: if they are minced, mixed with anise and fresh officinal storax, kneaded with honey and given to a man suffering from pleurisy to drink with boiled and purified fennel water, then this will go away.	—	Meat of sandgrouse breast and its fat: if they are minced with boiled smelling fennel, then this will be useful for a man suffering from pleurisy, and this will cure him.
45.5	Sandgrouse eggs: if they are taken, macerated in wine vinegar, given to a man suffering from abdomen pain and gripes to eat, then he will heal, with the permission of God, may He be exalted.	—	Sandgrouse eggs: if they are boiled, and macerated into vinegar, they will be useful against abdomen pain and gripes.
45.6	Sandgrouse gall: if it is mixed with maiden's milk, and rubbed on the eye affected with water, then this will make it disappear, with the permission of God, may He be exalted.	—	Sandgrouse gall: if it is rubbed on the eye of a man who is starting to suffer from water in his eye, then this will be very useful to him.
45.7	Sandgrouse brain: if it is mixed with saffron, a little of sarcocolla and egg white, applied in drops to the swollen and burning eye, then this will heal, with the permission of God, may He be exalted.	—	Sandgrouse brain: if it is mixed with saffron, ground with sarcocolla and egg white, applied in drops into the swollen and burning eye, then this will cure this, with the permission of God, may He be exalted.
45.8	Francolin fat: if it taken, mixed with pandang oil, and let fall in drops inside the aching ear, then it will heal with, the permission of God, may He be exalted.	—	*om.*

٤٦. النسر

	a	b	c
	ذكر منافع اعضاء النسر	—	باب منافع الدراج والنسر
46.1	*om.*	—	شحم الدراج اذا اذيف وقطر منه في الاذن سكن المها وان القي عليه دهن الكاذي كان اجود
46.2	مرارة النسر تذاف بقطران وماء المطر ويكتحل بها من في عينيه الماء الاصفر ويذهب منه حول العين فتزول باذن الله تعالى	—	مرارة النسر اذا اذيف بقطران وماء بارد واكتحل بها من به في عينة الماء وطلى منها حول العين زال ذلك عنه
46.3	يؤخذ شحم النسر يذاب على النار ويغمس فيه فتيلة ويجعل في الاذن يوم وليلة ساعة بساعة فانها يبرأ باذن الله تعالى وهو الصمم والطراش	—	شحم النسر اذا اذيف على النار لينه وغمس فيه فتيلة وجعلت في الاذن يوما وليلة مرة بعد مرة نفع الصمم
46.4	مرارة النسر تذاف بعسل وتقطر في العين فينفع من الجرب والغشاوة في العين باذن الله تعالى	—	مرارة النسر اذا اذيفت بعسل وقطرت في العين نفع ما بها من الحكة والجرب والغشاوة
46.5	يؤخذ دم النسر يخلط معه زنبق ويقطر في الحلق صاحب نفث الدم من	—	دم النسر اذا اذيف بدهن الزنبق وسعط به من به رمى الدم من الانف والحلق

46.1: (a) For this recipe, see also 45.8
(c) الاذن] الاذن الموجوعة *add.* C | عليه] عليه شىء من *add.* C
46.2: (a) تذاف] تذاب B | ويذهب] فيذهب B | فتزول] *om.* B
(c) منها] بها C
46.3: (a) ساعه بساعه فانها يبرأ] *om.* B | وهو الصمم والطراش] فانه يعافا من الصمم والطراش B
(c) النار] نار C | وجعلت] وتركت C | وليلة] وليلة يقلبها *add.* C | نفع الصمم] ازال الصمم وفتق السمع C
46.4: (a) تذاف] تذاب B | الجرب والغشاوة] الغشاوة والجرب B | فينفع] فينفعه B
(c) اذيفت] اذيبت C | وقطرت] وقطر منها C
46.5: (a) نفث] رمى B | من الحلق] والانف *add.* B
(c) ابرأه جدا] نفعه نفعا جيدا C

46. Vulture

	a	b	c
	Exposition of the useful properties of the parts of the vulture	–	**Chapter on the useful properties of the vulture and the francolin**
46.1	*om.*	–	Francolin fat: if it is mixed and applied in drops inside the ear, then this will calm its pain. And if some pandang oil is added to it, then this will be even better.
46.2	Vulture gall: if it is mixed with tar and rainwater, rubbed on the eyes affected by yellow water, and smeared all around the eyes, then this will disappear, with the permission of God, may He be exalted.	–	Vulture gall: if it is mixed with tar and cold water, rubbed on the eyes affected by water and rubbed all around them, then this will make it disappear.
46.3	Vulture fat: if it is taken, liquefied on the fire, a tampon is soaked in it, then put inside the ear for one day and one night—changing it every hour—then this will cure it, with the permission of God, may He be exalted. This is against deafness.	–	Vulture fat: if it is mixed and liquefied on the fire, a tampon is immersed in it, and put inside the ear for one day and one night, time after time, then this will be useful against deafness.
46.4	Vulture gall: if it is mixed with honey, applied in drops into the eye, then this will be useful against the scabies and the cataract of the eye, with the permission of God, may He be exalted.	–	Vulture gall: if it is mixed with honey, and applied in drops into the eye, then this will be useful against itch, scabies and cataract.
46.5	Vulture blood: if it is taken, mixed with lily, applied in drops inside the throat that spits out blood, then this	–	Vulture blood: if it is mixed with lily oil, inhaled by a man who bleeds from the nose and from the throat,

	الحلق فتزول عنه باذن الله تعالى		ابرأه جدا
46.6	لحم النسر يطبخ ويخلط معه ورس وملح وكمون كرماني وعسل نحل ويضرب الجميع ويسقي منه من لسعه حية او عقرب او شيء من الذبيب فيبرأ باذن الله تعالى	—	لحم النسر اذا طبخ مع ورس وملح وكمون كرماني وعسل وشرب منه صاحب اللسعة ونهش الهوام بماء حار ازال ذلك عنه
46.7	مخ النسر يذاف ويكتحل به من في عينيه رمد عتيق فانه يزول باذن الله تعالى	—	مخ النسر اذا اكتحل به من في عينيه الرمد المنكر والقديم ابرأه باذن الله تعالى
46.8	دماغ النسر يذاف بدقيق الحمص ويضمّد به العين وان كان بماء القرط الاخضر كان ابلغ	—	دماغ النسر اذا خلط بدقيق الباقلا وماء القرط الاخضر وضمد به العين التي تشتكي الضربان ازاله
46.9	اذا اردت ان تصف داء الجذام تاخذ مرارة النسر ودماغه ويخلط معها قطران وزيتا عتيقا ويسعط به داء الجذام فيذهب عنه باذن الله تعالى يجعل ذلك الدواء مثل الحمص ويسقي منه لصاحب اللسعة بالماء البارد ويحمي من اللبن والخل والجبن والسمك والعدس والله اعلم بالصواب	—	مرارة النسر ودماغه اذا خلطا بقطران خالص وزيت مغسول وشربها صاحب الجذام ومن سقط حواجبه وقشر وجهه فانه يبرأ
46.10	*om.*	—	مرارة النسر ودهن العنب اذا قم ثلاث ايام وسعط به من به الجذام ان كان قديما وقف وان كان حديثا اذهبه

46.6: (a) ويضرب الجميع] *om.* B | منه من لسعه] لمن لسعته B | حية او عقرب] العقرب او حية او B
(c) مع ورس] بورس C | صاحب...ذلك عنه] الملسوع بملء حار نفع من جميع النهش والهوام وازال ذلك عنه وسكن الالم C
46.7: (a) يذاف] يذاب B
(c) In L this recipe is at the end of the chapter: الرمد المنكر والقديم] رمد متكسّر وقديم C | ابرأه] ازاله عنها واباه منه وحسّن نظره وشد عصبه ونفع جميع ذلك C
46.8: (a) يذاف] يذاب B
(c) القرط الاخضر] القرط وهو الكبريت الاخضر C | الضربان] الضربان والالم *add.* C
46.9: (a) اذا اردت ان تصف داء الجذام] *om.* B | معها] معهم B | به] بهم B | داء] صاحب B | فيذهب] فيزول وينفع ايضا لمن يسقط حواجبه وجفون عينيه B | يجعل ذلك...اعلم بالصواب] *om.* B
(c) مرارة النسر ودماغه] واذا اخذ دماغه ومرارته C | وشربها] وشرب C | ومن...يبرأ عنه] الاتيون ويكون معجون اذهبه وان كان حديثا ان كان قديما اوقفه C
46.10: (c) *om.* C

§	Version A		Version B
	will cease, with the permission of God, may He be exalted.		then this will cure him well.
46.6	Vulture meat: if it is cooked, mixed with curcuma, salt, cumin, and honey—everything whipped—and given to a man who has been bitten by a snake, a scorpion or any kind of fly to drink, then he will recover, with the permission of God, may He be exalted.	—	Vulture meat: if it is cooked with curcuma, salt, cumin, and honey, then drunk with warm water by a man who has been stung or bitten by obnoxious insects, then this will make it cease.
46.7	Vulture marrow: if it is mixed, rubbed on the eye affected by a chronic inflammation, then this will cease, with the permission of God, may He be exalted.	—	Vulture marrow: if the eyes affected by acute and chronic ophtalmia are rubbed with it, then this will cure them, with the permission of God, may He be exalted.
46.8	Vulture brain: if it is mixed with chick-peas flour, and used to bandage the eyes, [then it will be useful]. And if it is mixed with fresh alfalfa, it will be even more effective.	—	Vulture brain: if it is mixed with broad beans flour and alfalfa water, used to bandage the eye suffering from pangs, then this will make them cease.
46.9	If you want to do something for the man affected by elephantiasis, take the gall of vulture and its brain, mix them with tar and old oil, let it be inhaled by the man suffering from elephantiasis, then it will disappear, with the permission of God, may He be exalted. Give this medicament the shape of a chick-pea, give it to the man who has been stung, forbid him to eat milk, vinegar, cheese, fish and lentils, and God knows what is right.	—	Vulture gall and its brain: if they are mixed with pure tar and washed oil, drunk by the man affected by elephantiasis, fall of eyebrows and desquamation of the face, then this will cure him.
46.10	*om.*	—	Vulture gall and grapes oil: if they are let to rest for three days, then inhaled by a man affected by elephantiasis then, if the elephantiasis is chronic, it will get better; if, instead, it is recent, then this will make it pass. It should be drunk kneaded with anise, avoiding sour milk and dry foodstuffs.

٤٧. الفواخت

	a	b	c
	ذكر منافع اعضاء الفواخت	—	باب منافع الفواخت
47.1	يؤخذ دم الفاختة جزء ومن دم حمام بري جزء ومن الزيت الصافي جزء ومن القطران جزء ومن دهن الجوز جزء ويخلط الجميع ويطلي به البرص فيذهب باذن الله تعالى	—	دم الفاخت اذا أخذ منه جزء ومن دم الحمام جزء ومن الزيت والقطران ودهن الجوز من كل واحد جزء وخلط الجميع وطلى به البرص ابرأه
47.2	زبل الفواخت يعلق على من يفزع في النوم او الطفل الذي يفزع ايضا في النوم فيسكن عنه باذن الله تعالى وهو صحيح مجرب	—	زبل الفاخت اذا علق على الطفل الذي يفزع ليلا اذهب فزعه

47.1: (a) ومن الزيت الصافي جزء ومن القطران] *om.* B

47.2: (a) يعلق] تعلق B

47. Collared Pigeon

	a	b	c
	Exposition of the useful properties of the parts of the collared pigeon	–	**Chapter on the useful properties of the collared pigeon**
47.1	Collared pigeon blood: one part of it, one part of wild pigeon blood, one part of purified oil, one part of tar, one part of nut oil, everything mixed up and rubbed on the leprosy, then this will go away, with the permission of God, may He be exalted.	–	Collared pigeon blood: if one part of is taken, with one part of pigeon blood, oil, tar, and nut oil—one part of each one—everything mixed up and rubbed on the leprosy, then this will cure it.
47.2	Collared pigeon excrement: if it is hung on a man who flails, or a child who is frightened during the sleep, then this will calm him, with the permission of God, may He be exalted. And this is true and tried out.	–	Collared pigeon excrement: if it is hung on a child who is frightened during the night, then the fear will disappear.

٤٨. الورشان

	a	b	c
	ذكر منافع اعضاء الورشان	—	—
48.1	يؤخذ دم الورشان يقطر في العين المطروفة او المضروبة فيذهب باذن الله تعالى	—	—

48.1: (a) المطروفة...فيذهب] فتبرأ الطرفة B | In B another recipe is added, with wood pigeon blood against the pain in the eye: وكذلك تفعل بخرخ الحمام البري وخذ ريشه من جناحه يكحل به العين المطروفة او المضروبة فيذهب.

48. Wood Pigeon

	a	b	c
	Exposition of the useful properties of the parts of the wood pigeon	–	–
48.1	Wood pigeon blood: if it is taken, applied in drops in the bulging and aching eye, then this will cease, with the permission of God, may He be exalted.	–	–

٤٩. الهدهد

	a	b	c
	ذكر منافع اعضاء الهدهد	—	باب منافع الهدهد
49.1	اذا اردت ان يكثر الحمام في البرج فبخره بفخذ الهدهد فانهم يكثرون فيه	—	اذا اردت ان تعمر برج الحمام فبخره بعش الهدهد فانه يعمر وتجتمع اليها الطير من كل جانب
49.2	تأخذ عين الهدهد اليمنى فتعلقها على من يشتكي السهر فانه ينام وان علقها على سريره الذي ينام عليه كان ابلغ	—	عينان الهدهد اذا علقتا على انسان او على سرير طفل فانه لا ينام حتى ينزعا عنه
49.3	مخالب الهدهد تحرق ويسقي للمرأة العقيم فتحبل باذن الله	—	مخاليب الهدهد تحرق وتذاف بشراب عتيق وتحمله المرأة بل يشربه فانها تحمل سريعا
49.4	اذا اردت ان تغلب من يخاصمك فخذ لسان هدهد وعلقه على عضدك الايمن فانك تغلب من يخاصمك باذن الله تعالى	—	لسان الهدهد اذا علق على عضدك الايمن لم يخصمك احد الا قهرته وغلبته
49.5	اذا اردت المرأة تخبرك بكل ما صنعته فخذ قلب هدهد واربطه في خرقة واجعله على صدرها وهي نائمة وهي تخبرك بكل ما صنعته في الدنيا	—	قلب الهدهد اذا جعل في خرقة كتان وجعل على صدر المرHاة وهي نائمة اخبرتك بما عملته في اليقظة
49.6	واذا اردت ان تبطل سحر الساحرات فبخر الموضع بلحم هدهد فما يفيد السحر ويبطل وان كان في البيت مسحورا برئ باذن الله تعالى	—	لحم الهدهد اذا بخرت به البيت ابطل السحر ولا يدخله سحر

49.2: (a) علقها على] علق من B

49.4: (a) يخاصمك] ولو كانوا جماعة تغلبهم B

49.5: (a) خرقة] خرقة كتان *add.* B | صدرها] من الجانب اليمن B | وهي] فانها B

49.6: (a) الساحرات] الساحر B | يفيد السحر] يحيق في السحر B | ويبطل] *om.* B

49. Hoopoe

	a	b	c
	Chapter on the useful properties of the parts of the hoopoe	–	**Chapter on the useful properties of the hoopoe**
49.1	If you want that pigeons increase in the pigeon house, then fumigate it with the leg of a hoopoe, and they will increase in number.	–	If you want that the pigeon house prospers, fumigate it with a hoopoe nest, then the pigeon house will prosper, and the birds will gather there from all parts.
49.2	Take the right eye of a hoopoe, hang it on a man suffering from insomnia, then he will sleep. And if you hang it on the bed where he sleeps, it will be even more effective.	–	Hoopoe eyes: if they are hung on a man's or on a child's bed, then they will not be able to sleep until the eyes are removed.
49.3	Hoopoe claws: if they are burnt, given to a woman to drink, then she will get pregnant, with the permission of God, may He be exalted.	–	Hoopoe claws: if they are burnt, mixed with old wine, and a woman carries it with her or drinks it, then she will quickly get pregnant.
49.4	If you want to subdue the one who disputes with you, take the tongue of a hoopoe, hang it on your right arm, then you will subdue whom disputes with you, with the permission of God, may He be exalted.	–	Hoopoe tongue: if it is hung on your right arm, none will face you in a quarrel without been overwhelmed and subdued.
49.5	If you want that a woman tells you everything she did, take the heart of a hoopoe, tie it in a piece of cloth and place it on her breast while she is asleep, then she will tell everything she has done in the world.	–	Hoopoe heart: if it is put in a linen cloth and placed on the breast of a woman while she is asleep, then she will tell everything she has done while she was awake.
49.6	If you want to neutralize the magic of the sorceresses, fumigate a place with hoopoe meat, then the magic will not be effective and will be void. And if the house is already enchanted, then this will come to an end, with the permission of God, may He be exalted.	–	Hoopoe meat: if a house is fumigated with it, then magic will not be able to enter it.

اذا اردت ان تخاصم انسانا فاجعل على اذنك ريشة من جناح الهدهد فانك تغلب كل من يخاصمه وتقوي على خصمك	—	اذا اردت ان تحاكم خصمك فخذ معك ريشة من جناح هدهد فانك تغلبه وتقوي عليه باذن الله	49.7
رأس الهدهد اذا علق على من يشتكي وجع الرأس ابرأه	—	يؤخذ جلد رأس الهدهد يعلق على من يشتكي الضربان والصداع الشديد فيبرأ باذن الله تعالى	49.8
قلب الهدهد اذا جفف وسحق وشربت بخمر عتيق زاد في قوة الجماع وانعاظ الباه	—	يؤحذ هدهد يجفف ويسحق ويشربه انسان قليل النكاح فانه يقوي شهوة النكاح	49.9
دم الهدهد اذا قطر في العين اذهب البياض منها	—	دم الهدهد يقطر في العين الرمدة فيبرأ باذن الله تعالى وينفع ايضا للبياض في العين	49.10
زبل الهدهد ومنقاره ومخاصيه اذا دق الجميع وخلط بسمسم مدقوق واستعمل منه امرأة ستة ايام متوالية قطع عنها النزيف	—	يؤخذ زبل الهدهد ومخصاه ومنقاره يدق الجميع ويخلط معهم سمسم ويشرب صاحب نزيف الدم فينقطع باذن الله	49.11
لسان الهدهد واطول ما في ريشة من جناحه الايمن اذا جعل في جلد غزال وربطه على فخذه الايمن رأيت عجبا في الجماع	—	اذا اردت ان تقوي على الجماع فخذ لحى الهدهد ولسانه واطول ريشة في جناحه واربطهم في خرقة وشدهم على فخذك الايمن فانك ترى عجبا	49.12
اذا أخذ هدهد وجعل في كور وبات ليلة في التنور صار رمادا ضعه في خرقة	—	اذا اردت ان تسكر الجماعة فخذ هدهدا واجعله في قدر وشد رأسها شدا	49.13

49.7: (a) معك] *om.* B | جناح هدهد] جناح الهدهد B
49.8: (a) فيبرأ] يبرأ B
49.9: (a) يؤحذ هدهد] قلب الهدهد B
49.11: (a) ويشرب] ويشربه B
49.12: (a) الايمن] الامن B
49.13: (a) قدر] قدرة B | ليلة] يوما وليلة B | يعود] يصير B | تلك] ذلك B | نسمه سكر واجميعهم] لوقته B

49.7 If you want to bring your opponent to trial, take with you a feather from the wing of a hoopoe, then you will defeat him, and you will be stronger than him, with the permission of God.

— If you want to defeat a man in a quarrel, put a feather from the hoopoe wing behind your ear, then you will subdue everyone who argues with you, and you will be stronger in your arguing.

49.8 Skin from the hoopoe head: if it is taken, hung on a man suffering from stabs and strong headache, then he will recover, with the permission of God, may He be exalted.

— Hoopoe head: if it is hung on a man suffering from headache, then he will recover.

49.9 If a hoopoe is taken, dried, ground, and given to drink to the man who has just little sexual intercourse to drink, then this will strengthen the sexual desire.

— Hoopoe heart: if it is dried, ground, and drunk with old wine, then this will increase the power of coitus and the sexual excitement.

49.10 Hoopoe blood: if it is applied in drops in the eye affected by inflammation, then this will heal, with the permission of God, may He be exalted. This is also useful for the glaucoma of the eye.

— Hoopoe blood: if it is applied in drops in the eye, then this will cure the glaucoma.

49.11 Hoopoe excrement, testicles and beak: if they are taken, ground together, mixed with sesame, given to a man affected by loss of blood to drink, then this will stop it, with the permission of God, may He be exalted.

— Hoopoe excrement, beak, and testicles: if they are ground together, mixed with ground sesame, and applied on a woman in the same quantity for six days, then this will stop the loss of blood.

49.12 If you want to give power to the coitus, take the hoopoe jawbone, its tongue, and the longest feather of its wing, wrap them in a piece of cloth and tie it on your right leg, then you will see wonders.

— Hoopoe tongue and the longest feather of its right wing: if they are put it in the skin of a gazelle, and tied on the man's right leg, then you will see wonders during the coitus.

49.13 If you want that a lot of people get drunk, take a hoopoe, put it in a cooking pot, close its opening firmly and put in a baking oven for one

— If a hoopoe is taken, put in a furnace, left there for one night—in the baking oven—it will become

واربطها ربطا جيدا واغمسها في الباطية التي يكون فيها النبيذ فكل من شرب منها سكر سكرا عظيما ولو شرب منه اهل بلد

وثيقا وتجعل في التنور يوما وليلة ثم اخرجه فانه يعود رمادا فخذ ذلك الرماد فشده في خرقة واجعله في باطية النبيذ فلو شرب من تلك الباطية الف نسمة سكر واجميعهم وهذا مليح عجيب

اذا اردت ان تحفر بئرا او تعرف هل الماء بعيد ام قريب خذ عيني الهدهد واكتحل بها قبل الطلوع الشمس وانظر الى الموضع الذي تريد محفرة فانك ترى بخارا يجري من الارض ان كان البخار بعيد منك فالماء بعيدا وان كان قريبا فقريب

—

49.14 اذا اردت تحفر بئرا وتعرف الماء قريب او بعيد فخذ عيني هدهد وعيني سرطان فجفف الجميع واسحقهم واكتحل بهم فانك تنظر الى الماء وهو قريب او بعيد ويكون الكحل قبل طلوع الشمس فانك تنظر الى تحت الارض وتنظر الى الماء وهو ينبع وهذا عجيب فان كان الماء بعيدا فهو مالح وان كان قريبا فهو حلو

من بلع قلب الهدهد وهو حار كما يخرج من جوفه فانه يرى في منامه كل شيء يصيبه

—

49.15 من أخذ قلب الهدهد بلعه وهو حار كما يخرج من جوفه رأى كل شيء يصيبه من خير او شر

مرارة الهدهد وماء القصب اذا سعط بها صاحب اللقوة في بيت المظلم نفعه

—

49.16 يؤخذ مرارة الهدهد تذاب بماء القصب الحلو ويسعط بها حلق صاحب اللقوة ويخبس في بيت مظلم فيبرأ ياذن الله تعالى

لسان الهدهد اذا سحق وسقى لانسان اذهب عنه سرعة النسيان

—

49.17 يؤخذ لسان الهدهد يجفف ويسحق ناعما ويسقي لمن يعتريه النسيان فانه يذكر كل ما نسيه ويعين على الحفظ والله اعلم

49.14: (a) بئرا] *om.* B | وتعرف] وتنظر B | قريب او بعيد] هل هو قريب منك او بعيد B | وعيني] وعين B | فجفف الجميع] فجففهم B | بهم] به B
49.15: (a) رأى] في منامه *add.* B
49.16: (a) *om.* B
49.17: (a) ناعما] *om.* B | لمن] من منه B

day and one night; then take it out—in the meanwhile the hoepoo has become ash—take this ash, tie it in a piece of cloth and put it inside a pitcher of wine, then even if one thousand people drank from this pitcher, all of them would get drunk, and this is witty and amazing.

ash; if this ash is put in a piece of cloth and tied up, plunged into the pitcher where the wine is, then everyone who drinks from it will get heavily drunk, even if the people of a whole town drank from it.

49.14 If you want to dig a well and know whether the water is close or far away, take the eyes of a hoopoe and the eyes of a crab, let everything dry, grind them, and rub this on your eyes, then you will see the water, either close or far; if the application takes place before the sunrise, then you will see the water underground, and it will spring out, and this is amazing. If the water is far, then it will be salty; if, instead, it is close then it will be fresh water.

— If you want to dig a well or to know whether the water is close or far, take the eyes of a hoopoe, rub your eyes with this before sunrise, look at the place where you want to dig, then you will see vapour coming out from the ground: if the vapour is far from you, then the water will be far; if, instead, the vapour is close, then the water will be close too.

49.15 If a man takes the heart of a hoopoe, swallows it while it is still warm as it comes out from the chest, then he will see everything that will happen to himself, either good or bad.

— The man who swallows the heart of a hoopoe while it is still warm, as it comes out from the chest, will see in his sleep everything that will happen to him.

49.16 Hoopoe gall: if it is taken, mixed with sugar cane sweet water, inhaled in the back side of the throat by a man affected by facial paralysis, and he is confined in a dark house, then he will recover, with the permission of God, may He be exalted.

— Hoopoe gall and sugar cane water: if a man affected by facial paralysis inhales this inside a dark house, this will be useful to him.

49.17 Hoopoe tongue: if it is taken, dried, ground into a fine powder, given to the man affected by forgetfulness to drink, then he will remember what he usually forgets and this will fix his memory, and God knows best.

— Hoopoe tongue: if it is ground, and given to a man to drink, then this will prevent him from forgetting things quickly.

فراخه اذا ذبحت وشقت جوفها وضمد
بها السرطان والورم الذي سمي داء
السرطان ابرأه واكثر ما يكون في الرأس

—

49.18 لداء السرطان يؤخذ فراخ الهدهد فتذبح
ويشق جدا ويضمد بها صاحب
السرطان فتذهب باذن الله

49.18: (a) *om.* B

49.18	Against cancer: the chicks of hoopoe have to be taken, slaughtered, minced, and used to bandage a man affected by cancer, then this will subside, with the permission of God.	–	Its chicks: if they are slaughtered, their abdomen split open, and used to bandage the cancer and the swelling called 'that with the crab', then this will cure it, and will increase what is inside the head.

٥٠. الخطاف

	a	b	c
	ذكر منافع اعضاء الواق	*om.*	باب منافع التوفر
	وهو الطير الاسود		
50.1	يؤخذ لحم الواق ويحرق ويعجن بماء المطر ويجعل مثل حب البندق فاذا حمّ ابن ادم يعلق عليه من ذلك الحب فتزول الحمى باذن الله تعالى	*om.*	اذا احرق هذا الطائر وصار رمادا وعجن وحبب مثل البنادق واستعمل منه المحمور واحده صحي لوقته
50.2	يؤخذ مرارة الواق يسعّط بها الانسان وهو ابن ثمانين سنة فلا يشيب ابدا وهو مليح عجيب	*om.*	ومرارة هذا الطائر اذا سعطها لانسان وقف عنه الشيب وسود شعره
50.3	واذا سعط به يجعل في شيء لبن حليب حار ولا يسود لسانه	*om.*	واذا اراد الانسان ان يسعط بهذا الدواء اجعل في شيء من اللبن الحليب واسود اسنانه
50.4	اذا اردت ان تبغض المرأة لمن يراها يؤخذ جناح هذا الطير فينتف ريشه ويؤخذ دم بقرة ومن بولها ويجعل الجناح في قارورة ويصبّ ذلك الدم والبول ويغمس الجميع بزيت طيب صافي فاذا اردت العمل فخذ منه وزن دانق وادهن به وجه المرأة فلا يراه احد الا بعضها	*om.*	واذا اردت ان تبغض المرأة لمن يراها خذ جناح هذا الطائر واجعله في وعاء واجعل عليه دم بقرة وشيئا من بولها وشيئا من دهن السمسم واتركه في الشمس عشرة ايام وادهن به وجه المرأة فكل من راها بغضها وكره منظرها

50.1: (a) ذلك] تلك B | فتزول الحمى] فيبرأ B
50.2: (a) وهو مليح عجيب] *om.* B
50.3: (a) *om.* B
50.4: (a) This recipe is attested only in B

50. Swallow

	a	b	c
	Exposition of the useful properties of the parts of the *wāq* bird	**om.**	**Chapter on the useful properties of the *twfr* [?]**
	that is a black bird.		
50.1	*Wāq* bird meat: if it is taken, burnt, kneaded with rain water, made in grains; when a man has fever, these grains have to be hung on him, and the fever will cease, with the permission of God, may He be exalted.	*om.*	If this bird is burnt and becomes ash, then this is kneaded, made into grains similar to pills, and one of them is given to a feverish man, then he will immediately heal.
50.2	*Wāq* bird gall: if it is taken, inhaled by a man—and he can even be in his eighties—then he will never become white-haired, and this is witty and amazing.	*om.*	Gall of this bird: if it is inhaled by a man, then the grey hair will fall, and the rest of the hair will turn black.
50.3	If it is inhaled, with the addition of some warm cow milk, then this will blacken his tongue.	*om.*	If a man wants to inhale this remedy, add some cow milk to it, but his teeth will become black.
50.4	If you want that a woman is hated by anyone who looks at her, take this bird, shave its feathers, take the blood and the urine of a cow too, put the wing in a long-necked flask, pour these blood and urine in it, and cover everything with pure and good oil. When you want to use it, take one *dāniq* of it, and rub the face of the woman, then nobody will be able to look at her without hating her.	*om.*	If you want that a woman is hated by anyone who looks at her, take this bird, put it in a vessel, add some cow blood, some of its urine, and some sesame oil, leave it in the sunlight for ten days, and rub the face of the woman with it, then everyone who looks at her will hate her, and will be disgusted by the sight of her.

50.5	الواق يطبخ ويجفف جميعه فاذا جف اسحقه واخلط معه جزء من بزر جرجير واجعل الجميع في بودقة وسدّ رأسها بالطين واوقد عليها سبعة ايام واخرجه وصب عليه شيئا يسيرا من دهن الآس واسقي لمن شيت وزن دانق فانه لا ينام	*om.*	اذا ذبح هذا الطائر وشق جوفه وسحق ناعما وخلط معه من بزر جرجير واوقد عليه في بودقة سبعة ايام
50.6	للسهر ايضا عين هذا الطائر ويشد في خرقة كتان ويشد على سرير فمن صعد على ذلك السرير لا ينام ابدا ما دامت الخرقة عليه	*om.*	واذا أخذت عينين هذا الطائر وربطها في خرقة كتان او ناووس وعلقتها على سرير فان صاحب السرير لا ينام ما دام معلقين عليه
50.7	عين هذا الطائر يجفف ويسحق ويذاب بدهن ورد واسقي منها ان شيت على اسمه واسم امه فانه يحبك حبا شديدا	*om.*	اذا أخذت عينين هذا الطائر وسحقتها وذر بهما بدهن ورد وشرب من ذلك بصف درهم من اردت احبك حبا شديدا مفرطا
50.8	يؤخذ دماغ الواق يذاف بدهن زنبق وحبّة مسك ويسعط به الانسان فلا يشيب ابدا	*om.*	دماغ هذا الطائر اذا اذيبته بمسك خالص وسعط به انسان ذكرا كان او انثى فانه لا شيب ابدا
50.9	اذا اردت ان لا تسكر فخذ رأس هذا الطائر الذكر منه والانثى فاحرقهما واسحقهما وخذ منه رمادهما شيئا يسيرا والقه في الباطية فلو شرب منه الف نفر لم يسكروا ابدا	*om.*	ودماغه ايضا اذا احرق وأخذ من رماده واطرح بنبيذ لا سكر منه احد

50.5: (a) This recipe is attested only in B
50.6: (a) This recipe is attested only in B
50.7: (a) This recipe is attested only in B
50.8: (a) الواق] هذا الطائر B | يذاف] يذاب B | وحبّة] وحب B | ذلك] تلك B | به] منها B
50.9: (a) فاحرقهما واسحقهما] فاحرقهم واسحقهم B | رمادهما] رمادهم B | منه...ابدا] لم يسكر منها كثير B

50.5	If the *wāq* bird is cooked and completely dried, then, once it has dried, it is ground and melted with one part of rocket seeds—everything put in a crucible, sealed with clay and put on the fire for seven days; then take it out, pour some myrtle oil on it, and give this to drink to whomever you want, then he will not sleep for the sake of insomnia.	*om.*	If this bird is slaughtered, its abdomen split, finely minced, mixed with some rocket seeds, cooked in a crucible for seven days, [then this will be useful].
50.6	Also for insomnia, eye of this bird: if it is taken, tied in a linen cloth, put in a bed, then whoever climbs in this bed will never sleep, as long as the eye remains there.	*om.*	If the eyes of this bird are taken, tied in a linen cloth or in a sarcophagus bandage, and hung on a bed, then the man who uses this [bed] will not sleep, as long as the eyes remain hung on it.
50.7	Eye of this bird: if it is taken, dried, ground, and mixed with rose oil, given to anyone you desire to drink—in his name and in the name of his mother—then he will passionately love you.	*om.*	If you take the eyes of this bird, ground them, and pour rose oil on them, if you give one dirham of it to the one you desire, then he will love you with extreme passion.
50.8	*Wāq* bird brain: if it is taken, mixed with lily oil and one grain of musk, and inhaled by a man, then he will never become grey-haired.	*om.*	Brain of this bird: if it is mixed with pure musk, and inhaled by someone—male or female—then this will never become grey-haired.
50.9	If you do not want to get drunk, take the head of this bird—both from the male and the female—burn them, grind them, take a little bit of the ash and put it inside a pitcher, and even if one drank one thousand glasses from it, then these would not be intoxicating.	*om.*	Its brain, also: if it is burnt, its ash is taken and added to some wine, then no one will get drunk with it.

50.10	*om.*	*om.*	اذا اذبح هذا الطائر واحرق وأخذ من رماده مثقالين ومن بزر السذاب مثقالين ومن الملح الهندي ومن الاهليلج الايلح والافتيمون الاقريطشي من كل واحد مثقالين ومن الملح الهندي نصف درهم ومن الايارج عشرة درهم يدق الجميع وينخل ويعجن بماء الفجل المغلى ويلت بشحم ماعز ويحبب مثل البندق ويسقي منه صاحب الصداع مثقالين بماء الفجل يسكن الصداع لوقته
50.11	*om.*	اذا اردت ان تمنع المرأة من الفسق اسقها دم الخطاف في نبيذ فانها تمتنع من الفسق	واذا اردت ان تمنع المرأة من العشق فاسقها من دم هذا الطائر ربع مثقال بنبيذ عتيق فانه نافع جدا
50.12	*om.*	فراخ الخطاف حين يستوي بريشها قبل ان ينهض يصير بعد ان يذبح في كوز فخار ويلقي عليه ملح جريش ويطين رأس الكوز ويصير في تنور قد خبز فيه ثم يترك حتى يحترق ثم يخرج من الكوز ويرفع ويؤخذ فيسحق ويذاف بدهن الجوز ويطلي على الحلق اذا ما عرضت له الاورام والخوانيق بريشة من داخل ويتغرغر بزيت الجوز فيسكن باذن الله تعالى	فراخ الهدهد اذا استوى ريشه اذبحه واجعله في كوز جديد وطين رأسه وادخل تنور الفرن حتى يحرق وسحقه وخذ منه وزن درهم واذبه بدهن الجوز وطلية به الحلق فانه يذهب الخوانيق
50.13	اذا اردت ان تبيض الشعر فاطليه بزبل خطاف مثل حناء فانه يبيض	فاذا اردت ان تبيّض شعر انسان فاطل رأسه بزبل الخطاف مثل الحنى واتركه عليه فانه يبيض	*om.*

50.12: (b) In T this recipe is after 50.14
(c) الخطاف] الهدهد L

50.10	*om.*	*om.*	If this bird is slaughtered, burnt, two *miṯqāl* of its ash are taken with two *miṯqāl* of rue seeds, with two *miṯqāl* each of Indian salt, myrobalan and clover dodder of Crete, half dirham of Indian salt and the dirham of *ayārağ* [?], everything is ground, sieved, and kneaded with boiled radish water, mixed with goat fat, made in pills, and two *miṯqāl* of this are given to a man suffering from headache with radish water to drink, then this will immediately calm the headache.
50.11	*om.*	If you want to keep a woman from a dissolute life, give her the blood of the swallow to drink with wine, and then she will keep aloof from a dissolute life.	If you want to prevent a woman from the ardour of love, give her one quarter *miṯqāl* of the blood of this bird with old wine to drink, then this will be very useful.
50.12	*om.*	Swallow chicks, when their feathers are of the same length, but before they leave the nest: if—after it has been slaughtered—it is put in a small clay jug, with the addition of crushed salt, the opening of the jug is closed with clay, then this is put in an oven in which bread has already been baked, then it is left there until it is burnt; then it is taken out from the jug, put away, ground, mixed with nut oil, and rubbed on the body—if this is affected by swellings and suffocation—with a feather from the inside, while the nut oil is used to gargle—then this will cease, with the permission of God, may He be exalted.	Swallow chicks: if their feathers are of the same length, then they have to be slaughtered, put in a new small jug, its opening closed with clay, and put in the backing oven until it is burnt, and ground; and if one dirham of it is taken, mixed with nut oil and rubbed on the back of the throat, then this will cure the suffocation.
50.13	If you want that the hair turns white, rub it with swallow excrement—as you do with the henna—and then the hair will turn white.	If you want that the hair of a man turns white, then apply the droppings of the swallow one his head, like one does with the henna, and this will turn white.	*om.*

50.14	اعلم ان في رأس الخطاف حصاية او في حوصلته او في فكل من قدر على تلك الحصاية وكان لايراه احد الا احبه واهابه من رجال والنساء	واعلم ان في رأس الخطاف حصاة فيها منافع كثيرة وكل خطاف فهو يبلع تلك الحصاة ان ظفر بها كانت له وسيلة الى من يحبه لم يمتنع منه	*om.*
50.15	يؤخذ خطاف فيحرق حتى يصير رمادا ويلقي عليه سكر نبات وزبد البحر ويتخذ منها كحلا فينفع من الغشاوة والجرب في العين والصفرة باذن الله تعالى والله اعلم	*om.*	*om.*
50.16	*om.*	زبل الخطاف اذا سقى منه من به حوارة أظفاها	*om.*
50.17	*om.*	وان بخرت به وطلى على الدبيلة يبرأ باذن الله تعالى	*om.*

50.14: (a) الخطاف] الخطاطيف B | حوصلته] حصاة B | وكان] فكان B

50.14	Know that inside the head of the swallow, or inside its craw, there is a small stone, then every one who gets hold of this small stone will not be seen by anyone but the one—woman or man—who loves and likes him.	Know that inside the head of the swallow there is a small stone that has many useful properties, and every swallow gulps down this stone; and this is a stone that, if one possesses it, there will be such a drive towards the one who loves him, that he will not be able to stay away.	*om.*
50.15	If a swallow is taken, burnt until it has become ash, some rock sugar is added to it, eye salve is made with it; then this will be useful against the cataract, scabies and the yellow colour in the eye, with the permission of God, may He be exalted, and God knows best.	*om.*	*om.*
50.16	*om.*	Swallow excrement: if it is given to the one who has gypsum, then this will slake it.	*om.*
50.17	*om.*	And if it is used for fumigation, and rubbed on the abdomen suffering from internal ulceration, then this will heal, with the permission of God, may He be exalted.	*om.*

٥١. السلوى

	a	b	c
	ذكر منافع اعضاء الالسلوى	السلوى	باب منافع الالسلوى
	هو طائر لطيف طويل الرجلين يشبه المرعة		
51.1	يؤخذ الالسلوى فيذبح ويجعل في قدر [. . .]	*om.*	اذا ذبحت وغسلت وجعلت في قدر واغلى عليها حتي تنهري ولا سقى منها شيء ورفعت في اناء فاذا اردت ان ترى العجب خذ من ذلك الدهن وصبه في سراج والق عليه زيتا واشعله بين جماعة فانه يرون بعضهم بعضا مثل الثيران
51.2	*om.*	*om.*	كبد الالسلوى اذا شوى على النار واكل منه صاحب وجع الكبد نفعه
51.3	[مرارة الالسلوى] يذاف بخل خمر والقى عليها زعفران واطل به البهق الاسود والابيض فيغير لونه	كبد السلوى يخلط معها زعفران ويذاف بخل ويطلي على البهق الاسود فيغير لونه ويرده الى اللون الطبيعي	مرارة الالسلوى اذا اذيفت بزعفران وخل خمر خالص وطلى به البهق الاسود غير لونه ورده الى لون البدن وينفع ايضا اللقوة
51.4	زبل الالسلوى اذاف بزيت ويطلي به القروح التي يكون في الجسد فتبرأ باذن الله تعالى والله اعلم	زبل السلوى يسحق ويسر على قروح منعقدة والمتأكلة يبرأ باذن الله تعالى	زبل الالسلوى اذا سحق ودر على القروح المتأكلة نفعها باذن الله سبحانه وتعالى

51: (c) السلوى [السلوا C

51.1: (c) *om.* C

51.3: (c) صاحب [به من C

51.4: (c) نفعها [ابرأها C

51. Quail

	a	b	c
	Exposition of the useful properties of the parts of the quail	**The quail**	**Chapter on the useful properties of the quail**
	This is a nice bird, with long feet, that resembles the sandgrouse		
51.1	If a quail is taken, slaughtered, put in a cooking pot [...]	*om.*	If it is slaughtered, washed, put in a cooking pot until it is well cooked, not taken immediately, but preserved into a vessel; then, when you want to see something amazing, take this oil, pour it in a lantern and add some oil, light it among a group of people, then they will see one another as bulls.
51.2	*om.*	*om.*	Quail liver: if it is roasted and then eaten, it will be useful against the liver complaint.
51.3	Quail gall: if it is mixed with wine vinegar, some saffron is added to it, then it is rubbed on the black and the white vitiligo, then this will change its colour.	Quail gall: if it melted with saffron, mixed with vinegar, and rubbed on the black vitiligo, then this will change its colour, and will revert to its natural hue.	Quail gall: if it is mixed with saffron and wine vinegar, rubbed on the black vitiligo, then this will change its colour and will turn it to the normal colour of the body; it is also useful against the facial paralysis.
51.4	Quail excrement: if it is mixed with oil, rubbed on the ulcers which are on the body, then they will heal, with the permission of God, may He be exalted, and God knows best.	Quail excrement: if it is ground, and poured on the festering and grangrenous ulcers, then this will cure them, with the permission of God, may He be exalted.	Quail excrement: if it is ground, and abundantly poured on the gangrenous ulcers, then it will be useful against them, with the permission of God, may He be praised and exalted.

٥٢. العصفور

	a	b	c
	ذكر منافع اعضاء العصفور	العصافير	باب منافع العصفور
52.1	يؤخذ عصفور دوري ذكر وينتف ريشه وهو بالحياة ثم اجعله على بيت الزنابير حتى يموت ثم تأخذ تقليه من ساعتك بسمن بقري حتى يذوب لحمه ويتهري فارفعه في إناء بريشة فاذا هممت بالجماع فخذ من ذلك الدهن بريشة فامسح محالك واحليلك فانك ترى العجب من كثرة الجماع	يؤخذ عصفورا ذكرا فينتف ريشه وهو حي ثم يوضع على عش زنابير حتى يلدغونه ويموت فاذا مات فاطبخه من ساعتك بسمن بقر حتى يذوب لحمه ويتهري ثم ارفعه في قارورة فاذا هممت بالجماع فامسح احليلك وجانبيك فترى منها عجبا ولذة شديدة	اذا اردت ان تقوي على الجماع خذ عصفورا ذكرا وانتف ريشه وهو حي ودعه على بيت الزنبور ويلدغه حتى يموت فاذا مات اطبخه سمن بقر واقليه فيه حتي ينهري وارفعه في قارورة فاذا هممت بالجماع فادهن منه الاحليل والمحالب ترى عجبا
52.2	اخر مثله يؤخذ عصفور فينتف ريشه وهو بالحياة وينقع في زيت طيب خالص صافي يوما وليلة واخرجه وانقعه في دهن زنبق مثله واخرجه واعصره عصرا جيدا فاذا احتجت الى النكاح فخذ من ذلك الدهن وادهن به رأس الاحليل فانه يهيج ويقوي على الجماع	يؤخذ العصفور يفعل به كما وصفت لك من ساعتك فتنقعه في زنبق جيد وتدعه يوما وليلة ثم تعصره حتى لا يبقي فيه شيئا من الدهن ثم تدهن به اعنى احليلك في وقت الجماع	اذا أخذت عصفور وانتفت ريشه وغمرته في الزيت حتي يموت ودعه يوما وليلة واخرجه من الزيت واعصره عصرا شديدا فاذا اردت الجماع ادهن احليلك تري عجبا
52.3	*om.*	واذا كان انسان لا يفند النبيذ ولا يحب يفارقه فخذ عصفورا دوريا ذكرا فاذبحه وخذ من دماغه فدقه بشيرج واطعمه اياه يبغض النبيذ	اذا اردت ان يبغض انسانا لشرب النبيذ اذبح عصفورا دوريا وادهن دماغه بشيرج واشويه وطعمه لمن يحب النبيذ فانه يبغضه ولا يعود يشتهيه

52.1: (c) بيت الزنبور [بيت الديناري الزنبور | C حتى يموت [حتى يلدغه ويموت | C بقر [البقر | C هممت بالجماع [اردت ان تجامع | C عجبا [عجبا في الجماع *add.* C

52.2: (a) زنبق [زيبق T

(c) حتى [الى ان C

52.3: (c) يبغض [بغض | C وطعمه [واطعمه | C ولا يعود [ولا يكاد C

52. Sparrow

	a	b	c
	Exposition of the useful properties of the parts of the sparrow	**The sparrows**	**Chapter on the useful properties of the sparrow**
52.1	Take a male domestic sparrow, pluck out its feathers while it is still alive, then place it on a hornet hive until it dies, then fry it immediately with cow fat until its meat melts and it is well cooked, and preserve it in a vessel together with a feather; and when you are concerned about the coitus, take this oil with that feather and apply it in your urethra and on its outer opening, then you will be amazed by the great number of copulations.	Domestic sparrow: if it is taken, its feathers plucked out while it is still alive, then it is placed on a hornet hive until [the insects] bite it to death; once it is dead, it has to be cooked immediately with cow fat until its meat melts and it is well done, and preserved in a long-necked flask; then when you are concerned about the coitus, apply this on the outer opening of your urethra and on your hips, then you will see wonders and have great pleasure.	If you want to give power to the coitus, take a male sparrow, pluck out its feathers while it is still alive, leave it on a hornet hive and let it be stung until it dies; once it is dead, cook it with cow fat and fry it until it is well done, and preserve it in a long-necked flask; when you are concerned about the coitus, rub the outer opening of the urethra and the ureter with it, and then you will see wonders.
52.2	Another similar recipe. If a sparrow is taken, its feathers plucked out while it is still alive, then its is macerated in purified pure good oil, taken out and macerated again in lily oil, taken out and squeezed well; then, if the need of coitus arises, take this oil and rub the top of the outer opening of urethra with it, then this will excite you and give power to coitus.	If a sparrow is taken and what I have just described to you is done to it, then it is well macerated in lily oil, and left there for one day and one night, then squeezed until no oil is left in it; then rub the oil on the outer opening of your urethra at the moment of coitus.	If a sparrow is taken, its feathers are plucked out, it is fried in oil until it dies and left there for one day and one night, then taken out from the oil and squeezed well; then when you desire the coitus, rub the outer part of your urethra with that oil and you will see wonders.
52.3	*om.*	If someone does not refuse wine and would not like to quit drinking it, then take a male domestic sparrow, slaughter it, take its brain, mince it with sesame oil, and whoever is fed with it will hate wine.	If you want that a man hates drinking wine, slaughter a domestic sparrow, mix its brain with sesame oil, roast it and feed it to the man who loves wine, then he will hate it and will never desire it again.

52.4	يؤخذ لحم العصافير فيدق جيدا ويطبخ بغيل ويلقي عليه خولنجان جزء ويرفع في اناء واسقي صاحب عسر البول بماء الكمون مغلى فيدر البول	لحم صدر العصافير يطبخ ثم يدق معه خولنجان وعسل ويورق ويرفع ويشرب منه وزن مثقال بماء الكمون مغلى مصفى لوجع المثانة وعسر البول	صدور العصافير اذا دقت والقي عليها عسل وخولنجان وجعل في اناء اذا شرب منه بماء الكمون المغلى فانه ينفع من عسر البول ووجع المثانة
52.5	*om.*	يؤخذ بيض العصافير وزن درهم ويصير في قدح نبيذ ويدهن به الجسد ويشرب فانه يهيج الجماع	*om.*
52.6	يؤخذ بيض العصافير يسلق ويلقي عليه بزر الجرجير مسحوقا ويوكل منه فانه يهيج شهوة النكاح ويزيد في الباه	يؤخذ بيض العصافير فيسلق ويؤكل مع الجرجير فانه يزيد الجماع	اذا أخذت بول العصافير وسلق واكل الجرجير فانه يقوي الجماع
52.7	*om.*	دماغ العصافير يذاف بماء السذاب وعسل ويشرب على الريق لاورام البواسير	*om.*
52.8	اخر مثله يؤخذ العصافير فتذبح على دقيق العدس حتى يسيل دمهم عليه فاعجنه عجنا جيدا واجعله مثل البندق فاذا اردت ان تجامع فخذ بندقة واسحقها ناعما واعجنها بزيت مغسول واطل بها تحت قدميك ولا فطا بقدميك الارض فانك ان وطئت الارض انقطع نكاحك	يؤخذ فتذبح ويسيل دمها على دقيق العدس ويجعل منه بنادق فاذا اردت الجماع فذوب منع بندقة بزيت فاطلي به رجليك ولا تطأ على الارض فاذا وطئت على الارض انقطع	اذا اذبح من العصافير ما شئت على دقيق واعجنه مثل بنادق واذا اردت الجماع فخذ بندقة واسحقها واعجنها بزيت واطلي بها قدميك فانك ترى عجبا واذا اطئت على الارض انقطع ذلك

52.6: (c) *om.* C
52.8: (b) In T this recipe is after 52.9
(c) واذا] فاذا C | واطلي] واطل C | اطيت] وطيت C

52.4	If the meat of sparrows is taken, minced well, cooked with the milk of a pregnant woman, one part of galangal is added to it, then it is preserved in a vessel and given to a man suffering from urine retention to drink with boiled cumin water, then the urine will easily flow.	Meat of sparrows chest: if it is cooked, then galangal and honey are ground with it, then it is made in slices, preserved, and one *miṯqāl* of this is drunk with boiled and purified cumin water, then this will be useful against bladder complaints and urine retention.	If some chests of sparrows are minced, galangal and honey are added to them, and they are put in a vessel; then when this is drunk with boiled cumin water, it will be useful against urine retention and bladder complaints.
52.5	*om.*	Sparrow eggs: if one dirham of them is taken, put in a goblet of wine, the body is rubbed with it and it is also drunk, then this will excite the coitus.	*om.*
52.6	Sparrows eggs: if they are taken, boiled, ground rocket seeds are added to them, and they are eaten, then this will excite the desire of coitus and will increase the sexual potency.	Sparrow eggs: if they are boiled, and eaten with rocket, then this will make the coitus more intense.	If sparrow urine is taken, boiled, and eaten with rocket, then this will give power to the coitus.
52.7	*om.*	Sparrow brain: if it is mixed with rue water and honey, and drunk on an empty stomach, then this will be useful against the swellings and the haemorrhoids.	*om.*
52.8	Another similar recipe. If some sparrows are taken, slaughtered over lentil flour until it becomes a paste, then this is well kneaded, and made in pills; then, if you want to copulate, take a pill, grind it and rub it under your feet—without touching the ground with them—but if you step on the ground, then your coitus will be interrupted.	If [some sparrows] are slaughtered, their blood leaks over lentil flour, then this is made in pills; then when you want to copulate, mix a pill with oil, and rub your feet with it without stepping on the ground; and if you step on the ground, the effect will cease.	If some sparrows—as many as you want—are slaughtered over flour, this is kneaded in the form of pills; then when you want to copulate, take one pill, pound it, knead it with oil and rub it on your feet, then you will see wonders, but if you step on the ground, then this will cease.

	(a)	(b)	(c)
52.9	خذ مرائر ثلاث عصافير الجميع واجعله في قارورة ومتى احتجت الى ذلك فخذ منه بريشة وامسح قدميك واحليلك فانك ترى من الجماع عجبا ولا تزال تجامع ما لم نشطا الارض فان وطيت الارض انقطع	يؤخذ ثلاث مرارات عصافير دوري ذكورا ويخلط معها زنبق خالص ونصف مثقال يبروج وحبات شهدانج تدق البيروج والشهدانج دقا ناعما ويخلط بالمرارات والزنبق ويصير في قارورة فاذا احتجت اليه فامسح باطن قدمك والاحليل والانثيين والوركين ولا تطأ على الارض لا تزال نشيطا فاذا وطئتَ على الارض انقطع	*om.*
52.10	خذ ادمغة العصافير ايام هيجانها جففها في ظل وخذ الحسك الرطب دقه واعصر مائه ثم يرفع في إناء فاذا اردت الجماع خذ من ذلك الدواء واذفه في العسل واشرب منه فانه يفعل فعلا عظيما لا يسكن حتى يربط رأس الاحليل	يؤخذ ادمغة العصافير يفتح ويجفف في الظل يؤخذ حنل رطب فيدق ويخرج ماؤه ويجعل في اناء فاذا هممتَ بالجماع فخذ من ادمغة العصافير وزن درهم ويصير في قدح بنبيذ ويدهن بالجسد ويشرب منه فانه يهيج الجماع ولا يسكن الانعاظ حتى يشرط رأس الاحليل فيخرج الدم فاذا خرج الدم هذا الانعاظ [...]	اخر مثله يؤخذ ادمغة العصافير ايام هيجانها فتجفف في الظل وترفع في إناء فاذا احتجت مثقال وافرجه بعسل او نبيذ واشربه فانه يقوي الظهر ويهيج النكاح ولا يرقد الاحليل حتى يشرط رأسه
52.11	ذرق العصافير اذا اذيب بلعاب ابن ادم وهو نايم وطلى به ثآليل ذهبت وينفع ايضا للحزاز باذن الله تعالى	*om.*	ذرق العصافير يذاف ببصاق ابن ادم ويطلي به ثآليل فانه يزياها من البدن واليدين باذن الله تعالى

52.9: (b) In T this recipe is after 52.9 | زنبق] زيبق T | والزنبق] والزيبق T
(c) *om.* C
52.10: (b) In T this recipe is after 52.9
52.11: (a) ثآليل] الثواليل S
(c) ثآليل] التواليل L | اذيب] ذوّبته C | وطلى] وطليت C | ذهبت وينفع] ذهبها ونفع C | للحزاز] للحزاز وابرأه C

52.9	*om.*	If the gall of three male domestic sparrows is taken, then pure lily oil, half *miṯqāl* mandrake, and some grains of Indian hemp—ground into a fine powder with the mandrake—are mixed with them, and finally this is put in a long-necked flask; when you need it, rub the soil of your feet, the outer opening of the urethra, the testicles, and the legs with this, without stepping on the ground, and then your ardour will not stop; but if you step on the ground, then it will cease.	Take all the gall of three sparrows, put it in a long-necked flask and when the need of it arises, take some of it with a feather, apply it on your feet and on the outer opening of you urethra, then you will see wonders, and you will not stop to copulate as long as you do not touch the ground, but if you walk on the ground, then this will cease.
52.10	Another similar one, sparrow brains: if they are taken when the birds are on heat, dried in the shade, preserved in a vessel; and then, when you need it, one *miṯqāl* of it has to be dissolved—either in honey or wine—and drunk, then this will strengthen the back, excite the coitus, and the penis will remain erected until its top rips open.	Sparrow brains: if they are taken, opened, dried in the shade, then some fresh *ḥanal* [?] is taken, ground so that its water comes out, and put in a vessel; then when you are concerned about the coitus, take one dirham of these sparrow brains, put it in a goblet of wine, rub the body with the wine and drink it, then this will excite the coitus, and the erection will not cease until the top of the urethra rips open and the blood comes out. And when the blood comes out, the erection [will come to an end].	Take some brains of sparrows when they are on heat, dry them in the shade, then take some fresh beard, ground it, squeeze its juice, and preserve it in a vessel; then when you need to have sexual intercourse, take this remedy, dilute it with honey and drink it: this will have a great effect and will not let you rest, until you tie up the outer opening of the urethra.
52.11	Sparrows droppings: if they are mixed with human saliva, rubbed on the warts, then these will disappear from the body and the hands, with the permission of God, may He be exalted.	*om.*	Sparrow droppings: if they are mixed with the saliva of a sleeping man and rubbed on the warts, then these will disappear. This is also useful against the impetigo, with the permission of God, may He be exalted.

٥٣. الخفاش

	a	b	c
	ذكر منافع اعضاء الخفاش	الخفاش	باب منافع الخفاش وهو الوطواط
53.1	يؤخذ رأس خفاش فاجعلها في وسادة واجعله تحت رأس انسان فلا يزال نائما ما دامت تحت رأسه واذا علقها عليه فلا يزول نائما حتى ينقلها عنه	من أخذ رأس الخفاش وخيّطه في المخدّة التي تحت رأسه وعلق على انسان لم ينم ما دام	من أخذ رأس الخفاش وجعله في وسادته التي ينام عليها وعلقه على انسان فانه لا ينام ما دام ذلك في وسادته او معلقا عليه
53.2	اذا اردت ان ترى الناس ولا يراك احد فخذ خفاش فاذبحه وخذ عينيه وعلقهم على عضدك الايمن ولا تتكلم فان تكلمت بطل فعله فطنوا بك	وان اردت ان لا يراك الناس فخذ عيني الخفاش جميعا في خرقة جديدة وعلق على عضدك الأيمن ولا تتكلم فان تكلمت فطن بك	عينين الخفاش اذا جعلتهما في خرقة ناووس وعلقتها على عضدك الايمن فلا يراك احد من الناس لم تتكلم
53.3	فانزعهم عنك واجعلهم على عضدك الايسر فانك ترى الناس ولا يروك	فاذا فطنوا بك فانزعها عنك واطرحها على الارض ثم خذها وشدها على عضدك الايسر فانك ترجع الى ان تبصر الناس وهم لا يبصروك وليكون الخفاش الذي تأخذ عينيه مذبوحا	واذا اردت ان اجاله فانزع تلك الصرة والقها علي الارض ثم خذها بعد ذلك والقها على عضدك الايسر فانك [ترى] الناس ولا يرونك وهذا عجيب
53.4	اذا كانت المرأة تموت اولادها فتأخذ خفاشا على اسمها فاذبحه وجففه فاذا كانت وقت الولادة فعلقه عليها فاذا ولدت فلا يموت الا بعد حين	تأخذ خفاشا فتذبحه وتعلقه على رقبة المرأة فلا يموت لها ولد	واذا اردت المرأة لا يموت لها ولد خذ خفاش وجففه فاذا جف علقه على المرأة في عنقها وهي حامل فانه لا يرجع يموت لها ولد

53: (a) خفاش] خشاف For the whole chapter, both in S and in B
53.1: (a) واجعله] *om.* B | رأس انسان] رأس الانسان C | ما دامت تحت رأسه] من رأس C
(c) رأس] من رأس C | وعلقه] او علقه C
53.2: (a) ولا يراك احد] ولا يران B | وخذ عينيه] *om.* B | فعله فطنوا] فعلهم يفطنوا B | عضدك الايسر] العضد الايسر B | ولا يروك] من ولا يروا B
(c) فانك...عجيب] فلا يراك احد من الناس ما لم تتكلم C
53.4: (a) فتأخذ] فخذ B | الا بعد حين] الاوقت ما ينقضي عمره B
(c) اردت] ان اردت *add.* C | فانه] فانها C

53. Bat

	a	b	c
	Exposition of the useful properties of the parts of the bat	**The bat**	**Chapter on the useful properties of the bat**
			that is the noctule.
53.1	Bat head: if it is taken, put inside a pillow, and this is placed under the head of a man, then he will sleep as long as this remains under his head. And if it is hung on him, then he will sleep until it is removed.	If one takes the head of a bat, sews it inside the cushion that is under his head, or hangs it on a man, then he will not sleep as long as this remains on him.	If one takes the head of a bat, places it inside a pillow where one sleeps and hangs it on someone, then he will not be able to sleep as long as this remains inside the pillow or hung onto him.
53.2	If you want to see people, but not to be seen by anyone, take a bat, slaughter it, take its eyes and hang them on your right harm and do not speak, because its effect will be void if you talk, and people will become aware of your presence since they will hear you.	If you do not want to be seen by people, take the eyes of a bat together in a new piece of cloth, and hang them on your right arm without uttering a word, since, if you talk, people will become aware of you.	Bat eyes: if you put them in a piece of cloth taken from a sarcophagus, hang them on your right arm, then nobody will see you, if you do not talk.
53.3	Then, remove them, and hang them on your left arm, and then you will see people, but they will not see you.	And when they become aware of you, throw the eyes on the ground, then take them again, and hang them on your left arm, and then you will see people without being seeing again. The bat, whose eyes you take, has to be slaughtered.	If you want it to overcome this, remove this purse and throw it on the ground, then take it again, and place it on your left arm, then you will see people, but you will not be seen by them, and this is amazing.
53.4	If a woman happens to lose her babies, take a bat in her name, slaughter it and hang it on her when she gives birth.	Take a bat, slaughter it, hang it on the neck of a woman, then no child of hers will die.	If you want that a woman does not lose her baby, take a bat, dry it, once it has dried, hang it on the neck of the woman while she is pregnant, and then she will never lose a baby again.

53.5	يؤخذ خفاش ويذبح ويطبخ في قدر ويؤخذ دهنه فاطلِ به عرق الانسان فيسكن باذن الله تعالى	*om.*	اذا أخذ الخفاش وذبح وطبخ بزيت او غيره من الادهان الى ان ينهري وادهن به صاحب الافساء ابرأه
53.6	يؤخذ ذرق الخفاش ويسحق ويعجن معه زرنيخ احمر ويلطخ به الشعر فلا ينبت ابدا	*om.*	ذرق الخفاش اذا مع زرنيخ احمر وشيء من نورة وخلط الجميع وطلى به الشعر لم ينبت مكانه من اي مكان شئت من الجسد
53.7	اذا اردت ان تجمع الحمام فخذ ثلثة من ذلك الطيور وهو الخفاش وعلقهم على شجرة طويلة فان الحمام تجتمعون اليها	تأخذ من الخفاش ثلاثة فتعلقهم على شجرة طويلة يجتمع عليها الحمام	اذا اخذ ثلاث طيور من الخفاش وعلقتهم علي شجرة طويلة فان الحمام يجتمع الى تلك الشجرة وهذا جلب الحمام
53.8	للكلف يؤخذ دم الخفاش فاطلِ به الوجه فيذهب الكلف باذن الله	دم الخفاش يطلي بها الكلف يذهبه	دم الخفاش اذا طلى به الكلف اذهبه
53.9	اذا اردت ان تطول الشعر فتاخذ رأس الخفاش يدق ناعما ويطلِ به راس الاقرع والقصير الشعر فانه يطول الشعر ويربيه ويحسنه	رأس الخفاش تدق وتطبخ ويلطخ به رأس الانسان القليل الشعر يكثر ويحسن نباته	واذا ذبح الخفاش واخذ رأسه واذيب ولطخ به رأس الاقرع انبت فيه الشعر وغزره وحسنه
53.10	يؤخذ مرارة الخفاش وشوك الغبيراء فاسحق الجميع واكحل به صاحب الغشاوة فيحد نظره ويقوي باذن الله تعالى	وماء شوك الغبيراء يخلط جميعا ويكتحل به للغشاوة في العين وظلمة البصر	مرارة الخفاش وشوك الغبيراء المدقوق ناعما وخلطا واكتحل من ذلك من في عينيه غشاوة اذهبها

53.5: (a) قدر] قدرة B | فاطلِ] اطلي B
(c) وادهن] فاذا انك دهنت C | الافسا] الفسا C
53.6: (a) معه زربيخ] بزرينج B | ويلطخ] ويطلي B | الشعر فلا ينبت] موضع الشعر فلا يعود يطلع B
(c) ارزنيخ] زربيح L | مع رزنيخ] مع شيء من زرنيخ C | من اي مكان شئت] شيء من الشعر في مكان C
53.7: (a) ذلك الطيور وهو الخشاف] ذلك الطيور وهو الخشاف B | وعلقهم] وعلقه B
(c) طيور] من اطيار C | وهذا] وهذا هو C
53.8: (c) *om.* C
53.9: (a) ويطلِ] ويطلي B
(c) *om.* C
53.10: (a) فاسحق] يسحق B
(c) الغبيراء] العنبر L | *om.* C

53.5	If a bat is taken, slaughtered, cooked in a cooking pot, its grease taken, and rubbed on the vein of a man, then he will be calmed, with the permission of God, may He be exalted.	*om.*	If a bat is taken, slaughtered, cooked with olive oil—or another kind of oil—until it is well done, then it is rubbed on the man suffering from winds, this will cure him.
53.6	Bat droppings of: if they are taken, ground, kneaded with realgar (red arsenic), spattered on the hair, then it will never grow again.	*om.*	Bat droppings: if they are taken with realgar (red arsenic) with some lime, everything is rubbed on the hair, then it will not grow there, on whatever part of the body you want.
53.7	If you want that the pigeons gather, take three of these birds—that is the bat—and hang them on a high tree, then the pigeons will gather there.	If you take three bats, hang them on a high tree, then the pigeons will gather there.	If three bats are taken and hung on a high three, then the pigeons will gather on this three, and this attracts pigeons.
53.8	Against freckles: take the blood of a bat, rub it on the face, then the freckles will disappear, with the permission of God, may He be exalted.	Bat blood: if it is rubbed on the freckles, then they will disappear.	Bat blood: if it is rubbed on the freckles, then they will disappear.
53.9	If you want that the hair becomes longer, take the head of a bat, mince it finely, and rub it on the head affected by the ringworm and with just a few hair, then this will strengthen it, increase it and make it nicer.	Bat head: if it is minced, cooked, the head of a man who has a few hair is spattered with it, then the hair will increase and grow nicely.	If a bat is slaughtered, its head is taken, liquefied and spattered on the head with ringworm, then this will make the hair grow, become stronger and nicer.
53.10	Bat gall: if it is taken with thorns of rowan, everything pounded, and rubbed on the eye of a man with cataract, then this will sharpen and strengthen his eyesight.	And with water of thorns of rowan—everything mixed together—it has to be rubbed on the eye affected by cataract and obscuration of the eyesight.	If the gall of a bat and finely ground thorns of rowan are mixed, and rubbed on the eye of a man affected by cataract, then this will disappear.

53.11	*om.*	ومن أخذ من شعر انسان وفتل منه خيطا ثم ربطه وتركه يطير لم ينم ذلك الانسان ما دام [عليه]	اذا اردت ان تعقد نوم الانسان فخذ من شعره وافتله خيطا وخذ خفاشا واعقد في عنقه ثلاث عقد على اسم الشخص فان عملت معه خيرا فاحبس عندك الخشاف والاهلك الشخص
53.12	دم الخفاش اذا طلى به بيت النمل مات فيه ولا يقربه نمل ابدا	الشعر في عنق الخفاش اذا جعل على جحر النمل رأس الخفاش فنى	اذا اردت ان يهلك النمل فخذ خفاشا فانتف ريش جناحه وسبيه في بيت النمل فلا يظهر منه نملة
53.13	رأس الخفاش اذا دفن في برج الحمام يعمر ويكثر الحمام فيه	وان دفن في برج حمام لم يذهب من ذلك البرج شيء من ذلك الحمام	*om.*
53.14	*om.*	دم الخفاش يستعمل في الاكحال النافع من الغشاوة في العين والظلمة في البصر	*om.*
53.15	رؤوس الخفاش اذا طبخ في اناء من نحاس او من حديد والقي عليها دهن زنبق غمره وطبخ حتى ينهري وأخذ ذلك الدهن وادهن به صاحب النقرس برأه وكذلك صاحب الرعشة والفالج والبهق	للفالج والنقرس والارتعاش يؤخذ رأس الخفاش فيطبخ في اناء النحاس او حديد بدهن زنبق جيد قدر ما يغمره مرات ثم يطبخ حتى ينهري ويصفي ذلك الدهن ويدهن به الفالج وصاحب النقرس والمرتعش والمتورم الجسد ومن به بهق نافع ان شاء الله تعالى	للنقرس العتيق والرعشة في اليدين والرجلين تأخذ خمس رؤوس من رؤوس الخفاش فاجعلهم في قدر نحاس واجعل عليهم غمرهم دهن زنبق واجعلهم في شمس حاده عشر ايام وان طبخ حتي نتهري كان ابلغ ويؤخذ دهنه ويدهن به الذي يكون به الارتعاش والنقرص والمفلوج ومن به بهق ومن في جسده الورم فيذهب الجميع باذن الله تعالى
53.16	اذا اردت طرد الحيات من المكان خذ قلب الخفاش وادفنه في ذلك المكان فلا يقربه شيء من الحيات	يؤخذ الخفاش فيذبح ويؤخذ قلبه فيدفن في البيت فلا يدخل ذلك البيت شيء من الحيات ولا من العقارب	اذا اردت ان تطرد الحيات من الدار فخذ خفاش فشق جوفه واستخرج قلبه وادفنه في بعض زوايا الدار فلا يقربها عقرب ابدا ولا حية

53.11: (a) واعقد] واربطه B | فان عملت...الشخص] وخليه يطير فلا ينام ذلك الشخص فان خفت عليه فاحبس الخشاف والا يهلك الشخص B
53.12: (a) يهلك] يهرب B | ريش] ريشه B | بيت] بيوت B | منه] منهم B
(c) بيت النمل] النمل C | فيه] جميع ما فيه C | نمل] *om.* C
53.13: (c) يعمر ويكثر] عمر وكثر B
53.15: (b) زنبق] زيبق T
(c) للنقرس] للنقرص S | اذا طبخ] طبخت رؤوس الخفاش اذا أخذ *add.* C | وطبخ حتى ينهري] الى ان تهتري وطبخت به C | وادهن] واندهن C
53.16: (a) *om.* B
(c) اذا اردت...الحيات] قلب الخفاش اذا دفن في مكان لا يقربه حية C

53.11	If you want to bind the sleep of a man, take his hair and twist it like a thread, take a bat and tie three knots on its neck in the name of that man; if you have done this well and kept the bat with you, then this will be the ruin of this men.	If someone takes the hair of a man, twists them making a thread, ties it on the bat, and let it fly, then this man will not sleep as long as this remains on it.	*om.*
53.12	If you want to destroy ants, take a bat, cut the feather of its wing and place them inside the anthill, then not a single ant will come out of it.	Hair on the bat's neck: if the head of the bat is placed on the anthill, then this will be destroyed.	Bat blood: if it is smeared on an anthill, then the ants inside it will die, and not a single ant will approach it again.
53.13	*om.*	And if it is buried under a pigeons loft, then no pigeon will leave the place.	Bat head: if it is buried under a pigeon house, then this will make the pigeon prosper and multiply.
53.14	*om.*	Bat blood: if it is used in an eye salve, then it will be useful against the cataract and the obscuration of the eyesight.	*om.*
53.15	Against chronic gout and tremor of hands and legs: take five heads of bat, put them in a copper cooking pot, add abundant lily oil, place it in the sunlight and leave it there for ten days, and if you cook them until they are well done, this will be even better. Take its oil and rub it on a man affected by gout, tremor, paralysis and vitiligo, swellings on his body, then everything will cease, with the permission of God, may He be exalted.	Against tremor and gout: the head of a bat has to be taken, cooked in a copper or iron vessel with good lily oil—an amount that can cover it several times—then cooked until it is well done, this oil has to be purified, and rubbed on the paralysis, on the man affected by gout, the paralyzed or the swollen one, and the one who is affected by vitiligo, and this will be useful, God, may He be exalted, willing.	Bat heads: if they are cooked in a copper or iron vessel—with the addition of abundant lily oil—until they are well done, this oil has to be taken and rubbed on a man suffering from gout, and then this will cure him. Likewise, this will also cure the man suffering from tremor, paralysis and vitiligo.
53.16	If you want to chase snakes away from the house, take a bat, split its abdomen, take its heart out, and bury it in a corner of the house, then not a single scorpion or snake will approach it again.	If a bat is taken, slaughtered, its heart taken, and buried in the house, then no snake or scorpion will enter this house.	If you want to chase snakes away from a place, take the heart of a bat and bury it in that place, then not a single snake will approach it.

53.17	اذا علقت عليك عين الخفاش منعت من العقرب والحية	*om.*	من عمل معه عيني الخفاش فلم يقربه العقرب ابدا
53.18	*om.*	مرارة الخفاش تمسح بها المرأة التي يعسر عليها ولدها حقوها تلد باذن الله تعالى	اذا عسر الطلق على المرأة فامسح حقوها بمرارة الخفاش فتلد سارعا باذن الله تعالى
53.19	خذ خيطا من النير على اسم المرأة وامها واعقد اربع عقد واحد من اليمين وثلاث من الشمال واربط بذلك فم الخفاش فيقطع عن المرأاة النزيف	للنزيف يؤخذ خيط نير قد نسجته امرأة ويعقد اربعة عقد من اليمنى وثلاثة من الشمال ويربط به فم الخفاش فيسكن عن المرأة	يؤخذ خيط من كتان قد غزلته امرأة وبنتها فتعقده اربع عقد من اليمنى وثلاثة من الشمال فاربط فم الخفاش على اسم المرأة فينقطع عنها النزيف باذن الله تعالى
53.20	اذا اردت ان تقطع العلة التي تكون تحدث للمرأة في الباطن يؤخذ قطع من شحم الخفاش يجعل في قطنة وتحمل به المرأة فانها تبرأ	واذا اردت المرأة ان ينقطع عنها هذه العلة تأخذ شحم الخفاش فتمسكه مرارا ينقطع عنها الدم	اذا كانت المرأة بها علة الاحشاء يؤخذ شحم من الخفاش وتحمل به المرأة فتهدي باذن الله تعالى
53.21	اذا اردت المرأة لا تحبل اذبح خفاشا وارم جوفه واجعل الخفاش في وسادة المرأة وهي نائمة فانها لا ترجع لتحمل بولد	وان اردت ان تحبك فخذ خفاشا واذبحه واخرج كلما في بطنه في قطنة وضعه تحت رأس المرأة فانها تحبك	يؤخذ خفاش ويذبح ويستخرج منه جميع ما في جوفه ويجفف ويجعل في الوسادة تحت رأس المرأة اذا حب معها الرجل فلا تحبل ابدا
53.22	دماغه اذا اذيب وطلى به تحت قدم الرجل فانه يزيد في النكاح ويقوي الجماع	يؤخذ دماغ الخفاش يمسح به قدمه يزيد في الجماع	ان اردت ان تقوي على الجماع فخذ دماغ الخفاش وادهن به تحت قدميك فانه عجيب

53.17: (a) *om.* B
(c) منعت] امنعت C | والحية] والحية فائدة *add.* C
53.19: (a) يؤخذ] تأخذ B | من كتان] *om.* B | قد غزلته] قد شجته B | فاربط] واربط B | فينقطع] ينقطع B
(c) واعقد اربع] *om.* C | بذلك] بهذا الخيط C | فيقطع] يقطع C
53.20: (a) شحم من الخفاش] من شحم الخشاف B | به] بها B | فتهدي] فتبرأ B
(c) *om.* C
53.21: (a) *om.* B
(c) لتحمل بولد] تضرب بولد ابدا C
53.22: (a) This recipe is attested only in B
(c) دماغه] دماغ الخفاش C | قدم] القدم C | فانه...الجماع] اهاج النكاح وزاد الباه وقوى الجماع C

53.17	If a man carries the eyes of a bat with him, then the scorpions will never approach him.	*om.*	If you hang the eye of bat on your body, then this will protect you from scorpions and snakes.
53.18	If the labour pains are difficult for a woman, wipe her groin with the gall of a bat, then she will quickly give birth, with the permission of God, may He be exalted.	Bat gall: if the groin of a woman who has a difficult labour is rubbed with it, then she will give birth, with the permission of God, may He be exalted.	*om.*
53.19	If a linen thread—that a woman and her daughter have already spun—is taken, four knots are tied from the right side and three from the left one, then this is used to sew the bat mouth in the name of a woman, then this will stop her bleeding, with the permission of God, may He be exalted.	Against the bleeding: a thread from the weft that a woman has already woven has to be taken, four knots have to be tied from the right side and three from the left, then the mouth of a bath has to be sewn with it, and then the bleeding will leave the woman.	Take a thread from the weft in the name of a woman and her mother, tie four knot first from the right side and then three from the left, sew the mouth of the bat with it, then this will stop her bleeding.
53.20	If a woman is affected by the illness of the bowels, take the fat of a bat, the woman should carry it, and then she will recover, with the permission of God, may He be exalted.	If you want that this illness leaves a woman, take the fat of a bat, she has to hold it for some times, and then the bleeding will leave her.	If you want that the disease which affects the woman inside her abdomen stops, a piece of bat fat has to be taken, put it in a cotton cloth, and the woman should carry it, and then she will recover.
53.21	If a bat is taken, slaughtered, everything that is inside its abdomen is taken out, dried, and put inside a pillow under the head of a woman when she makes love to a man, then she will never get pregnant.	If you want that she gets pregnant, take a bat, slaughter it, take out what is inside its abdomen wrapped in a cotton piece of cloth, and place it under the head of the woman, and then she will get pregnant.	If you want that a woman does not get to pregnant, slaughter a bat, extract what is inside its abdomen, and put it inside the pillow of the woman, while she is asleep, and then she will never get pregnant.
53.22	If you want to give power to the coitus, take the brain of a bat, and rub it under your feet, then this will be amazing.	Bat brain: if a man's feet are rubbed with it, then he will be greater in the coitus.	Its brain: if it is liquefied, and rubbed under the feet of a man, then he will increase in his sexual intercourse, and this will also give power to the coitus.

53.23	لعسر البول يؤخذ الخفاش ويطبخ حتى ينهرا ويُرفع في اناء فاذا احتجتَ الى النكاح فخذ من ذلك الدهن نقطة وامسح به الاحليل فانه يدرّ البول باذن الله تعالى	لعسر البول يطبخ الخفاش حتى ينهري ثم يؤخذ ذلك المرق فيمسح به الاحليل فيدر البول	اذا أخذ الخفاش وذبح وطبخ الى ان ينتهري ومسح بدهنه الاحليل والمحالب ادر لبول العسر
53.24	للقولنج يؤخذ الخفاش يسلق ويجعل في اناء واسع ويجلس فيه صاحب القولنج فيبرأ باذن الله تعالى	يؤخذ ذرق الخفاش فيلقي في الاتون ويقعد فيه من به القولنج يبرأ باذن الله تعالى	اذا أخذ خفاش والقي في قدر واغلي عليه وصب في اناء واسع واجلس فيه صاحب القولنج ابرأه
53.25	يؤخذ دم الخفاش ويجفف ويسحق ويداف بالعسل ويكتحل به صاحب الغشاوة والبياض والبرة في العين فيبرأ باذن الله تعالى	دم الخفاش ينفع من نزول الماء في العين اذا خلط بالعسل بعد ان يحرق ويكتحل به وان اردت ان تعقد النورة فالقي فيها من ذرق الخفاش قليل	دم الخفاش اذا احرق وسحق واذيف بعسل بلا نار واكتحل به من بعينيه بياض ابرأ
53.26	*om.*	وان اردت ان تسمّن البازي فخذ خفاشا واذبحه وجففه وخذ منه وتكون جميع ذلك قدر نصف مثقال يدق دقا ناعما ويصير في لقمتين او ثلاث وينزل حتى يرمي به فاذا رمى فعشّه بقدره	*om.*
53.27	من اراد ان يحفظ ويقل نسيانه فيأكل الخفاش مطبوخا فانه ويقوي الحفظ ويقل نسيانه باذن الله تعالى	*om.*	من اراد ان يجود الحفظ ويقل نسيانه فاليكل خفافيشا مشوية

53.23: (a) الى ذلك [الى النكاح B
(c) اذا تعسر [العسر | C به [بدهنه | C اذا ذبح الخفاش [اذا...وذبح C
53.24: (a) *om.* B
(c) من به [صاحب | C وجلس [واجلس | C وترك [وصب | C *add.* الى ان يطبخ جدا [واغلي عليه C
53.25: (a) *om.* B
(c) ثم اكتحل [واكتحل | C واذيب [واذيف C
53.27: (a) يزيد في الذهن ويقوي الحفظ ويذكر ويطرد النسيان [ويقوي...تعالى B
(c) من أكل خفاشا مشويا جاد حفظه لكل شيء ونقل نسيانه [من اراد...مشوية C

53.23	Against urine retention: if a bat is taken, cooked until it is well done and preserved in a vessel; then, when you need to have sexual intercourse, take a drop of this oil and rub it on the outer opening of the urethra, then the urine will flow easily, with the permission of God, may He be exalted.	Against urine retention: if a bat is cooked until it is well done, then this broth is taken and rubbed on the outer opening of the urethra, then the urine will flow easily.	If a bat is taken, slaughtered, cooked until it is well done, this oil is rubbed on the outer opening of the urethra and the ureter, then this will make the urine flow easily.
53.24	Against the colic: if a bat is taken, boiled, put in a large vessel, then a man affected by a colic sits on it, then he will heal, with the permission of God, may He be exalted.	If the droppings of a bat are taken, put inside an oven, then a man affected by a colic sits on it, then he will heal, with the permission of God, may He be exalted.	If a bat is taken, put in a cooking pot, boiled, poured into a large basin, and a man suffering from colic sits there, then this will cure him.
53.25	Bat blood: if it is taken, dried, ground, mixed with honey, and rubbed on the eye of a man affected by cataract, glaucoma, and sty, then he will heal, with the permission of God, may He be exalted.	The blood of the bat is useful against the water that leaks from the eye, if it is mixed with honey—after that it has been burnt—and applied on the eye. And if you want that lime congeals, add some bat droppings to it.	Bat blood: if it is burnt, ground, and mixed with honey—but not on the fire—and rubbed on the eyes affected by glaucoma, then this will heal.
53.26	*om.*	If you want that a hawk gains some weight, take a bat, slaughter it, dry it, take the amount of half *miṯqāl* of it, grind it into a fine powder, then it has to be made in two or three morsels, and pushed down its throat until it refuse it; and when it refuses this, then the hawk has reached its good size.	*om.*
53.27	The one who wants to have good memory and reduce his forgetfulness should eat a cooked bat, then he will strengthen his memory and reduce his forgetfulness, with the permission of God, may He be exalted.	*om.*	The man who wants to improve his memory and reduce his forgetfulness should eat roasted bats.

53.28	*om.*	*om.*	اذا اردت ان ترقد انسانا فخذ زغب خفاش واطرحه في قدح شراب واسقه لمن شئت فانه ينام من وقته وساعته
53.29	اذا اردت ان يسهر الانسان فخذ جلد رأس الخفاش واجعل في الوسادة التي ينام عليها فانه لا ينام ما دامت تحت رأسه	*om.*	جلد رأس الخفاش اذا جعل تحت رأس انسان وهو لا يعلم فانه لا ينام ما دام تحت رأسه
53.30	*om.*	زبل الخفاش يسحق ويعجن بالخل ويطلي به اللقوة فيبرأ	*om.*
53.31	يؤخذ زبل الخشاف ويسحق ويخلط معه زيت واطلِ به موضع الشعر فلا يطلع ابدا والله أعلم بالصواب	وان اردت ان لا ينبت الشعر في اي موضع شئت من البدن فخذ خفاشا وجففه واسحقه واخلط معه زيت وتدهن به اي موضع شئت من البدن فانه لا ينبت في شعر	زبله اذا اذيف بالزيت الطيب وطلى به اماكن الشعر فانه لا ينبت فيها شعر ابدا باذن الله تعالى

53.28: (c) اذا...انسانا] *om.* C | فخذ...وساعته] زغب خفاش اذا طرح في قدح شراب من شربه نام لوقته وساعته C
53.29: (a) جلد رأس] رأس B | لا ينام] ما ينام B
(c) جلد...جعل] واذا وضع جلد راس الخفاش C
53.31: (a) يؤخذ] *om.* B | واطلي] وأطلِ B | والله اعلم بالصواب] بحمد الله تحت منافع اعضاء الخفاش B
(c) زبله] زبل الخفاش C | اذيف] ذوب C | فيها شعر ابدا] فيها شيء من الشعر بعد ذلك ابدا C | In C another recipe is added, with bat droppings against the cataract: ذرق الخفاش اذا اكتحل به ازال الطغر والغشاوة والدمعة من العين والبياض الحادث

53.28	*om.*	*om.*	If you want that a man falls asleep, take the fuzz of a bat, throw it in a drinking bowl full of wine, give this to drink to whomever you want, then he will sleep from that very moment onward.
53.29	If you want that a man cannot find any sleep, take the skin from the head of a bat, put it inside the pillow on which he sleeps, then he will not sleep as long as it remains under his head.	*om.*	Skin of bat head: if it is placed under the head of a man—and he is not aware of it—then he will not sleep as long as this remains under his head.
53.30	*om.*	Bat excrement: if it is ground, kneaded with vinegar, and rubbed on the facial paralysis, then this will heal.	*om.*
53.31	Bat excrement: if it is taken, ground, mixed with oil, and rubbed on the part where the hair is, then it will never grow again, and God knows what is right.	If you want that the hair does not grow on any part of the body you want, take a bat, dry it, grind it, mix it with oil, rub with it any part of the body you want, and then no hair will grow there.	Its excrement: if it is mixed with good oil, and rubbed on a part of the body covered in hair, then the hair will never grow there again, with the permission of God, may He be exalted.

٥٤. ذكر منافع ابو تمرة

	a	b	c
	ذكر منافع ابو تمرة	—	—
54.1	يؤخذ هذا الطير يذبح ويشوي ويأكله صاحب القولنج فيبرأ باذن الله تعالى وان سمّطه وتحسي مرقته كان ابلغ والله اعلم بذلك	—	—
54.2	زبل هذا الطائر يذاف بدهن ورد ويطلي به الفالج فيبرأ باذن الله تعالى والله اعلم بالصواب	—	—

54.1: (a) يذبح] فيذبح B | وتحسي مرقته] وغلى وشرب مرقته B | ابلغ] انفع B
54.2: (a) يداف] يذاب B

54. *Abū Tamra* Bird

	a	b	c
	Exposition of the useful properties of the *Abū Tamra* bird	–	–
54.1	If this bird is taken, slaughtered, roasted, and fed to a man suffering from colic, then he will recover, with the permission of God, may He be exalted.	–	–
54.2	Excrement of this bird: if it is mixed with rose oil, and rubbed on the paralysis, then this will heal, with the permission of God, may He be exalted, and God knows what is right.	–	–

٥٥. الحمام

	a	b	c
	ذكر منافع اعضاء الحمام	الحمام	باب منافع الحمام
55.1	اذا كان الباز صعوبا نفورا فخذ فرخ حمام فاذبحه وشق حلقومه يوما وليلة فاذا كان بالغداة فاطعمه للباز بالبورق ويصلح ويقوي للحسّي	اذا كان البازي نفور مستصعب فخذ فرخ الحمام وشد حلقه وعلقه برأسه يوما فاذا كان من الغداة فاطعمه للبازي فان نفاره وصعوبته تذهب	اذا كان البازي نفورا خذ فرخ الحمام ابن يوم وليلة فاذا كان الغداة اطعم البازي ذلك الفرخ فانه يصلح ويزيل نفره
55.2	دماغ فرخ الحمام يذاب بالورق والسذاب ويطلي به بدن المحموم فيذهب الحمى باذن الله	دماغ الحمام يذاب بماء البورق وشراب ويسحق ويطلي به بدن المحموم فانه يسكن حماه واذا شرب منه بعسل وماء فانه ينفع من المليلة والصفاء	ادمغة الحمام اذا اذيبت بالبورق والسذاب وجففت وسحقت ناعما وعجنت بالخل وطلى بها جسد المحموم زالت حماه
55.3	للبرص يؤخذ زبل حمام ابيض يجفف ويسحق ويذاف بخل خمر ويطلي به البرص فيزول باذن الله تعالى	دم الحمام يجفف ويسحق ويعجن بالخل ويطلي به البرص يغير لونه والبرص ايضا يؤخذ من دم حمامة سوداء جزء ومن دم الفواخت جزء ومن الزفت جزء فيخلط جميعا ويطلي به البرص فيذهب ويغير لونه	دماغ الحمام اذا جفف وسحق وعجن بالخل وطلى به بدن الابرص ابرأه وغير لونه
55.4	صدور الحمام تطبخ ويلقي عليها بورق ويسقي صاحب وجع الكبد بعسل نحل فيزول باذن الله تعالى	لوجع الكبد يؤخذ جزء من خراء الحمام فيطبخ حتى ينهري ويخلط معه بورق ويسقي بعسل وماء	صدور فراخ الحمام تطبخ حتى تنهري ويلقي عليها بورق مسحوق ويسقي لمن به وجع الكبد بعسل وماء حار يبرأه

55.1: (a) This recipe is attested only in B
(b) In T another recipe is added, with a diet for the hawk based on pork meat: وان كان بالباز قروح في حلقه فاطعمه بالغداة لحم خنزير يذر عليه حيث الحديد يفعل ذلك ثلاثة ايام متوالية فانه يبرأ
(c) كان] كانت C | نفره] نفر منه C
55.4: (a) يؤخذ] *om.* B | زبل] دم B | ويداف] ويذاب B | بخل خمر] بالخل والسمن B

55. Pigeon

	a	b	c
	Exposition of the useful properties the parts of the pigeon	**Pigeon**	**Chapter on the useful properties of the pigeon**
55.1	If the hawk has some difficulty and is skittish, take a pigeon chick, split its throat and leave it open for one day and one night; when the morning comes, feed it to the hawk with natron, then the hawk will be fine and stronger.	If the hawk is scared and uncomfortable, take a pigeon chick, tie its body, hang it from its head for one day; then when the morning comes, feed it to the hawk, and then its fear and uneasiness will disappear.	When the hawk is skittish, take a pigeon chick which is one day and one night old, when morning comes feed the hawk with this chick, then he will be fine and its skittishness will come to an end.
55.2	Pigeon chick brain: if it is mixed with natron and rue, rubbed on the body of a feverish man, then the fever will cease, with the permission of God, may He be exalted.	Pigeon brains: if it they are mixed with natron water and wine, ground, rubbed on the body of a feverish man, then this will calm his fever. If it is drunk with honey and water, then it will be useful against the feverish heat and for purity.	Its brain: if it is mixed with natron and rue, dried, ground into a fine powder, kneaded with vinegar and rubbed on the body of a feverish man, then the fever will cease.
55.3	Against leprosy: if the excrement of a white pigeon are taken, dried, ground and mixed with wine vinegar, rubbed on the leprosy, then it will disappear, with the permission of God, may He be exalted.	Pigeon blood: if it is dried, ground, kneaded with vinegar, rubbed on the leprosy, then this will change its colour and the leprosy iself too. If one part of black pigeon blood, one part of collared pigeon blood, one part of pitch are taken, mixed together, rubbed on the leprosy, then this will go away and its colour will change.	Pigeon brain: if it is dried, ground, mixed with vinegar, and rubbed on the body affected by leprosy, then this will change its colour.
55.4	Pigeon chests: if they are cooked with the addition of some natron, given to a man suffering from liver complaint to drink with honey, then this will cease, with the permission of God, may He be exalted.	Against liver complaint: if one part of pigeon excrement is taken, cooked until it is well done, natron is mixed with it, and given to drink with honey and water, [then it will be useful].	Pigeon chicks chests: if they are cooked until they are well done, some ground natron is added to them, and this is given to a man suffering from liver complaint with honey and warm water to drink, then this will cure it.

55.5	اذا امسك الحشيمة على المطلقة فتبخر بزبل حمام فانها ترميها	زبل الحمام تبخر به المرأة التي يسقط البشيمة فتسقطها	زبل الحمام اذا بخرت به المطلقه التي امسكت البشيمة عليها ارمتها لوقتها
55.6	يؤخذ زبل حمام برّي يذاب بماء حار ويطلي به جسد صاحب وجع المفاصل فيذهب عنه باذن الله تعالى	زبل الحمام فيه حرارة شديدة وهو يطبخ في الحقن النافعة للقولنج ويلطخ ايضا على تشبيك المفاصل التي تكون من البرد يغسل الموضع بالماء الحار ويلطخ عليه خرء حمام فانه ينفعه نفعا بينا	واذا اذيف زبل الحمام بماء حار وغسل به المفاصل ابرأها من وجعها وتشكي وزبل الحمام البرّي اجود
55.7	لوجع الخاصرة والمثانة والحرقان في الاحليل يؤخذ زبل حمام جزء ومن الخولنجان جزء ويسحق الجميع ويعجن بعسل ويستعمل منه صاحب هذا المرض وزن مثقال بماء حار فيبرأ	ومن أخذ من ذرق الحمام جزء ومن الخولنجان جزء ويذاف ينحل ويعجن بالعسل ويشرب منه وزن مثقال لوجع الخاصرة وتقطير البول ووجع المثانة والحرقة في الاحليل ويزيد في الباه	اذا اخذ من زبل الحمام جزء ومن الخولنجان جزء ودق الجميع وعجن بعسل وشرب منه مثقال لوجع الخاصرة والحرقان التي في الاحليل ويزيد في الباه
55.8	يؤخذ زبل حمام واسطراطيقوس وحب النيل من كل واحد جزء يبخر به وكل من شمّ من ذلك البخور فلا ينام والله اعلم	يؤخذ زبل حمام ووشق وحب النيل من كل واحد جزء ويبخر فيطرد النوم والغشاوة	اذا أخذ زبل الحمام وشيطرج وحب نيل من كل واحد جزء وبخر به فكل من شم ذلك البخور فانه ينام
55.9	للغشاوة في العين يؤخذ حمام مسرول ابيض فيذبح ويؤخذ رأسه فيحرق حتى يصير رمادا ويسحق ناعما ويكتحل به من في عينيه عشاوة وفتزول باذن الله تعالى	يؤخذ حمام مسرول ابيض فيذبح ويؤخذ رأسه فيحرق بريشه حتى يصير رمادا ويسحق به للعمش نافع	الابيض المسرول اذا ذبح وأخذ رأسه واحرقت بريشها وصارت رمادا واسحق واكتحل به من في عينيه غشاوة او عمش ابرأه
55.10	*om.*	مرارة الحمامة البيضاء يكتحل بها للغشاوة في العين وظلمة البصر	*om.*

55.5: (a) فيبرأ] فيزول C
55.6: (a) This recipe is attested only in B
55.7: (a) جسد] *om.* B | وجع المفاصل...الاحليل] ينفعه وجع الخاصرة والمثانة والحرفان في الاحليل B
55.8: (a) This recipe is attested only in B
55.9: (a) واسطراطيقوس] واسطرنس S; واسطرقس B | وكل من] فمن B | فانه لا ينام] فلا ينام B
55.10: (a) غشاوة] غشاوة وعمش *add.* B

55.5	If a repudiated woman is taken by shyness, she has to be fumigated with pigeon excrement, then she will get rid of it.	Pigeon excrement: if a woman who happens to have nausea is fumigated with it, then then she will immediately drop it.	Pigeon excrement: if a free woman who is taken by shyness is fumigated with pigeon excrement, then she will instantly expel it.
55.6	Wild pigeon excrement: if it taken, mixed with warm water, rubbed on the body of a man suffering from joints pain, then this will cease, with the permission of God, may He be exalted.	Pigeon excrement: in it there is a strong hotness, and it is prepared in clysters that are useful for the colic: it is also spattered on the connection of the joints in which there is coldness, and the part is washed with warm water, and the pigeon excrement is spattered on it, then this will clearly be useful.	Pigeon excrement: if it is mixed with warm water, and used to wash the joints, then this will cure their pains. Wild pigeon excrement is even better.
55.7	Against the pain of the waist, of the bladder, and the burning of the outer opening of urethra: if one part of pigeon excrement is taken, with one part of galangal, everything ground, kneaded with honey, and one *miṯqāl* of it is applied on a man suffering from one of these diseases with warm water, then this will cure him.	If one part of pigeon droppings is taken with one part of galangal, mixed, dissolved, kneaded with honey, one *miṯqāl* of it has to be drunk against the pain of the waist, urine dripping, bladder complaints, and burning of the outer opening of the urethra, and this will also increase sexual desire.	Pigeon excrement: if one part of it is taken, with one part of galangal, everything ground, kneaded with honey, one *miṯqāl* of it has to be drunk against the pain of the waist and the burning of the outer part of urethra, and this will also increase sexual potency.
55.8	Pigeon excrement, aster, and ipomoea: if one part of each one is taken, and used for fumigations, then everyone who inhales this fumigation will not be able to sleep, and God knows best.	Pigeon excrement, sal ammoniac, and ipomoea: if one part of each one is taken, and used for fumigations, then this will ward off the sleep and the cataract.	Excrements of pigeon, pepperwort, and ipomoea: if one part of each one is taken, and used for fumigations, then everyone who breaths this fumigation will not be able to sleep.
55.9	Against cataract in the eye: if a pigeon with white legs is taken and slaughtered, its head is taken, and burnt until it becomes ash, ground into a fine powder, and rubbed on the eye affected by cataract, then this will cease, with the permission of God, may He be exalted.	If a pigeon with white legs is taken and slaughtered, its head is taken, burnt with its feathers until it becomes ash, and it is ground against rheum, then this will be useful.	Against the cataract, if a pigeon with white legs is slaughtered, its head is taken, burnt until it becomes ash, ground, and rubbed on the eye of a man affected by cataract and rheum, then this will cure him.
55.10	*om.*	White pigeon gall: if it is applied on the eyes, then this will be useful against the cataract in the eye and the obscuration of the eyesight.	*om.*

55.11

خذ من زبل الحمام جزء ومن زبل الخفاش جزء ومن دقيق الكرسنه جزء او من زبد البحر جزء ودق الجميع واذفه بلبن حليب ومخ بيضة واطل به كلف الوجه او البدن فانه يبرأ ويصلح البهق وعلة السوداء

وكذلك دم الحمام اذا دلك به الكلف يؤخذ خرء حمام وخرؤ الخفاش وجزء من دقيق الكرسنة واصول السوس جزئين والمقل الازرق جزء وزبد البحر جزء ويدق الجميع وينخل ويذاف باللبن الحليب ومخ البيض ويطلي به على الوجه نافع

للكلف في الوجه يؤخذ زبل الحمام ومن زبل الخشاف ومن دقيق العدس والكرسنه واصل السوس والمقل الازرق وزبد البحر من كل واحد جزء ويسحق الجميع ثم يعجن بلبن حليب ومخ البيض ويطلي به الوجه والجسد فيزول الكلف باذن الله تعالى

55.12

اذا أخذ من زبل الحمام جزئين ومن قثاء الحمار جزين ومن الفودنج وهو المرزنجوش جزء وثلاث بيضات وجزء من دهن ودقت الادوية وضربه الدهن والبيض ضربا جيدا وطلى به البدن نفع من الكلف والبهق والعلة السوداء

صفة دواء ينفع البهق وغلبه المرة السوداء او الصفراء ومن وجع الوركين يؤخذ خرء الحمام وزن مثقال ومن الفودنج النهري مثقالين ومن المرزنجوش مثقالين ويلت بيضات ودهن ورد مثقالين تدق الادوية كل واحد على حدة ويخلط على الدهن والبيض ويطلي به البدن نافع ان شاء الله

اخر مثله يؤخذ زبل الحمام جزء ومن قثاء الحمار جزئين ومن الفودنج النهري جزء ومن المرزنجوش مثقال ويسحق الجميع ويذاف بثلاث بيضات ودهن ورد وتضرب الجميع ضربا جيدا ويطلي به البدن فانه نافع للاستسقاء

55.13

om.

زبل الحمام اذا زبّل به الكرم اخصب

om.

55.14

اذا أخذ ما في جوف الحمام كما هو بلا غسل وطبخ بخل خمر وزعفران واكله صاحب الاستسقاء ابرأه

اجواف الحمام كما هي بطونها غير منقى ينفع من الاستسقاء واوجاع الجوف

يؤخذ اجواف الحمام المنسوبة ولا تغسلهم فاطبخ الجميع بخل خمر واطعم صاحب المرض فيبرئ باذن الله تعالى

55.15

اذا أخذ ما في اطراف الحمام من الرطوبة واكتحل به صاحب العين المطروقة ابرأه واذا قطر من ذلك في العين التي احتبس فيها الدم نفعها

الدم الذي يكون في اطراف اجنحة الفراخ الصغار يقطر في العين التي تكون قد اصابها طرفة او ضربة واجتمع فيها الدم نافع

اذا انظرت العين واحتبس فيها الدم فيقطّر فيها ثلاث قطرات من دم فرخ حمام فيبرأ باذن الله

55.11: (a) زبل...الخشاف] زبل حمام وزبل خشاف B | ومن دقيق] ودقيق B | والمقل الازرق] ومقل ازرق B | حليب] *om.* B | الكلف] *om.* B
55.12: (a) المرزنجوش] المردكوش S | *om.* B
(b) المرزنجوش] المرزنخوش T
(c) المرزنجوش] المردقوش L
55.14: (a) *om.* B
55.15: (a) In B this recipe is after 55.10 | فيبرأ] نافع B
(b) In T another recipe is added, with the fat of a different bird (*al-ǧarādī*): الجرادي يؤخذ شحم هذا الطائر ويذوب ويمسح به من كان به بواسير فانه ينفع نفعا جيدا

55.11 Against freckles on the face: if pigeon and bat excrement, lentil flour, vetches, liquorice roots, blue bdellium and meerschaum are taken—one part of each one—everything ground, then kneaded with cow milk and yolk, rubbed on the face and the body, then the freckles will disappear, with the permission of God, may He be exalted.

And likewise, pigeon blood: if the freckles are rubbed with it, one part of pigeon excrement and bat excrement, one part of vetches flour, two parts of liquorice roots, one part of blue bdellium, one part of meerschaum are taken, everything ground, sieved, mixed with milk and yolk, and rubbed on the face, then this will be useful.

Take one part of pigeon excrement, one part of bat excrement, one part of vetches flour, and one part of meerschaum, then grind everything, and mix it with cow milk and yolk, rub it on the freckles on the face or on the body, then these will heal, it also cures vitiligo and the disease of the black gall.

55.12 Another similar recipe. If one part of pigeon excrement, two parts of squirting cucumber, one part of river oregano, one *miṯqāl* of sage are taken, everything ground, mixed with three eggs, whipped and rubbed on the body, then this will be useful against the dropsy.

Preparation of the remedy that is useful against vitiligo, the excess of black or yellow gall, and the pain of the legs: if one part of pigeon, two *miṯqāl* of oregano, two *miṯqāl* of marjoram, two *miṯqāl* of crushed eggs and rose oil—every drug crushed by itself—are mixed with the oil and the eggs, rubbed on the body, then it will be useful, God willing.

If two parts of pigeon excrements, two parts of squirting cucumber, one part of oregano—that is marjoram—three eggs and one part of oil are taken, the simple drugs are crushed, the oil and the eggs are whipped, then it is rubbed on the body, this will be useful against freckles, vitiligo and the disease of the black gall.

55.13 *om.*

Pigeon excrement: if they are dropped on the vineyard, then this will become fertile.

om.

55.14 If the entrails of well-bred pigeons are taken, they are left unwashed and everything is cooked with wine vinegar, and given to a man affected by the illness to eat, then he will be cured, with the permission of God, may He be exalted.

Pigeon abdomens, just as they are, uncleaned: these will be useful against dropsy and pain in the abdomen.

If what is inside the abdomen of the pigeons is taken, left unwashed, cooked with wine vinegar and saffron, and given to a man suffering from dropsy to eat, then this will cure him.

55.15 If you look in the eye and see that the blood has coagulated in it, apply three drops of pigeon chick blood, and then this will heal, with the permission of God, may He be exalted.

Blood in the extremities of the wings of small chicks: if it is applied in drops in the eye already suffering from twinkling or pangs, and in which the blood coagulates, [then this will be useful].

If the wetness that can be found in the extremities of a pigeon is taken, and rubbed on the burning eye, then this will cure it. And if this is applied in drops in the eye affected by blood retention, this will be useful for it.

٥٦. الرخم

	a	b	c
	ذكر منافع الرخمة	الرخمة	باب منافع الرخم
56.1	زبل الرخمة يذاف بخل خالص حادق ويطلي به البرص فيغير لونه	زبل الرخمة يذاف بخل حادق عتيق ويطلي به البرص يبرأ	اذا اذيف زبل الرخم وطلى به مواضع البرص اذهبه
56.2	دم الرخمة يغلي في قلب فرخ حمام ويتغرغر به صاحب الخوانيق فيبرأ باذن الله تعالى	دم الرخمة يغلي مع قلب الحجل ويخلط معه فيه نافع	دم الرخمة اذا غلى بدهن الجوز وتغرغر به نفع لذاء العلة
56.3	وان مزج بعسل فكان ابلغ لوجع الحلق وضيق النفس	للخوانيق ووجع الحلق ويتغرغر به ايضا ويذاف بشيء من عسل وماء حار فيسكن وجع الحلق وذيف النفس	واذا خلط بعسل كان ابلغ وينفع ايضا لضيق النفس
56.4	لحم الرخمة يدق ويخلط معه خردل وسذاب ويبخر به المسحور والمعقود فيبرأ باذن الله	لحم الرخمة يدق ويخلط مع خردل وسذاب ويحبب ويبخر به المسحور والمعقو جيد مجرب	لحم الرخم اذا دق وخلط معه خردل وسذاب ودق الجميع وجفف بعد ان حبب وبخر به المعقود انحل عقد
56.5	للصداع دماغ الرخمة يذاف بدهن ورد ويدهن به الرأس ويزول ويسكن الصداع	دماغ الرخمة يذاف بدهن ويدهن به الرأس يسكن الصداع باذن الله نعالى	دماغ الرخم اذا اذيف بدهن ورد وادهن به صاحب الصداع ابرأه
56.6	عظم رأس الرخمة يعلق على من يشتكي الصداع فيبرأ باذن الله تعالى	عظم رأس الرخمة من الجانب الايمن يعلق على من به الصداع في صدفه الايسر يسكن	عظم الرخم الايمن اذا علق على من يشتكي الصداع ان كان من جانب الايمن علق العظم من الجانب الايسر وان كان من الايسر علق من الايمن

56. Egyptian Vulture

	a	b	c
	Exposition of the useful properties of the parts of the Egyptian vulture	**The Egyptian vulture**	**Chapter of the useful properties of the Egyptian vulture**
56.1	Egyptian vulture excrement: if it is mixed with pure acid vinegar and rubbed on leprosy, then this will change its colour.	Egyptian vulture excrement: if it is mixed with old acid vinegar and rubbed on the leprosy, then this will cure it.	If the excrement of an Egyptian vulture are mixed and rubbed on the area affected by leprosy, then this will go away.
56.2	Egyptian vulture blood: if it is boiled inside the heart of a pigeon chick, and a man suffering from suffocation gargles with it, then he will recover.	Egyptian vulture blood: if it is boiled with the heart of a sand grouse, and mixed with what it is inside it, then this will be useful.	Egyptian vulture blood: if it is boiled with nut oil and used to gurgle, then this will be useful for the one affected by the disease.
56.3	And if it is mixed with honey, it will be even more effective against the pain in the pharynx and breath difficulties.	Against the suffocation and the pain in the pharynx: if it is also used to gargle together with some honey and warm water, then the pain of the pharynx will go away and the breath will loosen up.	And if it is mixed with honey, it will be even better, and it will also cure breath difficulties.
56.4	Egyptian vulture meat: if it is minced, mixed with mustard seeds and rue, then an enchanted man or a man tied by magic knots is fumigated with it, then he will recover.	Egyptian vulture meat: if it is minced, mixed with mustard seeds and rue, made in pills, and used to fumigate an enchanted man or a man tied by magic, this will be good: tried out.	Egyptian vulture meat: if it is minced, mixed with some mustard seeds and rue, everything ground and dried after it has been made in pills, then a man tied in magical knots is fumigated with it, this will untie him.
56.5	Against headache: if the brain of an Egyptian vulture is mixed with rose oil and rubbed on the head, then the headache will subside.	Egyptian vulture brain: if it is mixed with essential oil and rubbed on the head, then the headache will subside.	Egyptian vulture brain: if it is mixed with rose oil and a man suffering from headache is rubbed with it, then he will recover.
56.6	Bone in the head of the Egyptian vulture: if it is hung on a man suffering from headache, then he will recover, with the permission of God, may He be exalted.	Egyptian vulture bone from its right side: if it is hung on a man suffering from headache close to his left ear, then this will subside.	Egyptian vulture right bone: when it is hung on a man suffering from headache—if the pain is on the right side, then hang it onto the left one; if, instead, the pain is on the left side, then hang the bone on the right side—[it will be useful].

56.7	للمجنون كبد الرخمة تشوي على نار لينة وتجفف وتسقي منها المجنون ثلثة ايام متواليات فيبرأ باذن الله تعالى	كبد الرخمة تشوي ةتجفف وتسحق وتذاف بخل ويسقي من به جنون ثلاثة ايام في كل يوم مرات فانه يذهب	كبد الرخم اذا شوى وجفف وسحق وشرب منه المجنون ثلاثة ايام متوالية ابرأته واذهبت جنونه
56.8	مخالب الرخمة اليمنى تعلق على من يشتكي القولنج فيبرأ باذن الله تعالى	مخاليب رجل الرخمة اليمنى تعلق على من به القولنج يبرأ باذن الله تعالى	مخالب الرخم اذا علق على من يشتكي القولنج ابرأه
56.9	*om.*	قلب الرخمة يغمس في قطران ويشد في جلد ذئب او جلد ابل من علق عليه لم يخف اللصوص	قلب الرخم اذا غمس في القراط وشد في جلد ايل او جلد ذيب وعلق على الأنسان لا يخاف لصا ولا سارقا واذا علقت في البيت كان محفوظا
56.10	عين الرخمة اليسرى تجفف وتسحق في هاون ويصب عليها دهن ورد وترفع في اناء وتأخذ العين اليمنى وتشد في خرقة فاذا اردت الدخول على السلطان فادهن قليل من ذلك الدهن وعلق العين اليمنى على عضدك الايمن فتقضي حوائجك باذن الله تعالى	يؤخذ عين الرخمة اليسرى في دهن وتجعل في اناء وتؤخذ عينها اليمنى وتصر في خرقة فاذا اردت ان تدخل على السلطان فادهن وجهك من ذلك الدهن وشد العين اليمنى في ذراعك فان حوائجك تقضي	عين الرخم اليسرى اذا جففت وسحقت وجعلت في اناء وصب عليها دهن ورد بقدر الحاجه ويؤخذ عينها اليسرى تصر في خرقة جديدة خضراء فاذا اردت الدخول على السلطان فانك تعظم عنده ويجلك ويقصي حاجتك
56.11	دماغ الرخمة يجفف ويسحق ويذاف بخل ويسقي منه صاحب الخنازير التي تكون في الرقبة فيبرأ باذن الله تعالى	دم الرخمة يخلط بزراوند مسحوق ويطلي به البرص [نافع]	دم الرخم اذا اذيف بخل خمر وشرب منه صاحب الخنازير ذهبت عنه
56.12	*om.*	*om.*	مخالب الرخم اليمنى اذا علقت على من يشتكي القولنج ابرأه

56.10: (c) ويؤخذ] واوخذ C | عينها اليسرى] تصرت العين اليمنى C | حاجتك...فانك] وادخل على عضده الايمن وشد العين من هذا الدهن وجهك ادهن فانك تعظم عنده ويجلك وهو قبول الاعظم النافع لقضاء الحوايج عند الملوك والاكابر *add.* C

56.11: (b) In T this recipes is after 56.9

(c) اذيف] اذيب C

56.12: (c) *om.* C

56.7	For the insane: if the liver of an Egyptian vulture is roasted on a soft fire, dried and given to an insane to eat—in the same quantity for three days—then he will recover, with the permission of God, may He be exalted.	Egyptian vulture liver: if it is roasted, dried, minced, mixed with vinegar, given to an insane for three days to drink—several times every day—then his insanity will go away.	Egyptian vulture liver: if it is roasted, dried, minced and fed to an insane man—in the same quantity for three days—then this will cure its insanity.
56.8	Egyptian vulture right talon: if it is hung on a man suffering from colic, then he will recover, with the permission of God, may He be exalted.	Egyptian vulture right talons: if they are hung on a man suffering from colic, then he will recover, with the permission of God, may He be exalted.	Egyptian vulture talon: if it is hung on a man suffering from colic, then he will recover.
56.9	*om.*	Egyptian vulture heart: if it is dipped in some tar, tied in a wolf or camel skin, then the one who hangs it on himself will not be afraid of thieves.	Egyptian vulture heart: if it is dipped in some alfalfa, tied in the skin of a stag or a wolf, and hung on a man, then he will not be afraid of thieves and raiders. And if it is hung inside a house, then this will be safe.
56.10	Egyptian vulture left eye: if it is dried, ground in a mortar, some rose oil is poured in it, and it is preserved in a vessel, then the right eye is taken and tied in a piece of cloth; and when you want to have a hearing with the sultan, rub yourself with a bit of that oil and hang the right eye on your right arm, and he will grant you your requests, with the permission of God, may He be exalted.	Egyptian vulture left eye: if it is taken in essential oil, put in a vessel, the right eye is taken and placed in a piece of cloth; then, when you want a hearing with the sultan, rub your face with this oil, and tie the right eye on your forearm, then your requests will be granted.	Egyptian vulture left eye: if it is dried, ground, put in a vessel, as much rose oil as you needed is poured on it, then the left eye is taken and put in a new piece of green cloth; then when you want a hearing with the sultan [rub yourself with it], then you will be mightier in his eyes, he will honour you, and grant your requests.
56.11	Egyptian vulture brain: if it is dried, ground, mixed with vinegar, and given to drink to a man suffering from scrofula which affects the neck, then he will recover, with the permission of God, may He be exalted.	Egyptian vulture blood: if it is mixed with ground aristolochia and rubbed on the leprosy, then this will be useful against it.	Egyptian vulture blood: if it is mixed with wine vinegar and a man suffering from scrofula drinks it, then the scrofula will disappear.
56.12	*om.*	*om.*	Egyptian vulture right talon: if it is hung on a man suffering from colic, then this will cure him.

56.13	*om.*	تأخذ الرخمة فتخنقها حتى تموت في يدك اليسرى فاذا ماتت فالقها اربعة اقساط زيتا حتى تنهري واقم المجذوم في ذلك الزيت ثلاثة ايام فانه يبرأ	*om.*
56.14	*om.*	يؤخذ دماغ الرخمة نيئا فيجفف ويسحق ويخلط معه بعض الادوية نافعة للخنازير	*om.*
56.15	يؤخذ ريشة من ريش جناح الرخمة فتجعل تحت رجل المطلقة تلد سريعا	يؤخذ ريشة من ريش الرخمة توضع بين رجلي المرأة فتلد سريعا	اذا وضعت ريشة من الرخم بين [رجلي] المطلقة وضعت الولد سريعا

56.15: (c) بين رجلي المطلقة] بين رجلي المطلقة C

56.13	*om.*	Take an Egyptian vulture, strangle it until it dies in your left hand; when it is dead, immerse it in four measures of oil until it is well cooked, then set the one affected by elephantiasis inside this oil for three days, and then he will recover.	*om.*
56.14	*om.*	Egyptian vulture brain: if it is taken raw, dried, ground, mixed with some drugs useful against scrofula, [then this will be useful against it].	*om.*
56.15	If one of the feathers from the wing of an Egyptian vulture is taken, put under the feet of a woman in labour, then she will quickly give birth.	If a feather of an Egyptian vulture is placed between the feet of a woman, than she will easily give birth.	If you put a feather of an Egyptian vulture between the feet of a woman in labour, then she will quickly give birth.

٥٧. الزرزور

	a	b	c
	—	الزرازير	—
57.1	—	تخلط مع السفطير وتصر مع الدماميل ينفع	—
57.2	—	لحم الزرازير يؤكل يزيد في الباه	—

57. Starling

	a	b	c
	–	**The starlings**	–
57.1	–	If they are mixed with *safṭīr* [?] and tied on the abscesses, then this will be useful.	–
57.2	–	If the meat of the starlings is eaten, then this will increase the sexual desire.	–

٥٨. الحدأة

	a	b	c
	ذكر منافع اعضاء الحدأة	الحدأة	باب منافع الحدأة
58.1	يؤخذ بيض الحدأة وزبل الوبر وورق الاراك فيدق ورق الاراك ويفقش عليه بيض الحدأة واجعل الجميع في قدر واسكر عليه من الزيت فهما اجيدت واطرح عليه زبل الوبر مدقوقا فاذا غلى الجميع فاخرج البيض فارميه وادهن بذلك الزيت البرص الفاضح فانه يغيره ويوقفه باذن الله تعالى	يؤخذ بيض الحدأة وزبل الوبر وورق الاراك يدق ورق الاراك ويفقس البيض في طبخه ويصير عليه الزيت ما احببت ويطرح عليه الورق والزبل مدقوقين ثم اخرج البيض وادهن به من به البرص الذي ينزل منه الدم	بيض الحدأة وزبل الاوز اذا جعل في طاجن والقي عليه من الزيت واغلي غليا جيدا وانزلته عن النار وطليت به البرص والبهق والوضح اذهبه
58.2	واما البرص الذي يسيل منه الدم والماء الاصفر فخذ بيض الحدأة فاقليه في الزيت الطيب المغسول قليا جيدا وأرم البيض وادهن بذلك الزيت مواضع البرص والجذام فانه يزول باذن الله تعالى	واما البرص الذي ينزل منه الماء الاصفر فخذ الحدأة فاقله بالزيت قليا جيدا وأرم بالبيض وادهن بذلك الزيت البرص	واما البرص الذي يسيل منه الماء الاصفر خذ له بيض حدأة واقليه في الزيت قليا جيدا واذهن به البرص فانه يغيره لونه ويوقفه
58.3	يؤخذ دم الحدأة يذاف بماء ورد يخلط معه مسك ويشرب على الريق فانه نافع من ضيق النفس باذن الله تعالى	دم الحدأة يذاف بماء ورد يخلط معه شيء من مسك ويشرب على الريق ينفع من السهر	دم الحدأة اذا اذيف بماء ورد ومسك وشربه على الريق من به ضيق النفس والبهر ابرأه جدا
58.4	يؤخذ مرارة الحدأة تجفف في الظل وتسحق ناعما واكحل بها من كان في عينه صنان وصفار ومن لسعه العقرب فانه يبرأ باذن الله	مرارة الحدأة تنفع تجفف في الظل وتسحق سحقا ناعما ويكتحل من لسعه العقرب في العين في جانب اللسعة وكذلك تفعل بلسعة الزنبور	*om.*

58.1: (b) ويفقش] وينقش T
(c) وزبل الاوز] وزبل الاوز وورق الاراك C | اذا جعل] اذا وضع C | والوضح] *om.* C | فانه يغيره لونه ويوقفه] فانه يوقفه ويغيره لونه C
58.3: (b) الحدأة] الخلد T
(c) اذا اذيف] اذا اذيب C

58. Kite

	a	b	c
	Exposition of the useful properties of the parts of the kite	*om.*	**Chapter on the useful properties of the kite**
58.1	Kite eggs, hyrax excrement, and miswak leaves: if these are taken, the leaves are pounded, the kites eggs broken on top of it, then this is put in a cooking pot, some oil is poured over this all; when it is well done, the pounded excrement of hyrax are added to it; once everything has boiled well, the eggs have to be taken out and thrown away; then if the abominable leprosy is rubbed with this, it will change [its colour] and will be cured, with the permission of God, may He be exalted.	Kite eggs, hyrax excrement, and miswak leaves: if the leaves are minced, the eggs broken on top of it, while it is cooking; an amount of oil of your choosing is added to this, the pounded excrement and the leaves are added, then the eggs are taken out, and a man affected by leprosy that suppurates blood is rubbed with it, [then he will be cured].	Kite eggs and goose excrement: if they are put in a frying pan, some oil is poured on it, then it is left to boil well, removed from the fire and rubbed on the leprosy and the vitiligo, then this will cure them.
58.2	As for the leprosy from which yellow water and blood suppurate, take the eggs of a kite, fry them well with good oil, throw the eggs away and rub this oil on the parts affected by leprosy and elephantiasis, then this will make them cease.	As for the leprosy that suppurates yellow water, fry it well with oil, add the eggs, and rub this oil on the leprosy.	As for the leprosy that suppurates yellow water: against it, take the eggs of a kite, fry them well with oil, and rub this oil on the leprosy, then this will change its colour and will cure it.
58.3	Kite blood: if it is diluted with rose water, mixed with some musk, and drunk on an empty stomach, this will be useful against breathing difficulties, with the permission of God, may He be exalted.	Kite blood: if it is mixed with some musk, and drunk on an empty stomach, then this will be useful against insomnia.	Kite blood: if it is diluted with rose water and musk, then given to a man suffering from breath difficulties and breathlessness to drink, this will effectively cure him.
58.4	Kite gall: if it is taken, dried in the shade, ground into a fine powder, and the eyes affected by pus and festering matter or the man stung by a scorpion are rubbed with it, then this will cure these, with the permission of God, may He be exalted.	Kite gall: it will be useful, if dried in the shade, ground into a fine powder, and rubbed on the eyes of the man who has been stung in the eye by a scorpion, on the side of the sting. The same is done with the sting of the hornets.	*om.*

مرارتها اذا جفت في الظل وسحقت وأخذ منها وزن درهم ورد على سلة الحاوي ماتت الحيات التي فيه

وكذلك اذا جففت وسحقت اذا ذريت منها على الحية ماتت

58.5 يؤخذ مرارة الحدأة تجفف في الظل وتسحق ناعما وتذر على الحيات فتموت واذا اردت ان تعلم صحة ذلك فخذ مرارة الحدأة وجففها في الظل واسحقها وذرها في سلّة الحواي فان جميع الدبيب الذي معه يموت باذن الله تعالى

مخ الحدأة اذا غلى بماء الكمون وشربه بعسل وسنبل من اصابه الاسهال والزحير نفعه وكذا البواسير

مخ الحدأة يقلو بماء الكراث وعسل لمن به اسهال وزحير وبواسير

58.6 مخ الحدأة يغلي بماء الكراث والسعد ويسقي منه صاحب الزحير فيبرأ باذن الله تعالى وان جعلت فيه سنبل الطيب وقرنفل كان ابلغ

58.5: (c) مرارتها] مرارة الحدأة C | جفت] جففت C | فيه] فيها C

58.6: (c) غلى] اغلي C | وشربه] وشرب منه C | والزحير] الاسهال المفرط C | وكذا البواسير] الاسهال C | البواسير وكذا من اصابه الزجير وكذا من اصابه البواسير C

58.5	Kite gall: if it is taken, dried in the shade, ground into a fine powder, and thrown on a snake, then this will die. And if you want to know whether this is true, take the gall of a kite, dry it in the shade, grind it, and strew it in the basket of a snake charmer, then all the reptiles that are with him will die, with the permission of God, may He be exalted.	Likewise, if it is dried, ground, and scattered on a snake, then this will die.	Its gall: if it is dried in the shade and ground, one *dirham* of it is taken, and thrown into the basket of a snake charmer, then the snakes inside it will die.
58.6	Kite marrow: if it is boiled with leek and sedge, given to a man affected by dysentery to drink, then he will recover, with the permission of God, may He be exalted. And if some nardus and clove are added to it, then this will be even more effective.	Kite marrow: cooked with leek water and honey, for the man suffering from diarrhoea, dysentery, and haemorrhoids.	Kite marrow: if it is boiled with cumin water, and drunk with honey and hyacinth by a man suffering from diarrhoea and dysentery, then this will be useful to him. And the same goes for the haemorrhoids.

٥٩. الغراب

	a	b	c
	ذكر منافع الغراب	الغراب الاسود والابقع والغداف	باب منافع الغراب
59.1	يؤخذ غراب اسود جميعه ويحرق ويعجن يسير من رماده بيزيت طيب واطل به رأس الاقرع فينبت الشعر باذن الله تعالى	*om.*	الغراب الاسود اذا حرق وسحق وعجن بزيت وطلى به المواضع التي تريد نبات شعرها انبتها
59.2	يؤخذ قلب غراب اسود يجفف ويسحق ويسقي منه انسان في شهر تموز فانه يمسك عنها لعطش ولا يشرب في ذلك الشهر ماء اكثر من مرتين او ثلاثة	*om.*	قلب الغراب الاسود اذا سحق وجفف واذيف بالماء وشرب منه انسان في شهر تموز او آب لا يصيبه في ذلك الشهر عطش فان الغراب لا يشرب الماء في تموز
59.3	*om.*	يؤخذ غراب اسود يطعم الخبز ينثر ريشه ثم اذبحه وصيره في إناء وسد رأسه وادفنه في زبل رطب واتركه اربعين يوما واخرجه فانك تجد فيه مثل الدود الاسود والابيض فيصير ذلك الدود في طست في الشمس حتى يموت واعزل كل واحد من الدود على حدة ثم خذ من الدود الابيض ثلاثا ومن الاسود ثلاثا واسحق ذلك بسيرج طري ويسعّط به صاحب البرص ويدلك موضع البرص ويدهن من هذا فانه يذهب	اذا أخذ غراب اسود واطعم الحنطة حتى ينتف ريشه وقيل يطعم الخبز وهو الاصح ثم يذبح ويجعل في اناء ويطين عليه ويدفن في الزبل اربعين يوما ثم يظهره يجد فيه دودا بيضاء وسوداء جعل ذلك الدود في طشت نحاس واتركه في الشمس حتى يموت الدود اعزل كل جنس على حده وخذ من الدود الاسود ثلاثا ومن الابيض ثلاثا واسحقهم بشيرج طري وسعط منه صاحب البرص واطله بالباقي فانه يذهب عنه
59.4	*om.*	وان اذاف هذا الدهن شعر اسود لم يبيض	واعلم ان هذا الدهن اذا اصاب الشعر الاسود بيضه

59.1: (c) انبات شعرها انبتها [انبات الشعر بها C

59.2: (c) اذا سحق وجفف [اذا جفف وسحق C | انسان [احد C

59.3: (b) ثلاثا [ثلثا T

(c) غراب اسود [غرابا اسودا C | الحنطة [القمح C | وقيل يطعم الخبز وهو الاصح [*om.* C | يجد [فانك تجد C | دودا بيضاء وسوداء [دودا ابيض واسود C | طشت نحاس [طست من نحاس C | ومن الابيض ثلاثا [*om.* C | حتى يموت الدود اعزل كل جنس على حده [الى ان يموت فاذا مات اعزل الاسود وحده والابيض وحده C | بشيرج طري [بشيء من الشيرج الطري C | منه [به C | فانه يذهب عنه [فان ذلك يذهب عنه ويزيل الاوي عنه C

59. Crow

	a	b	c
	Exposition of the useful properties of the crow	**The black crow, the spotted crow and the raven**	**Chapter on the useful properties of the crow**
59.1	If a whole black crow is taken, burnt, its ash kneaded with good oil, and rubbed on a head affected by ringworm, then the hair will grow there, with the permission of God, may He be exalted.	*om.*	If a black crow is burnt, ground, kneaded with oil, and rubbed on the area where you want the hair to grow, then this will make it grow.
59.2	Black crow heart: if it is taken, dried, minced and given to a man in July to drink, then this will withhold his thirst, and during this month he will not drink water more than two or three times.	*om.*	Black crow heart: if it is minced, dried, mixed with water, and a man drinks it in July or August, then he will not be thirsty during these months, since the crow does not drink water in July.
59.3	*om.*	If a black crow is taken and fed with bread, its feathers will fall out; then slaughter it, put it in a vessel, its opening has to be sealed, and the vessel has to be buried in fresh manure and left there for forty days, and finally taken out. Then you will find black and white worms in it, these worms have to be placed in the sun in a large copper basin until they die; then each kind of worm has to be taken out separately; take three white worms and three black worms, grind them with fresh sesame oil and make it inhale to a leper and rub it on the area affected by leprosy, and then it will disappear.	If a black crow is taken, fed with common wheat until its feathers fall out—it is said that if it is fed with bread the crow will be better—slaughtered, put in a cooking pot, then it is covered with clay and buried in the manure for forty days; then, when it is dug out, white and black worms appear in it; if these worms are put in a large copper basin and left in the sunlight until they die, then the extremities of each worm are cut and three pieces from the black one and three from the white one are taken, ground with fresh sesame oil, then it is inhaled by a leper, and the remaining part is rubbed on him, then the leprosy will leave him.
59.4	*om.*	If this oil is applied on black hair, it will not turn white.	Know that if this oil touches black hair, it will become white.

59.5	وان أخذ من الدود الاسود بل الابيض وسحقته واسقيه انسانا سقط شعره جميع ولا يكاد ينبت ابدا	وان أخذت من الدود وسخنته بالماء وسقيت منه انسانا يتساقط شعره كله ولم ينبت ابدا	*om.*
59.6	لحم الغراب وحوصلته اذا جففا جميعا وسحقا وخلط بعسل وشربه صاحب البرص والبهق في كل يوم ثلاثة قراريط بماء الحلبه نفعه	لحم الغراب وحوصلته تسحق ويخلط معه عسل ويشرب من به بهق في كل يوم ثلاث قراريط بماء الحلبة المغلى المصفى	يؤخذ لحم الغراب وحوصلته يجفف الجميع ويسحق ويخلط معهما عسل نحل ويسقي منه صاحب البهق كل يوم ثلاث قراريط بماء الحلبة فيذهب عنه باذن الله تعالى
59.7	مرارة الغراب اذا اذيف بدهن زنبق ودهن سوسن وطلى به الاحليل عند الجماع فانه يهيج هيجا عظيما	مرارة الغراب تخلط مع دهن سوس ويطلي به الاحليل في وقت الجماع فمن فعل ذلك وجامع امرأته لم ير في عينه مثل الذُباب	يؤخذ مرارة الغراب يذاف بدهن الزنبق او السوسن واطل به الاحليل عند الجماع فان المرأة تحبك حبا شديدا
59.8	مرارة الغراب ومرارة الديك الاسود اذا أخذ من كل واحد جزء واذيف الجميع واكتحل به صاحب الغشاوة ابرأها	الغراب الاسود ومرارة الديك من كل واحد جزء يخلط جميعا ويكتحل به نافع	يؤخذ دم غراب ومرارة ديك ويخلط الجميع واكحل من في عينه ضباب او غشاوة
59.9	*om.*	مرارة الغراب تدق بدهن لوز ويسعّط من به برد في رأسه ينفعه	*om.*
59.10	*om.*	*om.*	للنوم يؤخذ حنك الغراب الجانب الايمن فيشد في ثوب الانسان فلا يزول ناعما ما دام ذلك في ثوبه
59.11	اذا اردت ان احد يبغض شرب الخمر خذ دم الغراب على اسم من تريد واسقيه له في نبيذ فانه يبغض ولا يكاد يراه	واذا اردت ان تبغض انسانا الشراب فخذ دم غراب ابقع فصيره في نبيذ واسقه اياه ينفعه ولا يعود الى شربه	اذا اردت ان تبغض النبيذ فخذ دم غراب على اسم الشخص واسقه له في النبيذ فلا يعود يذكر مسكرا ابدا

59.5: (c) الاسود بل الابيض] الدود الابيض C | واسقيه انسانا سقط] وسقيه لاحد اسقط شعره C
59.6: (a) ثلاث] ثلث T
(c) اذا جففا جميعا وسحقا] اذا جففا وسحقا جميعا C | وشربه صاحب] وشرب منه من اصابه C | نفعه] نفعه من ذلك جدا C
59.7: (a) السوسن] السوسان S
(b) لم ير] لم يرى T
(c) اذا اذيف] اذا اذيفت C | بدهن زنبق ودهن سوسن] بدهن الزنبق ودهن السوسن C | فانه يهيج هيجا عظيما] هيجه وانعظ انعاظا عظيما C
59.8: (c) اذا أخذ] مرارة الغراب ومرارة الديك الاسود اذا أخذ] مرارة الغراب ومرارة الديك C | من كل واحد] واذا أخذت مرارة C | من كل مرارة C | واذيف الجميع] وخلط C | صاحب] من في عينه C | ابرأها] ابرأها وجلي الغشاوة C | المرارتين C
59.11: (c) خذ دم] فخذ من دم C | في نبيذ] في الخمر C | ولا يكاد دياه] فلا يكاد ينظر اليه ابدا C

59.5	*om.*	And if you take the worms, grind them with water, and give this to a man to drink, then all his hair will fall and will never grow again.	And if you take the black or the white worm, grind it and give it to a man to drink, then all his hair will fall and will never grow again.
59.6	Crow meat and its craw: if they are taken, everything is dried, ground, melted with honey and given to a man affected by vitiligo to drink—three carats everyday along with fenugreek water—then the vitiligo will go away.	Crow meat and its crop: if they are ground, dried, mixed with honey, and drunk by a man affected by vitiligo—three carats everyday—along with boiled and purified fenugreek water, [then this will be useful to him].	Crow meat and its crop: if they are dried, ground, melted with honey, and given to a man affected by leprosy and vitiligo to drink—three carats everyday together with fenugreek water—then this will be useful to him.
59.7	Crow gall: if it is taken, mixed with lily or iris oil, and rubbed on the outer opening of the urethra at the moment of coitus, then the woman will passionately love you.	Crow gall: if it is mixed with liquorice oil, rubbed on the outer opening of the urethra at the moment of coitus, then the one who does so and has sexual intercourse with his woman will not see in his eye something like flies.	Crow gall: if it is mixed with lily oil and iris oil, and rubbed on the outer opening of the urethra at the moment of coitus, then this will excite you very much.
59.8	Crow blood and rooster gall: if they are taken, everything mixed and rubbed on an opaque eye and an eye affected by cataract, [then it will be useful].	Black crow and rooster gall: if one part of each one is taken, everything is mixed and applied on the eye, then this will be useful.	Crow gall and rooster gall: if one part of each one is taken, everything mixed, and rubbed on the eyes of a man affected by cataract, then this will cure it.
59.9	*om.*	Crow gall: if it is ground with almond oil and inhaled by someone with the cold humour in his head, then this will be useful to him.	*om.*
59.10	For the sleep: if the right side of the palate of a crow is taken and fastened inside a man's cloth, then he will not stop sleeping as long as this remains inside his cloth.	*om.*	*om.*
59.11	If you want that someone hates wine, take the blood of a crow in his name, give him this to drink with wine, and then he will never drink [wine] again.	If you want that someone hates wine, take the blood of a spotted crow, pour it in the wine and give this to drink to him, and then he will not drink again.	If you want that someone hates the drinking of wine, take the blood of a crow in the name of the person you want, and give him this with wine to drink, then he will hate it and will not even be able to look at it.

59.12	*om.*	بيض الغراب الابقع اذا طرح في النورة وطلى به البدن لم تعمل النورة شيئا	*om.*
59.13	*om.*	دم الغراب الابقع يجفف ويحشي به البواسير ينفع لمن قد فسد سمعه	*om.*
59.14	اذا جفف الغراب وخلط معه عنزروت واذيف بماء السذاب والعسل [و]الشهد بشمعة ولطخ به داخل الاذن وخارجه فانه يحد البصر ويقويه	يؤخذ دم غراب ويخلط معه عنزروت ويذاف بماء السذاب وعسل ويلطخ به المنخرين من داخل وخارج	دم الغراب يخلط معه عنزروت ويذاف الجميع بماء السذاب وشيء من عسل ويلطخ به الاذن من داخل ومن برّا فيزول الضربان باذن الله تعالى
59.15	قلب الغراب ورأسه اذا خففا وسحقا وطرحا في نبيذ وشربه انسان احبك حبا شديدا جدا	قلب الغراب ورأسه يطرح منه في النبيذ فلا يشرب منه انسان الا احبك وكرمت عليه	يؤخذ قلب الغراب ورأسه يجفف الجميع ويسحق ناعما وخذ مقدار درهم على اسم من تريد ان يحبك واجعله في نبيذ واسقيه ذلك الشحص فانه يحبك حبا شديدا
59.16	ذرق الغراب اذا جعل في صوفة وترك تحت لسان من به السعال واكل بعده بصلا مشويا على الريق عند النوم حتى ياوي الى فراشه فانه يبرأ	ذرق الغراب يصير في صوفة مغسولة عند رأس من به السعال ويأكل بصلا مشويا على الريق وحين ياوي الى فراشه ليال متوالية فيذهب عنه السعال	يؤخذ ذرق الغراب يجعل في صوفة بلا غسل ويجعل تحت رأس من يشتكي السعال وخذ بعد ذلك بصلا مشويا على الريق وعند النوم ثلاثة ايام متوالية فيزول باذن الله تعالى
59.17	واذا اردت ان يخرج نصلا من انسان فخذ فرخ غراب شق جوفه والصقه على موضع النصل فانه يخرج بلا اذى	واذا انكسر في بدن انسان نصل او سهم او عضو فخذ دماغ عقعق فيصير على قطنة وألصقه على الموضع فان الذي فيه يخرج باذن الله تعالى	اذا انكسر نصل النشاب في الجسد تأخذ منفحة غراب فتجعلها في قطنة والصقها على الجرح فيخرج النصل بلا كلاب ولا اذى ان شاء الله تعالى

59.14: (c) جفف الغراب] جفف شيء C | عنزروت] غردت C | واذيف] واذيب C | والعسل الشهد بشمعة] وشيء من الشهد C | وخارجه] وظاهرها C | السمع] البصر L | فانه يحد السمع ويقويه] فتق سمع الاصم وقوى السمع C
59.15: (c) في نبيذ وشربه] في النبيذ وشرب منه C
59.16: (c) من به السعال] من اصابه السعال C | حتى] حين C
59.17: (c) واذا اردت...بلا اذى] فرخ الغراب اذا شق جوفه والصقه على مكان الذي فيه النصل من جميع البدن فانه يخرجه C | In C another recipe is added, with crow chicks to open locks: واذا أخذت فرخ الغراب من عشه صغيرا وربط بحل ربطا جيدا تحت الشهرة التي أخذ الفراخ منها فان اياه ياقي من عشه يعود يضعه بحل الحبل فانه يحل فاذا أخذت ذلك العود ووضعته على الاقفال والضباب فانها ينفتح

59.12	*om.*	Spotted crow eggs: if they are added to lime, then the lime will have no effect.	*om.*
59.13	*om.*	Spotted crow blood: if it is dried, and the haemorrhoids are stuffed with it, then it will be useful for the one whose hearing is damaged.	*om.*
59.14	Crow blood: if it is mixed with sarcocolla, everything mixed with rue water and some honey, spattered on the external and internal part of the ear, then the stabs will cease, with the permission of God, may He be exalted.	Crow blood: if it is mixed with sarcocolla, diluted with rue water and honey, spattered in the nostrils, [it will be useful].	If a crow is dried, mixed with sarcocolla, honey and honeycomb wax, then spattered outside and inside the ear, this will sharpen the hearing and will make it more acute.
59.15	Crow heart and its head: if they are taken, minced finely, one dirham of it is taken in the name of the one you want to be loved by, put in wine and given to this person to drink, then he will passionately love you.	Crow heart and its head: if they are thrown in some wine, and if a man drinks from it, then he could not help loving you.	Crow heart and its head: if it is dried, minced, thrown in some wine, and given to a man to drink, then he will love you with great passion.
59.16	Crow droppings: if they are taken, put in a woollen piece of cloth that has not been washed, and this is put under the head of a man suffering from cough; after this, a roasted onion is eaten on an empty stomach for three days at the moment of sleeping, then the cough will go away, with the permission of God, may He be exalted.	Crow droppings: if they are put in a woollen piece of cloth that has been washed next to the head of a man affected by cough, and he eats a roasted onion on an empty stomach; then after he has slept into his bed for a number of nights, the cough will go away.	Crow droppings: if they are put in a woollen piece of cloth, and this is put under the tongue of a man affected by cough, then he eats a roasted onion on an empty stomach at the moment of sleeping and eventually he goes to bed, then this will cure him.
59.17	If the arrowhead of an archer breaks inside the body, take the rennet of a crow, put it in a piece of cotton, make it adhere to the wound, then the arrowhead will come out without any pain or suffering, God, may He be exalted willing.	If an arrowhead, or an arrow, or some kind of body penetrates in the body of a man, take the brain of a magpie, put it in a piece of cotton, make it adhere to the part, and then what is inside it will come out, with the permission of God, may He be exalted.	If you want that an arrowhead comes out from a man, take a chick of crow, split it and make it adhere to the zone where the arrowhead is, then this will come out without any suffering.

59.18	دم الغراب يذاف بخل عنصل ويسقي منه صاحب الطحال ووجع الكبد فيبرأ باذن الله تعالى	مرارة الغراب تذاف بخل العنصل وتشرب على الريق لوجع الطحال والورم	*om.*
59.19	*om.*	*om.*	مرارة الغراب اذا طلى به جسد المسحور ابطل السحر عنه
59.20	*om.*	لحم الغراب يطبخ ويجفف ويدق ويخلط مع صبر وزعفران ويكتحل به العين التي فيها جرب وحرارة وظلمة	*om.*
59.21	مرارة الغراب تذاف بكفور واسق منها انسانا وزن حبّة في نبيذ فلو شرب من ذلك النبيذ الف انسان ما سكر وهو مليح عجيب	قلب الغراب ولسانه يدقان ويلقيان في النبيذ فلا تسقي من ذلك النبيذ احدا الا احبك وشكرك	واذا خلط معها كافور وشرب منها انسان وزن حبة فانه لا يسكر ابدا ولو شرب منه ما عسى ان شرب
59.22	من أخذ شحم الغراب فيذيبه ويذافه بدهن زنبق وادهن به وجهك واجعل منه وزن حبة تحت قدميك وادخل على السلطان فيكون لك عنده قبول باذن الله تعالى	ومن أخذ شحم بطن الغراب فذوبه بدهن ودهن به وجهه ويديه وأتى سلطانا رفع قدره ويجله	شحم بطنه اذا اذيف بدهن زنبق ودهن به انسان ودخل على السلطان فانه يعظم عنده ويقضي حاجه
59.23	زبل الغراب الفرخ الصغير يذاف بخل خمر ويسقي منه صاحب الطحال فيبرأ باذن الله تعالى	*om.*	واذا اذيف بالخل وشرب منه صاحب الطحال ابرأه

59.19: (c) مرارة الغراب...عنه] واذا طليت المسحور بمرارة غراب بحل عنه السحر باذن الله عز وجل C

59.21: (c) معها كافور] شيء من كافور C | فانه لا يسكر] لم يسكر C | ان شرب] ان يشرب شحم C

59.22: (c) شحم بطنه] شحم بطن الغراب C | اذا اذيف] اذا اذيب C | ودهن به انسان] واندهن به احد C | ودخل على...حاجة] فانه قبول لدخول الملوك والاكابر وذي الحاجة C

59.23: (c) واذا اذيف] واذا اذيب C | صاحب] من اصابه C

59.18	Crow blood: if it is mixed with red squill vinegar, and given to a man suffering from liver and spleen complaints to drink, then he will recover, with the permission of God, may He be exalted.	Crow gall: if it is mixed with red squill vinegar, [it will be useful] if drunk on an empty stomach against spleen complaint and swelling.	*om.*
59.19	*om.*	*om.*	Crow gall: if it is rubbed on the body of someone that has been enchanted, the enchantment will be annulled.
59.20	*om.*	Crow meat: if it is cooked, dried, minced, mixed with aloe and saffron, rubbed on the eye affected by scabies, stinging, and obscuration of the eyesight, [then it will be useful].	*om.*
59.21	Crow gall: if it is mixed with camphor, one grain of it is given to a man with wine to drink , and if the man drinks some of this wine, then he will not get drunk, and this is witty and amazing.	Crow heart and its tongue: if they are minced, thrown into some wine, then no one will be able to drink this wine without loving you and being thankful to you.	And if it is melted with camphor and a man drinks one grain of it, then he will never get drunk again, and if he drank it, he would not manage to drink at all.
59.22	Take some crow fat, liquefy it and mix with lily oil, rub your face with this and put it one grain of it under your feet, then go to see the sultan and you will be received, with the permission of God, may He be exalted.	The one who takes the fat from the abdomen of a crow, mixes it with essential oil, rubs his face and hands with it, and enters in the presence of the sultan, then his power will be increased and he will be exalted.	Fat of its abdomen: if it is mixed with lily oil, and a man who goes to see the sultan is rubbed with it, then he will become more important and his requests will be satisfied.
59.23	Excrement of a crow's little chick: if it is mixed with wine vinegar and given to a man suffering from spleen complaints to drink, then he will recover, with the permission of God, may He be exalted.	*om.*	And if it is mixed with vinegar and a man suffering from spleen complaints drinks it, then he will recover.

59.24

رأس الغراب الابقع اذا سلق واستوي وأكل منه صاحب الصداع برئ صداعه لوقته

ومن كان به صداع عتيق فليأخذ رأس غداف أبقع فيطبخ حتى ينضج فان انضج فاخرج الدماغ وكله يسكن عنه

يؤخذ رأس غراب ابقع يلقي في قدر لطيفة واغليه بقليل ماء حتى يتهرا واطعمه لصاحب الصداع والشقيقة والضربان فيبرأ باذن الله تعالى

59.25

مرارته الاسود اذا طلى بها الشعر سوده وحسنه وغزره باذن الله تعالى

مرارة الغداف تسود الشعر اذا طليت عليه وله في ذلك خاصية كثيرة

مرارة الغراب الاسود يطلي بها الشعر فيسود باذن الله تعالى

59.24: (b) الغداف [الغذاف T

(c) من اصابه الصداع المزمن [صاحب الصداع برئ C

59.25: (b) الغداف [الغذاف T

(c) واذا طلى الشعر بمرارة الغراب سوده وحسنه وغيره والله اعلم [مرارته...تعالى C

59.24	Spotted crow head: if it is put in a fine cooking pot, boiled with a little water until it is well done, fed to a man suffering from headache, migraine and stabs, then he will recover, with the permission of God, may He be exalted.	The one who is affected by chronic headache should take the head of a spotted raven, cook it until it is well done; then, when it is well done, all the brain has to be taken out, and the headache will go away.	Spotted crow head: if it is well cooked in boiling water, and a man suffering from headache eats it, then its headache will immediately subside.
59.25	Black crow gall: if it is rubbed on the hair, then they will become black and nicer, with the permission of God, may He be exalted.	Black crow gall: if it is rubbed on the hair, then this has in it a great peculiar property about it.	Black crow gall: if it is rubbed on the hair, this will blacken it, make them nicer and thicker.

٦٠. البوم

	a	b	c
	ذكر منافع اعضاء البومة	البومة	باب منافع البوم
60.1	اعلم ايّها الطالب ان للبومة بيضتان الواحدة تنبت الشعر والاخرى تمنعه ان ينبت فاذا اردت ان تعرف التي تضرّ من التي تنفع تأخذ البيضة وتشقها وتدخل فيها ريشة فان خرجت بلا شعر وهي للقرع وان خرجت وفيها الشعر فهي لنبات الشعر فاحفظ بهما	اعلم ان البومة لها بيضان واحدة تنبت الشعر اذا طلى به الموضع الذي الشعر فيه والاخرى تحلق الشعر فاذا اردت ان تعلم انها تحلق الشعر او انها تنبته فادخل في احداهن ريشة فان خرجت صحيحة غير منحلقة فهي تنبت الشعر وان اخرجت منحلقة فهي تحلق الشعر	اعلم ان للبوم بيضتان واحدة منها تنبت الشعر والاخرى تحلقه اذا اردت ان تعرف الواحدة من الاخرى ادخل في البيضة ريشة فان حلق شعر الريشة فانها تعرف
60.2	*om.*	*om.*	قلب العوة وتسمى المصاصة نوع من البوم اذا جعل في قطعة من جلد ذئب فان من لبسه لم يقدر عليه لص ولم يخاف من احد ليلا ولا نهارا ولا يقربه شىء من الهوام
60.3	*om.*	*om.*	شحم البوم من اذابه واكتحل به ودخل مكانا ليلا فانه ابرأه مضيا
60.4	دم البوم يذاف بزيت مغسول وادهن به الرأس فلا يثبت فيه قملة ولا حصّة ولا صيبان ولا شىء يؤذي الشعر باذن الله تعالى	دم البومة يخلط بزيت ودهن بها الرأس فيقتل القمل والصبيان	دم البومة اذا خلط بالزيت واندهن به الرأس احد قتل القمل والصبيان

60.1: (c) بيضتان [بيضان C | واحدة [واحدهما C | من الاخرى [منهما C | فان حلق شعر [فهي التي تحلق الشعر C | فانها تعرف [فخذ منهما ما والاخرى تنبت تحتاج C

60.2: (c) This recipe is attested only in C

60.3: (c) This recipe is attested only in C

60.4: (c) This recipe is attested only in C

60. Owl

	a	b	c
	Exposition of the useful properties of the parts of the owl	**The owl**	**Chapter on the useful properties of the owl**
60.1	Know, oh student, that the owl lays two eggs, one of the two makes the hair grow, the other one prevents it from growing. If you want to distinguish the harmful from the useful one, take one egg, split it and plunge a feather in it: if it comes out without hair, then this is the egg that provokes baldness, if instead it comes out with its hair, then this egg is for the growth of hair.	Know that the owl lays two eggs, one of them makes the hair grow—when the part with hair is rubbed with it—while the other shaves it. When you want to know whether it shaves the hair or makes it grow, dip a feather in one of the two eggs, and if it comes out whole, then this is the one that makes hair grow; if , instead, it comes out 'shaved', then this is the one that shaves the hair.	Know that the owl lays two eggs, one of them makes the hair grow, while the other one shaves it. When you want to distinguish one from the other, plunge a feather in the egg and if the feather is shaved, then you will be able to tell them apart.
60.2	*om.*	*om.*	Heart of *'awwa*—also called barn owl (*maṣāsa*), a variety of owl—if it is put in a piece of wolf skin, then the man who wears it will be completely safe from thieves, he will not be afraid of anyone, by night nor during the day, and no pest will ever touch him.
60.3	*om.*	*om.*	Owl fat: if it is liquefied, a man rubs it on the eyes, and enters a place at night, then this will definitely cure him.
60.4	Owl blood: if it is mixed with boiled oil, rubbed on the head, then no lice, nits, nor anything harmful for the hair will remain there, with the permission of God, may He be exalted.	Owl blood: if it is mixed with oil, and rubbed on the head of someone, then this will kill the lice and the nits.	Owl blood: if it is mixed with oil, and rubbed on the head of someone, then this will kill lice and nits.

60.5	اذا اردت ان تخبرك المرأة بكل ما عملته في عمرها من خير وشر فخذ قلب بومة فصرّه في خرقة واجعله على صدر المرأة وهي نائمة فانها تخبرك بكل شيء عملته في عمرها واذا رايتها اختلّ عقلها فأزغه عنها ولا تهلك	قلب البومة ان أخذه انسان وصيره على قلب امرأة نائمة اخبرك بكل شيء فعلته	قلب البومة اذا جعل على يد اليسرى للمرأة النائمة تكلمت بما فعلته في اليقظة
60.6	يؤخذ دم بومة وهو حار فيلطخ به وجه من به اللقوة وعنقه فيزوله باذن الله تعالى	يؤخذ دم بومة كما تذبح وتلطخ به صاحب اللقوة وعنقه فانه يبرأ	*om.*
60.7	عيني البومة الواحدة يصلح للنوم والاخرى للسهر فاذا اردت ان تعرف بعضهم من بعض فخذ إناء فاجعل فيه ماء وارم فيه العينين فالذي تطف على وجع الماء وهي التي تصلح للسهر والتي ترسخ اسفل الإناء تصلح للنوم	عيني البومة واحده منها تصلح للسهر والاخرى للنوم واذا اردت ان تعلم انها للنوم فاجعل واحدة في الماء فان رسبت فهي للنوم وان ارتفع فهي للسهر	*om.*
60.8	فمن اراد ان ينوّم انسانا يأخذ العين فيجعلها تحت رأسه والذي يريد ان يحرمه ينام فعلّقها عليه وهو لا يدري فانه لا ينام ما دامت معلقة عليه	*om.*	*om.*
60.9	مرارة البومة وعود من شجرة الطرفاء فيحرق ويؤخذ رماده يخلط الجميع ويشرب منه الذي يبول في فراشه بعسل وماء حار عند النوم فانه يبرأ باذن الله تعالى	مرارة البومة تخلط مع رماد الطرفاء ويشرب عند النوم يخلط مع رماد الطرفاء بعسل وماء حار لمن يبول في الفراش فيذهب ذلك منه	*om.*

60.5: (c) This recipe is attested only in C

60.5	If you want that a woman tells you everything she did in her life—both the good and the bad—take the heart of an owl, tie it into a piece of cloth, and place it on the woman's breasts while she is asleep, then she will tell you everything she has done in her life. And when you see that her mind starts to be confused, remove it and she will not die.	Owl heart: if a man takes it, and places it on the heart of a sleeping woman, then she will tell everything she has done.	Owl heart: if it is placed on the left hand of a sleeping woman, then she will tell you everything she has done when she was awake.
60.6	Owl blood: if it is taken while it is still warm, spattered on the face and the neck of a man affected by facial paralysis, then the paralysis will go away.	Owl blood: if it is taken when the owl is slaughtered, and a man affected by facial paralysis spatters himself and also his neck with it, then he will heal.	*om.*
60.7	One of the owl's eyes is good for the sleep, the other one provokes insomnia. When you want to distinguish one from the other, take a vessel, fill it with warm water, and put the eyes inside it: the one that floats on the surface of the water is good for insomnia, while the one that sinks to the bottom of the vase is good for the sleep.	One of the two owl's eyes is good for insomnia, while the other one is for the sleep. When you want to know which one is for the sleep, put one in the water, if it sinks to the bottom, then it is for the sleep; if, instead, it goes up to the surface, then this is for insomnia.	*om.*
60.8	If one wants to make someone sleep, then the eye should be taken and put under his head. And the one who wants to prevent someone from sleeping should hang the eye on him—but the man should not be aware of this—then he will not sleep as long as the eye remains hung on him.	*om.*	*om.*
60.9	Owl gall and a branch of tamarisk: if they are burnt, their ash taken, mixed up, given to drink with honey and hot water at the moment of sleeping to a man who wets the bed, then he will recover, with the permission of God, may He be exalted.	Owl gall: if it is mixed with tamarisk ash, and given to a man who wets his bed to drink, at the moment of sleep mixed with tamarisk ash with honey and warm water, then this will leave him.	*om.*

60.10	يؤخذ لحم البومة وشحمه فيطبخ ويلقي عليه بورق وقليل خل خمر ويسقي لصاحب القروح ويجفف ويذرّ منه على القروح التي يكون في الجسد فتزول باذن الله تعالى	ولحم البومة وشحمه يخلط مع بورق وورس يسلق بخل ويجفف فاذا جفف سُحق وذرّ على قرحة تكون في البدن فانه يجففها	*om.*
60.11	يؤخذ دم البوم فيذاف بدهن بنفسج ويقطر في انف صاحب الشقيقة والضربان يبرأ باذن الله	دماغ البومة يذاف بدهن بنفسج ويقطّر في الاذن والأنف من الجانب الذي يشتكي الانسان فيه الشقيقة	*om.*
60.12	*om.*	دماغ البومة الذكر اذا اكتحل به انسان اورثه الغشاوة	*om.*
60.13	*om.*	دم البوم اذا جفف وسقى انسان منه اورثه القولنج	*om.*
60.14	*om.*	مرارة البوم اذا شربت في النبيذ المتخذ من فم الصرفان افسدت عليه ريته واورثه بخرا شديدا	*om.*

60.10	Owl meat and owl fat: if they are taken, cooked with the addition of natron and a bit of wine vinegar, given to a man affected by ulcers to drink–and also dried and sprinkled on the ulcers of the body–then these will cease, with the permission of God, may He be exalted.	Owl meat owl and fat: if they are cooked with natron and curcuma, boiled with vinegar, and dried; once this has dried, it is sprinkled on the ulcer on the body, and then this will dry it.	*om.*
60.11	Owl blood: if it is mixed with sweet violet oil, and applied in drops inside the nose of a man affected by migraine, then he will recover.	Owl brain: if it is mixed with sweet violet oil, applied in drops in the ear and in the nose, from the side in which a man suffers from migraine, [then he will heal].	*om.*
60.12	*om.*	Male owl brain: if it is rubbed on the eyes of a man, then the cataract will leave him.	*om.*
60.13	*om.*	Owl blood: if it is dried, and given to a man to drink, then the colic will leave him.	*om.*
60.14	*om.*	Owl gall of: if it is drunk with wine poured from an opening made of lead, then this will weaken his lungs and cause an intense foul breath.	*om.*

٦١. الديك

	a	b	c
	ذكر منافع اعضاء الديك	الديك	—
61.1	يؤخذ عرف الديك الابيض يبخر به المجنون الذي يصرع فانه يبرأ باذن الله تعالى	ان بخرت المجنون بعرف الديك نفعه	—
61.2	*om.*	وان احرق وسحق وسقى منه من يبول في الفراش نفعه وذهب عنه البول	—
61.3	مرارة الديك الابيض يذاف بدهن زنبق ويسقي لصاحب خفقان القلب والرجفان فانه يبرأ باذن الله	مرارة الديك الابيض تشرب لخفقان القلب مع شيء من زنبق وماء حار	—
61.4	*om.*	وان اردت ان تخبر المرأة بكل عملته وفعلته فخذ عين ديك واجعله في مجمرة وضعه على فخذها اذا نامت	—
61.5	*om.*	خصية الديك تحرق وتسقي منها من يبول في القراش فيذهب ذلك عنه	—
61.6	*om.*	واذا اردت ان تغلب خصمك فخذ مخالب الذيك رجله اليمنى فامسكها معك فانك تغلب خصمك	—
61.7	مخالب رجل الديك اليسرى اذا علقت على انسان احبّوه النساء وان كان الديك يأكل القمح كان ابلغ	ومخالب رجله اليسرى يعلقه الانسان عليه فتحبه النساء وليكن الديك مما يغلف قمحا او شعيرا ولا يأكل من القذر	—

61.3: (b) زنبق] زيبق T
61.6: (b) مخالب] مخاليب T
61.7: (a) مخالب] مخاليب S
(b) مخالب] مخاليب T

61. Rooster

	a	b	c
	Exposition of the useful properties of the parts of the rooster	**The rooster**	–
61.1	White rooster comb: if it is taken, and an insane who has an epileptic seizure is fumigated with it, then he will recover.	If an insane is fumigated with the comb of a rooster, then this will be useful to him.	–
61.2	*om.*	And if it is burnt, ground, and given to drink to the one who wets the bed, then this will be useful to him, and the urine [in bed] will leave him.	–
61.3	White rooster gall: if it is mixed with lily oil, given to a man suffering from heart palpitations and convulsions to drink, then he will recover.	White rooster gall: it should be drunk against palpitations of the heart with some lily and warm water.	–
61.4	*om.*	If you want that a woman tells you everything she did, then take the eye of a rooster, put it on a incense burner and place it on her leg, while she is asleep.	–
61.5	*om.*	Rooster testicle: if it is burnt, given to a man who wets the bed, then this will leave me.	–
61.6	*om.*	If you want to defeat your adversary, take the talons of a rooster from its right leg, keep them with you, and then you will defeat your adversary.	–
61.7	Rooster left talon: if it is hung on a man, then the women will love him. And if the rooster has eaten corn, this will be even more effective.	Talon from its left leg: if a man hangs it on himself, then the women will love him. The rooster must have eaten either corn or barley corn, but not filth.	–

— دم الديك نافع للشرى يخلط مع ورس ويعجن بالخل ويطلي به مواضع الشرى فينفعها

يؤخذ دم الديك اذا ذبح يذاف بدهن زنبق ويضرب الجميع بخل خمر واطل به البدن الذي يكون عليه الشرى فيذهب عنه باذن الله تعالى 61.8

— يؤخذ للمبطون لحم الديك فيطبخ حتى ينضج ويدق في هاون ويلقي عليه العفص والسماق ويخلط ويسقي للمبطون

يؤخذ ديك فيذبح ويسمط ويجعل في قدر ويجعل عليه غمره ماء ويسلق حتى يتهرّي ويلقي عليه عفص اخضر وسُمّاق من كل واحد جزء ويسقي للمبطون فانه يبرأ باذن الله تعالى 61.9

— يؤخذ من بطون الديوك حجارة منها بيضاء ومنها اغبر فاذا اصبت منها شيئا وأخذته وعلقته على المجنون برئ

يؤخذ في جوف الديك حجر منها لونه ابيض ومنها لونه اغبر يؤخذ ذلك الحجر ويعلق على المجنون فيبرأ باذن الله 61.10

— وان علقه انسان عليه زاد في باه وكثرة الجماع

وان علقه على انسان على نفسه عند الجماع نفعه نفعا بليغا 61.11

— ويطرد منه الشيطان وكل ريح سوء

وينفع ايضا من الشياطين والوسوسة 61.12

— وينفع للصبيان الذين يفزعون في النوم

ويعلق ايضا على الصغار الذين يفزعون في النوم 61.13

— الديك الاحمر الصادق اذا طبخ على هذه الصفة ينفع من القولنج واحتباس البطن

يؤخذ الديك الاحمر يذبح ويسمط ويشق جوفه ويخرج كل ما فيه ويحشي جوفه ملحا ويغلي غليانا جيدا ويلقي عليه حمص اسود وكمون كرماني وشبّ يماني ويسقي منه الذي يكون قد هلك من القولنج فيبرأ باذن الله تعالى 61.14

61.8	Rooster blood: if it is taken when it is slaughtered, mixed with lily oil, everything whipped with wine vinegar, rubbed on the body affected by scabies, then this will cease, with the permission of God, may He be exalted.	The blood of rooster is useful against the scabies if it is mixed with curcuma, kneaded with vinegar, and rubbed on the parts afflicted by scabies, then it will be useful for them.	–
61.9	If a rooster is taken, slaughtered, prepared, and put it in a cooking pot, abundant water is added to it, and it is left to boil until it is well-cooked, then nutgalls and fresh sumac are added to this—one part of each one—and this is given to a man affected by an intestinal ailment to drink, then he will recover, with the permission of God, may He be exalted.	For the constipated man: if the meat of a rooster is taken, cooked in an oven until it is well done, nutgalls and sumac are added to it, mixed, and given to the constipated man to drink, [it will be useful to him].	–
61.10	Stone inside the abdomen of roosters—some of them are white and some of them are dust-coloured—if this stone is taken, and hung on an insane man, then he will recover, with the permission of God, may He be exalted.	If the stone inside the abdomen of roosters—some of them are white and some of them are dust-coloured—then you take it, dissolve some of it, and place it on the insane man, then he will heal.	–
61.11	And if a man hangs this stone on himself at the moment of coitus, this will be extremely useful for him.	And if a man hangs it on himself, this will increase the sexual desire and the number of copulations.	–
61.12	This is also useful against the devils and the obsessions.	This will chase the devils and every evil spirit away from him.	–
61.13	And also, if it is hung on the children who are frightened in their sleep.	And it is useful for the children who are frightened in their sleep.	–
61.14	If a red rooster is taken, slaughtered, prepared, its abdomen quartered, and everything is taken out of it, then it is stuffed with salt, and boiled well, black chick-peas, cumin and Yemeni alum are added to it, and it is given to a man who has suffered from colic to drink, then he will recover, with the permission of God, may He be exalted.	Genuine red rooster: if it is cooked following this description, then it will be useful against colic and the constipation of the abdomen.	–

—	خصية الديك ودماغه يزيد في الباه وتحرك شهوة الجماع	يؤخذ مخاصي الديك ودماغه يجفف الجميع ويسحق ويذاف بعسل النحل والعقه عند الجماع فانه يزيد في الباه ويقوي الشهوة	61.15
—	الديك الابيض الافرق اذا كان في قافلة لم يفترس منها الاسد شيئا	الديك الابيض الافرق اذا كان في قافلة لم يعد واعليها اسد ولا وحش ولا سارق	61.16
—	*om.*	وكذلك اذا كان في الدار ديك ابيض افرق يطرد جميع الشياطين وكان مباركا	61.17

61.15	Rooster testicles and brain: if they are taken, dried, ground, mixed with honey, and licked at the moment of coitus, then this will increase the sexual potency and strengthen the desire.	Rooster testicles and brain: they will increase the sexual desire and excite the desire of coitus.	–
61.16	White rooster with a split on the collar: if there is one of them in a caravan, then this will not be attacked neither by a lion, nor by a wild animal, and not by a bandit either.	White rooster with a band on the collar: if there is one of them in a caravan, then the lions will not prey on it.	–
61.17	Likewise, if there is a white rooster with a band on the collar living in a house, then this will scare devils away and the house will be blessed.	*om.*	–

٦٢. الدجاجة

	a	b	c
	ذكر منافع اعضاء الدجاجة	*om.*	—
62.1	يؤخذ بيض الدجاجة يستخرج دهنه ويطلي به النقرس فيسكن وجهه باذن الله تعالى	*om.*	—
62.2	*om.*	يؤخذ دجاجة سوداء ليس بياض ولا غيره تذبح ويخرج ما في بطنها ويحرق بالنار فاذا صار رمادا يؤخذ ذلك الرماد ويخلط معه فلفل مثله مسحوق منخول ويشرب منه ثلاثة ايام بماء الكمون للقولنج نافع	—
62.3	يؤخذ شحم الدجاج يذاب على النار ويقطر في الأذن الوجعة يسكن وجعها باذن الله	لوجع اذان الصبيان يؤخذ شحم الدجاجة يذاب على النار فاذا ذاب خلط معه ماء البصل ويصير على النار فاذا اذاب حتى يفتر ويقطّر في اذان الصبي فيسكن عنه الوجع	—
62.4	*om.*	لحم الدجاجة وشحمه يطبخ مع القرط ويدق ويحبب مثل البندق ويدخن به صاحب الربو والسعال وعسر النفس ويستقبل الدماغ في فمه حتى يصير الى رأسه فانه عجيب مجرب	—
62.5	يؤخذ قانصة الدجاجة فتقشر ويؤخذ الداخلاني يشوي ويطعم لمن يبول في الفراش فيمنعه من ذلك	يؤخذ لمن يبول في الفراش داخل قانصة الدجاجة فتشوي ويطعم فيذهب عنه ذلك	—

62. Hen

	a	b	c
	Exposition of the useful properties of the parts of the hen	***om.***	**–**
62.1	Hen egg: if it is taken, its oily part extracted, and rubbed on the gout, then its pain will subside, with the permission of God, may He be exalted.	*om.*	–
62.2	*om.*	Against the earache of the children: if the fat of a hen is taken, melted on the fire, once it has melted it is mixed with onion water and put on the fire; then, once it has melted to the point that it becomes lukewarm, it is applied in drops inside the ears of a child, then the pain will subside.	–
62.3	Hen fat: if it is taken, liquefied on the fire and applied in drops inside the aching ear, then its pain will subside.	If a black hen, without any white spot or any other signs, is taken, slaughtered, what is inside her abdomen is taken out, burnt with fire; then, when it becomes ash, this ash is taken, mixed with the same amount of ground and sieved pepper, and drunk for three days with cumin water, then this will be useful against ulcers.	–
62.4	*om.*	Hen meat and its fat: if they are cooked with alfalfa, minced, made in small balls similar to a pill, and the a man affected by asthma, cough, breath difficulties and whose brain turns is fumigated with this inside his mouth until the smoke reaches its head, then this will be amazing: tried out.	–
62.5	Hen gizzard: if it is taken, peeled, its two external parts are taken, and given to eat to a man who wets the bed, then this will prevent him from doing so.	For the one who wets the bed, the external part of the gizzard of a white hen has to be taken, roasted, and given to him to eat, then this will leave him.	–

يؤخذ دجاجة بيضاء وتطبخ بعشر بيضات وكف سمسم مقشر صحيحا طبخا ناعما فاذا نضج أكل وشرب المرقة فانه يزيد في الباه ويزيد شهوة الجماع —

يؤخذ دجاجة سوداء كلها او بيضاء 62.6
كلها تذبح ويسمط ويجعل في قدر ويجعل عليها غمرها ماء وقليل مصطكى ودار فلفل ودار صيني فاذا نضجت القي عليه عشر بصلات كبار ويترك حتى يتهرّي الجميع وياكلها الذي يريد النكاح الكثير فانه يقوي على ذلك امر عظيم حتى انه لو اراد ينكح ماية جارية لنكحها من قوة الفعل وهو مليح

مرارة الدجاجة يطلي بها الكلف فانه يذهب باذن الله تعالى —

مرارة الدجاجة يلطخ بها الكلف الاسود 62.7
فيزول باذن الله تعالى

دجاجة الابيض يؤخذ الرطب يطبخ مع مخ البيض شيء من زعفران وينصب على الدماميل وعلى كل ورم مده فيفنحه —

يؤخذ زبل الدجاجة فيخلط معه بيضة 62.8
ويضرب الجميع والقي عليه يسير من زعفران ويلطخ به الاورام الحادة فيفتح من غير حديد

يؤخذ ثلاث بيضات وتنقع في الخل ثلاثة ايام وتصيرها في الشمس فاذا حصلت طلى بها البهق والنمش فانه يذهب —

يؤخذ ثلاث بيضات فتنقع في الخل 62.9
ثلاثة ايام وتشال من الخل تجفف في الشمس ويطلي به البهق الابيض والاسود فيذهب باذن الله تعالى

يؤخذ من داخل القانصة فيحرق ويخلط مع الزعفران ويسحق ناعما ويعجن بماء المطر وماء الكريرة الرطبة ويطلي به النمش ويقف صاحبه في الشمس يفعل هذا ثلاثة ايام فانه يذهب بالكلف والنمش —

يؤخذ قانصة دجاجة وتقشر ويؤخذ 62.10
الداخلاني فيحلقا ويسحق ناعما ويعجن بماء الكسفرة واطلِ به النمش الذي يكون في الوجه وعلى اليدين وعلى الرجلين وعلى البدن فيذهب باذن الله تعالى لو ان جلس صاحبه في الشمس فيزول الكلف والاثر ولا يبقي منه شيء

62.6	If a hen—either completely black or white—is taken, slaughtered, prepared and put in a cooking pot, covered with abundant water with the addition of some mastic, long pepper and cinnamon; then when it is well-cooked ten big onions are added to this, and they are left to cook until they are well done, then this is given to eat to a man who wants to have a lot of sexual intercourse; then he will be able to mate with one hundred girls thanks to the faculty of this action, and this is witty.	If a white hen is taken, well cooked with ten eggs and one handful of crushed sesame; when it is well done, if it is eaten and its broth drunk, then this will increase the sexual desire and the power of coitus.	–
62.7	Hen gall: if the black freckles are spattered with it, then they will go away, with the permission of God, may He be exalted.	Hen gall: if the freckles are rubbed with it, then they will go away, with the permission of God, may He be exalted.	–
62.8	Hen excrement: if it is taken, mixed with an egg, everything whipped with the addition of some saffron, and the acute swellings are spattered with it, then they will open without any incision.	If a white hen is taken fresh, cooked with yolk and some saffron, applied on the abscesses or on any swelling, this will make it subside and open.	–
62.9	If three eggs are taken, macerated in vinegar for three days, dried in the sunlight, and rubbed on the black and on the white vitiligo, then this will go away, with the permission of God, may He be exalted.	If three eggs are taken, macerated in vinegar for three days, placed in the sun, once this is done, they are rubbed on the vitiligo and the discoloured spots, then these will go away.	–
62.10	Hen gizzard: if it is taken, peeled, its two external parts are taken apart, ground into a fine powder, kneaded with fumitory water, and rubbed on the discoloured spots which are on hands, feet and the whole body, then they will disappear, with the permission of God, may He be exalted. And if the man affected by it sits in the sun, then the freckles and the signs on the skin will disappear, and nothing of them will remain.	Hen gizzard: if its external part is taken, burnt, mixed with saffron, ground into a fine powder, kneaded with rain water and fresh coriander water, then the discoloured spots are rubbed with it, and the man afflicted with them is left in the sun—and this is done for three days—then the freckles and the discoloured spots will disappear.	–

يؤخذ فروخ فيذبح ويدق بريشه وعظامه
وحرقة دقا ناعما ثم يجمع فيصير لُقمة
واحدة ويدخل في حلق الدابة ويوجر
برطلين نبيذ فانه يذهب عنه الحمر

62.11 لحمر الدواب يؤخذ فرخ لطيف يذبح
ويدق لحما وهو بريشه وجميع كما في
جوفه ويطعم للدابة التي بها الحمر فيزول

62.11 Against the erysipelas which affects the beasts: if a little chick is taken, slaughtered, its meat minced while it has still his plumage and everything as it is in its stomach, then given to the animals affected by erysipelas to eat, then this will cease.

If some chicks are taken, slaughtered, finely minced with their plumage and bones, put together and made in a single piece, then inserted in the body of an animal and given to drink this with two *raṭls* of wine, then the erysipelas will disappear.

—

٦٣. النعامة

	a	b	c
	ذكر منافع اعضاء النعامة	النعامة	—
63.1	للمجنون يؤخذ قشر بيض النعام يدق ويخلط معه سنبل ويذاف بسمن بقري واطعمه للمجنون فانه يفيق من جنونه ويدهن منه رأسه	ان القى قشر بيض النعامة في قدر مع الماء ثم وضعت القدر على البلح غلت وان ضرب بعسل وسمن بقر ويطعم للمجنون ويجعل منه على وسط رأسه نفعه	—
63.2	اذا كان القضيب يضرب على الانسان فيؤخذ دماغ النعام فيدهن به القضيب يبرأ باذن الله تعالى	دماغ النعامة جيد لوجع الاحليل وعسر البول	—
63.3	وينفع ايضا لمن يبول الدم يذاف بدهن الجوز ويدهن به القضيب في الحمام	ولمن يبول الدم يذاف بدهن جوز وشيء من خولنجان ويشرب في الحمام وهو حار	—
63.4	لوجع الكبد يؤخذ دم النعام يذاف بماء الحلبة المغلى ويقطر عليه دهن زنبق ويشرب في الحمام على الريق فانه نافع لوجع الكبد والجوف	لوجع الكبد يؤخذ ماء الحلبة مغلى مصفى يذاف فيه شيء من مخ النعام ويقطر عليه دهن الزنبق ويشرب في الحمام على الريق	—

63. Ostrich

	a	b	c
	Exposition of the useful properties of the parts of the ostrich	**The ostrich**	–
63.1	For the insane: if the shell of ostrich eggs is taken, crushed, melted with hyacinth, mixed with cow fat, and given to the insane to eat, then he will overcome his insanity, and this will leave his head.	If the shell of ostrich eggs is put in a cooking pot with water, then you place the pot on small unripe dates, they will ripen; and if it is whipped with honey and cow fat, then given to the insane to eat, and put on the middle of his head, then this will be useful to him.	–
63.2	If the penis of a man aches, then the brain of an ostrich has to be taken, and the man penis has to be rubbed with it, then it will heal.	The brain of the ostrich is good against the pain of the urethra and urine retention.	–
63.3	It is also useful to a man who urinates blood, if mixed with nut oil and rubbed on the penis in the bath.	For a man who urinates blood: if it is mixed with nut oil and some galangal, then drunk in the bath while it is still warm [it will be useful].	–
63.4	Against liver complaints: if ostrich blood is taken, mixed with boiled fenugreek water, lily oil is added in drops to it, and this is drunk in the bath on an empty stomach, then this will be useful against the pain of the liver and the abdomen.	Against liver complaints: if boiled and purified fenugreek water is taken with the marrow of an ostrich, lily oil is added in drops to it, then it has to be drunk in the bath on an empty stomach.	–

٦٤. الاوز والبط

	a	b	c
	ذكر منافع اعضاء البطة	الاوز والبط	—
64.1	مرارة البطة تذاف بدهن بنفسج ويسعّط بها صاحب الشقيقة في الرأس فيبرأ باذن الله	مرارة الاوز اذا اذيف بدهن بنفسج وسُعّط به من به شقيقة في الرأس نفعه	—
64.2	دم البط تذاف بماء وملح ويشرب في الحمام على الريق فيفتت الحصاة ويدر البول	دمه اذا اذيف بملح وشرب على الريق نفع من وجع المثانة	—
64.3	لوجع اجنب الخاصرة يؤخذ لحم البط وشحمه وكبده يدق الجميع دقا ناعما ويلقي عليه حلبة وسنبل الطيب ودار صيني من كل واحد جزء ويسحق الجميع ويسقي لصاحب هذا العلة فيبرأ باذن الله تعالى	شحمها وكبدها يؤخذ منها خمس اواقي يدق ناعما ويلقي عليه قطنية مدقوقة منخولة وسنبل ودار صيني من كل واحد جزء ويشرب بماء السذاب المغلى المصفى لتقطير ووجع الخاصرة وحرقة البول	—
64.4	*om.*	بيض البط يعجن بسمن بقر وعسل ويضمد به الخاصرة	—
64.5	يؤخذ بيض البط يسلق ويعجن بزيت مغسول ويلقي عليه حلبة وورس وكراويا من كل واحد جزء ويعجن الجميع ويذر عليه سذاب اخضر ويؤكل على الريق فيزيد في شهوة الجماع ويقوي الظهر والجماع وينفع ايضا من عسر البول	وان عجن بزيت ورشّ عليه مُري ويلقي عليه كراويا ويقطع عليه سذاب رطب ويؤكل فيزيد في شهوة الجماع وينفع من عسر البول	—

64.1: (b) This recipe is attested only in G

64.2: (b) This recipe is attested only in G

64.3: (b) شحمها وكبدها] لحمه وشحمه وكبده G | قطنية] حلبة G | وحرقة البول] *om.* G

64.4: (b) يعجن] اذا طبخ G | ويضمد به الخاصرة] واطعم للمبرسم بفعه G

64.5: (b) وان...عسر البول] بيض البط الصيني اذا طبخ بزيت ورشّ عليه شيء من مُري وكراويا وسذاب رطب واكل زاد في الباه G

64. Goose and Duck

	a	b	c
	Exposition of the useful properties of the parts of the duck	**The goose and the duck**	–
64.1	Duck gall: if it is mixed with sweet violet oil, and inhaled by the man suffering from migraine, then he will recover.	Goose gall: if it is mixed with sweet violet oil and inhaled by the man affected by migraine in the head, it will be useful to him.	–
64.2	Goose blood: if it is mixed with water and salt, drunk in the bath on an empty stomach, then this will crumble the stones, and will make the urine flow copiously.	Its blood: if it is mixed with salt and drunk on an empty stomach, this will be useful against the pain of the bladder.	–
64.3	Against the pain of the hips, take the meat, the fat and the liver of a duck, mince all of them finely and add one part of fenugreek, nard and cinnamon to it, grind everything and give it to drink to the man suffering from this disease, then he will recover, with the permission of God, may He be exalted.	Its meat and its liver: if five ounces of this are taken, finely minced, then ground and sieved legumes, hyacinth and cinnamon are added to it—one part of each one—drunk with boiled and purified rue water, then this will be useful against urine dripping, waist pain, and burning urine.	–
64.4	*om.*	Duck eggs: if they are cooked with cow fat and honey, and used to bandage the waist, they will be useful.	–
64.5	Duck eggs: if they are taken, cooked in boiling water, kneaded with washed oil, fenugreek, curcuma and caraway are ground over it—one part of each one—everything is kneaded, green rue is thrown on it, and this is eaten on an empty stomach, then this will increase the desire of coitus and strengthen the back.	If they are kneaded with oil, some vinegar sauce [or bitter water] is sprinkled on them, caraway is added, and fresh rue cut over it, and eaten, this will increase sexual desire and will be useful against urine retention.	–

—	يؤخذ من بطون البط حجارة كثيرة تنفع لاستطلاق البطن وكثرة الاختلاف واذا سحقت وسقى المبطون او علق عليه منها	يؤخذ في بطون البط حجارة وهي مختلفة الالوان تؤخذ وتسحق سحقا ناعما ويسقي منها المبطون فيبرأ باذن الله تعالى وان علقت عليه كان ابلغ	64.6
—	ذكر البط وخصيته اذا أكل يزيد في الباه	*om.*	64.7
—	لسانه اذا أكل نفع من تقطير البول	لسان البط يجفف ويسحق ويلعق بعسل نحل فانه ينفع من قطار البول	64.8
—	في اطراف اجنحة الاوز والديوك عظاما طوالا فما كان في طرف الجناح الايسر [ينفع] من حمى الربع اذا علقه على الانسان عليه	في اطراف اجنحة البط عظما طويلا يؤخذ ذلك العظم ويبخر به المحموم قيبرأ باذن الله وان علق عليه كان اجود	64.9
—	وكانوا علماء فارس يجعلون هذا العظام في ثيابهم التي يلبسونها فتقطع عنهم الاوجاع	وكانت حكماء الفرس والقبط يعلقوا هذه العظام في ثيابهم وكانت تطرد عنهم جميع اعلال الحمى وكذلك يؤخذ في اجنحة الديوك منها	64.10
—	مخ الاوز يذاف بدهن ويفتّر ويكمّد به الرأس ينفع من الصداع	مخ البط يذاف بدهن بنفسج ويدهن به الرأس الذي يعتريه الصداع فيذهب عنه باذن الله تعالى	64.11
—	زبل الاوز اذا أخذ يابسا يسحق ويشرب ينفع من السعال اليابس	يؤخذ زبل البط اليابس يسحق ويشرب منه من يشتكي السعال اليابس فيزول باذن الله تعالى	64.12

64.6: (b) من بطون البط] في بطن الاوزة G | لاستطلاق] من استطلاق G | وكثرة الاختلاف] *om.* G | المبطون او علق عليه منها] منها او علق عليه منها G
64.7: (b) البط] الاوز G | يزيد] زاد G
64.8: (b) This recipe is attested only in G
64.9: (b) في اطراف] يؤخذ في اطراف G | والديوك] الذكور G | كان] يكون G | من حمى الربع اذا علقه على الانسان عليه] نفع من اذا علق على الانسان الحمى الربع G
64.10: (b) وكانوا] وكان G | هذا العظام] ذلك G | التي يلبسونها فتقطع عنهم الاوجاع] دائم G
64.11: (b) مخ] دهن G | يذاف] اذا اذيف G | ويفتّر ويكمّد] وفتّر وكمّد G | ينفع] نفع G
64.12: (b) زبل...اليابس] ذرق الاوز اليابس اذا سحق وشرب نفع من السعال G

64.6	Stones inside the abdomen of goose, they are of different colours: if they are taken, crushed finely, and given to the man affected by an intestinal ailment to drink, this will be useful. And if they are hung on the abdomen, it will be even more effective.	Many stones can be taken from the abdomens of ducks, they are useful against bowel movement and the abundance of controversy [?], if they are crushed and a constipated man is given them to drink, or if they are hung on him.	–
64.7	*om.*	Goose penis of and its testicles: if they are eaten, this will increase the sexual desire.	–
64.8	The tongue of the duck is useful against urine dripping, if it is dried, ground, and licked with honey.	Its tongue: if it is eaten, this will be useful against urine dripping.	–
64.9	On the outermost part of the duck's wing there is a long bone, if that bone is taken and used to fumigate a feverish man, then he will recover, with the permission of God. And if it is hung on him, this will be even more effective.	In the outermost part of the left wing of geese or roosters there are long bones, the extremity of the left wing is useful against quartan fever, if a man hangs it on his body.	–
64.10	There were Persian and Coptic wise men who used to hang these bones on their cloths, because this repels all kinds of fever. You can find such a bone in the wings of male ducks.	There were Persian learned man who used to put this bones inside the cloths they wore, and this would make their pains cease.	–
64.11	Duck marrow: if it is mixed with sweet violet oil, rubbed on the head of a man affected by headache, then it will go away, with the permission of God, may He be exalted.	Duck marrow: if it mixed with oil, warmed up and applied as a hot compress on the head, this will be useful against the headache.	–
64.12	Duck dry droppings: if they are taken, ground, and given to a man suffering from dry cough to drink, then this will go away.	Duck excrement: if it is taken dry, ground and drunk, this will be useful against the dry cough.	–

—	دماغ البط الصيني جيد لوجع الرأس يذاف بماء السذاب والبورق ويسحق ويكمد به الرأس	دماغ البط الصيني يذاف بماء السذاب الاخضر ويلقي عليه بورق مسحوق وتكمد به الرأس فهو نافع من الشقيقة والصداع ووجع الرأس باذن الله تعالى	64.13
—	واذا اذيف بماء الرازيانج المغلى المصفى يشرب للبواسير واوجاع الارحام في الحمام على الريق	*om.*	64.14

64.13: (b) للبواسير...جيد لوجع] اذا اذيف بماء السذاب والبورق بماء الرازيانج المغلي المصفي وشرب نفع من البواسير G

64.13	Chinese duck brain: if it is mixed with green rue water, ground natron is poured on it, and this is applied as a compress on the head, this will be useful against migraine, headache, and the pain of the head.	Chinese duck brain: it is good against the pain in the head, if it is mixed with rue water and natron, ground and applied as a compress on the head.	–
64.14	*om.*	If it is mixed with boiled and purified fennel water, it is to be drunk against haemorrhoids and uterus pains, in the bath on an empty stomach.	–

٦٥. الكركى

	a	b	c
	ذكر منافع اعضاء الكركى	الكركى	—
65.1	يؤخذ لحم الكركى وشحمه ويجعل في قدر ويجعل عليه غمرة ماء يطبخ حتى يظهر دسمة ثم يقطف الدسم فيقطر منه في الاذن الثقيلة السمع فيبرأ باذن الله تعالى	لحمه وشحمه يطبخ ويصفي دسمه ويقطر منه في الاذن لمن ثقل سمعه وهو فاتر [نفعه]	—
65.2	يؤخذ مرارة الكركى وزن قراط يضاف بدهن زنبق ويسقي منه لصاحب اللقوة فتذهب باذن الله تعالى ويدهن منه الوجه بعد خروجه من الحمام ويذاف اليه ماء السلق الاخضر ويدهن به الوجه	يؤخذ مرارة الكركى وزن القيراط يذاف بزيبق ويسقي منه من به اللقوة بعد ان يخرج من الحمام ثلاثة ايام متوالية يؤخذ ايضا مرارة الكركى تذاف في بماء اصول السلق مصفى غير مغلى	—
65.3	دماغ الكركى اذا اذيف بماء الحلبة ويطلي به اليدين والرجلين الوارمة فينفشّ الورم	دماغ الكركى يذاف بماء الحلبة ويطلي به الورم الذي يكون في اليدين والرجلين من الجماعين نفعه	—
65.4	*om.*	عين الكركى اليمنى تسحق ويكتحل بها فلا ينام	—
65.5	*om.*	خصية الكركى تسحق ويدر عليها ملح اندراني ويجفف ويسحق ويلت معها زبد البحر وخرء الضب وسكر طبرزد من كل واحد جزء ويكتحل به من البياض الحادث في العين [نفعه]	—

65.1: (b) لمن ثقل سمعه [الثقيلة السمع G | وهو فاتر] *om.* G

65.2: (b) بزنبق [بزيبق T | ويسقي منه من به [ويسعط به صاحب G | ثلاثة [ثلثة G | متوالية] *om.* G | يؤخذ ايضا مرارة الكركى تذاف في ماء [ويسعط ايضا بمرارته مذافا بماء G | مصفى [المصفى G

65.3: (b) دماغ الكركى [دماغه G | يذاف [اذا اذيف G | ويطلي [وطلى G | يكون] *om.* G | من الجماعين [من التخمة G

65.4: (b) عين الكركى [عينه G | فلا ينام [للسهر G

65.5: (b) خصية الكركى [خصيته G | اندراني [دراني G | ويسحق [ثم يسحق G | ويلت معها [مع G | من البياض الحاديث في العين [البياض في العين G

65. Crane

	a	b	c
	Exposition of the properties of the parts of the crane	**The crane**	–
65.1	Crane meat and its fat: if they are taken, put in a cooking pot, abundant water is poured on them, then they are cooked until the grease comes up to the surface; then the grease is skimmed, and applied in drops inside the ear that is hard of hearing, then this will cure it.	Its meat and fat: if are cooked, their grease purified, and applied in drops inside the ear of a man who is hard of hearing—that is that he has a weak hearing—it will be useful to him.	–
65.2	If one carat of crane gall is taken, mixed with lily oil, and given to a man suffering from facial paralysis to drink, then this will cease. Rub it on the face after the bath, mix it with water of green beet and anoint the face with it.	Its gall: if one carat of it is taken, mixed with lily oil, and a man sufferings from facial paralysis inhales it after he has left the bath—this for three days in the same quantity—it will be useful; and also if crane gall is mixed with beet roots water, purified but not boiled.	–
65.3	Crane brain: if it is mixed with fenugreek water, and rubbed on the swollen hands and feet, then the swelling will subside.	Crane brain: if it is mixed with fenugreek water and rubbed on the swelling that affects hands and feet, it will be useful against it.	–
65.4	*om.*	Crane right eye: if it is ground and rubbed on the eye, then this will not let one sleep.	–
65.5	*om.*	Crane testicle: if it is ground, and rock salt is added to it, then it is dried and ground, some meerschaum is crushed with it, together with lizard excrement and hard white sugar—one part of each one—and this is rubbed on the eye of a man affected by the glaucoma of the eye, it will be useful against this.	–

65.6	لوجع الكلى والمثانة قانصة الكركى تجفف وتسقي منها صاحب وجع الكلى بماء الحمص الاسود مغلى فيبرأ باذن الله تعالى	قانصة الكركى تجفف تذاف بخل عنصل ويشرب منه من به وجع في طحاله ينفعه	—
65.7	مخ الكركى يذاف بخل عنصل وعسل ويسقي منه صاحب الطحال فيزول باذن الله تعالى	*om.*	—
65.8	*om.*	مرارته اذا اذيفت بماء المزرنجوش وسعط به صاحب اللقوة في الجانب الملقو [نفعه]	—
65.9	للورم قب الانف يؤخذ زبل الكركى ويضاف اليه زبل عرقون يعجن الجميع بماء الهليون ويبلّ فيه فتيلة ويجعلها في الانف فينفع من كل قرحة والناسور برئ الجميه باذن الله تعالى وقدرته	زبل الغرانيق اذا سحق وبلّ به فتيلة وجعلت في الانف نفع من كل قرحة فيه	—

65.6: (b) قانصة...ينفعه [قانصته تجفف وتسحق ويوخذ منها وزن درهمين ويشرب لوجع الكليتين والمثانة مع الحمّص المطبوخ G

65.8: (b) In G another recipe is added, with the inhalation from the other side causing seven days of blindness: ويسعّط في الجانب الاخر بدهن الجوز ولا يرى ضوء سبعة ايام

65.9: (b) This recipe is attested only in G

65.6	Crane gizzard against the pain of the kidneys and of the bladder: if it is dried, and given with black chickpeas water to a man who suffers from kidney complaint to drink, then he will recover.	Crane gizzard: if it is ground, mixed with red squill vinegar, and drunk by a man suffering from spleen complaint, it will be useful against it.	–
65.7	Crane marrow: if it is mixed with red squill vinegar and honey, given to a man who suffers from spleen pain to drink, then this will go away.	*om.*	–
65.8	*om.*	Its gall: if it is mixed with marjoram water, and inhaled by a man suffering from facial paralysis from the side affected by the paralysis, it will be useful to him.	–
65.9	Crane droppings against the swelling of the nostrils: if they are taken, mixed with the of *ʿaraqūn* droppings [?], everything kneaded with asparagus water and used to moisten a compress, then this compress is inserted in the nose, this will be useful against all the ulcers and fistulae and will cure them all, with the permission and the power of God, may He be exalted.	Crane droppings: if they are crushed, a compress is moistened with it, and then inserted in the nose, this will be useful against any sore inside it.	–

٦٦. الحبارى

	a	b	c
	ذكر منافع اعضاء الحبارى	الحبارى	باب منافع الحبارى
66.1	*om.*	*om.*	وهي عكس الدجاجة فان الحبارى اذا خافت سلحت فقد جعل الله سلحها سلاحا والدجاجة اذا خافت كتمت قال الشاعر ∴ وهم تركوك اسلح من حبارى رأت صتعر واسرد من النعام ∴
66.2	لحم الحبارى وشحمه يدق ويخلط معه سنبل وملح ويحبّب ويجفف في الظل فاذا حقن الانسان فيحقن بحبة واحدة فتسهله باذن الله تعالى	الحبارى وشحمه يدق ويخلط معه ملح وسنبل ويحبب ويجفف في الظل ويرفع الاسهال منه الديزج وزن خمس حبّات بماء فاتر	لحم الحبارى اذا دق وخلط بسنبل وملح وحبب وجفف في الظل فاذا احتفن الانسان واستعمل بندقة من ذلك اسهلته اذا اذيبت البندقة بجلاب غبار[ية] كان ابلغ في الاسهال
66.3	للبياض في العين يؤخذ داخل قانصة الحبارى تجفف وتسحق ويخلط معها ملح اندراني وخبز محروق اجزاء متساوية ويكتحل بها البياض في العين فيذهب باذن الله تعالى	داخل قانصته اذا تجفت وتسحق ويخلط معها ملح اندراني وخبز محرق اجزاء سوية ويكتحل به البياض في العين فيذهب باذن الله تعالى	قانصة الحبارى اذا جففت وسحقت وخلط بها ملح اندراني وخبز محروق اجزاء مستاوية واكتحل به من في عينيه البياض ابرأه باذن الله تعالى
66.4	ذرق هذا الطائر وهو الحبارى اذا ذرق على طائر اهرأه	*om.*	*om.*

66: (c) In L there is no dedicated chapter for this bird, the recipes 66.2 and 66.3 are at the end of the chapter on the owl (Ch. 60).

66.1: (c) The verse has a pun on two different meanings of the root *s-l-ḥ*, that is 'to expel excrements' and 'to fight'.

66.2: (b) الحبارى] لحمه G | معه ملح] بزعفران G | ويرفع الاسهال] ويرفع ويسقي الاسهال G | الديزج] الدززنج T
(c) لحم الحبارى] لحمه وشحمه C | الانسان] انسان C | واستعمل بندقة] ببندقة C | اسهلته] اسهله C | اذا اذيبت] وتذوب C | [ية] غبار] عبار L | بجلاب
غبار[ية]] بجلاب السكر الحات C | كان ابلغ] فانه بلغ C

66.3: (b) تجفت وتسحق] جففت وسحقت G | اندراني] دراني G | محرق] محترق G | سوية] سوى T | فيذهب] *om.* G
(c) وخبز] في خبز C | مستاوية] متوالية C | به من في عينيه البياض] بذلك من بعينه بياض C

66. Bustard

	a	b	c
	Exposition of the useful properties of the parts of the bustard	**The bustard**	**Chapter on the useful properties of the bustard**
66.1	*om.*	*om.*	This bird is the opposite of the hen: the bustard fights when it is afraid, since God gave it the droppings as weapon, whereas the hen just hides away when she is afraid. And the poet said: 'these weak people are more armed than a bustard that sees thyme, and is more leathery than an ostrich'.
66.2	Bustard meat and its fat: if they are minced, mixed with hyacinth and salt, made in pills and these are dried in the shade; then, when someone is constipated, give him a single pill as suppository, then this will purge him, with the permission of God, may He be exalted.	Bustard meat and its fat: if they are minced, mixed with salt and hyacinth, made in pills, and these are dried in the shade, it will relieve from diarrhoea, with five grains of sulphur and lukewarm water.	Bustard meat: if it is minced, mixed with hyacinth and salt, made in pills, and these are dried in the shade; then, when a man has a constipation, use one of these pills to purge him. And if you liquefy the pill with medlar julep, it will be even more effective as purge.
66.3	Against glaucoma in the eye, external part of a bustard gizzard: if it is taken, dried, ground, mixed with rock salt and burnt bread in the same quantity, and the glaucoma is rubbed with it, then it will go away, with the permission of God, may He be exalted.	External part of its gizzard: if it is dried, ground and mixed with rock salt and burnt bread in the same quantity, rubbed on the eye affected by glaucoma, then this will go away, with the permission of God may He be exalted.	Bustard gizzard: if it is dried, ground, rock salt and burnt bread in the same quantity are mixed with it, and it is rubbed on the eye affected by glaucoma, then this will cure it.
66.4	If the droppings of this bird—that is the bustard—are expelled against another bird, this will harm it.	*om.*	

٦٧. الصقر

	a	b	c
	—	—	فصل
67.1	—	—	كف الصقر اذا جعل في فراش لم يكد يقربه برغوث ما دام تحت النائم
67.2	—	—	ومن نقب الكف نقبين احداهما بالظل والثانية بالعرض أمن من السلطان ولم يخش من سواء ابدا
67.3	—	—	واذا بخر به الالعازة اسقط شعرها واذا دام عليه منع انبتها وهذا الخاصة في العانة دون البدن

37: (c) This chapter is attested only in C

67. Saker Falcon

	a	b	c
	–	–	**Section**
67.1	–	–	Saker falcon claw: if it is placed inside the bed, then the fleas will not be able to approach it, as long as the claw remains under the person who sleeps there.
67.2	–	–	The one who pierces its claw twice—the first time in the shade, while the second in the light—will be safe from the sultan, and he will not be afraid of anyone, without distinction.
67.3	–	–	If the pubes is fumigated with it, then the hair will fall; and if it is left there, the hair will be prevented from growing again. This is valid for the pubic zone, but not for the rest of the body.

٦٨. الطاؤوس

	a	b	c
	om.	الطاؤوس	باب منافع الطاؤوس
68.1	مرارة الطاؤوس يداف بشراب سكنجين وماء حار ويسقي للمبطون فينفع للاورام الحاسية	مرارته جيدة للمبطون يشربها بسكنجبين وماء حار	مرارة الطاؤوس اذا اذيبت بشراب سكنجبين وماء حار فانها تنفع المبطون والورم
68.2	يؤخذ دم الطاؤوس يخلط معه عنزروت وملح ويعجن الجميع بالخل ويدهن به الورم الحاشي فيفنح بلا الم	ودم الطاؤوس يخلط معه عنزروت وملح ويعجن بخل ويلطخ على الاقدام يحلل لذات الجنب	دم الطاؤوس اذا خلط بنزروت وملح وعجن بالخل الحادق وطلى به الورم الحاشى فتحد وادامه
68.3	لذات الجنب يؤخذ لحم الطاؤوس وشحمه يطبخ ويحسا لصاحب وجع دات الجنب فيبرأ باذن الله تعالى	لحم الطاؤوس يسحق وتحسّى مرقته من به ذات الجنب نفعه	لحم الطاؤوس وشحمه اذا طبخ الجميع وشربه صاحب وجع دات الجنب ابرأه
68.4	مخ الطاؤوس يداف بماء السذاب والعسل ويسقي منه صاحب القولنج وينفع ايضا من الارياح الغليظة والله اعلم بالصواب	مخ الطاؤوس يذاف بماء السذاب وعسل ويشرب فينفع من اوجاع المعدة والقولنج	مخه اذا اذيب بماء السذاب والعسل وشربه من به البواسير في مقعدة نفع ايضا صاحب القولنج والارياح الغليظ باذن الله تعالى

68: (a) In S the whole chapter is written in the margin, probably by the same hand
(c) الطاؤوس] الطاوس L
68.1: (b) يشربها] اذا شربها G
(c) اذا اذيبت] اذا ذوبت C | بسكنجبين] سكنجبيل L C | تنفع] نفع C | والورم] والمورّم C
68.2: (b) ويلطخ…الجنب] ولطخ به القروح الرطبة نفعها G
(c) اذا خلط] اذا اختلط C | بنزروت] بعنريث وملح L | بعنبروت] عنزروت C | بالخل الحادق] بخل خمر الحاذق C | الحاشي] الورم الحاثي L | فتحد واداماه] اذهبه C
68.3: (b) لحم الطاؤوس] لحمه وشحمه G
(c) صاحب] من اصابه C
68.4: (b) مخ الطاؤوس] مخه G | يذاف] اذا اذيف G | وعسل] والعسل G | ويشرب فينفع] نفع وشرب G
(c) مخه] مخ الطاؤوس C | والعسل] وعسل C | من به] من اصابه مرض C | في مقعدة] في معدة C | نفع ايضا صاحب القولنج] وينفع وجع القولنج C

68. Peacock

	a	b	c
	om.	**The peacock**	**Chapter on the useful properties of the peacock**
68.1	Peacock gall: if it is mixed with oxymel and warm water, and given to a man affected by intestinal ailments to drink; then it will be also useful against the swelling of the organs.	Its gall is good against intestinal ailments, if it is drunk with oxymel and warm water.	Peacock gall: if you dilute it with oxymel and warm water, then this will be useful to a man affected by intestinal ailments and swellings.
68.2	Peacock blood: if it is taken, mixed with sarcocolla and salt, everything kneaded with vinegar and rubbed on the intumescence, then this will open without any pain.	Peacock blood: if it is mixed with sarcocolla and salt, then spattered on the feet, then it will be soothing for a man affected by pleurisy.	Peacock blood: if it is mixed with sarcocolla and salt, kneaded with sour vinegar and rubbed on an intumescence, then this will either cut it open, or make it chronic.
68.3	Against pleurisy: if the meat and the fat of a peacock are taken, cooked and sipped by a man suffering from pleurisy, then he will be cured, with the permission of God may He be exalted.	Peacock meat: if it is cooked, and its broth is given to a man affected by pleurisy to sip, then this will be useful to him.	Peacock meat and fat: if they are cooked and given to a man suffering from pleurisy to drink, then this will cure him.
68.4	Peacock marrow: if it is mixed with rue water and honey, given to a man suffering from colic to drink, [it will be useful]. It is also useful for the putrid winds, and God knows what is right.	Peacock marrow: if it is mixed with rue water and honey, it will be useful against stomach ailments and colic.	Its marrow: if it is diluted with rue water and honey, and given to a man suffering from them to drink, it will be useful against the haemorrhoids of the backside; it is also useful against colic and the putrid winds, with the permission of God, may He be exalted.

٦٩. الكروان

	a	b	c
	ذكر منافع اعضاء الكروان	الكروان	باب منافع الكروان
69.1	لحم الكروان وشحمه فيطبخ ويسقي مرقته فيزيد في شهوة ويقوي على الجماع والنكاح	لحمه وشحمه اذا أكل زاد في شهوة الجماع والباه	لحم الكروان وشحمه اذا أكل طبخا زاد قوة الجماع وشهوته
69.2	اخر يؤخذ دماغ الكروان ودم سقنقور ويخلط ويستعمل فله فعل جيد	يؤخذ من ادمغة الكروان ويخلط معه لحم السقنقور مما يلي خاصرته وزن استار ويؤخذ وقت الحاجة ملعقة فانه يحرّك الباه تحريكا جيدا شديدا	دماغه اذا اذيب بدم سقنقور واذيب الجميع بماء حار زاد في الانعاظ
69.3	يؤخذ خصى الكروان تجفف وتسحق ويخلط بعسل فهو جيد ان شاء الله تعالى	*om.*	خصوته تسحق وتخلط بعسل وتلعق تزيد في الباه وتقوي الجماع باذن الله تعالى

69:(c) الكروان] الكيروان L C
69.1: (b) اذا أكل] اذا طبخ وأكل G | شهوة الجماع] *om.* G
(c) طبخا] مطبوخا C | وشهوته] وشهاه وانعظ C
69.2: (b) يؤخذ...شديدا] اذا أخذ من ادمغتهم جزء ولحم السقنقور جزو ومما يلي خاصرته جزء ويعجن بعسل وسمن بقر من كل واحد جزء ويرفع ويؤخذ منه في وقت الجماع لعقة ويحرّك الجماع ويزيد زيادة شديدة G
(c) دماغه] دماغ الكيروان C
69.3: (c) خصوته] خصوتا الكيروان C | وتلعق تزيد] ويلعق فان ذلك يزيد C | الجماع] شهوة الجماع ويزيد في الانعظ *add.* C

69. Curlew

	a	b	c
	Exposition of the useful properties of the parts of the curlew	**The curlew**	**Chapter on the useful properties of the curlew**
69.1	Curlew meat and fat: if they are cooked and their broth is given to drink, then the desire of a man will be increased, and he will become stronger in the sexual intercourse and in the copulation.	Its meat and its fat: if they are eaten, then this will increase the desire for coitus and sexual potency.	Curlew meat and its fat: if they are eaten once cooked, the power and the desire of coitus will increase.
69.2	Another one: if curlew brain and skink blood are taken and applied to him, this will have a positive effect.	Curlew brains: if they are taken, mixed with one *astār* of skink meat from its waist, and a spoonful of it is taken in the moment of need, this will extremely excite the coitus.	Its brain: if it is mixed with skink blood, everything mixed up with warm water, then this will increase the erection.
69.3	Curlew testicles: if they are taken, dried, ground and mixed with honey, then this will be good, God willing.	*om.*	Its testicles: if they are ground, mixed with water, and taken as pills, this will make the coitus more intense, with the permission of God, may He be exalted.

٧٠. العقاب

	a	b	c
	ذكر منافع اعضاء عقاب الماء	العقاب	باب منافع العقاب
70.1	مرارة هذا العقاب تجفف وتسحق وتداف بالماء ويطلي بها ثدى المرأة فتدر اللبن باذن الله	مرارة العقاب اذا طليت ثدى المرأة التي انقطع لبنها من ورم الثدى يحلل الورم ويغزر اللبن ويسكن الوجع	مرارة العقاب اذا طليت به المرأة ثديها الذي ينقطع لبنها در لبنها لوقته
70.2	دم هذا العقاب تجفف وتسحق ناعما ويخلط معه هليلج اصفر ويكحل به العين الرمدة ويلطخ من خارج العين وينفع ايضا لجرب الجفون	دم العقاب يجفف يخلط معه اهليلج اصفر ويسحق سحقا ناعما ويكتحل به للعين الجربة ويطلي عليها من خارج	دم العقاب اذا جفف وسحق وخلط معه اهليلج اصفر مسحوقا ناعما ثم سحق الجميع واكتحل به من في عينيه وجفونه جرب نفعه نفعا بليغا
70.3	[...]	شحم العقاب يذاف بزيت ويدهن به من وجع النقرس	شحم العقاب اذا جمع واذيب بزيت مغسول ودهن به المفاصل ورجلين من يشكي وجع النقرس نفعه نفعا جيدا
70.4	—	دماغ العقاب يذاف بماء الفجل الحديث ويفتّر ويشرب لذات الجنب في الحمام وهو حار	دم العقاب اذا اذيب بماء الفجل وفتر على النار وشرب في الحمام نفع من ذات الجنب وان خلط بعسل كان ابلغ في المنفعة
70.5	—	*om.*	اذا لسعت انسان عقرب يشقها نصفين ويلقيها عليها على موضع اللسعة تبرأ لوقتها باذن الله تعالى

70: (a) and (c) العقاب] العقرب There is only one recipe in which the ingredient is actually a scorpion, see 70.5
70.1: (b) مرارة العقاب...الوجع] مرارته اذا طلى بها ثدي المرأة التي قطع لبنها عاد وحلّل الورم الذي فيه وسكّن الوجع G
(c) الذي ينقطع] عند انقطاع C | در لبنها] ادر اللبن C
70.2: (b) دم العقاب] دمه G | يجفف يخل] وخلط اذا جفف G | ويسحق] *om.* G | ويكتحل] وكحّل G | للعين] *om.* G | الجربة] الجربة بزيت G
(c) معه اهليلج...الجميع] مع ذلك شيء من الاهليلج الاصفر المسحوق ناعما C | في عينيه وجفونه] من بعينيه C
70.3: (b) شحم العقاب...النقرس] شحمه اذا ذوّب بالزيت ودهن به المفاصل والنقرس نفعهما G | النقرس] لنفس T
70.4: (b) دماغ العقاب...حار] دماغه اذا اذيف بماء النُجَل الحديث وفُتّر وشرب في الحمام حار نفع من ذات الجنب G
(c) بماء...النار] بماء الفجل الحار C | نفع...الجنب] من به وجع ذات الجنب ابرأه C
70.5: (c) تبرأ] فانها تبرأ C

70. Eagle

	a	b	c
	Exposition of the useful properties of the parts of the water eagle	**The eagle**	**Chapter on the useful properties of the eagle**
70.1	Gall of this eagle gall: if it is dried, ground, mixed with water, and rubbed on a woman's breast, then the milk will flow copiously, with the permission of God, may He be exalted.	Eagle gall: if it is rubbed on the breast of a woman whose milk has stopped to flow because of a swelling of the breast, then the swelling will subside, the milk will be abundant, and the pain will cease.	Eagle gall: if it is rubbed on the breast of a woman whose milk has stopped to flow, then the milk will instantly flow copiously.
70.2	Blood of this eagle blood: if it is dried, ground into a fine powder, mixed with yellow myrobalan, rubbed on the eye affected by inflammation, spattering it from outside; this will also be useful against the scabby eyelid.	Eagle blood: if it is dried, mixed with yellow myrobalan, ground into a fine powder, rubbed on the eye affected by scabies and rubbed from outside, it will be useful.	Eagle blood: if it is dried, ground, mixed with yellow myrobalan, ground into a fine powder, then everything is crushed and rubbed on the eye and the eyelid affected by scabies, this will be very useful against it.
70.3	[...]	Eagle grease: mixed with oil and rubbed on the gout pain, it will be useful.	Eagle grease: if it is collected, mixed with washed oil, rubbed on the joints and the feet suffering from gout pain, then this will be very useful against it.
70.4	–	Eagle brain: if it is mixed with fresh radish water, made tepid and given to drink to a man suffering from pleurisy into a warm bath, it will be useful.	Eagle brain: if it is mixed with radish water, made tepid on the fire and drunk in the bath, this will be useful against pleurisy. And if it is mixed with honey, this will be even more effective in its usefulness.
70.5	–	*om.*	If a scorpion stings a man, split it in two and apply it on the area of the sting, then this will be instantly cured, with the permission of God, may He be exalted.

70.6	—	مخ العقاب يذاف بعسل وويصير على الجرح الذي يكون في الرأس يلحمه	*om.*

70.6: (b) مخ العقاب...يلحمه] مخه اذا اذيف بعسل وخلط معه صبر وجعل على الجرح في الرأس الحمه G

70.6	–	Eagle marrow: if it is mixed with honey and applied on a wound on the head, this will cicatrize it.	*om.*

٧١. الزمج

	a	b	c
	—	الزمج	—
71.1	—	الزمج يصير في الاكحال التي تنفع من الغشاوة وظلمة البصر	—

71.1: (b) الزمج يصير] تجعل الزمج مرارة G | التي تنفع] النافعة G | البصر] *om.* G

71. *Zummağ* falcon

	a	b	c
	—	**The *zummağ* falcon**	—
71.1	—	The *zummağ* falcon is used in the eye salves that are useful against the cataract and the obscuration of the eyesight.	—

٧٢. الباشق

	a	b	c
	—	الباشق	—
72.1	—	مرارته تنفع من الخفقان العارض من المرة السوداء يسقي منها وزن نصف درهم بماء البارد يبرأه	—

72.1: (b) مرارته...يبرأه] مرارته اذا سقى منها وزن نصف درهم بماء الباذنجويه نفع من الخفقان العارض من المرأة السوداء G

72. Sparrow Hawk

	a	b	c
	–	**The sparrow hawk**	–
72.1	–	Its gall is useful against the manifest palpitations due to the black gall: if half dirham of it is drunk with cold water, then this will cure them.	–

٧٣. اليؤيؤ

	a	b	c
	—	طير اليؤيؤ	—
73.1	—	دماغ اليؤيؤ يجفف يسحق مع سكر الطبرزد ويخلط معه بعر الضبّ ويكتحل به من البياض في العين يزيله	—
73.2	—	مرارته تذاف بماء الشهدانج ويسعط من به المصداع فينفعه	—

73.1: (b) دماغ اليؤيؤ...يزيله [دماغ اليؤيؤ اذا جفف وسحق مع سكر طبرزد وبعر ضبّ وكحل به البياض في العين اذهبه G
73.2: (b) تذاف [اذا آذيفت G | ويسعط [وسعط G | المصداع [المصروع G | فينفعه [نفعه G

73. Merlin

	a	b	c
	–	**The merlin**	–
73.1	–	Merlin brain: if it is dried, ground with hard white sugar and lizard droppings, and rubbed on the eye affected by the glaucoma, then this will go away.	–
73.2	–	Its gall: if it is mixed with Indian hemp water, and inhaled by a man affected by headache, then this will be useful to him.	–

٧٤. الباز

	a	b	c
	—	الباز	—
74.1	—	لحمه ينفع من اوجاع الرأس اذا أكل لوجع يقال له وجع البيضة	—
74.2	—	مرارة الباز تسعط لمن يبقي حبة او حبتين للشقيقة يذاف بلبن الجارية ويسعط	—

74: (b) الباز] البازي T G

74.1: (b) لحمه...البيضة] لحمه اذا طبخ وأكل نفع من اوجاع الرأس ويسمى وجع البيضة G

74.2: (b) مرارة...نفعه] مرارته اذا سعّط منه وزن حبة للشقيقة مذاف بلبن جارية نفعه G

74. Hawk

	a	b	c
	–	**The hawk**	–
74.1	–	Its meat: it is useful against the kind of headache called 'egg ache', if it is eaten.	–
74.2	–	Hawk gall: if one or two grains of it are inhaled by a man still affected by migraine with the milk of a young girl, then this will be useful to him.	–

٧٥. الشقراق

a	b	c
—	الشقرّاق	—
—	مرارته يتخذ منه دواء لسواد الشعر على هذا الصفة يؤخذ ملح وعفص تخلط معه المرارة ويلقي عليه دهن الشيرج بقدر ما يغمر ويعجنه ناعما معتدلا ويعلف به الرأس فانه يسود به الرأس تسويدا جيدا حسنا	—

75.1

75: (b) الشقراق] *om.* G

75.1: (b) مرارته...حسنا] مرارة الشقراق مع ملح وعفص يحرقان ويسحقا ويعجنا بالمرارة مع دهن الشيرج ويطلي به الشعر فيسوّده G

75.Green Woodpecker

	a	b	c
	–	**The green woodpecker**	–
75.1	–	From its gall, a remedy for black hair is extracted, following this procedure: salt and gall nuts have to be taken, the gall has to be mixed with them, enough sesame oil to cover it has to be poured on this, then it has to be kneaded in a nice and moderate way, and it has to be applied on the head, and then it will become nicely black.	–

٧٦. دجاج الحبش

	a	b	c
	—	دجاج الحبش	—
76.1	—	يطلي به الوجه والبدن يقلع كل أثر فيه من النمش والكلف والثآليل الظاهرة ويخلط معه ورس مسحوقا وبورق احمر يحسّن اللون ويصفيه	—

76.1: (b) الثآليل] التواليل T

76. Guinea Fowl

	a	b	c
	–	**The Guinea fowl**	–
76.1	–	If the face and the body are rubbed with it, this will erase every sign of discoloured spots, freackles, and the superficial warts; if some ground curcuma and red borax are mixed with it, then this will make the colour [of the skin] nicer and will purify it.	–

٧٧. الشفانين

	a	b	c
	—	الشفانين	—
77.1	—	يؤخذ شحمه الذي في جوفه فيذاف بدهن شيرج ويقطّر منه في الاذن الذي عرض لها الصمم فيذهب باذن الله تعالى	—
77.2	—	من أخذ فرخين من فراخ هذا الطير فاخرج قليبهما وحفظهما عنده لم تزل النساء تحبه ما داما القلبان عنده ولا يعلمها بمكانهما	—
77.3	—	لورم العين يقطر في العين دم السفنين حارا يوضع على العين من خارج بقطنة مبلولة ببياض البيض مع شيء من دهن الورد	—
77.4	—	وبيض الشافنين يخلط معه عسل وشيء من بورق وكله من به وجع في كبده فينفع	—

77: (b) الشفانين] وهو طير المشتري *add.* G
77.1: (b) يؤخذ] *om.* G | فيذاف] اذا ذوّب G | ويقطّر] وقطر G | الذي...فيذهب] نفع من الصمم G
(c) For this recipe, see also 78.4
77.2: (b) فراخ] *om.* G | فاخرج] فاخذ G | النساء] امرأته G | داما] دام T | القلبان] ذلك G | بمكانهما] بهما G
77.3: (b) الورم...حارا] دمه الحار او دم الحمامة G | يوضع] اذا وضع G | من خارج] الرمدة G | بقطنة] في قطنة G | الورد] مع شيء من دهن الورد] مع دهن ورد وشراب
نفعها G
77.4: (a) For this recipe, see also 78.7
(b) وبيض الشافنين] بيضه G | يخلط معه] اذا طبخ وخلط G | وشيء من] *om.* G | من به وجع في كبده فينفع] نفع من وجع الكبد G
(c) For this recipe, see also 78.7

77. Turtledove

	a	b	c
	–	**The turtledoves**	–
77.1	–	If the fat from its abdomen is taken, mixed with sesame oil, and applied in drops inside the ear that is affected by deafness, then this will go pass, with the permission of God, may He be exalted.	–
77.2	–	Women will not stop loving the man who takes two chicks of this bird, then takes out their hearts and keeps them with himself, as long as the hearts remain with him and he does not reveal the position of the two hearts.	–
77.3	–	Against the swelling of the eye: if warm turtledove blood is externally applied in drps in the eye with a cotton piece of cloth soaked in egg white, with some rose oil [it will be useful].	–
77.4	–	Turtledove eggs: if some honey and some natron are mixed with them and the man who suffers from pain in his liver eats this, then this will be useful.	–

77.5 — لوجع الارحام يؤخذ شفنين ويسحقون ويذاف بدهن ورد ويبلّ به صوفة وتمسكها المرأة معها فيسل عنها وجع الارحام —

77.6 — دم الشفنين الذكر ان أخذه انسان وطلى به احليله وجامع امرأة لم يقدر عليها احد غيره وان مات ماتت زوج بعده —

77.5: (a) For this recipe, see also 78.8
(b) لوجع الارحام يؤخذ] om. G | شفنين ويسحقون ويذاف] اذا سحق واذيف G | ويبلّ] وبلّ G | وتمسكها المرأة معها فيسل عنها] وتحمّلت بها المراة نفعها G من
(c) For this recipe, see also 78.8
77.6: (a) For this recipe, see also 78.9
(b) دم الشفنين] دمه G | ان أخذه انسان وطلى] اذا طلى G | احليله] الاحليل G | احد] om. G | وان ماتى ماتت زوج بعده] om. G | In G another recipe is added, with turtledove gall: مرارته اذا خلط معها الشيلثا واذيف
منه قدر عدسة بماء الشهدانج وسعط به لريح الباذنجان نفعه
(c) For this recipe, see also 78.9

77.5	—	Against womb pain: if the droppings are taken, mixed with rose oil, a woollen cloth is soaked in it, and a woman carries it with her, then the womb pain will leave her.	—
77.6	—	Male turtledove blood: If a man takes it and rubs it on the outer opening of his urethra and has sexual intercourse with his woman, then nobody apart from that man will be able to have intercourse with her. And if he dies, his partner will die after him.	—

٧٨. اليمام

	a	b	c
	om.	حمامة البحر	باب منافع اليمام
78.1	الشخص لا يبول ويمرض حتى تنزع الشوكة من البول فيتخلص باذن الله تعالى	في جناحها شوكتان ان أخذت واحدة وغرسها في موضع قد بال فيه انسان مرض ذلك الانسان ولم يزل مريض حتى تنزع الشوكة من ذلك الموضع	*om.*
78.2	وان غرزت تلك الشوكة في بناء فلا يتم ذلك البناء والله اعلم	وان وضعت احدى الشوكتين في دار لم يتمّ كل من في تلك الدار	*om.*
78.3	*om.*	*om.*	اذا أخذ شحم اليمام واذيب بشيرج وقطر في الاذن الثقيلة السمع فتح الشدد ونفع السمع
78.4	*om.*	*om.*	اذا أخذ قلب اليمام على اسم من تريد واسم امه وجففته عندك وعلقته عليك فلا يزال ذلك الشخص يحبك ما دام عندك ولا يعلم به
78.5	يؤخذ دم يمام ودم حمام فاجعلهما على العين وهما حاران يسكن عنه الضربان ويجعل على العين بياض بيضة ودهن ورد وسذاب ويخلط الجميع ويغمس في قطنة ويجعل على العين فيبرأ باذن الله تعالى	*om.*	اذا أخذت دم الحمام ودم اليمام وحار ولطخت به العين وغسلت داخل العين بياض البيض نفعه

78.1: (a) In S this recipe is after 78.9
(b) أخذت واحدة وغرسها] أخذ منهما واحدة وجعلت G | ذلك الانسان] *om.* G | ولم يزل مريض] ولا يزال مريضا G | الشوكة من ذلك الموضع] *om.* G
78.2: (a) In S this recipe is after 78.9
(b) دار] بناء G | كل من في تلك الدار] *om.* G | In G another recipe is added, with lark meat against the colic: لحم القنابر اذا طبخ واكل وتحسى مرقة نفع من القولنج ولين الطبيعة
78.3: (c) أخذ شحم اليمام] *om.* C | ونفع السمع] *om.* C
78.4: (c) ذلك] *om.* C
78.5: (c) دم الحمام ودم اليمام وحار] قلب اليمام ودم الحمام دم يمام وهو حار C | نفعه] نفعها C

78. Wild Pigeon

	a	b	c
	om.	**The sea pigeon**	**Chapter on the useful properties of the wild pigeon**
78.1	A man will not urinate and be ill until the thorn is removed from the urine, then he will get rid [of the disease], with the permission of God may He be exalted.	Inside its wings there are two thorns, if you take one of them and plant it in the place where a men has urinated before, then this man will become ill, and hid disease will not cease until the thorn is removed from this place.	*om.*
78.2	If this thorn is thrusted inside a building, this building will not be completed, and God knows best.	And if you put one of these two thorns inside a house, then nobody in this house will be complete.	*om.*
78.3	*om.*	*om.*	If wild pigeon fat is taken, mixed with sesame oil, and applied in drops inside the ear that is hard of hearing, then this will open it and it will be useful for the hearing.
78.4	*om.*	*om.*	If the heart of a wild pigeon is taken in the name of the man you desire and in the name of his mother, then you let it dry close to you, and hang it on your body, then this man will love you as long as you wear it, but he should not be aware it.
78.5	If wild pigeon blood and domestic pigeon blood are taken while they are still warm, and applied on the eye, then this will calm the stabbing pain; and if they are applied on the eye with some egg white, rose oil and rue—everything mixed together—and a cotton cloth is dipped into it and placed on the eye, then this will be cured, with the permission of God, may He be exalted.	*om.*	If you take domestic pigeon blood and wild pigeon blood while they are still warm, spatter them on the eye, and wash the external part of the eye with egg white, this will be useful to it.

78.6	لوجع الكبد يؤخذ بيض اليمام يسلق ويخلط معه عسل وشيء من بورق يأكله من به وجع الكبد فيبرأ باذن الله تعالى	*om.*	اذا سلق بيض اليمام والقي عليه عسل وبورق وأكل من به وجع الكبد ابرأه
78.7	يؤخذ زبل اليمام ويداف بدهن ورد وينقع فيه صوفة وتتحمل به المرأة فيسكن عنها وجع الثنّة فبرئ باذن الله تعالى	*om.*	زبل اليمام اذا سحق واذيفه بدهن ونقعت فيه صوفة وحملها من النساء من يشتكي وجع الارحام ابرأها
78.8	يؤخذ دم يمام ذكر واطلِ به الاحليل عند الجماع وجامع امرأة فلا يقدر عليها احد غيرك وان متّ فلا يتزوج ابدا	*om.*	[دم اليمام اذا] طلى به الاحليل عند الجماع وجامع امرأة فلا تستطع ان تجامع احد غيرك
78.9	زبل اليمام ودم الحمام بري يبخر به المحموم يبرأ	*om.*	*om.*

78.6: (c) اذا سلق بيض اليمام] بيض اليمام اذا سلق C | عسل وبورق] العسل والبورق C
78.7: (c) واذيفه] واذيبه C | بدهن] بدهن الورد C
78.8: (c) فلا تستطع] فانها لا تستطع C

78.6	Against liver complaint: if wild pigeon eggs are taken, cooked in boiling water, mixed with honey and some natron, given to the man who has liver complaint to eat, then he will heal, with the permission of God, may He be exalted.	*om.*	If wild pigeon eggs are cooked in boiling water, honey and natron are poured over it, and they are given to eat to the man who has liver complaint, then this will cure him.
78.7	If wild pigeon excrement is taken, mixed with rose oil, a woollen cloth is soaked in it, and a woman carries it, then this will calm the pain of the womb and will cure her, with the permission of God, may He be exalted.	*om.*	Wild pigeon excrement: if it is taken, ground and mixed with oil, a woollen piece of cloth is soaked into it, and the women who suffers from womb disease carries it, then they will cure her.
78.8	If the blood of a male wild pigeon is taken, rub it on the outer opening of the urethra at the moment of coitus and have a sexual intercourse with a woman, then she will not be able to copulate with anyone else but you; and if she is related to you, she will never be given in marriage.	*om.*	Wild pigeon blood: if it is rubbed on the outer opening of the urethra at the moment of coitus, and one has sexual intercourse with a woman, then she will not be able to have intercourse with anybody else but you.
78.9	Wild pigeon excrement and *barrī* pigeon blood: if a feverish man is fumigated with it, then he will heal.	*om.*	*om.*

٧٩. الحية

	a	b	c
	ذكر منافع اعضاء الحية البرصاء	الحية	باب منافع الحية
79.1	اذا اردت ان تهرب العصافير من اوكارها بخر الوكر بسلخ حية فلا يقربه عصفور ابدا	ان بخّرتَ عش عصافير بسلخ حية هربوا منه	قشر الحية اذا بخرت به عش العصافير نفروا منه ولا يعودون اليه
79.2	اذا جعل جلد الحية في ثياب فلا يقربها السوس ابدا	وان جعلت سلخ حية في ثياب لم يسوس	اذا جعل جلد الحية في الثياب لم يقربها سوس
79.3	يؤخذ جلد الحية يعجن بالتمر ويطعم لصاحب الثآليل فيذهبوا باذن الله	يؤخذ سلخ حية يعجن ثلاث مرات ويطعم لمن به ثآليل فتسقط وتذهب وان أكله انسان ليس له الثآليل لم يخرج به ابدا	جلد الحية اذا دق وعجن بالتمر وأكله صاحب الثآليل ذهبت عنه
79.4	ناب الحية اذا علق على من يشتكي الحمى فتذهب عنه باذن الله	قلبها ان علق على من به حمّى الربع ذهبت	ناب الحية اذا علق على المحموم ابرأه
79.5	وان علق على من يشتكي وجع الاسنان سكن وجعها	نابها الاسير ان علق على من به وجع الاسنان سكن	*om.*

79.1: (b) عش] اعشاش G | هربوا منه] هربت الحية G
(c) يعودون] يعودوا C
79.2: جعلت] جعل G | سلخ حية] سلخها G
(c) سوس] ارضة C
79.3: (a) الثآليل] التواليل I
(b) الثآليل] التواليل T | *om.* G
(c) الثآليل] التواليل L
79.4: (b) This recipe is attested only in G | In G this recipe is after 79.5
(c) الحية] الحية السوداء C
79.5: (b) This recipe is attested only in G

79. Snake

	a	b	c
	Exposition of the useful properties of the parts of the white snake	**The snake**	**Chapter on the useful properties of the snake**
79.1	If you want that the sparrows flee from their nests, fumigate the nest with a the skin of a snake, then no sparrow will approach it again.	If you fumigate the nest of the sparrows with the skin of a snake, then they will flee from it.	Snake slough: if you fumigate the nest of the sparrows with it, then they will flee, and will not return to it.
79.2	If the skin of a snake is put among some clothes, then the moths will never approach them.	If the skin of a snake is put among some clothes, they will not be eaten by the moths.	If the skin of a snake is put among some clothes, then the moths will not approach them.
79.3	Snake skin: if it is taken, kneaded with dates, and given to eat to the man affected by warts, then they will go away, with the permission of God.	Snake skin: if it is kneaded three times, and fed to the man affected by warts, then these will fall and go away; if, instead, it is fed to a man who does not have warts, then he will never have them.	Snake skin: if it is ground, kneaded with dates, and it is given to eat to the man affected by warts, then the warts will leave him.
79.4	Snake fang: if it is hung on the man suffering from fever, then this will leave him, with the permission of God.	Its heart: if it is hung on the man affected by quartan fever, then this will go away.	Snake fang: if it is hung on the feverish man, then this will cure him.
79.5	If, instead, it is hung on the man who suffers from toothache, then his pain will be calmed.	Its left fang: if it is hung on the man affected by toothache, then this will be calmed.	*om.*

79.6	يؤخذ الافعى ويجعل في قدر فخار ويطين رأسها تجعل في التنور ليلة واحدة واخرجها وخذ جميع ما فيها واسحقه واعجنه يدهن شبث وادهن به البواسير الظاهرة تبرأ	للبواسير يؤخذ افعى فتصيره في قدر نحاس ويطيّن رأسها وتصير في اتون الكلس ثم يخرج يتفتح رأس القدر ويخرج ما فيها من الغظام ويسحق ويعجن بدهن ويطلي به البواسير الظاهرة باذن الله تعالى	اذا أخذ الافعى وترك في قدر فخار وطين علبة وجعلت في تنور ليلة كاملة واخرجت وأخذ ما فيها وسحق وعجن بدهن زيت او غيره ودهن به صاحب البواسير نفعها وقطع ذلك
79.7	للبواسير ايضا يؤخذ جلد حية يقطع مثل الاظافير ويسحق ناعما ويعجن بدقيق الشعير واطعمه لصاحب البواسير فيذهبوا باذن الله تعالى	يؤخذ سلخ حية فيقطع صغارا مثل الاظفار ويسحق ويؤخذ منه وزن درهمين ومن دقيق الشعير وزن درهمين ويهيأ منه اقرصه ويجعل في مستوقد حتى ينضج وياكله صاحب البواسير فيذهب باذن الله تعالى	جلد قشر الحية اذا قطع صغار مثل قلامة العظافير وسحق ناعما وأخذ منه شريحة ومن دقيق الشعير درهمين وعجن بزيت وجعل مثل القرص وشويته في الفرن واطعمته لصاحب البواسير الظاهرة نفعها
79.8	اخر لاسترخاء الاجفان العين والدمعة يؤخذ سلخ الحية يجعل في خرقة كتان ويحرق الجميع وخذ من ذلك الرماد فيداف بشراب نبيذ ثم يجفف ويسحق ناعما ويكتحل به صاحب المرض فانه يجفف وينشفّ الدمعة ويقوي الناظر	للدمعة في العين والاسترخاء في الاجفان يؤخذ سلخ حية فيحرق بالنار في خرقة ويؤخذ رماد ويذاف بشراب ويكتحل به فانه ينشف الدمعة ويقوي البصر	جلد الحية اذا ربط في خرقة واحرق واذيف رماده بماء السذاب وجفف وسحق ناعما واكتحل به من في عينه دمعة او استرخاء الجفن قوى بصره خلا الغشاوة
79.9	*om.*	وان وطئت المرأة الحبلي على حية اسقطت	*om.*
79.10	يؤخذ خرؤ الحية يدق وينخل ويدر على القوبة فيبرأ باذن الله تعالى	*om.*	زبل الحية اذا اذيف وعجن ودر على القوبة التي تعتري الادمي في المقعدة ويسيل منه الدم بزيت وقيل انها للارياح الباطنة

79.6: (a) للبواسير] *om.* G | فتصيره] صغير ويجعل G | نحاس] فخار G | وتصير] وتجعل G | رأس القدر] القدر وتروّح ما في G | الغظام] الطعام T | ويسحق...الظاهرة] تسحق وتعجن بدهن ويطلي به البواسير G
(c) وجعلت] وترك C | بدهن زيت] بزيت C
79.7: (b) فيقطع] ويقطع G | مثل الاظفار] *om.* G | وزن...فيذهب] فينفعه البواسير به من وياكله ويخبز قرص منه ويجعل شعير دقيق درهم ووزن درهم وزن G
(c) جلد قشر الحية] قشر الحية C | العظافير] العصافير L | وجعل] وقطع وجعل C
79.8: (b) للدمعة...البصر] يحد البصر ويحد الدمعة ينشف فانه ويكتحله بشراب يذاف رماده ويؤخذ خرقة في يحرق الحية سلخ G | In G another recipe is added, with snake vertebra against the haemorrhoids: خرزة الحية تدق وتنخل وتذر على البواسير تجفّ
79.9: (b) المرأة الحبلي] امرأة حبلي G | اسقطت] اسقطت حملها *add.* G
79.10 (c) وعجن] وسحق وعجن C | الادهي] الانسان C | بزيت] *om.* C | وقيل...الباطنة] *om.* C

79.6	If a viper is taken, put in an earthenware pot, its opening is sealed with clay, then it is put in a backing oven for one night, then taken out, everything inside it is taken, ground, kneaded with dill oil, and rubbed on the external haemorrhoids, then they will be cured.	Against haemorrhoids, a viper should be taken, put in a copper pot, its opening is sealed with clay, put it in a lime kiln; then it is taken out, the pot is open, and the bones inside it are taken, ground, kneaded with oil, and rubbed on the external haemorrhoids, with the permission of God, may He be exalted.	If a viper is taken, left in an earthenware pot, the pot is sealed with clay, and put in a baking oven for a whole night, then it is taken out, and what is inside it is taken, ground, kneaded with oil or another grease, and rubbed on the man who suffers from haemorrhoids, then this will stop.
79.7	Also against haemorrhoids, if the skin of a snake is taken, cut like the nails, ground finely, kneaded with barley flour, and given to the man who suffers from haemorrhoids to eat, then these will cease, with the permission of God, may He be exalted.	Snake skin: if it is taken, cut into small pieces like the nails, and ground, then two dirhams of it are taken with two dirhams of barley flour, shaped in the form of bread loaves, then put in the fireplace until they are well cooked, then these are given to the man suffering from haemorrhoids to eat, then this will go away, with the permission of God, may He be exalted.	Skin, snake slough: if it is cut in small pieces, like nail clippings, finely ground, a chip of it is taken with two dirhams of barley flour, kneaded with oil, and made into a flat loaf, then baked in the oven, and given to the man who suffers from external haemorrhoids to eat, then this will be useful against them.
79.8	Another [recipe] against the flaccidity of the eyelids and lachrymation, snake skin: if it is taken, put in a linen cloth, and everything is burnt, then take some ash, and mix it with wine, then dry it, grind it finely, and rub it on the man affected by the disease, then the lachrymation will dry, and the eyesight will be strengthened.	Against the lachrymation in the eye and the flaccidity of the eyelids, snake skin: if it is taken, burnt with fire in a piece of cloth, its ash is taken, mixed with wine, and applied on the eye, then this will absorb the lachrymation and strengthen the eyesight.	Snake skin: if it is tied in a piece of cloth, burnt, its ash is mixed with rue water, dried, finely ground, and rubbed on the eye affected by lachrymation or flaccidity of the eyelid, then this will strengthen the eyesight, with the exception of the cataract.
79.9	*om.*	If a pregnant woman steps over a snake, then she will miscarry.	*om.*
79.10	Snake excrement: if it is ground, sieved, and applied on the tetter, then this will heal, with the permission of God, may He be exalted.	*om.*	Snake excrement: if it is mixed, kneaded, and poured together with oil on the tetter which affects the man in the backside and from which blood flows; and it is said that these are the inner winds.

79.11	اذا وقع جلد الحية في الماء واللبن الحليب واطعم للبازي مع اللحم كان ابلغ وان كان اللبن وحده فانفع وان كان من شحم الحية فابلغ	للقمل الذي يكون في الباري يؤخذ سلخ الحية فيبل بلبن حليب ويطعم الباز مع اللحم السلحفاة فانه يبرأ	اذا ان يجود الباز ويصلحه تأخذ سلخ حية فتبله بلبن حليب واطعمه للباز مع لحم وان كان من اللحم الحية وكان اجود
79.12	اذا أخذ قرن الحية وعلق على المحموم اذهب حماه	قرن من قرون الحية ذات القرون ان علق على من به حمى الغبّ زالت عنه	يؤخذ من قرون هذا الحية وعلّق على من يشتكي الحمى فتزول باذن الله تعالى
79.13	سلخ الحية اذا عجن بالزيت وطلى به داء الثعلب نبت الشعر	سلخ الافعى يحرق في كوز ويؤخذ منه ويعجن بزيت يطلي به للحمى	يؤخذ سلخ الافعى يحرق ويعجن بالزيت ويطلي به داء الثعلب فينبت فيه الشعر
79.14	دم الافعى اذا خلط ببورق وملح مسحق ولطخ به البرص اذهبه	دم الافعى يخلط معه بورق وملح به موضع البرص يغير لونه	دم الافعى يخلط معه بورق وملح ومر ويلطخ معه البرص فيزول باذن الله تعالى
79.15	اذا أخذ الافعى وقطع من عند رأسه وذنبه وطبخ بالماء والشب والقي عليه في اجزاء الصبح سنبل وقرنفل وخولنجان حتى يستوي وياكل لحمه وشرب مرقته صاحب الجذام فانه يبرأ منه	للجذام يؤخذ الافعى فيقطع من رأسها ومن ذنبها اصبع من كل ناحية ويطبخ بالماء والملح والشبّ ويلقي فيها الخولنجان والقرنفل ويؤكل لحمه وتسحّي من مرقتها تنفعه نفعا بينا	يؤخذ افعى تقطع من عند رأسه الى اسفل مقدار ثلاث اصابع ومن عند ذنبها ثلاث اصابع ويجعل في قدر ويجعل عليها غمرها ماء ويدر عليها يسير ملح وشب وقرنفل ويغلا غلياتا جيدا ويطعم لصاحب الجذام فيقف عنه باذن الله تعالى
79.16	*om.*	سلخ الحية يبخر به مع مقل وقشور اصول الكِبر وزراوند طريان وقشر البلاذر فيبرأ البواسير الظاهرة	*om.*

79.11: (b) للقمل...يبرأ] سلخ الحية يبل بلبن حليب ويطعم للباز الذي يكون به قمل مع لحم السلحفاة ينفعه G
(c) كان ابلغ] كان حسنه C | وان كان...فابلغ] وقطع وجعل C
79.12: (b) قرن...القرون] قرن الحية G | ان] اذا G | زالت عنه] نفعه G
(c) اذا أخذ...وعلق] قرن الحية اذا علق C
79.13: (b) ويؤخذ منه] *om.* G | للحمى] داء الثعلب فينبت الشعر G
(c) سلخ] مخ C | نبت] انبت C
79.14: (b) يخلط] اذا خلط G | وملح به موضع] وملح وطلى به G | يغير لونه] نفعه G
79.15: (b) للجذام] *om.* G | الافعى...ويطبخ] الافاعي ويُقطع من رؤوسها ومن اذنابها كل جانب اربع اصابع ويطبخ الاوساط G | ويلقي فيها] *om.* G | الخولنجان والقرنفل] والقرنفل والخولنجان G | ويؤكل لحمه] *om.* G | وتسحّي...بينا] ثم يتسحّي المجدوم مرقتها فينفعه G
(c) الافعى] الحية الانثى C | وذنبه] وعند ذنبه C | بالماء] بالماء والملح C | وياكل] فاذا أكل C | لحمه...منه] من اصابه الجذام ذلك وشرب مرقته ابرأه وأوقفه C
79.16: (b) سلخ الحية...الظاهرة] سلخ الحية اذا بخّر به البواسير مع مقل وقشور اصول الكِبر وزراوند طويل وتمر البلاذر اذهبه G

79.11	If you want that a hawk improves and gets better, take a snake slough, moisten it with cow milk, and give it to the hawk to eat with meat; and if it snake meat, then it is even better.	Against the lice of the hawk, snake slough: if it is taken, moistened with cow milk, fed to the hawk with turtle meat, then he will heal.	If a snake skin is soaked in water and milk, and fed to the hawk with meat, it will be more effective; if it is just with milk, it will be more useful; while, if it is with snake fat, it will be more effective.
79.12	Horn of this snake: if it is taken, and hung on the man suffering from fever, then this will cease, with the permission of God, may He be exalted.	Snake horn from a horned snake: if it is hung of the man suffering from tertian fever, then this will leave him.	If a snake is taken, and hung on the feverish man, then his fever will cease.
79.13	Viper slough: if it is taken, burnt, kneaded with oil, and rubbed on the alopecia, then the hair will grow there.	Viper slough: if it is burnt in a small jug, then taken, kneaded with oil, and rubbed, then this will be against fever.	Snake slough: if it is kneaded with oil, and rubbed on the alopecia, then the hair will grow.
79.14	Viper blood: if it is mixed with natron, salt and myrrh, and spattered on the leprosy, then this will cease, with the permission of God, may He be exalted.	Viper blood: if it is taken with natron, and the area of the leprosy is treated with it, then this will change its colour.	Viper blood: if it is mixed with natron and ground salt, and the leprosy is spattered with it, this will make it go away.
79.15	If a viper is taken, three fingers from the head and three fingers from the tail are cut, then it is put in a cooking pot, covered with abundant water, a bit of salt, alum and clove are added, it is then boiled well, and given to the man who suffers from elephantiasis to drink, then this will leave him, with the permission of God, may He be exalted.	Against elephantiasis, if a viper is taken, from its head and from its tail one finger is cut from each extremity, then it is cooked with water, salt, alum, galangal and clove; then its meat is fed and its broth sipped, then this will be very useful to him.	If a viper is taken, its head and its tail are cut away, then it is cooked with water and alum, hyacinth, clove, galangal are poured on it in the same quantity; then its meat is given to eat, and its broth is given to drink to the man affected by elephantiasis, then he will be cured.
79.16	*om.*	Snake slough: if it is fumigated with bdellium, fresh peelings of liquorice roots and aristolochia, and cashew peelings, then this will cure the external haemorrhoids.	*om.*

79.17	يؤخذ حية تحرق ويؤخذ رمادها فيخلط معه بورق ويدر على الخنازير فتذهب باذن الله تعالى والذي يكون في الحلق يعجن بخل ويطلي بها الحلق فيذهب	المتعلقة الحية يحرق ويؤخذ من رمادها ويخلط معه بورق ويقطع الخنازير التي تكون في البدن والرأس	اذا احرقت الحية وأخذ رمادها وخلط ببورق مسحوق ودر على الخنازير ابرأها والذي يكون [في الحلق] يعجن بخل خمر حادق ويطلي به الرأس يذهب
79.18	*om.*	يؤخذ من رماد الحية المحروقة ويعجن بماء السذاب ويطلي به البهق [نفعه]	*om.*
79.19	بيض الحية يجعل في هاون ويلقي عليه بورق ويسحق الجميع ويعجن بالخل واطل به صاحب البرص فيغيّر لونه ويوقفه باذن الله تعالى	يؤخذ بيض الحية فيلقي في هاون ويخلط معه بورق ويطلي به البرص الحديث يقلع	بيض الحية اذا جعل في هاون ومعه بورق وزيت وخل خمر ومرهم وطلى به البرص الحادث ابرأه وغير لونه
79.20	شحم الأفعى يداف بدهن ورد ويغمس فيه قطنة ويتحمل به صاحب البواسير فتذهب عنه باذن الله تعالى	شحمها اذا ذوّب ودهن به البواسير نفعها	*om.*
79.21	*om.*	يؤخذ رماد الحية بماء قشور الجوز الرطب وماء عروق الجوز ويطلي به مواضع الوضح يغير لونه ويحسن	*om.*
79.22	*om.*	شحم الافعى يخلط معه شيء يسير من ملح مسحوق وبورق مرزنجوش مدقوق منخول ويُذاف بماء السلجم ويطلي على البواسير مرة واحدة فتصلح الظاهرة والباطنة	*om.*

79.17: (b) المتعلقة الحية] سلخها G | يحرق...والرأس] سلخها اذا حُرق وخلط مع رماده البورق وعجن بخل وطلى به الحزاز اذهبه G
79.18: (b) يؤخذ...المحروقة] ورماد سلخ الحية G | ويعجن] اذا عجن G | ويطلي به] وطلى بها G
78.19: (b) يؤخذ...يقلع] بيض الحية اذا دق مع بورق وخل وطلى به البرص نفعه G
(c) *om.* C
79.20: (b) This recipe is attested only in G
79.21: (b) يؤخذ رماد الحية] الحية اذا حرقت وعجن رمادها G | ويطلي] وطلى G | مواضع الوضح] البرص G | يغير لونه ويحسن] نفعه G
79.22: (b) شحم الافعى] شحمها G | يخلط...السلجم] مع ملح مسحوق وورق المرزنجوش المدقوق المنخول ويُذوب الشحم G | ويطلي...والباطنة] وطلى به البواسير نفعه G

79.17	If a snake is taken and burnt, its ash is taken, mixed with natron, and applied copiously on the scrofula, then this will go away, with the permission of God, may He be exalted; also the one on the back of the throat, if if this is kneaded with vinegar and rubbed on the back of the throat, then it will go away.	Snake slough: if it is burnt, its ash taken and mixed with natron, then this will stop the scrofula that is on the body and on the head.	If a snake is burnt, its ash taken, mixed with ground natron, and copiously applied on the scrofula, then this will cure it; and also the one on the back of the throat, if the ash is kneaded with acid wine vinegar, and rubbed on the head, then this will go away.
79.18	*om.*	If the ash of the burnt snake is taken, kneaded with rue water, and rubbed on the leprosy, then this will be useful against it.	*om.*
79.19	Snake egg: if it is put in a mortar, natron is added to them, everything is ground with vinegar, then rub it on the man affected by leprosy, then this will change its colour, and will cease, with the permission of God, may He be exalted.	Snake eggs: if they are put in a mortar, natron is mixed with them, and the recent leprosy is rubbed with it, then this will eradicate it.	Snake eggs: if they are put in a mortar with natron, oil, wine vinegar and an ointment, and rubbed on the recent leprosy, this will cured it, and will change its colour.
79.20	Viper fat: if it is mixed with rose oil, a cotton cloth is soaked in it, and the man suffering from haemorrhoids carries it, then they will cease, with the permission of God, may He be exalted.	Its fat: if it is liquefied, and rubbed on the haemorrhoids, then this will be useful against them.	*om.*
79.21	*om.*	If the ash of the snake is taken with the water of nut peelings, and rubbed on the areas of the leprosy, then this will change its colour, and make it nicer.	*om.*
79.22	*om.*	Viper fat: if it is mixed with a little bit of ground salt, natron, ground and sieved marjoram, mixed with turnip water, and rubbed once on the haemorrhoids, then this will cure both the external and internal ones.	*om.*

اذا أخذت الحية وجعلت على لوح [وقطع] بطنها بسكين وذبحت وبقى مع رأسها اربعة اصابع وجعلت قدر نحاس ولقى عليها من الزيت قدر رطل ومن الماء رطلين واغلى عليه حتى يذهب الماء ويبقي الزيت خذه واتركه في قرورة واذا اردت استعمله خذ من ذلك الزيت بريشة واطلى رأس الاقرع فانه ينبت الشعر ويسوده وكذا صاحب داء الثعلب اذا طلى به انبت الشعر وسوّده وحسّنه

[الحية] اسود يؤخذ ويمد على لوح ويهيج بطنه بسكين ويذبح ويلقي من رأسه اربع اصابع ومن ذنبه مثل ذلك ويصير في قدر نحاس ويلقي عليه من الماء رطلين ومن الزيت رطل ويطبخ حتى يذهب الماء ويبقي الزيت واحذر ان يصيب يدك فان اصابها نبت فيها الشعر وارفعها في قارورة فان احتجتَ اليه فاطل منه بريشة على موضع داء الثعلب فانه ينبت الشعر

79.23 يؤخذ الحية السالخ يجعل على لوح ويقشّر جوفه من خارج ويقطع من عند الرأس اربع اصابع ومن عند ذنبه مثل ذلك ويجعل في قدر نحاس واجعل عليه من الزيت الطيب رطل ومن الماء رطلين واغليه حتى يذهب الماء ويبقي الزيت فارفعه في قارورة فاذا احتجتَ اليه فخذ منه بريشة واطل به داء الثعلب فانه ينبت فيه الشعر وايّال أن يصب به الجسد فانه ينبت فيه الشعر وهذا عجيب ومليح

79.23: (b) الاسود سالخ [الاسود G | يؤخذ ويمد [اذا مُد G | لوح [وضح G | ويهيج [يمسح G | ويلقي...ويصير [ويرمي من رأسه ومن ذنبه مقدار اربع اصابع G | ويلقي...رطل [مع رطلين ماء ورطل زيت G | ويبقي الزيت [ثم يصفي منه الزيت G | واحذر...الشعر [فاي شيء اصابه الزيت نبت فيه الشعر وارفعه في قارورة واطلي منه بريشه مواضع تريد نبت الشعر فيها فتنبت G
(c) حتى [الى ان C | في قرورة [في اناء C | واطلى رأس [واطل منه رأس C

79.23 If a snake is taken, placed on a slab, its abdomen is peeled from the outside, then it is cut four inches from its head and the same measure from its tail, it is put in a copper cooking pot, one *raṭl* of good oil and two of water are added to it, then it is left to boil until the water evaporates while the oil remains, then it is stored inside a long-necked flask; when you need it, take the oil with a feather and rub the alopecia with it, and the hair will grow; as soon as the body is touched, then the hair will grow, and this is amazing and witty.

If a black [snake] is taken, placed on a slab, its abdomen is opened with a knife, it is slaughtered, then four fingers from its head and the same from its tail are cut, it is put in a copper cooking pot, two *raṭls* of water and one of oil are poured on it, and it is cooked until the water has gone while the oil remains—pay attention that it does not touch your hand, because the hair would grow there—store it inside a long-necked flask, and when you need it, apply it with a feather on the area of the alopecia, and the hair will grow.

If a snake is taken, put on a slab, its abdomen cut open with a knife, then it is slaughtered leaving four fingers from its head, then it is put in a copper cooking pot and one *raṭl* of oil and two of water are poured on it, then is left to boil until the water is gone and the oil remains, take this oil, and store it inside a long-necked flask; when you want to use it, pick up this oil with a feather and apply it on the scabby head, then the hair will grow and become black; likewise for the man affected by alopecia, if he is rubbed with it, then the hair will grow, and become black and nicer.

٨٠. العقرب

	a	b	c
	ذكر منافع العقرب البري	العقارب	باب منافع العقرب
80.1	يؤخذ العقرب البري يجعل في كوز ويشوي في النار حتى يبقي رمادا ويؤخذ من رماده جزء ومن اصل الكبر جزء ويداف الجميع بعسل ويسقي منه صاحب الحصاة وبرد الكلى يبرأ	للحصاة في المثانة يؤخذ عقربا فيسحق في كوز ويؤخذ منها جزء وخولنجان جزء ومن اصل الكبر جزء ويشرب بطلاء وعسل فانه يفتت الحصاة من المثانة	اذا احرقت العقرب وأخذ رمادها وأخذت منه جزأ ومن اصول الكبر جزأ وخلطا ويسقي بالعسل لصاحب الحصاة وبرد الكلى والحصاة السوداء التي في المثانة ابرأ ذلك
80.2	*om.*	يؤخذ عقربا كبيرة سوداء فتجفف وتدق وتعجن بخل ويطلي على موضع البرص فيذهب باذن الله تعالى	العقرب الاسود اذا جفف وسحق وعجن رماده بالخل والخمر وطلى به البرص الفاضح ابرأه
80.3	يؤخذ عقرب فيلقي في الزيت حتى يموت وخذ ذلك الزيت واعجن به ذراريح واطل به المشش الذي يكون في رجل الدواب فيزول باذن الله تعالى	لمشش الدواب تلقي العقارب في الزيت حتى تموت ثم يؤخذ ذلك الزيت فيعجن به ذراريح مدقوقة منخولة ويضمد به المشش الذي في ايدي الدواب فتحله ويذهب به	اذا أخذ عقربا وغليته في زيت وعجنت بالزيت ودقيق الرازيانج اي السمر وضمدت به رجل الدابة التي اصابها المشش ابرأته
80.4	يؤخذ عقرب ويغلي في سمن حتى يذوب ورفع في اناء فاذا لسعت انسانا عقرب فالطخ موضع اللسعة من ذلك الدهن فيسكن المها باذن الله تعالى وهو يكون في خزائن الملوك	يؤخذ عقربا تطبخ بالسمن حتى تنهري ويرفع ذلك السمن فان لسع انسانا عقرب فيذهن ذلك الموضع بشىء من السمن ينفعه ويسكن وجهه	اذا غليت العقرب في زيت الى ان ينهري ورفعت الزيت في اناء فاذا لسع انسان ادهن لسعه من ذلك الزيت فانه يسكن الالم

80.1: (b) للحصاة...منها] العقرب اذا احرق في كوز وأخذ من رماده G | اصل] اصول G | فانه يفتت الحصاة من المثانة] فيفتّت الحصاة G
(c) العقرب] *om.* C | لصاحب...ذلك] في المثانة التي وبرد الحصاة صاحب نفع C

80.2: (b) يؤخذ...فيذهب] العقرب الكبيرة السوداء اذا جففت وسحقت وعجنت بخل وطلى به البرص نفعه G
(c) الفاضح] *om.* C

80.3: (b) المشش...ويذهب به] يذهبه الدواب ايدي في المشش به ويضمّد مدقوقة ذراديح الزيت بذلك ويعجن تموت ختى زيت في عقرب ملقى G
(c) وغليته] وغليتها C | الرازيانج اي السمر] الرازنانج وهو التمر C

80.4: (b) يؤخذ...ينفعه] العقرب اذا طبخت بسمن حتى تتهّرا ويرفع ذلك السمن فاذا لسعت العقرب انسانا دهن اللسعة من ذلك ينفعه G | ويسكن وجهه] *om.* G
(c) ينهري] يتهري C | السعة] اللسعة C

80. Scorpion

	a	b	c
	Exposition of the useful properties of the land scorpion	**The scorpions**	**Chapter on the useful properties of the scorpion**
80.1	Land scorpion: if it is taken, put it in a small jug, roasted on the fire until it becomes ash; then one part of this ash and one part of mustard roots have to be taken, everything mixed with honey, and given to the man who suffers from stones and kidney coldness to drink, then he will heal.	Against the stones in the bladder: if a scorpion is taken, ground in a small jug, one part of this, one part of galangal and one part of mustard roots are taken, and drunk with tar and honey, then this will crumble the stones in the bladder.	If a scorpion is burnt, one part of its ash and one part of mustard roots are taken, mixed and given with honey to drink to the man who suffers from stones, kidney coldness, and black stones in the bladder, then these will be cured.
80.2	*om.*	Big black scorpion: if it is dried, crushed, kneaded with vinegar, and rubbed on the area of the leprosy, then this will go away, with the permission of God, may He be exalted.	Black scorpion: if it is dried, ground, its ash is kneaded with vinegar and wine, and the infamous leprosy is rubbed, then this will cure it.
80.3	If a scorpion is taken, thrown into some oil and left there until it dies, then take this oil, knead some blister beetle with it, and rub it on the pustules on the feet of the animals, then they will cease, with the permission of God, may He be exalted.	Against the pustules of the animals: if the scorpions are thrown in some oil until they die, then this oil is taken, some crushed and sieved blister beetles are kneaded with it, and the pustules on the forelegs of the beasts are bandaged with it, then this will dissolve them, and send them away.	If a scorpion is taken, boiled in oil, kneaded with the oil and powder of fennel—that is the *samar* [?]—and the feet of the beasts affected by pustules are bandaged with it, then this will cure them.
80.4	If a scorpion is taken, boiled in fat until it melts, then it is stored in a vessel; and when a scorpion stings a man, spatter the area of the sting with this oil, then the pain will cease with the permission of God, may He be exalted. This can be found in the treasures of the kings.	If a scorpion is taken, cooked with fat until it is well done, then store this fat away; and if a scorpion stings a man, then this area has to be rubbed with some of this fat, then it will be useful against it, and will calm its pain.	If you boil the scorpion in oil until it is well done, and store this oil in a vessel; then if a scorpion stings a man, rub its sting with that oil, and then the pain will calm down.

	(c)	(b)	(a)
80.5	يؤخذ عقرب ويحرق حتى يصير رمادا ويؤخذ منه جزء ومن خرؤ الفار جزء ويسحق ويخلط الجميع بعسل ويطلي به اجفان العين فانه ينبت الشعر ويخلط الجفن ينفع العين باذن الله تعالى	يؤخذ العقارب المحرقة فتخلط مع عسل وخرء فار فيكتحل به في العين نافع من اسنان الاجفان وغلظها	اذا وقع شعر جفن العينين احرق عقربا وخذ من رماده جزء ومن خرو الفار جزء ومن العسل جزء بغير فار واخلط الجميع واكحل منه من لا في جفنه شعر فانه ينبت شعر الاجفان وعينه
80.6	اذا اردت ان تهرب العقارب من الدار فخذ عقربا تجففه وتبخر به الدار فانهم يهربون من رائحها ولا يرجع يقرب الموضع عقرب ابدا	وان بخّرتَ البيت بالعقارب هربت منه العقارب	اذا اردت ان لا يبقي في المكان عقرب بخره بعقرب فلا يبقي ذلك المكان عقرب
80.7	اذا لسعت العقرب لانسان فتأخذ عقربا فتشق جوفها وتضمدها اللسعة فيسكن المها باذن الله تعالى	تؤخذ العقرب فتسرج وتشق بطنها ويضمد به الملسوع وتضمد بها ايضا من عضة الكلب فيفرج الموضع ويخرج ما فيه من السم	*om.*
80.8	يؤخذ عقرب يشق جوفها ويضمد بها عضة الكلب الكلب فيبرأ باذن الله تعالى	*om.*	اذا شققت العقرب وضمدت بها عضة الكلب الكلب ابرأتها
80.9	يؤخذ اربع [او] خمس عقارب فتجعل في خرقة كتان وتجعل الخرقة في الشمس حتى تجف فاذا جفت الخرقة والعقارب سحقهما ناعما فاخلط معها عنزروت ومقل ازرق وسندروس وحبة مسك ويبخر به المجنون او المكان الذي يكون فيه فيبرأ باذن الله	يؤخذ عقربا فتصير في خرقة من ثوب جديد وتصير في السمن حتى تجف ثم تسحق ويخلط معها صندروس ومقل ازرق وشعير فارسي وحبة مسك ويخلط جميعا وتبخر به المصروع الذي يصرع في رأس كل شهر	اذا أخذت ثلاث عقارب وتركت في الشمس الى ان تجف وخلطت بشيء من سندروس ومقل ازرق وحبة مسك وبخرت به المصروع والمكان الذي يصرع فيه زال ذلك العارض

80.5: (b) خرء الفار] وجزوفان T | يؤخذ...وغلظها] العقرب اذا احرقت وخلط مع رمادها عسل وجزء الغار وكحّل به العين نفعها من غلظ الاجفان G
(c) العينين] العين C | واخلط] ثم اخلط C | وعينه] ويحسنه C
80.6: (b) بخّرت] بخر G | بالعقارب] بعقرب G
(c) فلا...عقرب] ابدا عقرب هناك يبقي لا رايحتها شم اذا فانه C
80.7 (b) فتشرح] فتسرج G | تؤخذ...السم] العقرب اذا شرّح بطنها وضمد بها اللسعة سكن وكذلك كلب الكلب تنفع من عضته G
80.8: (b) For this recipe, see 80.7
80.9: يؤخذ...شهر] تؤخذ عقرب تجعل في خرقة كتان جديدة وتجعل في الشمس حتى تجف وتسحق مع بسندروس ومقل ازرق وصعتر فارسي ومسك ويبخّر به المصروع عند الهلال تنفعه G
(c) وخلطت بشيء] واخلط مع ذلك شيء C

80.5	If a scorpion is taken, burnt until it becomes ash, one part of it and one part of mouse excrement are taken, ground, everything mixed with honey, and rubbed on the eyelids, then the hair will grow there; and if it is applied on the eyelids, this will also be useful to the eye itself, with the permission of God, may He be exalted.	If burnt scorpions are taken, mixed with honey and mouse excrement, and applied on the eye, then this will be useful against the 'teeth of the eyelids' and their hardness.	If the hair of eyelids does not grow, burn a scorpion, take one part of its ash, one part of mouse excrements, one part of honey and one part of excrement of another animal, melt everything together, and rub it on the eyelids, then the hair of the eyelids and of the eye will grow again.
80.6	If you want that the scorpions flee from the house, take a scorpion, dry it, and fumigate the house with it, then they will flee from its smell, and not a single scorpion will approach the place again.	If you fumigate the house with a scorpion, then the scorpions will flee from it.	If you want that not a single scorpion remains in a place, fumigate it with a scorpion, and then not a single scorpion will remain there.
80.7	If a the scorpion stings a man, take a scorpion, split its abdomen open, and bandage with it the sting, then the pain will cease, with the permission of God, may He be exalted.	If you take the scorpion, split its abdomen open, and bandage with it the man who has been stung—and also the bite of the dog—then that area will split open, and the poison in it will come out.	*om.*
80.8	If a scorpion is taken, its abdomen split open, and the bite of the rabid dog is bandaged with it, then this will cure it, with the permission of God, may He be exalted.	*om.*	If you split a scorpion, and bandage with it the bite of a rabid dog, then this will cure it.
80.9	Take four or five scorpions, put them in a linen piece of cloth, and leave them in the sun until they dry; once the piece of cloth and the scorpions are dry, grind them finely and mix with sarcocolla, blue bdellium, sandarac and a grain of musk, fumigate with it the possessed man or the place where he has been, then he will heal, with the permission of God, may He be exalted.	If a scorpion is taken, put in a piece of cloth from a new garment, left in the sun until it dries, ground with sandarac, blue bdellium, Persian barley and a grain of musk, and the epileptic man who has seizures at the beginning of every month is fumigated with it, then this will be useful to him.	If you take three scorpions, leave them in the sun until they dry, mix them with some sandarac, bdellium and a grain of musk, then fumigate with it the epileptic man and the place where he has had his attack, then this condition will cease.

80.10	*om.*	*om.*	اذا أخذت ثلاث عقارب وربطها في خرقة كتان وتركتها في الزيت حتى تجف ثم انزع واسحقها جيدا واخلطها بسندروس ومقل ومسك نافع للمصروع ايضا
80.11	اذا كانت المرأة لا يعيشها ولد يؤخذ عقرب على اسم المرأة واسم امها فتشد في خرقة ويجعل على عضدها او في عنقها وهي حامل فيسلم الجنين باذن الله تعالى ويخرج سالما	واذا كانت المرأة لا يعيش لها ولد فخذ عقربا وصيرها في خرقة وعلقها على المولود فانه يسلم	اذا كانت المرأة لا يعيش ولدها خذ عقربا واربطها في خرقة وعلقها في عنق المولود فانه يعيش
80.12	*om.*	وان كامت المرأة لا يعيش تسقط فينقش عقربا في خاتم ولبسه وهي حامل سلم ولدها	واذا كانت المرأة سقط اولادها خذ عقربا واجعلها في عنقها وهي حامل فانها تمسك الولد باذن الله تعالى
80.13	*om.*	*om.*	اذا أخذت فصا اخضرا ونقشه عليه صورة عقرب وجعلت في خاتم واعطيته للمرأة في اصبعها فانه يسهل عليها الولادة

80.10: (c) ومقل] *om.* C | نافع للمصروع ايضا] فانه يبرأ المصروع C
80.11: (b) واذا...يسل] يؤخذ عقرب ميتة وتجعل في خرقة كتان وتعلق على مولود فيسلم G
(c) *om.* C
80.12: (b) وان...ولدها] وتنفع الحامل اذا علقت عليها G
(c) سقط اولادها] تسقط الاولاد C
80.13: (c) وجعلت] وجعلته C

80.10	*om.*	*om.*	If you take three scorpions, and tie them in a linen piece of cloth, leave them in oil until they dry; then take them out, grind them well, and mix with sandarac, bdellium and musk: then this will be useful to the epileptic man too.
80.11	If no child survives to a woman, take a scorpion in the name of this woman and her mother, fasten it on the upper arm or onto her neck while she is pregnant, then the foetus will be safe, with the permission of God, may He be exalted, and will come out healthy.	If no child of a woman lives, taken a scorpion, put it in a piece of cloth, and hang it on the baby, and this will be healthy.	If no child of the woman lives, take a scorpion, wrap it in a piece of cloth, and hang it on the neck of the baby, and then this will live.
80.12	*om.*	If the woman keeps having miscarriages, engrave a scorpion on a seal, give her this to carry while she is pregnant, and then the baby will be healthy.	If a woman keeps losing her babies, take a scorpion and put it on her neck while she is pregnant, and then she will be able to keep the baby, with the permission of God, may He be exalted.
80.13	*om.*	*om.*	If you take a green stone, engrave on it the image of a scorpion, mount it on a seal [ring], and put it on the finger of a woman, then this will ease her delivery.

٨١. بقر بني اسرائيل

	a	b	c
	—	ام قيس	—
		وهى دابة صغيرة لها قرنان تكون في الرمل ويرى في موضعها مثل الطمع	
81.1	—	فاذا اردت ان تأخذها فاعرف موضعها واطرح فيه نملة فانها تخرج لتأخذها فاذا صارت في يدك فشق ظهرها وادخل فيه الميل واكتحل من بعينه بياض ثلاث مرات يذهب باذن الله تعالى	—

81: ام قيس] بقر بني اسرائيل G | دابة] وتعرف ببقرة حوشب ويقال بها ام قيس وام عويف add. G | ويرى في موضعها مثل الطمع] om. G
81.1: (b) ان تأخذها فاعرف] في اخراجها فابصق G | نملة فانها تخرج لتأخذها فاذا صارت في يدك] قملة فاذا خرجت G | من بعينه بياض ثلاث مرات] به من البياض في العين ثلث مرات فهو يذهب G | يذهب] G | In G another recipe is added, with the ladybird used against the ringworm: ويدكك بها موضع القرع ينبت فيه الشعر

81. Ladybird

	a	b	c
	–	**The ladybird**	–
		It is small beast and has two horns, it lives in the sand, one searches for it in its holes like a coveted thing.	
81.1	–	If you want to take it, discover where its hole is, throw an ant inside it and [the ladybird] will come out to grab it; when it is in your hand, split its back, dip a small brush into it and apply it on the eye affected by glaucoma for three times, then this will disappear, with the permission of God, may He be exalted.	–

٨٢. الحرذون

	a	b	c
	ذكر منافع الحرذون	الحرذون	باب منافع الحرذون
82.1	*om.*	*om.*	اذا احرقت جلده وطلى به الجسد لم يناله الم من ضرب ولا قطع ولو فرقت بين رأسه وجسده
82.2	لحم الحرذون يشد في خرقة حرير ويعلق انسان على العضد فانه يقوي على الجماع ويزيد في الباه وفي شهوة الجماع	يؤخذ لحم الحرذون تعلقه على عضدك فيزيد في الباه والقوة ويحرق الشهوة	لحم الحرذون اذا علقه انسان على عضده فانه يزيد في جماعه ويقوي الباه
82.3	يؤخذ حرذون يقطع ذنبه ويؤخذ دمه ويخلط معه دهن زنبق ويبل به فتيلة ويوقد في سراج فيصير ذلك البيت كانه الفضة وخاصّيته اذا كان الحرذون اسودا	يأخذ حرذون ويقطع ذنبه وتأخذ من دم ذنبه جزء فتخلطه بزنبق وبل فيه فتيلة وتصيرها في سراج فيصير البيت يلمع مثل الفضة	اذا قطع ذنب الحرذون وأخذ دمه وخلط بدهن زنبق خلطا جيدا واغمست فيه فتيلة واوقدت في سراج صار البيت يلمع كانه فضة جلية وان كان الحرذون اسود كان ابلغ
82.4	اذا اردت ان تخلا الدار من السكان فخذ زبل الحرذون مع زبل الذيك وبخر به الموضع فلا يسكن ابدا	[زبل] الجردون اسود وزبل الديك اجزاء سواء يبخر به البيت فلا يسكنه احد	بعر الحرذون مع زبل الديك اذا خلطا وبخر بهما المنزل فانه يخلوا ويخرب ولا يسكنه احد

82: (a) الحرذون] الجراذون السماني I
(b) الحرذون] الجردون T; الجراذين G
(c) الحرذون] الحردون بالحاء المهملة L; الجردون C
82.1: (b) In G another recipe is added, with lizard blood against leprosy and scabies: دمه اذا خلط معه دقيق الحمص ولطخ به البهق والجرب نفعه
(c) *om.* C
82.2: (b) يؤخذ...الشهوة] لحمه اذا علق على عضد انسان الايمن زاد في باهه وجماعه G
(c) ويقوي] وقوة C
82.3: (b) زنبق] بزيبق T | يأخذ...الفضة] دم ذنبه مع زنبق وبُل به قتيلة وتسرج في بيت لمع البيت مثل الفضة وليكر اسودا G
(c) جلية] مجلية C | كان ابلغ] فابلغ C
82.4: (b) زبل] ويكون T | اسود] *om.* G | وزبل] مع زبل G | اجزاء سواء] *om.* G | يبخر] اذا بخّر G | فلا] لا G
(c) بعر] خرء C | مع زبل] وزبل C | بهما] به C | يسكنه احد] يسكنه ابدا احدا C

82. Lizard

	a	b	c
	Exposition of the useful properties of the lizard	**The lizard**	**Chapter on the useful properties of the lizard**
82.1	*om.*	*om.*	If you burn its skin, and the body is rubbed with it, then this will not suffer from the pain of any stroke or cut, even if you severed the head from the body.
82.2	Lizard meat: if it is tied inside a silk cloth, and a man hangs it on his harm, then this will give power to his coitus, increase his sexual desire and appetite for the coitus.	Lizard meat: if it is taken, you hang it on your arm, then this will increase the sexual desire and power, and will create a burning desire.	Lizard meat: if a man hangs it on his arm, then it will improve his coitus, and strengthen its sexual desire.
82.3	If a lizard is taken, its tail is cut, its blood taken, and melted with lily oil, a wick is moistened with it, and lit in a lantern, then this house will become like silver, in particular if the lizard is black.	If a lizard is taken, its tail cut, one part of the blood from its tail is taken, mixed with lily oil, a wick is moistened in it, and put in a lantern, then the house will glow like silver.	If the tail of the lizard is cut, its blood is taken, mixed with lily oil, these two are well mixed, then a wick is soaked in it, and lit in a lantern, then the house will glow like shiny silver; and if the lizard is black, then it is even more effective.
82.4	If you want that a house becomes empty of its inhabitants, take the desert lizard with rooster, dung and fumigate that place with it, then it will never be inhabited again.	Lizard dung and rooster dung in equal parts: if the house is fumigated with it, then no one will be able to live there.	Lizard droppings with rooster dung: if these are mixed, and the house is fumigated with them, then it will become empty, will be destroyed, and nobody will be able to live there.

82.5	يؤخذ زبل الحرذون يخلط معه عنزروت ويسحق الجميع ويضاف اليه مسك خالص ويكتحل به من في عينه بياض وغشاوة فتزول باذن الله تعالى	وخلط معه العنزروت وشيء من مسك ويكتحل به صاحب العين الذي [له] غشاوة وظلمة ينفع نفعا بينا	بعر الحرذون اذا خلط بعنزروت ومسك عراقي واكتحل به من في عينيه غشاوة اذهبها عنه وبرئ وازال الظلمة
82.6	من دهن نفسه يشحم الحرذون ثم القى نفسه على التمساح لم يضرّه شيء	شحمه اذا دهّن به انسان والقى نفسه على التمساح في البحر صاده واذا انقلب على ظهره لم يتحرك	*om.*
82.7	*om.*	دم الحرذون يذاف بماء البورق ويطلي به الكلف فينفع ويصفي اللون ويحسنه وينفي النمش الذي يكون في الوجه	*om.*
82.8	*om.*	لحم الحرذون يطبخ بشهدانج ويجفف ويدق ويشرب منه مثقال او مثقالين هي اجود مع كأس من شراب يزيد في الباه ويهيج الجماع والشهوة	*om.*
82.9	*om.*	ولحم الجردون يذاف ويدهن به من وجع الصلبة والكليتين [ينفع] ويزيد الباه حرارة	*om.*
82.10	*om.*	*om.*	اذا اردت ان تمسك النار ولا تحرق ولا تؤذيك خذ حرذونا اغله وخذ دسمه وادهن به يديك وامسك النار فلا تؤذيك

82.5: (b) وخلط...بينا] زبلها ايضا اذا خلط معه عنزروت ومسك وكحل به العين نفع من الغشاوة والظلمة G
(c) بعر...خلط] والجردون خرء الفار واذا خلط C | عنه وبرئ] *om.* C
82.6: (b) This recipe is attested only in G | In G another recipe is added, with lizard blood against leprosy: دم الحرذون البحري اذا اخذ وهو حار مع ما البليلج والاملج وطلى على البرص نفعه; along with a remark in which the lizard is identified either with a crocodile or with a skink: قال قوم انه الاسقنقور وقال قوم هو التمساح
82.7: (b) دم...الوجه] دمه اذا اذيف بماء البورق وطلى به الكلف اذهبه G
82.8: (b) لحم...والشهوة] لحمه اذا ملح ودق وشرب منه وزن مثقال مع شراب زاد في الباه وهيج الجماع G
82.9: (b) ولحم...حرارة] شحمه اذا ذوب به الصلب نفع من وجعه G
82.10: (c) ولا تحرق] ولم تحترق C | دسمه] دهنه C | يديك] يدك C | فلا] فانها لا C

82.5	Lizard dung: if it is taken, melted with sarcocolla, everything is ground, mixed with pure musk, and applied in the eyes of the man who suffers from leucoma and cataract, then these will cease with the permission of God may He be exalted.	And if it is mixed with sarcocolla and some musk, and applied in the eye of the man suffering from cataract and obscuration, then this will be very useful.	Lizard dung: if it is mixed with sarcocolla and Iraqi musk, applied in the eyes of the man suffering from cataract, then this will eliminate it, and will cure and stop the obscuration.
82.6	The man who rubs himself with desert lizard fat, and then throws himself on a crocodile, then nothing will harm him.	Its fat: if a man rubs himself with it, and throws himself on the sea crocodile, then he will catch it; and if it is turned on its back, it will not be able to move.	*om.*
82.7	*om.*	Lizard blood: if it is mixed with natron water, and rubbed on the brown spots, then it will be useful, will purify the colour and make it beautiful, and it will clean the freckles on the face.	*om.*
82.8	*om.*	Lizard meat: if it is cooked with Indian hemp, dried, crushed, one *miṯqāl* or two are drunk—it is better with a glass of wine—then it will increase sexual desire and excite the coitus.	*om.*
82.9	*om.*	Lizard meat: if it is mixed, and rubbed on the man suffering from back and kidneys pain, then it will be useful, and it will also increase sexual desire greatly.	*om.*
82.10	*om.*	*om.*	If you want to hold fire in your hands without that it burns or consumes you, take a lizard, boil it, take its grease, and rub your hands with it, then hold the fire, and it will not consume you.

82.11	شحم الحرذون يذاب على النار ويدهن به الصلب فانه يقوي الظهر وينفع الكليتين ورخو المثانة	صلب الحرذون البحري يؤخذ الخرزة الوسطى من ظهرها فيعلقه الانسان على صلبه في وقت الجماع فيزيد في شهوته	شحم الحرذون اذا اذيب ودهن به الصلب والوركين زاد في شهوة الجماع كالسقنقور وهو يشبه الحردون بل هو اكبر
82.12	*om.*	خصية الحرذون البحري اما الخصية اليمنى فان أخذها انسان فجففها وشرب منها او شق غيره وزن قراط بماء السذاب قطع المنى ونشفه	*om.*
82.13	*om.*	واما خصيته اليسرى فخذها وجففها واسقى منها انسانا وزن قراط بماء الحمص الاسود المغلى المصفى وكأس من شراب وجزء من سمن البقر يدر المنى ويحرك الجماع ويسخن الكلى ويزيد في الانعاظ	*om.*
82.14	*om.*	وقال بعض الحكماء ان طبخ السقنقور واطعم لاناس بينهم عداوة او بغضا اصطلحوا وتالفت قلوبهم	اذا بخر من لحمه جماعة بينهم عداوة فانه يتحاببوا ويصطلحوا وتزول عداوتهم

82.11: (b) صلب [صلب خرز G | يؤخذ [اذا أخذت G | الخرزة [الجوزة T | الخرزة فيعلقه الانسان [ظهرها انسان وعلقها ظهره G | في [om. G | فيزيد [زاد G
(c) اذيب [ذوب C | كالسقنقو...اكبر [كالسقنقور وكان اعظم من السقنقور C

82.12: (b) خصية...ونشفه [خصية الحوذون البحري اليمنى اذا جفف وشرب منها وزن قيراط بماء سذاب قطع المني وييسّه G

82.13: (b) واما...الانعاظ [خصيته اليسرى اذا شرب منها قيراط بما الحمص الاسود المغلى المصفى مع شراب وسمن بقر ادر المنى وحرّك الشهوة G | In G other two recipes dealing with the bite of the skink are added: الحرذون البحري الذي هو السقنقور اذا عض انسانًا وسبق الاسقنقور وبال مات المعضوض; and وان بال المعضوض قبل الاسقنقور او الشحم مات الاسقنقور وسلم المعضوض من ساعته

82.14: (b) This recipe is attested only in G
(c) *om.* C

82.11	Lizard fat: if it is mixed on the fire, and rubbed on the spine, then this will strenghten the back, and will be useful to the kidneys and the weakness of the bladder.	Sea lizard spine: if a vertebra is taken from its middle, and the man hangs it on his spine at the moment of coitus, then this will increase his sexual desire.	Lizard fat: if it is mixed, and rubbed on the spine and the legs, then this will increase the desire of coitus; like the skink, that is similar to the lizard, but it is bigger.
82.12	*om.*	Testicle of the sea lizard: as for the right one, if a man takes it, dries it, and drinks or splits one carat of it with rue water, then this will stop and dry the sperm.	*om.*
82.13	*om.*	As for the left testicle, take it, dry it, give one carat of it to a man to drink with boiled and purified water of black chickpeas, a glass of wine, and one part of cow fat, then this will make the sperm flow, will excite the coitus, warm the kidneys, and improve the erection.	*om.*
82.14	*om.*	Some wise men say: if the skink is cooked, and given to eat to some people who harbour enmity and hatred among themselves, then they will reconcile with one another, and their hearts will be harmonized.	If its meat is fumigated amidst a group of people who harbour enmity among themselves, then they will reconcile, make peace, and their enmity will cease.

٨٣. الجعل

	a	b	c
	—	الجعل	—
83.1	—	يؤخذ الجعل الكبير الذي في رأسه شوكة ويصب عليه دهن بزر ويغليه حتى ينهري ويخرج الدهن فيخرجه فيدهن المشش والنملة	—

83: الجعل] العجل T | الجعل الكبير G

83.1: (b) الجعل] العجل T | الجعل الكبير] *om.* G | شوكة] مثل الشوكة G | ويصب عليه دهن] ويجعل في مغرفة حديد مع G | حتى...والنملة] الى ان يتهرا ويحمّر ثم يؤخذ ويدهن المشش في الدواب فيذهنه ويقلع البواسير ايضا والنملة G

83. Dung Beetle

	a	b	c
	–	**The dung beetle**	–
83.1	–	Take the large dung beetle that has a thorn inside its head, pour on it some seeds, boil it until it breaks in pieces and the oil comes out, then take it and rub it on the excrescences that grow on the beasts of burden and on the small swelling.	–

٨٤. العضاية

	a	b	c
	ذكر منافع العضاية وهي الحرباء	العضاية	باب منافع العضاية
84.1	يؤخذ رأس عضاية ودمها فيصرها في خرقة وتجعلها على فخذ المرأة وهي نائمة فانها تخبرك بكل ما صنعته في الدنيا فاذا رأيتها قد اختل عقلها فازيل الخرقة عنها والا فهي تتوسوس	تأخذ رأس العضاية وذنبها فصيره خرقة نضيفة من كتان وتجعله على فخذ امرأة وهي نائمة فتحبر بما صنعت كل شيء عملت	اذا أخذت رأس عضاية وذنبها وجعلتها في خرقة كتان وربطت الخرقة على فخذ امرأة نائمه اخبرتك بكل ما صنعت في اليقطة فاذا اردت ان تحبل علقها اتركها عليها وربما جنت من ذلك ولحقها مرض الوسواس
84.2	*om.*	تأخذ عصابة فتحرق ختى يصير رمادا ثم تأخذ رمادها فاغليه بزيت وادهن من ذلك الزيت الموضع اللذي تباشر منه الشعر ينبت باذن الله تعالى	*om.*
84.3	لنبات الشعر يؤخذ فتحرق حتى تصير رمادا وخذ الرماد فاغليه بالزيت وخذ ذلك الزيت فاطلِ به مواضع القرع فينبت فيه الشعر باذن الله تعالى	عضاية اذا احرقت ويُغلي رمادها بزيت ويدهن به القرع نبت الشعر	اذا احرقت عضاية وصارت رمادا واغليته بزيت ودهن بها المواضع التي تناثر شعرها انبت الشعر
84.4	يؤخذ ذنب العضاية ويصر في خرقة ويجعلها فتيلة ويعملها في سراج ويقد	تأخذ عضاية فتعملها في خرقة فتجعله فتيلة في دهن زنبق واسرج به في سراج	*om.*

84: (b) العضاية] العطاية T
(c) العضاية] العظايا L; العظاية C
84.1: (b) العضاية] العطاية T | تاخذ...عملت] رأسها وذنبها اذا جعلا في خرقة كتان وجعلت على فخذ امرأة نائمة اخبرت بكل ما عملت واذا خلطت فارفعها G
(c) في خرقة كتان] في خرقة من كتان C | فاذا اردت...مرض الوسواس] فاذا اردت ان حبله اتركه عنها C
84.2: (b) *om.* G
84.3: (b) العضاية] عصابة T | تأخذ...ينبت] العضاية اذا احرقت ويغلي رمادها بزيت ويدهن به القرع نبت الشعر G
84.4: (b) العضاية] عضابة T | زنبق] زيبق T | تأخذ...سودا] ذنبها اذا جعل في خرقة في دهن زنبق وجعل فتيلة واسرج في جديد فان اهل البيت يرون وجوههم سودا G

84. Chameleon

	a	b	c
	Mention of the useful properties of the chameleon	**The chameleon**	**Chapter on the useful properties of the chameleon**
	that is *al-ḥirbā'*		
84.1	Chameleon head and its blood: if they are put in a piece of cloth that is placed on the leg of the woman while she is asleep, then she will tell you everything she has done in the world. And if you see that she is mentally deranged for the fact that this is hanging on her, then remove it or not, otherwise she will become obsessed.	Take the head of the chameleon and its tail, put them in a clean linen cloth, place it on the leg of a woman who asleep, and then she will tell everything she has done.	If you take the head and the tail of the chameleon, put them in a linen cloth, the cloth is tied to the leg of a sleeping woman, then she will tell you everything she has done when she was awake. And if you want that the woman gets pregnant, hang the piece of cloth on her and leave it there, but she may become mad or affected by obsession.
84.2	*om.*	Take the chameleon, burn it until it becomes ashes; then take its ashes and boil it with oil, rub this oil on the area from which hair has been shaved off, and then it will grow, with the permission of God may He be exalted.	*om.*
84.3	For hair growth: the chameleon has to be taken, burn it until it becomes ash, boiled with oil, this oil taken and rubbed on the areas affected by the ringworm, then the hair will grow there, with the permission of God, may He be exalted.	If you burn a chameleon and boil its ash with oil and anoint the ringworm with it, then the hair will grow again.	If the chameleon is burnt until it becomes ash, boiled with oil and rubbed on the zone where the hair falls off, then it will grow again.
84.4	Chameleon tail: if it taken, made into a wick, put it in a lantern with lily oil, and this is lit among a group	Take its tail, put it in a piece of cloth, make it into a wick with lily oil, light it on in a lantern, and then	*om.*

فاذا كان من في البيت يرون وجوههم سوداء

بدهن زنبق بين جماعة فانها يرون وجوههم سوداء

84.5

اذا أخذت ذنب العضايه وجعل في خرقة مثل فتيلة وتركت في قدرة وصب عليها دهن الزنبق ورفعت ذلك لوقت الحاجة اذا اردت ان تكون محبوبا لمن يراك خذ شيئا يسيرا من هذا الدهن وادهن به من اردت ان يحبك فانه لا يصير عنك ساعة وقيل انه يتبعك في اي مكان غبت فيه

تأخذ عضايتين متساويتين تقنكهما وتخرج ما في بطونهما فترمي به ثم تصير في قارورة واسعة الرأس وتشد رأس القارورة فاذا اردتَ مودّة انسان فامسح اصبعا في القارورة ثم امسح في اي موضع شئت من الانسان الذي تريد مودته يتبعك ويحبك حبا شديدا

اذا اردت ان تكون محبوبا فخذ غضايتين فشق فوادهما واخرج جميع ما فيهما واجعلهما في قارورة وصب عليهما زيتا طيبا او دهن زنبق وارفعه عندك فاذا احتجت الى ذلك فادهن اصبعك من ذلك الدهن واجعله على اي امراة شئت فانها تتبعك وهذا مليح

84.6

اذا أخذت غضاية واحرقتها وادفتها بدهن بان وحملتها المرأة في صوفة فانها لا يشتكي وجع الارحام ابدا

العضاية الخضراء اذا احرقت وسقيت بها دهبا بان وتبطل بها قطن تحمّلها المرأة التي بها وجع الارحام [نفع]

يؤخذ عضاية خضراء يحرق ويداف رمادها بدهن بان ثم اجعل في قطنة وتتحمل به المرأة فانه ينفع من برودة الأحشاء ووجع الرحم

84.7

اذا أخذت دم الغضاية ولطخت بها موضع داء الثعلب وموضع القرع انبت الشعر

دم العضاية اذا ذبحت يطلي به موضع ذاء الثعلب والقرع ينبت فيه الشعر

يؤخذ عضاية تذبح ويؤخذ دمها يجفف ويسحق ويذاف بدهن ورد ويطلي به الشعر فانه ينبت باذن الله تعالى

84.8

اذا أخذت شحم الغضاية واذفته بدهن البان وقطرته في الاذن الكثيرة الضربان التي يسيل منها الماء الاصفر سكن الضربان وان كان فيها الدود قتلها

شحم العضاية يذاف بها بلسان ويقطر في الادن الكثيرة الرطوبة [نفع]

يؤخذ شحم العضاية يداف بدهن البان ويقطر في الاذن فانه جيدا للصمم وان كان فيها دود قتله

84.5: (b) عضايتين] عصابتين T | تأخذ...شديدا] اذا اردت محبة احد يؤخذ عضايتين متسادتين يقتلا ويخرج في بطنهما ويجعلا في قارورة وشدّ رأسها فاذا اردت محبة احد فامسح منها صبعك وامسح من تريد فهو يتبعك G
(c) اذا أخذت...وجعل] اذا جعل ذنب C | في قدرة] في المسرجة C | وصب...الزنبق] وصبت عليها شيئا من دهن الزنبق C | لمن] عند من C | من اردت] من يريده C | ساعة] ابدا C | وقيل] وربما قيل C | في اي مكان غبت فيه] حيث كنت او سرت C
84.6: (b) العضاية] العطاية T | وسقيت...الارحام] العضاية الخضرا اذا احرقت وعجن رمادها بان وبل به قطنة وتحمّلت بها المرأة نفعها من وجع الارحام G
(c) وادفتها] واذبتها C | الارحام] الرحم C | ابدا] *om.* C
84.7: (b) العضاية] العطاية T | دم...الشعر] دمها اذا طلى به داء الثعلب نبت الشعر G
(c) اذا...بها] الغضايه اذا لطخت به C
84.8: (b) [نفع] | شحم...[نفع]] اذا ذوّب بدهن بلسان وقطر منه الاذن نفع من وجعها G
(c) واذفته] واذبته C | وقطرته] وقطرت منه C | الضربان] وأزال الألم منه *add.* C | وان...قتله] *om.* C

of people, then they will see their faces black.

the people in the house will see their faces black.

84.5 If you want to be loved, take two chameleons, split them and extract everything that is inside their body, put them in a long-necked flask, pour some good oil or lily oil, and store it; once you need this, rub with it any woman you desire, then she will follow you, and this is witty.

Take two similar chameleons, kill them and remove what is inside their bellies, put it in a long-necked flask with a large opening; and when you want the love of a man, rub your finger inside the bottle, then rub them on any part of the man whose love you want, and he will follow you and deeply love you.

If you take the tail of a chameleon, put it in a piece of cloth like a compress, then leave it in a pot and store it until the moment in which you need it. When you want to be loved by anyone who sees you, take some of this oil, and rub with it the man you want to be loved by, then he will not leave you for a moment, and it is said that he will follow you wherever you will go.

84.6 Green chameleon: if it is taken, burnt, its ash mixed with ben oil, then put in a cotton cloth that has to be carried with her by the woman, then this will be useful against the cold in the bowels and womb pain.

Green chameleon: if it is burnt, some ben oil is poured on it, then a cotton cloth is moistened with it, and a woman suffering from womb pain carries it with her, this will be useful.

If the chameleon is taken, burnt, mixed with ben oil and a woman carries it with her in a woollen cloth, then she will never suffer from womb pain.

84.7 If the chameleon is taken, slaughtered, its blood taken, dried, made into a powder, mixed with rose oil, and rubbed on the hair, then it will grow, with the permission of God, may He be exalted.

Chameleon blood: if [the chameleon] is slaughtered, and this is rubbed on the areas affected by alopecia and ringworm, then the hair will grow there.

If the blood of a chameleon is taken and spattered on the zone affected by alopecia and ringworm, then this will make the hair grow.

84.8 Chameleon fat: if it is taken, mixed with ben oil, applied in drops inside the ear, then this will be good against deafness; and if there are worms inside the ear, then this will kill them.

Chameleon fat: if it is mixed with balsam of Mecca oil, and applied in drops inside the ears with a lot of moistness [in them], then this will be useful.

If you take the fat of the chameleon, mix it with ben oil, apply it in drops inside the ear suffering from sharp pains, and from which yellow water flows, then this will calm the pain; and if there are worms [in the ears], then this will kill them.

٨٥. الذراريح

	a	b	c
	—	الذراريح	—
85.1	—	يؤخذ خمس ذراريحات تصيرها في مغرفة ويلقي عليها زيت ويطبخ حتى ينهري ثم انزلها عن النار وصفى الزيت وادهن به الموضع الذي تريد ينبت فيه الشعر فانه ينبت باذن الله تعالى	—

85: الذراريح [الذراريح T

85.1: (a) يؤخذ] *om.* G | ذراريحات] واحدات G | تصيرها] اذا جعلا G | ويلقي...فيه الشعر] ويدهن ذلك الزيت ويصفي ثم يتهروا حتى وطبخوا مع زيت حديد به موضع القرع G | Between Ch. 88 and Ch.93 , in T there is another recipe, with green blister beetle against the spots on the face: دراريح المقاني الدراريح الخضر التي تكون على المقاتي تؤخذ وتنقع في خل وعسل ويطلا بها الكلف في الوجه يذهب

85. Blister Beetle

	a	b	c
	–	**The blister beetles**	–
85.1	–	If five blister beetles are put in a ladle, some oil is poured on them, and they are cooked until and they are well done; then this is removed from the fire, the oil is purified, and rubbed on the areas in which you wish the hair to grow, then the hair will grow, with the permission of God may He be exalted.	–

٨٦. شحمة الارض

	a	b	c
	—	شحمة الارض	—
		وهي دود اذا مسستها تجتمع مثل الجوزة	
86.1	—	يؤخذ من ذلك الدود فيجفف يسقي منه المرأة اذا عسر عليها الولادة قدر باقلاة ويذاف بنبيذ ويشربه المرأة فتلد من ساعتها	—

86: الجوزة...وهي] تقلّصت مسستها اذا وهى G
86.1 (b): ساعتها...يؤخذ] فتلد بنبيذ باقلاة قدر منها وتشرب وتسحق تجفف ولادتها المرأة على عسر اذا G | For this recipe, see also 90.4

86. White Worm

	a	b	c
	–	**The white worm**	–
		this is the worm that, when it is touched, contracts [becoming] like an almond.	
86.1	–	If this worm is taken, dried, given to a woman to drink when she has difficulties in giving birth—in the quantity of a broad bean, mixed with wine—then she will immediately give birth.	–

٨٧. سامّ أبرص

	a	b	c
	ذكر منافع سامّ أبرص	سام أبرص	باب منافع الوزغ
	وهو الوزغة		
87.1	يؤخذ الوزغ فيجعل في مشاقة كتان او في خرقة ويجعل في سراج ويصب عليه زيت واعطه لمن شئت يمسكه فانه لا يزال يضرط وكانت الملوك يدخرونه عندهم لمرض القولنج وهذا عجيب	يؤخذ ذنب سام أبرص فاجعله في خرقة وصيرها فتيلة واجعلها في سراج جديد واعطيه مع انسان يمسكه فلا يراه احد	اذا أخذت سام أبرص وعملته في فتيلة واوقدتها بزيت ومسكها انسان فانه لا يبرح يضرط ما دامت الفتيلة بيده
87.2	وقيل ان الوزغة اذا علقت على امرأة حامل لم يسقط اولادها باذن الله تعالى	*om.*	اذا علق سام ابرص على حامل فانها لا تسقط
87.3	*om.*	وان القي في جُحر حية مفتولا هربت منه	واذا قتلت سام أبرص وجعلته في جحر الحية هربت منه ولا تاوي اليه
	—	وزغ البساتين	—
87.4	لخروج الشوك من الجسد يؤخذ وزغ البساتين يجفف ويسحق ويضمّد به مواضع الشوكة فتخرج بلا الم وكذلك نصول النشاب من الجسد	اذا شق وضمدت به المواضع التي فيها نصول النشابين والشوك خرجت	اذا أخذت وزغ البستان وجففته وسحقته وضمدت به مواضع النصل والشوكة اخرج ذلك بلا الم ولا اذي باذن الله تعالى

87.1: (b) يؤخذ...احد] ذنبه اذا جعل في خرقة وصيّر فتيلة في سراج جديد وحمله انسان فلا يزال يضرط ما دام في يده G
(c) سام أبرص وعملته] الوزغ وجعلته C | ومسكها انسان...يضرط] واوقدها احدٌ فانه لا يكاد ان يمسك ضراط C
87.2: (c) سام أبرص] الوزغ C | حامل] المرأة الحامل C
87.3: (b) This recipe is attested only in G
(c) قتلت سام أبرص] قتلتها C | في حجر] في وكر C | هربت منه] هربت من وقتها C
87.4: (b) وزغ] دمع T | وضمدت] وضمد G | نصول النشابين والشوك خرجت] نصل الشوك او الشوك اخرج ذلك G
(c) النصل والشوكة] نصل النشاب والشوكة C | ولا اذي] *om.* C

87. Gecko

	a	b	c
	Exposition of the useful properties of the gecko (*sāmm abraṣ*)	**The gecko**	**Chapter on the useful properties of the gecko**
	that is *al-wazaġ*.		
87.1	Gecko: if it is taken, put it in a linen scrap or in a cloth, then it is placed in a lantern as wick, some oil is poured on it, and [the lantern] is given to hold to whomever you want, then he will not stop breaking winds. There are some kings who store this away against colic, and this is amazing.	Gecko tail: if it is taken, put inside a piece of cloth, a wick is made of it and put in a new lantern and a man holds it, then he will not stop breaking winds, until this lantern remains in his hand.	If you take a gecko, make a wick of it, light it with oil and a man holds it, then he will not stop breaking winds, until the wick remains in his hand.
87.2	It is said that if you hang a gecko on a pregnant woman, then she will not lose her babies, with the permission of God, may He be exalted.	*om.*	If a gecko is hung on a pregnant woman, then she will not lose her baby.
87.3	*om.*	If a gecko is vigorously throw in a snake nest, then the snakes will flee.	If you kill a gecko and throw it into a snake nest, then the snake will flee and will not seek shelter there anymore.
	–	**Gecko of the gardens**	–
87.4	To extract thorns from the body: a garden gecko has to be taken, dried, pulverised, and used to bandage the parts in which the thorns have penetrated, then this will extract them without pain; this is equally useful to pull arrowheads out of the body.	If it is split and used to bandage with it the parts in which arrowheads or thorns have penetrated, then this will pull them out.	If you take a garden gecko, dry it, powder it and bandage with it the zones where arrowheads and thorns have penetrated, this will pull them out without any pain or suffering, with the permission of God may He be exalted.

87.5	*om.*	قلب الوزغ اذا علق على امرأة حامل تسقط	*om.*

87.5: (b) اذا] ان G | امرأة] *om.* G | تسقط] اسقطت G

87.5	*om.*	Gecko heart: if it is hung on a pregnant woman, then she will miscarry.	*om.*

٨٨. الذباب

	a	b	c
	om.	**الذباب**	باب منافع الذباب
88.1	*om.*	اذا علقت ذبابة حية على انسان في خرقة رقيقة ويوسع عليها اسكن عنه وجع العين	اذا أخذت ذبابه بالحياة وجعلتها في خرقه وعلقتها على من يشتكي التخم برئ
88.2	*om.*	خرؤه اذا اذيف بطلاء وسقى لمن قد عسر عليها الولادة ولدت	اذا أخذت الذباب بخمر خالص وشربته حامل عسر عليها خروج الولد ولدت سريعا
88.3	يؤخذ رؤوس الذباب فيدلك بها جفن العين الذي ينبت فيه الشعر فيزول باذن الله تعالى	رؤوس الذباب اذا دلك الشعرة في العين ذهبت	اذا أخذت رؤوس الذباب ودلكت به الشعر التي في العين ازال ذلك وابرأه
88.4	*om.*	الذباب اذا شرح وضمّد به العين الوارمة نفعها	*om.*
88.5	يؤخذ الذباب يحرق في خرقة ويأخذ ايضا اصول القصب يحرق ويخلط الجميع في خرقة ويداف الجميع بالزيت العتيق او بوسخ السراج وأطل به موضع الشعر فانه يطول الشعر ويحسّنه	*om.*	اذا احرق الذباب في خرقة مع اصول القصب وخلط الجميع وعجن بالزيت وطلى به الشعر طوله وغزره وحسنه
88.6	*om.*	*om.*	اذا اذيف الذباب بشراب وشيء من عسل ولطخت به صوفة وحملته من يشتكي وجع الارحام ابرأه

88: (b) This chapter is attested only in G, in T there is only the chapter heading
88.1: (c) التخم] التخمة C
88.2: (c) بخمر...سريعا] وادبته بالخمر الخالص وشربت منه من تعسر عليها الولادة ووضعت سريعا C
88.3: (c) اذا...ودلكت به] رؤوس الذباب اذا دلكت به C
88.5: (c) وخلط الجميع] وخلط ذلك C
88.6: (c) اذا اذيف] اذا اذيب C | ولطخت به] وعمل منه C | وجع الارحام] وجع الرحم C

88. Fly

	a	b	c
	om.	**The fly**	**Chapter on the useful properties of the flies**
88.1	*om.*	If a fly is hung alive on a man, well wrapped in a piece of fine cloth, and applied on the eyes, then the eye pain will cease.	If a fly is taken alive, put inside a piece of cloth and hung on the man who suffers from indigestion, then he will recover.
88.2	*om.*	Its excrement: if it is melted with liquid pitch and given to drink to the woman who has had some difficulties in giving birth, then she will deliver.	If some flies are taken with pure wine, and given to drink to a woman who has some difficulties in giving birth, then she will quickly deliver.
88.3	If some fly heads are taken, rubbed on the eyelid where the hair grows, then this will cease to grow, with the permission of God, may He be exalted.	If the hair of the eye is rubbed with some fly heads, then it will disappear.	If some fly heads are taken, and rubbed on the hair of the eye, then this will disappear.
88.4	*om.*	If some flies are made into pieces and used to bandage the eye, then this will be useful to the swollen eye.	*om.*
88.5	If some flies are taken, burnt inside a piece of cloth, some sugar cane roots are taken too; then this is burnt and mixed together with old oil or lantern soot, and rubbed on the place where the hair grows, then this will become longer and nicer.	*om.*	If some flies are burnt inside a piece of cloth with sugar cane roots, everything mixed, kneaded with oil, and rubbed on the hair, then it will become longer, more abundant and nicer.
88.6	*om.*	*om.*	If some flies are melted with wine and honey, spattered on a piece of woollen cloth that has to be carried by the woman who suffers from womb disease, then she will be cured.

٨٩. الذباب الاخضر

	a	b	c
	—	—	باب منافع الذباب الاخضر
89.1	—	—	اذا أخذ رؤوس الذباب الاخضر وجعلت في فتيلة واشغلتها بين جماعة فانهم ينظرون انفسهم بلا رؤوس

89. Spanish Fly

	a	b	c
	–	–	**Chapter on the properties of the Spanish flies**
89.1	–	–	If the heads of some Spanish flies are taken, placed inside a lantern wick, and this is lit among a group of people, then they will see each other without their heads.

٩٠. الزنبور

	a	b	c
	الزنبور	الزنبور	—
90.1	ومن خاصيّة هذه الديابة اذا طرحت في الزيت ماتت	ان طرح في زيت مات	—
90.2	واذا طرحت في الخل عاشت كانها لم تمت	وان طرح في خل عاش	—
90.3	فراخ الزنبور التي تكون في اوكارها اذا قليت بالزيت وطرح عليها كروايا وسذاب يابس واكلها لانسان زاد في قوة الجماع	فراخها اذا قليت بزيت مع سذاب وكراويا وأكلت زاد في الباه	—
90.4	فاذا عسر على المرأة الولادة يسحق مقدار باقلاية وتشربها المرأة بشراب عتيق تلد سريعا	*om.*	—

90: (b) This chapter is attested only in G
90.1: (a) In S this recipe is after 90.3
90.2: (a) In S this recipe is placed after 90.3
90.4: (b) For this recipe, see also 86.1

90. Hornet

	a	b	c
	The hornet	**The hornet**	–
90.1	Among its occult properties, there is that this beast dies if you throw it into some oil.	If it is thrown into some oil, it will die.	–
90.2	Whereas, if you throw it into some vinegar, it will live, as if it cannot die.	Whereas, if it is thrown into some vinegar, it will live.	–
90.3	Hornet grubs, that can be found in their nests: if they are fried with some oil with the addition of some caraway and dry rue, then given to a man to eat, then this will increase his sexual power.	If some of its grubs are fried in some oil with rue and caraway, and this is eaten, then this will increase the sexual potency.	–
90.4	If a woman has difficulties in giving birth, the measure of a broad beans of hornets has to be ground, and given to her with some old wine to drink, then she will immediately give birth.	*om.*	–

٩١. جمل اليهود

	a	b	c
	—	جمل اليهود وهو الحرباء	—
91.1	—	يؤخذ يذبح ويشق بطنه ويرمي ما فيه ثم يملّح ويجعل في كوز جديد حتى يجف ويبخّر به المسحور والمعقود فيبطل	—
91.2	—	واذا أخذ منه مقدار لوزة مع مثله شحم خنزير وبخر به المصروف عن اهله بطل عنه	—
91.3	—	يؤخذ ويشق بطنه ويرمي بما فيه ويجعل في قدر جديد مع ماء غمره ويلقي عليه يبروح وبزر سذاب وجاوشير جندبادستر وبزر العنب وفاشرشين ومقل اليهود وحلتيت وملح وزرنار ودرونج من كل واحد جزء مدقوق ثم يجعل في قارورة ويمسح المجنون اذا تلك بمقدار ما يحمله اصبعك فان شيطانه يهرب ويستعيث	—
91.4	—	رجل الحرباء اذا جعلت في بان خالص يومين ثم اخرج وعلقت في رقبة المصاب نفعه	—

91: (b) This chapter is attested only in G
91.3: (b) جند بادستر] جند بيذستر G

91. Mantis

	a	a	c
	–	**The mantis,**	–
		that is *al-ḥirbāʾ*	
91.1	–	Take it, slaughter it, split its abdomen and remove what is inside it, then add some salt and put it inside a new jug until it dries; then fumigate with it the man who has been bewitched and tied by magic: and [the magic] will cease.	–
91.2	–	If you take the quantity of an almond of it and the same quantity of pork fat, fumigate with it the man who has been alienated from his family, then this will cease.	–
91.3	–	Take it, split its abdomen and remove what is inside it, put it inside a new jug with enough water to cover it, add some mandrake, rue seeds, bisabol myrrh, castoreum, grape seeds, white bryony, bdellium of the Jews, asafoetida, salt, *zarnār* [?], leopard's bane—one part of each one, ground—then put it inside a long-necked flask, and wipe the possessed man with it—if this substance is in the quantity that you can collect with your fingers—then his evil spirit will flee and will be destroyed.	–
91.4	–	The foot of the mantis is useful when you put it in ben oil for two days, then take it out, and hang it on the neck of a wounded man.	–

٩٢. النمل

	a	b	c
	ذكر منافع النمل	النمل	—
92.1	يؤخذ النمل بالزيت على نار لينة ويقطر منه في الاذن التي يكون تضرب فيسكن ضربانها باذن الله تعالى	اذا طبخ بزيت وقطّر منه في الاذن سكن دويها	—
92.2	*om.*	بيضه اذا دق وخلط بدهن كاذي ودهنّ من يشتكي راسه سكن	—
92.3	*om.*	بيضه اذا جفف وسحق وسقى انسان فلا يزال يضرّط حتى يسقي شيرج او يستفّ كمون كرماني مقلي	—
92.4	*om.*	اذا اردت ان تخرج ماء فانظر الى قرية النمل فان رايت النمل غلاظا سودا ثقيل المشي فالماء قريب	—
92.5	*om.*	وان رأيت النمل خفيف المشي سريع فالماء منها على اربعين ذراعا والماء الاول يكون عذبا طيبا والثاني مالحا	—
92.6	*om.*	وان علّق خرقة من خرق الحائض حول بيدر لم تقربه النمل	—
92.7	*om.*	وان طافت امرأة حائض حول بيدر لم تدخله النمل	—
92.8	*om.*	وان جعل على بيت الذر كمون مدقوق معجون بماء هرب	—

92. Ant

	a	b	c
	Exposition of the useful properties of the ants	**The ants**	–
92.1	If the ants are taken with oil, put on a light fire, applied in drops inside the ear suffering from pangs, then these will cease, with the permission of God, may He be exalted.	If they are cooked with oil, and applied in drops inside the ear, then its buzzing will stop.	–
92.2	*om.*	Its eggs: if they are crushed, mixed with pandang oil, and rubbed on the man who suffers from headache, then this will cease.	–
92.3	*om.*	Its eggs: if they are ground, given to a man to drink, then he will not stop breaking winds, until he is given some sesame oil to drink, or until he swallows some roasted cumin.	–
92.4	*om.*	If you want to find water, observe an anthill: if you see that the ants are thick, black and that they plod, then the water is near.	–
92.5	*om.*	If you see, instead, that the ants walk briskly, the water is forty arms far, and the first water will be fresh, while the second will be salty.	–
92.6	*om.*	If a piece of cloth soaked with menstrual blood is hung around a barn, then the ants will not approach it.	–
92.7	*om.*	If a menstruating woman walks around a barn, then the ants will not enter it.	–
92.8	*om.*	If some crushed cumin kneaded with water is put on the anthill of the small ants, then the these will flee.	–

—	وكذلك الكبريت والمرتج ان جعل في بيت النمل هلكن	om.	92.9
—	وان اردت اصراف قوم مجتمعين فانثر عليهم وحولهم بيض النمل	om.	92.10
—	وان دلك ابط الغلام قبل الاحتلام ببيض النمل الاحمر الصغار لم ينبت عليه الشعر ابدا وكذلك عانته	om.	92.11
—	وان أخذت حبة قمح من نملة بابهامك وسبّابتك وعلق على امرأة لم تحبل	om.	92.12
—	وان خطّت الجرة بتراب ابيض لم يقربها النمل	om.	92.13

92.9	*om.*	Likewise, if you put some sulphur or some silver foam in a house, then the ants will be destroyed.	–
92.10	*om.*	If you want the dispersion of a whole group of people, scatter ant eggs upon and around them.	–
92.11	*om.*	If the armpit of a boy who has not yet reached the puberty is rubbed with the eggs of the small red ants, then the hair will never grow on him. The same goes for his pubes.	–
92.12	*om.*	If you pick a wheat grain from an ant with your thumb and your index finger, and hang it on a woman, then she will not get pregnant.	–
92.13	*om.*	If a jar is marked with white earth, then the ants will not approach it.	–

٩٣. الخنفساء

	a	b	c
	om.	الخنفساء	—
93.1	*om.*	يؤخذ من وسطها الى اسفل فيخلط مع شحم الخنزير جزء ومن شحم الدجاجة سوداء جزءئ ويخلط الجميع في قارورة ويؤخذ منه فيقطر في الاذن التي فيها الوجع والضربان ويسد بعده بقطنة يفعل ذلك اياما متوالية	—
93.2	لجرب العين يؤخذ خنفساء وهي بالحية تقطع من الموخر ودسّ فيها الميل ويكتحل به من في عينه جرب ولاينظر في الليل شيء ينفع ذلك	يؤخذ الخنفساء حيّة فيقطع موخرها ثم تدخل الميل فيها ويكتحل به من لا ينظر بالليل والجرب في العين يبرأ	—
93.3	يؤخذ خنفساء واثقب ظهرها والطخ باللذي تخرج من الثقب القوبة فتزول باذن الله تعالى	*om.*	—
93.4	يؤخذ خنفساء تغلي بدهن جوز وتقطّر في الاذن التي يكون فيها الصمم فتبرأ باذن الله تعالى	[الاذن] الثقيل السمع تطبخ الخنافس بدهن الجوز ويقطر الاذن ينفه	—
93.5	وكذلك اذا كان في الاذن هواء او ريح او ماء يؤخذ خنفساء تقشر ويؤخذ لحمها يعصر في الاذن فتهدي باذن الله تعالى	*om.*	—

93.1: (b) من وسطها...متوالية] يؤخذ اسفل خنفساه من وسطها مع شحم خنزير وشحم دجاجة سودا من كل واحد جزء ويجعل في قارورة ويقطر منه في الاذن الوجهة فيذهب G

93.2: (b) يؤخذ] *om.* G | فيقطع] يقطع G | من لا ينظر بالليل] للعشاوة G | يبرأ] *om.* G | In G another recipe is added, to dye the inside of an ivory box red: وان اردت ان يحمّر داخل حقه حاج ويبقي خارجها لبيض فاجعل فيها خنافيس وطبق عليهم فانهم نفسون فيه فيحمّر

93.4: (b) الاذن...ينفعه] الخنافس اذا طبخت بدهن الجوز وقطر منه في الاذن الثقيلة السمع نفعها G

93. Scarab

	a	b	c
	om.	**The scarab**	–
93.1	*om.*	If the part from its middle to its back is taken, mixed with one part of pig fat, one part of black hen fat, everything mixed in a long-necked flask; then it is taken, and applied in drops inside the ears suffering from sharp pains, and these are filled after this with some cotton–this has to be done for a number of days in a row–[then this will cease].	–
93.2	Against the scabies of the eye: if a scarab is taken while it is still alive, its back is ripped open, an eye probe is dipped inside it, and it is applied on the eye of the man affected by scabies, and who cannot see during the night, then this will be useful to this.	If the scarab is taken alive, its back is cut, then an eye probe is dipped inside it, and the man who cannot see at night and has scabies in the eye applies it, then he will heal.	–
93.3	If a scarab is taken, its back pierced, and the tetter is spattered with the substance that comes out, then the tetter will cease, with the permission of God, may He be exalted.	*om.*	–
93.4	If the scarab is taken, boiled with nut oil, and applied in drops inside the ear affected by deafness, then it will be cured, with the permission of God, may He be exalted.	Ear that is hard of hearing: if the scarabs are cooked with nut oil, and applied in drops inside the ear, then this will be useful against it.	–
93.5	Likewise, if there is air, wind or water inside the ear, if a scarab is taken, peeled, its flesh is taken, and squeezed inside the ear, then this will be well cured, with the permission of God, may He be exalted.	*om.*	–

93.6	*om.*	خذ خنفساء وقشر جلدها واعصرها في الاذن فانها تبرأ	—
93.7	*om.*	اذا كثرت البق والبعوض في موضع فتذبحه فدخنه بعورتين وينضح في الموضع ماء وملح او بدقيق حمص للبراغيث	—
93.8	*om.*	للبراغيث ومن ارد ان لا يتأذي بالبراغيث فليحفر في البيت حفرة ويدهن اعلاه بدم تيس فاذا فعل هذا اجتمعت اليه البراغيث الى تلك الحفرة	—
93.9	اذا اردت ان تشتري دابة رخيصة فادخل في اذنها خنفساء فتمرض الفرس فاشتريها أنت رخيصة فاذا اشتريتها نحها من اذنها تصب العافيه	اذا ادخلت خنفساء في دُبر اي حيوان كان مرض فاذا اخرجت قام صحيحا وهي حيلة لمن يشتري الدواب حتى يشتريه بشيء يسير	—

93.6: (b) خذ...تبرأ] الخنفساه اذا تشرّ جلدها وعصرت في الاذن سكن عنه ضربانها G
93.7: (b) *om.* G
93.8: (b) *om.* G | In T another recipe is added, with squirting cucumber leaves against the fleas: وان سلق ورق قثاء الحمار بالماء ونضح في البيت قتل البراغيث
93.9: (b) This recipe is attested only in G | In G another recipe is added, with the heads of seven scarabs in wine to induce the menstruation: رؤوس الحنافس الملس السود سبعة تنفع في شراب الصرف وتشربه المرأة الذي قد اختبس عنها الطمث فيدر

93.6	*om.*	Take a scarab, peel its skin, squeeze it inside the ear, then this will heal.	–
93.7	*om.*	If the bedbugs and the mosquitos multiply in a certain place, then slaughter it [the scarab], fumigate the place with its genitals, and sprinkle the place with water and salt, or chickpea flour.	–
93.8	*om.*	Against the fleas: the one who does not wish to be troubled by fleas has to dig a hole in the house, rub its upper part with ram blood, and when he does this, then the fleas will gather in this hole.	–
93.9	If you want to buy a beast for a low price, put a scarab inside its ear: then the horse will fall ill, and so you can buy it for a low price. Once you have bought it, take the scarab out of its ear, and this will be healthy again.	When you put a scarab inside the buttocks of any animal, then it will be sick; when you take it out, then he will be healthy again, and this is the stratagem for the one who wants to purchase animals for a small price.	–

٩٤. الفسافس

	a	b	c
	—	الفسافس	—
94.1	—	اذا دقت وشممت من به الصداع سكنه	—
94.2	—	وان بخر بواحدة من في حلقه علقة اخرجها	—
94.3	—	وينفع من اليرقان اذا خلط مع الخمر وشرب وينفع من عسر البول	—
94.4	—	وان سحقت وذيفت بعسل وطليت على الحلق نفعت من الخوانيق	—
94.5	—	وان طبخت في رأس رمانة حلوة مع دهن وقطر في الاذن الوجعة سكن الوجع	—
94.6	—	وان جففت وسقى منها امرأة قد عسر عليها الولادة نفعها	—
94.7	—	وان طليت على الثدى ادرّ اللبن	—
94.8	—	والصراصير وبنات [الارض] وردان اذا سحقت اجوافها وطبخت مع دهن وقطر في الاذن نفعت	—

94. Bedbugs

	a	b	c
	–	**The bedbugs**	–
94.1	–	If they are ground and sniffed by someone affected by headache, then this will make it cease.	–
94.2	–	If one of them is used to fumigate the one who has a leech in his body, then this will extract it.	–
94.3	–	They are useful against jaundice, if mixed with wine; this is also useful against urine retention.	–
94.4	–	If they are ground, mixed with honey, and rubbed on the body, then this will be useful against suffocation.	–
94.5	–	If they are cooked with essential oil inside a sweet pomegranate, and applied in drops inside the aching ear, then the pain will cease.	–
94.6	–	If they are dried, and a woman who has difficulties in giving birth takes them, this will be useful to her.	–
94.7	–	If they are rubbed on the breasts, this will make the milk flow copiously.	–
94.8	–	Cockroaches, worms, and roaches: if their abdomens are crushed, cooked with essential oil, and applied in drops inside the ear, then this will be useful to it.	–

٩٥. القمل

	a	b	c
	—	القمل	—
95.1	—	اذا أخذت باقلاة مسوسة ونزع ما فيها من السوسة وجعل فيها قملة رأس وتسد عليها بشمع وتعلق على من به صداع فانه سكن	—
95.2	—	واذا اردت ان تعلّم ان المرأة حامل بذكر او انثى فان لب من لبنها في كف انسان واطرح قملة من الرأس فان خرجت فهي حامل بانثى وان لم تخرج منه فانها حامل بذكر والله اعلم	—

95. Lice

	a	b	c
	–	**The lice**	–
95.1	–	If you take some broad beans eaten by moth worms, remove these and put the head of a louse inside the bean, seal it up with bee wax, and hang it on the man suffering from headache, then this will cease.	–
95.2	–	When you want to sort out whether a woman is pregnant with a boy or a girl, prepare some of her milk into the palm of a man's hand and throw a louse in it; if the louse comes to the surface, then she is pregnant with a girl, if, instead, it does emerge, then she is pregnant with a boy.	–

٩٦. الحلم

	a	b	c
	ذكر منافع الحلم وهي دودة يقال لها القردان	الحلم	—
96.1	يؤخذ القردان الكبار مما شئت فيجعل في طشت نحاس ويجففوا في الظل وان كان في الشمس فهو ابلغ فاذا جف فخذ منه جزء من المسك العراقي حبّة ويسحق الجميع ناعما ويكتحل به صاحب البياض في العين فيزول باذن الله تعالى	اذا شققت ظهره وادخلت فيه مرود واكتحل به قطع الشعر من العين وان طُرحت في ماء في طشت وجفف في الظل وسحق مع جزين زبد البحر وجزء عسل ونصف جزء كافور وبخل وذرّ به بياض العين يذهب به	—
96.2	يؤخذ هذا الدودة فتقتل واطلِ بدمها الشعر التي تنبت في العين فتزول باذن الله تعالى	وان قطع الحلم ودلك الشعرة في جفن العين بعد تنفيه منه من نباته	—

96. Flea

	a	b	c
	Exposition of the useful properties of the flea (*ḥalam*), that is a worm also called *al-qirdān*	**The flea**	–
96.1	Take as many big fleas as you want, put them in a large copper basin and let them dry in the shade—in the sun is even better—once they have dried, take one part of them, one grain of Iraqi musk, pound everything into a fine powder and rub it on the eye suffering from glaucoma, then this will cease, with the permission of God, may He be exalted.	If you split its abdomen, dip a probe for the kohl inside it, and apply this on the eye, then this will cut the hair of the eye. If it is thrown in a large basin, dried in the shadow, ground with two parts of meehrschaum, one part of honey, half part of camphor with vinegar, and the glaucoma is rubbed with it, then this will disappear.	–
96.2	Take this insect, kill it, and rub its blood on the hair that grows on the eye, and it will disappear, with the permission of God, may He be exalted.	If the flea is cut and rubbed on the hair of the eyelid, then this will prevent its growth.	–

٩٧. العنكبوت

	c	b	a
	—	العنكبوت	منافع العنكبوت
97.1	—	*om.*	يؤخذ العنكبوت يغلي بدهن ورد ويجعل على ضرس فيسكن وجعه باذن الله تعالى
97.2	—	يؤخذ العنكبوت الذي ينسج في البيت فيصيره في خرقة وتعلقه على الذي به الحمى الربع او الحمى الغب فيذهب عنه باذن الله تعالى	*om.*

97. Spider

	a	b	c
	Useful properties of the spider	**The spider**	–
97.1	If a spider is taken, boiled with rose oil, and applied on the molar, then its pain will cease, with the permission of God, may He be exalted.	*om.*	–
97.2	*om.*	If the spider that weaves nets in the house is taken, is placed in a piece of cloth, and hung on a man affected by quartan fever or by intermittent fever, then this will leave him, with the permission of God, may He be exalted.	–

٩٨. الكنج

	a	b	c
	ذكر منافع الكنج	الكنج	—
	وهي دابة تشبه الحرباء وهي تتلون على الوان المواضع التي يكون فيها		
	وهذه الدابة اذا تفحت على ابن ادم اظلم بصره		
98.1	يؤخذ دم الدابة يخلط معه بلسان ويطلي به الخنازير اليابسه فتزول باذن الله تعالى	اذا خلط دمه مع دهن بلسان وطلى به الخنازير ابرأها	—
98.2	يؤخذ من دماغ هذه الدابة جزء ومن أصول الكبر جزء ومن ماء الذراريح جزء ويجمع ذلك كله واسحقه واطل به الخنازير فتذهب باذن الله تعالى	*om.*	—
98.3	يؤخذ في دماغ هذه الدابة حصاة يسحق ويخلط بدهن زنبق ويسعط به صاحب اللقوة من الجانب الذي يكون فيه العوج فيبرأ باذن الله تعالى	في دماغه حصاة اذا أخذها انسان وسحقها واذافها بدهن زنبق وسعّط بها للقوة نفع	—
98.4	يؤخذ مرارة هذه الدابة تداف بالماء ويطلي بها الوضح فيزول باذن الله تعالى	مرارته اذا خلط معها موبرح [؟] وسحقها وطلى بها البرص غير لونه	—

98. *Kanǧ*

	a	b	c
	Exposition of the useful properties of the *al-kanǧ*.	**The *kanǧ***	–
	It is a beast that resembles the chameleon, and it has the ability to change its colours according to the place in which it is.		
	When this animal hisses against a man, then his eyesight will grow dark.		
98.1	If the blood of this animal is taken, mixed with balsam of Mecca, and rubbed on the dry scrofula, then it will disappear, with the permission of God, may He be exalted.	Its blood: if it is mixed with balsam of Mecca oil, and the scrofula is rubbed with it, then this will cure it.	–
98.2	Take one part of the brain of this animal, one part of mustard, one part of Spanish fly water, mix all of them together and rub it on the scrofula, and then it will disappear, with the permission of God, may He be exalted.	*om.*	–
98.3	If the stone which is inside the brain of this animal is taken, crushed, and mixed with lily oil, made snuffed by the man suffering from facial paralysis, from the side where the unevenness is, then this will disappear, with the permission of God, may He be exalted.	In its brain there is a stone: if someone takes it, grinds it, and mixes it with lily oil, this will be useful, when inhaled against the facial paralysis.	–
98.4	Gall of this animal: if it is taken, diluted with water, and rubbed on the leprosy, then this will disappear, with the permission of God, may He be exalted.	Its gall: if some *mwbrḥ* [?] is mixed with it, and smeared on the leprosy, then this will change its colour.	–

وزبله اذا عرق موضعه وجمع وخلط معه زبد البحر وسكر وملح وسحق وذر في العين اذهب البياض —

98.5 يؤخذ زبل هذه الدابة اذا وجد يجفف ويسحق ويخلط معه زبد البحر وسكّر نبات وملح اندراني يسحق الجميع واكحل به صاحب البياض في العين فيذهب باذن الله تعالى

98.5: (b) زنبق] زيبق T

98.5 The excrement of this beast (when it is possible to find it): if it is taken, dried, pounded, and mixed with meerschaum, rock candy and rock salt, then all this is made into a powder, and rubbed on the eyes of a man suffering from glaucoma, then this will disappear, with the permission of God, may He be exalted.

If the place in which its excrement can be found is watered, the excrement is collected; meerschaum, sugar, and salt are mixed with it, then ground and poured in the eye, then this will remove the glaucoma.

٩٩. الخراطين

	a	b	c
	الخراطين	الخراطين	—
	وهي دودة تخرج من الارض الندية التي على شطوط والانهر وهي دودة طويلة		
99.1	تغلي في الزيت حتى تحترق واسحقه ويضرب الزيت حتى يصير كالمرهم واجعلها في صوفة ويتحمل بها صاحب البواسير فتذهب باذن الله	غليت في الزيت وسحقت وسقيت الخل حتى يصير كالمرهم واحتمل منه بصوفة صاحب البواسير نفعه	—
99.2	يؤخذ هذه الدودة تدق ويخلط معها قطران ويطلي بها البثرة التي تكون في العين فتبرأ	وان دق ناعما وسحق مع حناء وشيء من قطران وطلي البثر الحاد في الجسد نفعه	—
99.3	يؤخذ هذه الدودة وتجعل في قارورة ويصب عليها زيت وتدفن في الزبل سبعة ايام واخرجها وارم الدودة وخذ الزيت واغليه حتى يذهب رائحته واجعل في قارورة واترك عليها شقايق النعمان ويدفن ايضا في الزبل سبعة ايام اخرى ثم اخرجها وادهن به الشعر فانها يسوّد ولا يسيب ابدا	وان أخذ من الحراطين وصيرت في قارورة والقي عليها زيتا ودفنت القارورة سبعة ايام واخرجت وربي الحراطين والقى على الزيت دق الغار الطري جزء واغلى [على] النار حتى تذهب رايحته وطرح عليه شقايق النعمان ودُفن سبعة ايام ثم اخرج صار خضبا حسنا يسود الشعر ويطول سواده	—
99.4	يؤخذ هذه الدودة يدق ويخلط بالسمن العتيق ودهن ورد ويترك على الورم الحادّ فيذهب والله أعلم	وان سحقت واديف بسكنجبين نفعت من اليرقان وان خلطت بعد دفنها بشمع ودهن ورد تفعت الاورام الحادة	—

99: (a) الخراطين] الخراطيم S
(b) الخراطين] الخراطير T

99. Earthworm

	a	b	c
	The earthworms	**The earthworms**	–
	This is a worm that comes out from the moist ground along the river banks, and is a long worm.		
99.1	If it is boiled with oil until it is burnt, then pounded and the oil whipped until it becomes like an ointment; and if it is put in a woollen cloth, and carried by a man suffering from haemorrhoids, then these will disappear, with the permission of God.	If it is boiled in oil, ground, moistened with vinegar until it becomes like an ointment, and a man suffering from haemorrhoids carries it in a woollen cloth, then this will be useful for him.	–
99.2	If this this worm is taken, crushed, mixed with pine tar, and rubbed on the pustules that are on the eye, then these will be cured.	If it is ground into a fine powder with henna and a bit of asphalt, rubbed on the acute pustules on the body, then this will be useful to this.	–
99.3	If this worm is taken, put inside a long-necked flask, some oil is poured on it, the flask buried in the manure for seven days, then it is taken out and the worm thrown away; then the oil is taken and boiled until it loses its smell, put in a flask with some red anemones on top of it, and buried again for other seven days; then it is taken out and the hair is rubbed with such oil, then they will turn black and will never turn white again.	If some earthworms are taken, put in a long-necked flask, some oil is poured on them, and the bottle buried in the manure for seven days; then the earthworms are taken out and thrown away, one part of liquid pulverized laurel is added to the oil, then boiled on the fire until its smell has gone, red anemones are added to it, then buried again for seven days; once it is taken out, this becomes an excellent dye that makes the hair black, and makes their blackness longlasting.	–
99.4	If this worm is taken, made into a powder, mixed with old fat and rose oil, and applied on an acute swelling, then this will subside, and God knows best.	If they are made in powder, mixed with oxymel, they will be useful against the jaundice; if, instead, they are mixed after having been buried with wax and rose oil, then they will be useful against the acute swellings.	–

١٠٠. حوت الماء

	a	b	c
	ذكر منافع حوت الماء	—	—
100.1	وهذه الحوت تؤخذ في ناحية تُنيس ويخرج من عينيه ودك عظيم يؤكل به الخبز ويوقد به السرج	—	—
100.2	مرارة هذه الحوت يصبغ بها الصوف فلا يقص ابدا	—	—
100.3	يؤخذ مرارة هذه الحوت وخردل احمر مسحوق واسحق الجميع بالخل واطل به البرص فانه يذهب	—	—

100. Sperm Whale

	a	b	c
	Exposition of the useful properties of the sperm whale	–	–
100.1	This fish can be found in the region of Tunis, a superb grease comes out from its eyes, this is eaten with bread, and used to light lamps.	–	–
100.2	Gall of this whale: if some wool is dyed with its gall, then this will never be cut.	–	–
100.3	Gall of this whale: if it is taken with some ground seeds of red mustard, everything ground with vinegar and rubbed on the leprosy, then this will go away.	–	–

١٠١. السرطان النهري

	a	b	c
	ذكر منافع السرطان النهري	السرطان النهري	—
101.1	يحرق ويداف بالماء ويلطخ الاورام الحاشية فيفتحها بلا حديد ويفشّها باذن الله تعالى	اذا سحق وضمد به الاورام الحاشة حللها واخرج نصول النشاء اذا بقيت في البدن	—
101.2	السرطان يحرق ويؤخذ رماده يكتحل به من في عينه الماء فيزول باذن الله تعالى	يحرق في كوز فخار ويؤخذ رماده يكتحل به في العين الذي نزل فيه الماء فيبرأ باذن الله تعالى	—
101.3	ويحرق ايضا ويؤخذ رماده يسقي لمن عسر البول فيزول باذن الله تعالى	رماد السرطان النهري يسقي منه من احتبس بوله يدر باذن الله تعالى	—
101.4	السرطان يسحق ويحشي به البواسير فيذهب باذن الله تعالى	رماد السرطان النهري كذلك اذا سحق وحشي به الباسور حيث كان من البدن نفع نفعا بينا	—
101.5	لسلس البول يؤخذ سرطان فاغليه بزيت حتي يحترق واسحقه ويسقي منه لصاحب عسر البول فانه يسلسه ويدره باذن الله	ولمن لم يمكنه ان يحبس بوله بيض السرطان النهري يؤكل بعد ان يُشق السرطان فيزيد في الباه	—
101.6	يحرق السرطان ويؤخذ رماده ويلتّ بدهن كادي ويخلط معه شبّ يماني ويجعل في صوفة وتحمله المرأة فينقطع النزيف باذن الله تعالى	*om.*	

101. River Crab

	a	b	c
	Exposition of the useful properties of the river crab	**The river crab**	**–**
101.1	If it is burnt, diluted with some water, spattered on the suppurative swellings, then these will open without any incision and will subside, with the permission of God, may He be exalted.	If it is burnt and used to bandage the suppurative swellings, then this will dissolve them. It also extracts the points of the arrows, when they are stuck inside the body.	–
101.2	If the crab is burnt, its ash is taken, and applied on the eye of the man who has water in it, then this will cease, with the permission of God, may He be exalted.	If it is burnt in a clay pot, and its ash applied on the eye from which water drps, then this will heal, with the permission of God, may He be exalted.	–
101.3	Again, if it is burnt and its ash is given to a man who suffers from urine retention to drink, then this will cease, with the permission of God, may He be exalted.	River crab ash: if it is taken by someone who retains urine, then this will flow again, with the permission of God, may He be exalted.	–
101.4	If the river crab is crushed and stuffed in the haemorrhoids, then they will subside, with the permission of God, may He be exalted.	River crab ash: likewise, if it is ground and stuffed in the haemorrhoids—wherever they may be on the body—then it will clearly be useful.	–
101.5	For the flowing of urine: if a river crab is taken, boiled with oil until it burns, pounded and given to a man suffering from urine retention to drink, then this will make the urine flow more easily, with the permission of God, may He be exalted.	And for someone who cannot retain urine: river crab eggs, eaten just after that the river crab has been split, then his sexual desire will increase.	–
101.6	If the river crab is crushed and stuffed in the haemorrhoids, then they will subside, with the permission of God, may He be exalted.	*om.*	–

101.7	رماد السرطان بخنطيانة وكندر ويسقي منه لمن عضه الكلب الكلب اربعين يوما متوالية فيسلم	*om.*
101.8	يشوي السرطان النهري ويؤكل فانه زيد في الباه	*om.*
101.9	يؤخذ هذا السرطان النهري ويطبخ مع السعتر ويُطعم لصاحب مرض السل فانه يبرأ باذن الله	*om.*
101.10	رماد السرطان مع الطين الرومي يسقي لمن يطرح الدم فيبرأ باذن الله تعالى	*om.*

101.7	Ash of river crab: with gentian [*ḥinṭīāna*] and incense, given to a man bitten by a rabid dog to drink for forty days in a row, then he will recover.	*om.*	–
101.8	If the river crab is roasted and eaten, then this will increase the sexual potency.	*om.*	–
101.9	If this river crab is cooked with wild thyme and given to a man suffering from consumption to eat, then he will recover.	*om.*	–
101.10	Rive ashr crab: if it is given to drink with Byzantine [*Rūmī*] clay to a man affected by a loss of blood, then he will recover, with the permission of God, may He be exalted.	*om.*	–

١٠٢. السرطان البحري

	a	b	c
	om.	السرطان	—
102.1	اطراف السرطان يدق وتتحلل ويخلط بالاثمد ويكتحل بها من في عينه بياض فيزول	يدق وينخل ويخلط بالاكحال النافعة للبياض في العين والغشاوة والحرارة ينفع نفعا بينا	—
102.2	يحرق السرطان ويعجن رماده بالماء ويضمد على موضع النصل فيخرجه من الجسد بلا حديد وكذلك الشوكة	السرطان البحري اذا احرق وأخذ رماده وعجن بالماء وضمد به مواضع النصول والشكوك الذي في البدن اخرجها	—
102.3	اذا جفّف السرطان ويشرب بالماء فانه يخرج بحبّ القرع من الجوف وقيل بشراب سكنجبين [كان ابلغ]	*om.*	—

102. Sea Crab

	a	b	c
	–	**The crab**	–
102.1	Sea crab extremities: if they are crushed, ground, mixed with antimony, and rubbed on the eyes affected by glaucoma, then this will disappear.	If it is crushed, sieved, mixed with some eye salves useful against glaucoma in the eye, the cataract, and the reddening, then this will clearly be useful.	–
102.2	If the sea crab is burnt, its ash kneaded with water and used to bandage the part where an arrowhead has penetrated, then this will come out without any incision. It is equally useful for the thorns.	If the crab is burnt, its ash is taken, kneaded with water, and used to bandage the parts where arrowheads and thorns have penetrated in the body, then this will extract them.	–
102.3	If the sea crab is dried and drunk with some water, this will remove the pustules of the ringworm from the abdomen. It is said that, with some oxymel, it is even more effective.	*om.*	–

١٠٣. الحوت

a	b	c
ذكر منافع الحوت يسمى باطس	—	—
103.1 يتخذ من هذا الحوت لعوق ينفع لعضة الكلب الكلب وهذا صفته يؤخذ من كبد هذا الحوت سبعة دراهم ومن الفَرْك الحلوا المقشور ثمانية دراهم ومن حب السفرجل ثلاثة دراهم ومن الصبغ العربي ثلاثة دراهم ومن البقلة الحمقاء جزء ومن لب الشاهترج مثل وزن الجميع يسحق الجميع ويعجن بعسل نحل ويضرب حتى يصير مثل المرهم ويرفع في اناء ويسقي لمن عضه الكلب الكلب وزن مثقال بنبيذ صرف فانه يهدي باذن الله تعالى	—	—
103.2 وهذا حوت عظيم لا يقوي به المركب واهل الجزائر يعرفونه ويحملونه معهم خرق الحيض لاجله فاذا شم هذا الرائحة القذيرة فلا يقرب المركب وهو عجيب الخلقة	—	—

103. Whale

	a	b	c
	Exposition of the useful properties of the whale called *bāṭus*	–	–
103.1	From this huge whale, an electuary is prepared, that cures the bite of the rabid dog, and this is the way of preparing it. Take seven dirhams of the liver of such whale, eight dirhams of peeled sweet bdellium, three dirhams of quince seeds, three dirhams of Arabic amaranth, one part of purslane, and fumitory in the same quantity of all the other ingredients; grind this, knead it with bee honey and whip it until it becomes like an ointment, store it in a vessel and give one *miṯqāl* of it to drink to the man bitten by a rabid dog together with some pure wine; then he will be guided on the right way [of healing], with the permission of God, may He be exalted.	–	–
103.2	This is an enormous and mighty whale, and even a great ship is powerless against it. The people of the islands are aware of this and prepare a piece of cloth soaked with menstrual blood for this reason; when the whale sniffs this filthy smell, then it does not approach the ship, and this is a wonder of the creation.	–	–

١٠٤. السلحفاة

	a	b	c
	ذكر منافع السلحفاة	السلحفاة	باب منافع السلحفاة
	وهي الفكرونة		السلحفاة التي تكون في الانهار وهي التي ترى في البيوت
104.1	اذا اطبخ هذا السلحفاة بالخل مثل السكباج وأكله صاحب الاستسقاء برئ باذن الله تعالى	*om.*	*om.*
104.2	من أكل لحم السلحفاة لم يحيك فيه السحر	*om.*	*om.*
104.3	السلحفاة الذكر اذا امتنعت منه الانثى يعمد الى حشيشة يقال لها اسطوخدس فيأخذ منها ورقة ويلقي على الأنثى فيطيعه	*om.*	*om.*
104.4	السلحفاة البحرية اذا اكتحل بها انسان بدمها عمى	*om.*	*om.*
104.5	واذا طرحت لجاة بحرية في قدر الحمام فمن اغتسل بذلك الماء ورمت عيناه	*om.*	*om.*
104.6	دم اللجاة اذا طلى به البهق الاسود غيّر موضعه	*om.*	*om.*
104.7	مرارة اللجاة اذا خلطت بالعسل واكتحل بها انسان يشتكي من الغشاوة برئ باذن الله	تحلل القصول الغليظة وتنفع من اوجاع الارحام وتدر البول وتحلل وتجفف وتحد النظر وتنقي البرص من الوجه	*om.*

104.4: (a) اسطوخدس] اسطوخس S

104. Turtle

	a	b	c
	Exposition of the useful properties of the turtle,	**The turtle**	**Chapter on the useful properties of the turtle,**
	that is *al-fakarūna*.		the turtle that lives in the rivers, that is the one you may see in the houses.
104.1	If this turtle is cooked with some vinegar, such as the *sakbāǧ* [meat cooked in vinegar], and it is fed to a man suffering from dropsy, then he will recover, with the permission of God, may He be exalted	*om.*	*om.*
104.2	The one who eats turtle meat will not be bound by magic.	*om.*	*om.*
104.3	Male turtle: when the female refuses him, he makes use of a herb called *asṭūḫūdus* [French lavender]; he takes one leaf, flings it at the female, and then she submits to him.	*om.*	*om.*
104.4	Sea turtle: if the eyes of someone are rubbed with its blood, then he will become blind.	*om.*	*om.*
104.5	If a sea turtle is thrown in a basin for the bath, then the eyes of the one who washes himself with this water will swell.	*om.*	*om.*
104.6	Turtle's blood: if it is rubbed on black leprosy, then this will change its condition.	*om.*	*om.*
104.7	Gall of sea turtle: if it is mixed with honey and rubbed on the eyes of a man who suffers from cataract, then he will recover, with the permission of God, may He be exalted.	It loosens the hard umbilical hernia, it is useful against the pains of the womb, makes the urine flow, loosens, dries, and sharpens the eyesight, and cleanses leprosy away from the face.	*om.*

104.8	كبد اللجاة تشوي ويطعم لصاحب وجع الكبد يبرأ باذن الله تعالى	*om.*	*om.*
104.9	ذنب السلحفاة تجفف وتحمله معك فلا ينبح عليك كلب	ذنبها اذا جفف وحمله انسان بيده لم ينبح عليه الكلاب ما دام معه	اذا أخذ الذكر منها وامسكه انسان في يده لم تنبح عليه كلب
104.10	يؤخذ السلحفاة تذبح وتجفف وتسحق ويداف بدهن زنبق وادهن به الظهر الجانب فانه يقوي على الجماع ويزيد في شهوة النكاح	وان اخذ سلحفة وذبخت وسحقت وذيفت بدهن ورد وزنبق وطلى بها قدما الرجل زاد في الجماع	واذا أخذت السلحفاة وجففت وسحقت واذيفت بدهن وطلى بها الاحليل عند الجماع فانه لا يجامع امرأة الا احبته واقتصرت عليه
104.11	يؤخذ ذنب السلحفاة ويعمل خاتم فاذا لبسته كنت محبوبا الى الخُلق واذا جامعت امرأة احتبك حبا شديدا	وان جعل فص خاتم من ذنب السلحفاة وكل رجل لبسه وجامع امرأته احبته حبا شديدا وبعض الناس يصير الذنب خاتما ويلبسه يفعل ذلك	*om.*
104.12	*om.*	مرارتها اذا خلطت مع بورق وقطران وطلى به الشعرة التي تنبت في العين ابرأها وقطعها	*om.*
104.13	اذا كتبتَ كتابا بمرارة السلحفاة في قرطاس تبين في الليل من غير سراج	وان كتب بها قرأ الكتابة في الليل من غير سراج وان سعط به المصروع نفع	مرارة السلحفاة اذا كتبت بها في قرطاس واخرجته بالليل بان لك من غير مصباح
104.14	تأخذ دم السلحفاة تبلّ منه قتيلة وتجعلها في سراج دهن واعطه لمن شئت وقُل له اسرجه وامسكه فلا يزيل يضرط ما دام في يده وهو عجيب	*om.*	دم السلحفاة اذا بللت خرقة واوقدت منها فتيلة في سراج جديد واعطتيها لمن شئت فانه اذا امسكه في يده لا يزال يضرط ما دام في يده حتى تنطفي

104.9: (c) اذا أخذ الذكر منها] الذكر من ذلك اذا C
104.10: (a) وزنبق] وزيبق T
(c) اخذت] اذبحت C
104.13: (c) اذا كتبت] اذا كتب C | بالليل] في الليل C
104.14: (c) دم السلحفاة] دمه C

104.8	Turtle liver: if it is roasted and fed to a man who suffers from liver complaint, then this will cure him, with the permission of God, may He be exalted.	*om.*	*om.*
104.9	If you dry and carry with you the tail of a turtle, then no dog will bark at you.	Its tail: if it dried, and a man carries it with him, then the dogs will not bark at him, as long as this remains on him.	Turtle penis: if it is taken and a man holds it in his hand, then the dogs will not bark at him
104.10	If the turtle is taken, slaughtered, dried, ground, diluted with lily oil and rubbed on the loins, then this will give power to the coitus and increase the sexual desire.	If a turtle is taken, slaughtered, ground, mixed with rose and lily oil, and rubbed on the feet of a man, then he will become more potent in the coitus.	If a turtle is dried it, ground, diluted with essential oil and rubbed on the outer opening of the urethra at the moment of coitus, then the man will not be able to have sexual intercourse with any other woman but with the one who loves and desires only him.
104.11	Take the turtle's tail to make a seal [ring] out of it: and when you wear it, you will be loved for your character; and when you have sexual intercourse with a woman, she will passionately love you.	If the tail of the turtle is made into the gem of a seal [ring], then every man who wears it and has sexual intercourse with a woman, then she will passionately love him: some people turn its tail into a seal [ring], wear it, and obtain this effect.	*om.*
104.12	*om.*	Its gall: if it is mixed with natron and tar, and the hair growing on the eye is rubbed with it, then this will cure and cut it.	*om.*
104.13	If you write something with turtle gall on a sheet of papyrus, the writing will be visible in the night without the help of any lantern.	And if one writes with it, then the writing can be read in the night without the help of any lamp. And it is useful to the epileptic man, if he inhales it	Turtle gall: if you write something with it on a papyrus sheet and bring it in the open during the night, then the writing will become visible without the help of any light.
104.14	Take the blood of the turtle, moisten a wick with it, put this in an oil lantern, give this lantern to carry to whomever you want, saying him: "Light it and hold it!"; then he will not stop breaking winds as long as he holds it in his hand, and this is amazing.	*om.*	Tortoise blood: if a piece of cloth is moistened with it, then lit as a wick in a new lantern and given to whomever you want; then, when he holds it in his hand, he will not stop to break winds as long as it remains in his hand, to the point that he dies.

104.15	اذا أخذت صغير على اسم من تريد وكان مجذوما فاحرق السلحفاة واسق صاحب الجذام من رمادها بنبيذ عتيق فانه يوقفه عنه	واخذ سلحفاة على اسم مجذوم وسحقت بعد ان تحرق وتكون صغيرة وتسفي بشراب عتيق للمجذوم جفف القروح ولحمها	للجذام يؤخذ سلحفاة صغيرة على اسم المجذوم ثم تحرق ويؤخذ رمادها يسحق ويسقي للمجذوم بشراب عتيق فيقف عنه باذن الله تعالى
104.16	*om.*	*om.*	يؤخذ رماد السلحفاة فيدلك به البدن الوارم والحرة فتزول باذن الله
104.17	دم السلحفاة وكبدها اذا دق الجميع والقى عليه ملح وحلبة وكمون وكرسنه وهو الكسيس من كل واحد جزء مسحوق وعجن الجميع وحبب واستعمل منه من يشتكي وجع المقعدة كل يوم حبة عي الريق نفع جميع اوجاع المقعدة	وكبدها اذا دق وخلط مع ملح مر نفع من وجع المقعدة اذا شرب منه كل يوم حبة	يؤخذ لحم السلحفاة وكبدها ومنفحتها يدق ويخلط معه ملح وحلبة وكمون وكرسنه اجزاء متساوية ويسحق ويعجن ويحبب ويرفع في اناء ويشرب منها كل يوم وزن حب على الريق بماء حار فانه ينفع لكل الاوجاع المقعدة باذن الله تعالى
104.18	*om.*	رماد قحفها اذا دلك بخل وزيت وشرب في الحمام نفع من وجع الكبد والطحال	*om.*
104.19	*om.*	واذا أخذ دم سلحفاة برية او بحرية وعجن به دقيق شعير وعمل حبا كالحمص وسقى للمصروع غدوة وغشية نفع نفعا بليغا	*om.*
104.20	دماغ السلحفاة اذا اذيف بالزيت وطلى به البرص والنقرس سكنه	*om.*	دماغ السلحفاة يعجن بالزيت ويطلي به النقرس
104.21	بيض السلحفاة اذا سلق واكله صاحب السعال المقرح نفعه نفعا جيدا	*om.*	للسعلة اذا أكل نفع من السعال العتيق

104.15: (c) صغير] سلحفاة صغيرة C | وكان مجذوما] وكان به الجذام C

104.16: (a) يؤخذ...فتزول] رماد السلحفاة اذا عجن بزيت ودهن به صاحب القرحة والورم ابرأه B

104.17: (c) دم السلحفاة] وشحمه *add.* C | وهو الكسيس] *om.* C | من يشتكي وجع المقعدة] من وجع المقعدة C | كل...المقعدة] *om.* C

104.20: (c) دماغ السلحفاة] دماغ السلحفاة البحرية C | اذيف] اذيب C

104.15	Against leprosy: take a small turtle in the name of the person affected by leprosy, burn it, pound its ash and give it to drinkto the man affected by leprosy together with some old wine, and then this will leave him.	If the turtle is taken in the name of a man affected by leprosy, ground after that it has been burnt and its quantity reduced, given with old syrup to the man affected by leprosy to drink, then this will 'fry' the sores and their flesh	If a small one is taken in the name of anyone you want who is affected by leprosy, then the tortoise is burnt and its ash given to the one affected by leprosy to drink together with some old wine, then the leprosy will leave him.
104.16	Turtle ash: if a swollen and burning body is rubbed with it, then it will stop burning, with the permission of God, may He be exalted.	*om.*	*om.*
104.17	Turtle meat, liver, and rennet: if they are taken, minced and mixed with salt, fenugreek, cumin and vetches in equal parts; then ground, kneaded and stored in a vessel; then one grain of it is taken every day on an empty stomach with some hot water, then this will be useful against all the pains of the backside, with the permission of God, may He be exalted.	Its liver: if it is chopped up, bitter salt is mixed with it, it will be useful against the pain of the backside, if one grain of it is taken every day.	Turtle blood and liver: if they are crushed, with the addition of ground salt, fenugreek, cumin and vetches—that is *kasīs*, one part of each one—kneaded, made in grains and given to a man who suffers from backside pain, one pill every day on an empty stomach, this will be useful against all the pains of the back.
104.18	*om.*	Ash of its skull: if it is mixed with vinegar and oil, and drunk in the bath, then it will be useful against the liver and bladder complaint.	*om.*
104.19	*om.*	Blood of wild or sea turtle: if it is kneaded with wheat flour, made in grains of the dimension of a chickpea, and given to drink to the epileptic man, in the morning and in the evening, then this will be greatly useful for him.	*om.*
104.20	Turtle brain: kneaded with oil and rubbed on the gout [it is useful for it].	*om.*	Turtle brain: if it is mixed with oil and rubbed on the leprosy and on the gout, then they will disappear.
104.21	Against cough: if it is eaten, it will be useful against the chronic cough.	*om.*	Turtle eggs: if they are boiled and eaten, then this will be very useful against the ulcerous cough.

104.22	خف السلحفاة اذا احرق وسحق وعجن بعسل وملح ورفع في اناء وأخذ منه جزء واذيف بخل وشراب وشرب في الحمام منه بماء حار من يشتكي وجع الطحال اذهبه ونفعه	*om.*	فخذ رأس الساحفاة يجفف ويسحق ويعجن بعسل وملح يؤخذ جزء منه يداف بخل ويشرب في الحمام على الريق فانه ينفع ويذهب الطحال
104.23	اذا أخذت صفار بيض السلحفاة وجفف ورفع في اناء وأخذ منه وزن دانقين وشرب منه صاحب السعال الشديد بخمر سكن عنه وان شرب منه بلبن حليب كان ابلغ	بيض السلحفاة اذا أخذت صفرته وجفف وسقى منه وزن درهمين بنبيذ لمن به سعال شديد يسكن يفعل اذا شرب بلبن حليب	للسعال الشديد يؤخذ صُفرة بيض السلحفاة يغلي بزيت ثم يرمي الزيت ويأخذ الصفرة ويسحقها واسقِ منها صاحب السعال ينبيذ او عسل فيزول السعال ويسقي بلبن حليب
104.24	دم السلحفاة اذا اذيف بدهن لبان وخلط في هاون والقى عليه زيت ورفع على النار لينة وجعل وجعل في مكحلة وأخذ منه بريشة من ريش البط وهو فاتر وجعل منه في رأس الاحليل ودهن منه الحالب ادر البول المتعسر لبوله	*om.*	دم السلحفاة يداف بدهن زنبق ودهن بلسان ويسحق في هاون ويرفع في اناء على النار ويؤخذ منه بريشة ويدخل في رأس القضيب فيدر البول باذن الله تعالى
104.25	*om.*	واذا شرب بيض السلحفاة البرية نفع من الصرع فهذا ما انتهى الينا من ذلك	*om.*

104.22: (c) وملح] والملح C | في اناء] فاذا احتج اليه لوقت حاجته *add.* C | واذيف] وذوبه C | بماء حار] بالماء الحار C | ونفعه] وابرأه منه C
104.23: (c) عنه] وان استعمله C | وان شرب منه] واستعمل منها من افرط به السعال بخمر سل عنه السعال C | ورفع...سكن] C
104.25: (b) Here ends the text of T, with the following formula: تم الكتاب وبالله المستعان
(c) بدهن لبان] بدهن لسان C | وخلط] ومرهم C

104.22	Take the head of the turtle, dry it, crush it and knead it with honey and salt, take one part of it, mix it with vinegar and drink it in the bath on an empty stomach, then this will be useful for the spleen.	*om.*	Turtle paw: if it is burnt, ground, kneaded with honey and salt, and stored in a vessel, then one part of it is taken, mixed with vinegar and wine, given to drink to the man suffering from spleen complaint in the bath on an empty stomach, then the pain will cease.
104.23	Against violent cough: the yolk of turtle eggs, boiled with oil, then this oil is taken away and the yolk is taken apart, crushed and given to the man suffering from cough to drink, together with wine or honey, then the cough will cease. It can be drunk with cow milk as well.	Turtle eggs: if their yolk is taken, dried, one dirham of it is given with wine to the man affected by severe cough to drink, then this will cease; it has this affect also when drunk with milk.	If the yolk of turtle egg is dried and stored it in a vessel, two *dāniq* of it are taken, and if a man suffering from violent cough drinks it with wine, then the cough will cease. If you drink it with cow milk, it is even better.
104.24	Turtle blood: if it is mixed with lily oil and balsam of Mecca's oil, ground in a mortar and boiled in a vessel on the fire; a bit of it is taken with a feather and applied inside the tip of the penis, then the urine will flow copiously, with the permission of God, may He be exalted.	*om.*	Turtle blood : if it is mixed with frankincense oil, ground in a mortar, with the addition of some oil, put on the fire to melt and then in a kohl jar; then a bit of it is taken with a goose feather while it is still lukewarm, and applied on the top of penis's opening and rubbed in the urethra, this will make the retained urine flow copiously.
104.25	*om.*	Wild turtle eggs: if they are drunk, they will be useful against epilepsy.	*om.*

١٠٥. الحلزون الانهار

	a	b	c
	ذكر منافع الحلزون الذي يكون على الانهار	—	*om.*
105.1	اذا أبطأ الحيض على المرأة تأخذ حلزونة تدق ناعما ويخلط معها قنّة و شونيز من كل واحد جزء وتتحمل به المرأة فيدر الطمث	—	*om-*
105.2	لوجع الرحم يؤخذ الحلزون الذي يكون في الحجارة يدق ناعما ويخلط معه سذاب ويذاف بعسل نحل واجعله في صوفة وتتحمل به فتصلح	—	*om-*
105.3	لوجع الكبد يؤخذ الحلزون النهري يدق ويلتّ بعسل نحل وورس ويسقي منه صاحب وجع الكبد فيبرأ باذن الله تعالى	—	اذا أخذت الحلزون البحري واحرقته ودقته ناعما وتحلته ولينته بعسل ودهن زنبق وشرب صاحب الكبد بماء حار ابرأه باذن الله تعالى

105.1: (a) شونيز] شونير S

105.3: (c) اذا...واحرقته] اذا احرقته الجردون البحري C | بعسل ودهن زنبق] بالعسل ودهن الزنبق C

105. River Snail

	a	b	c
	Exposition of the useful properties of the river snail	–	*om.*
105.1	When the monthly period of a woman is late, take a snail, crush it into a fine powder and mix it with galbanum and black [cumin] seeds, one part of each one; then the woman has to carry this with her, and then the menstruation will flow abundantly.	–	*om.*
105.2	Against the pain of the womb: take the snails that dwell among the stones, crush them into a fine powder, mix them with rue, dilute this with bee honey and put it in a woollen cloth; the woman should carry it, and then she will recover.	–	*om.*
105.3	Against liver complaint: if the river snails are crushed, mixed with bee honey and curcuma, given to a man suffering from liver complaint to drink, then he will recover, with the permission of God, may He be exalted.	–	If sea snails are burn, ground into a fine powder, dissolved in water, tempered with honey and lily oil, and given to drink to someone suffering from liver complaint, then he will recover, with the permission of God, may He be exalted.

١٠٦. الصدف

	a	b	c
	ذكر منافع الصدف	الصدف	باب منافع الصدف
106.1	*om.*	ينفع اللؤلؤ خفقان القلب والفزع العارض من السوداء	*om.*
106.2	*om.*	ولحم الصدف اذا طبخ وطبخ مع المرقة عسل وشراب وشرب منه من به زحير عن قروح نفعه	*om.*
106.3	*om.*	وشحمه ينفع من قروح وان ضمد برأس الصوف والاورام التي تحدث في الاذنيين نفع وينفع من البثر الاحمر	*om.*
106.4	يقشّر عنه جلده ويحرق ويحلّ بنبيذ ويسقي لامرأة فانها لا تحلب ابدا	واذا أخذ قبل ان يتكامل جوهره واستخرج ماؤه يمزج بشراب وسقيت منه امرأة لا تحمل حملت وولدت	الصدف اذا قشر جلده اعني براه الاسود وحل وسحق وخلط بشراب عتيق وشربته المرأة التي لا تحبل وجمعها الرجل حملت تلك الليلة
106.5	يؤخذ الصدف يحرق ويسحق ويذر على الخنازير	والذي يكامل اذا طلى به الخنازير المتأكلة ابرأها	الصدف اذا احرق وسحق وذر عليه الخنازير ابرأها
106.6	لوجع رحم المرأة يؤخذ الصدفة يحرق ويعجن ويشرب منه المرأة مقدار درهم فتصلح	*om.*	واذا احرق وعجن بدهن زنبق وسحق وشربته المرأه التي تشتكي وجع الارحام ابرأها
106.7	*om.*	لحم الصدف اذا اذيف مع العسل وضمد به موضع عضة الكلب الكلب نفعه	*om.*

106.4: (c) الصدف [*om.* C | وشربته [وشربت منه C | الليلة [وجمعها...الليلة [وجمعها...عز وجل باذن الله عز وجل ثم جامعها بعدها حملت من وقته C

106.5: ويذر [ودر L

106.6: (c) واذا احرق [الصدف اذا احرق C | وعجن [وسحق C

106. Pearl Oyster

	a	b	c
	Exposition of the useful properties of the pearl oysters	**The pearl oysters**	**Chapter on the useful properties of the pearl oysters**
106.1	*om.*	The pearl is useful against the manifest palpitantions of the heart due to the black gall.	*om.*
106.2	*om.*	Oyster flesh: if it is cooked, then some honey and syrup are cooked with its stock, and a man who suffers from dysentery due to the ulcers eats it, this will be useful for him.	*om.*
106.3	*om.*	Its fat is useful for the ulcers; and if it is used to bandage with wool the swellings that appear on the ear, this will be useful against this; and it is also useful against the red pustules.	*om.*
106.4	If their shell is peeled off, burnt, dissolved in some wine and given to a woman to drink, then she will never get pregnant.	If its precious stone is taken before it has completely formed, its water taken out, blended with syrup, and a woman who does not get pregnant drinks it, then she will get pregnant and give birth.	If the skin of the pearl oyster—that is the black external part—is peeled, dissolved, ground, mixed with some old wine, and given to the woman who does not get pregnant to drink before she mates with a man, then she will get pregnant that same night.
106.5	If the pearl oyster is burnt, ground, and applied on the scrofula [it will be useful against it].	If the corrosive scrofula is rubbed with a pearl that has completed its formation, then this will cure it.	If the pearl oyster is burnt, ground and applied on the scrofula, then this will heal it.
106.6	Against the pain of the womb which affects the women, the pearl oyster has to be taken, burnt, kneaded, and one dirham of it has to be given to a woman to drink, and then she will recover.	*om.*	If it is burnt, kneaded with lily oil, ground and given to a woman suffering from womb pain to drink, then this will cure her.
106.7	*om.*	Pearl oyster flesh: if it is mixed with honey, and used to bandage the part where the bite of the rabid dog is, then this will be useful against it.	*om.*

106.8	*om.*	واذا احرق وأخذ رمده واخلط بالقطران وطلى به موضع الشعر الزائد الذي ينبت في الاجفان بعد ينفد ابرأه	*om.*
106.9	*om.*	واذا طبخ بالماء والملح نفع من السموم والهوام	*om.*
106.10	*om.*	واذا احرق واخلط بشحم الاوز وضمد به الثديين نفع من اللبن المحترق فيها وحلله	*om.*
106.11	*om.*	وان سحق مع الكسفرة وذيف بعسل وطلى به ومسكته امرأة نفع من البثر والثآليل والجرب الكائن في الرحم	*om.*
106.12	*om.*	*om.*	الصدف النهري اذا دق بلحمه دقا جيدا والقي عليه سمن بقري الى ان يغمره ويمرهم فيه ويجعل في خرقة لطيفة قدر صلب المرأة وتلصق عليها الى ان تجمد على ظهرها فانها تحبل اذا ابطا حبلها
106.13	*om.*	الدلنيس هو صدف يأكله الناس في الشام وغيره	*om.*
106.14	*om.*	مطبوخ بالماء والملح ينفع من رطوبة المعدة والاستسقاء	*om.*
106.15	*om.*	زبد البحر اذا كحّل به العين نفع من البياض وينشف من الدمعة	*om.*

106.12: (c) سمن بقري] السمن البقري C

106.8	*om.*	If it is burnt, its ash mixed with tar, and rubbed on the part of the eyelids where the superfluous hairs grows, after it has been pulled out, then this will cure it.	*om.*
106.9	*om.*	If it is cooked with water and salt, it will be useful against the poisons and the poisonous insects.	*om.*
106.10	*om.*	If it is burnt, mixed with goose fat, and used to bandage the breasts, it will be useful against the milk 'burnt' inside them, and this will dissolve it.	*om.*
106.11	*om.*	If it is ground with fumitory, mixed with honey, used as an ointment, and a woman holds it, then it will be useful against pustules, warts, and the scabies which is in the womb.	*om.*
106.12	*om.*	*om.*	If the river pearl oyster shells are crushed into a fine powder together with their flesh, with the addition of enough cow grease to cover them and let them float in it; then put in a fine piece of cloth of the size of a woman's spine, and applied on her back until it hardens, then she will get pregnant, even though this has been difficult for her before.
106.13	*om.*	*Dalīnas* shell: it is an oyster that the people from Syria and others eat.	*om.*
106.14	*om.*	Cooked with water and salt, it is useful against the moistness in the stomach and the dropsy.	*om.*
106.15	*om.*	Meerschaum: if it is applied on the eye, it will be useful against the leucoma, and will stimulate the lachrymation.	*om.*

١٠٧. العلق

	a	b	c
	منافع العلق	العلق	باب منافع العلق
107.1	يؤخذ العلق يجعل في كوز رصاص ويترك حتى يموت ثم يحرق ويسحق ناعما ويعلق به الشعر فينبت سريعا باذن الله	اذا أخذ وترك في كوز حتى يموت ثم سحق ويطلي به اصول الشعر بعد ان يذيف منعه من النبات	اذا جعلت العلق في كوز حديد وتركته الي ان يموت وسحقته واخرجته وان احرقته كان ابلغ وعلقت به الشعر فانه يطوله ويغزره ويحسنه
107.2	*om.*	وان اخذ وخلط مع علق حي مدقوق واضيفه اليه من زبد البحر بالجميع الاحليل كبّره وغلظه وان علق على الصُدغين نفع	اذا أخذ العلق الحي ودق في هاون وطليت به الاحليل غلظه وكبره
107.3	*om.*	*om.*	اذا أخذت شيئا من العلق وشيئا من احليل حمار وجعلته في اناء ودفنته بالزبل الي ان ينهري ثم اطهرته والقيته في قدر والقيت عليه ماء وسلقت فيه حنطة واظهرتها وجففتها وعلقت منه دجاجة سوداء ثم ذبحتها وأخذت من شحمها ورفعته علي النار وسلقت الدجاجة الي ان تنهري ودخلت الحمام ودهنت احليلك من شحم الدجاجة واكلت اللحم وشربت المرق رايت من غلظه ما لا يعبر عنه
107.4	اذا بخّر بالعلق دكان زجاج تكسر جميع ما فيها	وان بخّر بالعلق دكان الزجاج كسّر زجاجه	اذا اردت ان تكسر ما في حانوت الزجاج فلا يبقي فيه شيء الا انكسر فتبخر فيه شيء من العلق

107.1: (c) ويعلق] ويعلف S | في كوز حديد] في كوز جديد C | واخرجته] *om.* C | فانه يطوله ويغزره ويحسنه] طوله وغزره ويحسنه C
107.2: (c) اذا أخذ] اذا أخذ اي اعلق *add.* C | الحي] *om.* C | في هاون] في الهاون C
107.3: (c) اذا أخذت شيئا من العلق] اذا أخذت العلق C | وجعلته] وتركته C | بالزبل] في زبل حامي C | واظهرتها وجففتها] واظهرتها ثم انك جففتها C | تنهري] تهتري C | احليلك] الاحليل C | ما لا يعبر عنه] ما لا يكاد يعبر عنه C | عنه] وهو دواء نافع جدا *add.* C
107.4: (c) في حانوت] ماء بحانوت C | فلا يبقي...من العلق] فالحكمة فيه انك بخره بشيء من العلق فانه ينكسر ولا يبقي فيه شيء من الزجاج الا انكسر او انصدع C

107. Leech

	a	b	c
	The useful properties of the leeches	–	**Chapter on the useful propertiesof the leeches**
107.1	If the leeches are taken, put in a lead jug and left there until they die, then burnt, ground into a fine powder and hung on the hair, then the hair will quickly grow, with the permission of God.	If they are taken and thrown in a jug until they die, then ground, and smeared on the roots of the hairs, after that this has been mixed, then it will prevent their growth.	If the leeches are put in an iron jug, left there until they die, ground, taken out—it is even better if you burn them—and hung on the hair, then the hair will become longer, thicker, and nicer.
107.2	*om.*	If they are taken, mixed with living leeches ground, everything mixed with meerschaum, then applied on the outer opening of the urethra, this will make it bigger and thicker.	If the leeches are taken alive, pulverized in a mortar, and rubbed on the outer opening of the urethra, then this will made your penis thicker and bigger.
107.3	*om.*	*om.*	If some leeches and a some penis of the donkey are taken, put in a vessel and buried it in the manure until they decompose; then they are dug out, some wheat is cooked in it, then taken out, let dry and hung on a black hen; then the hen has to be slaughtered, its grease taken, let simmer on the fire, and used to cook the hen until it is well done; then enter the bath and anoint your penis with the grease of the hen, eat its meat and drink its broth, then you will see that your penis becoming of a size that you could have never imagined.
107.4	If a glass shop is fumigated with leeches, then everything inside it will break.	If a glass shop is fumigated with leeches, then the glass there will break into pieces.	If you want that what is inside a glass shop breaks, then do leave inside the shop nothing but breakable stuffs and fumigate the place with some leeches.

107.5	*om.*	وان جففف علق النهر وسحق مع عسل وطلي به الوركين وقت الجماع وجدت المرأة لذلك لذة عظيمة	*om.*
107.6	واذا بخّر موضع البق بالعلق ماتوا جميعهم بقة	*om.*	اذا بخرت مكانا من العلق فانه لا يبقي فيه بق

107.5: (b) In T there is a recipe with lice, see also 86.2

107.6: (c) اذا بخرت فيه بق [اذا بخرت المكان الذي فيه من البق بشىء من العلق قتله ولم يبقي به شىء من البق ابدا C

107.5	*om.*	If the river leeches are dried, ground with honey, rubbed on the legs at the moment of coitus, then the woman will have great enjoyment.	*om.*
107.6	If the leeches are fumigated in the place where the bugs are, then all of them will die.	*om.*	If a place is fumigated with some leeches, then no bug will remain there.

١٠٨. الضفدع

	a	b	c
	om.	الضفادع	باب منافع الضفدع
108.1	اذا طليت داخل القدر بشحم ضفدع وجعلتها على النار فلا تغلي ابدا	اذا طليتَ داخل قدر بشحم الضفادع وصيرت على النار لم يغلي ما طبخ فيها ابدا	اذا أخذت الضفدع ووضعته في قدر وطليت داخله بدهنه وصيرتها على النار فانها لا تغلي ابدا ولا يطبخ فيها شيء
108.2	واذا دهنت يدك بشحم ضفدع وادخلتَها في النار فلا تحترق	وان دهنتَ يدك بشحم ضفدع وطليت من دمها وادخلتها النار لم يحرق	اذا ادهنت يدك بدهن ضفدع وادخلتها في النار لا توديك وهذا الدهن يذخره الطرقيون عندهم
108.3	يؤخذ ضفدع بالحيه اذا خرج من الماء فامسحه بالثآليل فانها تذهب باذن الله تعالى	*om.*	اذا أخذت ضفدعا وهو حي حال خروجه من الماء وسحقت به على الثآليل ذهبتها
108.4	يؤخذ ضفدع ويشق جوفه ويؤخذ قلبه ولسانه واجعله في خرقة واجعل معه بصل النرجس فاذا نامت المرأة فاجعله على صدرها فانها تخبرك بكل ما صنعته في اليقظة	*om.*	قلب الضفدع ولسانه وبصل نرجس اذا جعل الجميع في خرقة ووضع على قلب امرأة نائمة اخبرتك بكل ما صنعته في يقظتها وقيل تخبرتك بكل من جامعها
108.5	الضفدع الذي لا يقرب الماء هو الخسن الجلد اذا أخذ وجعل في قرورة حتى يموت وهو من السموم القاتلة والملوك يدخرون عندهم خزائنهم	*om.*	الضفدع الذي لا يقرب الماء وهو الخشن الجلد الذي هو من السم القاتل

108.1: (c) اذا أخذت...على النار] اذا أخذت قدر وطليت وخله بدهن الضفدع ورفعت على النار C
108.2: (c) وهذا الدهن يدخره الطرقيون عندهم] وهذا مما يعمل الشياطين C
108.3: (c) اذا أخذت...من الماء] اذا أخذت ضفدعا وهو بالحية حال ظهوره من الماء C
108.5: (c) الذي هو من السم القاتل] الخشن الجلد هو السم القاتل C

108. Frog

	a	b	c
	om.	**The frogs**	**Chapter on the useful properties of the frog**
108.1	If the external surface of a pot is rubbed with frog grease, and [the pot] is put on the fire, then it will never boil.	If you rub the external surface of a pot with frog grease, and put it on the fire, then what is cooking inside it will never boil.	If the frog is put in a pot whose external surface has been rubbed with frog grease, and the pot is put on the fire, then this will never boil, and it will be impossible to cook something in it.
108.2	If you anoint your hand with frog grease and then you stretch it on the fire, the hand will not burn.	If you rub your hand with frog grease, smearing it with its blood as well, and put it in the fire, then it will not burn.	If you anoint your hand with frog grease, and then stretch it in the fire, then this will not consume your hand. For this reason, the street tricksters use to hoard this grease.
108.3	If the frog is taken while it is alive, at the very moment in which it comes out from the water, and wiped on the warts, then these will disappear, with the permission of God, may He be exalted.	*om.*	If the frog is taken while it is alive—at the very the moment in which it comes out from the water—and you grind it on the warts, then these will disappear.
108.4	If the frog is taken, its abdomen split, its heart and its tongue are taken out and put in a piece of cloth together with narcissus bulb, then applied on the breast of a woman while she is asleep, then she will tell you about everything she has done when she was awake.	*om.*	If the heart of the frog, its tongue and the bulb of a narcissus are put in a piece of cloth to be placed on the heart of a sleeping woman, then she will tell you about everything she did when she was awake. Moreover, it is said that she will tell you about all the men with whom she has had sexual intercourse.
108.5	The frog that does not gets close to the water has a rough skin, if this frog is taken and put inside a long-necked flask until it dies, then this will become a deadly poison. The kings use to keep this in their treasures.	*om.*	The frog that does not get close to the water has a rough skin, which is a deadly poison.

108.6	اذا جعل في قارورة وصب عليه زيت الى ان يغمره وترك فيه الى ان يموت ودهن الشعر الابيض بهذا الدهن سوده لوقته	*om.*	فاذا أخذ هذا الضفدع وجعل في قرورة وصبّ عليه شيء من دهن يغمره ويترك حتى يموت ويدهن بذلك الدهن الشعر فانه يبيّض
108.7	اذا ذبحت ضفدعا وطليت بدمها مواضع الشعر حلقها وهو ابلغ في الفعل من النورة	وان ذبحت ضفدعة وطليت من دمها على موضع الشعر الذي في الإبطين والعانة وشعر الاذن ذلك جسم خروجه	دم الضفدع اذا طلى به الشعر حلقه ولا ينبت ابدا وانما يصلح لمثل شعر العانة وشعر الإبط والاذن
108.8	اذا شققت بطون الضفادع وضمدت بها النقرس اذهب داؤه	الضفادع الزرق تشق ويضمد بها النقرس الذي قد ظهر في القروح والنفخ ينفعه	يؤخذ ضفدع ازرق اللون يشق جوفه ويضمد به النقرس فيزول
108.9	اذا أخذت ضفدعا على اسم من تريد ان تعقد لسا[ن] واسم امه وخطت فمه بخيط إبريسم وعملت الضفدع في كوز جديد وشددت رأسه انقطع كلام هذا الشخص	ومن أخذ ضفدعا كبيرا على اسم رجل شيء الخلق فحيّط فمه بحيط ابرسيم وصيره في كوز كبير جديد وشد رأسه انقطع كثيرة كلامه وحسنت اخلاقه	لعقد اللسان يؤخذ ضفدع على اسم انسان واسم امه ويخيط فمه بخيط إبريسم واجعل في كوز جديد وشدّ رأسها فان ذلك الشخص ينقطع كلامه ويقصر لسانه ويقل يده وتحسن اخلاقه
108.10	عظم الضفدع اذا وضع على قدر وهو يغلي سكن غليانه	وان أخذ عظم الضفدع الكبير ووضعه على قدر يغلي على النار سكن غليانها	اذا أخذ عظم ضفدع وجعل على قدر وهي تغلي سكن غليانها باذن الله تعالى
108.11	اذا اردت ان تقطع عن المرأة شهوة الجماع شق ضفدعا من ظهره الى فمه على اسم المرأة واسم امها وابسطها على الارض وامر المرأة ان تتخطاه وتنام على وجهها ومر بهذا الضفدع على ظهرها فانها لا تشتهي بعد ذلك نكاحا ابدا	*om.*	*om.*

108.6: (c) وترك [وتركت C

108.7: (c) بدمها [بدمه C

108.8: (c) اذا شققت بطون الضفادع [بطن الضفدع اذا شققته C

108.9: (c) إبريسم [إبرسم L

108.6	If such a frog is put inside a long-necked flask with the addition of enough oil to cover it, and left there until it dies, and the hair is rubbed with this oil, then it will become white.	*om.*	If the frog is put inside a long-necked flask with the addition of enough oil to cover it, and left there until it dies, and the white hair is rubbed with such oil, then it will instantly become black.
108.7	Frog blood: if it is rubbed on the hair, this will be removed and will not grow anymore. And this is equally suitable for the hair of the pubic region, the armpit, and the hear.	If a frog is slaughtered, its blood smeared on the area of the hair on the abdomen, the pubic zone, and the hair in the ear, then this will pull it out.	If a frog is slaughtered and its blood rubbed on the area where the hair is, then it will be removed. This will work better if you do it in the sunlight.
108.8	If a blue frog is taken, its stomach split and used to bandage the gout, then the gout will cease.	Blue frogs: if they are split, used to bandage the gout which appears in the wounds and in the swellings, then this will be useful against it.	If the abdomen of the frog is split and used to bandage the gout, then this disease will go away.
108.9	For the tying of the tongue: if a frog is taken in the name of a man and his mother, its mouth is sewn with a silk thread, the frog is put inside a new jug and covered with a lid, then that man will not be able to speak, his tongue will be shortened, his hand will become smaller, and his temperament will improve.	If a big frog is taken in the name of someone, its mouth is sewn with a silk thread, then it is put in a new big jug and its opening is closed, then his words will be cut off and his temperament improved.	If you take a frog in the name of the man whose tongue you want to tie—and in the name of his mother as well—then sew the frog's mouth with a silk thread, put the frog inside a new jug and cover it with a lid, then this man will not be able to speak.
108.10	If the bone of a frog is taken and put in a cooking pot while it is boiling, then it will stop boiling, with the permission of God, may He be exalted.	If the big bone of a frog is taken and placed over a pot that is boiling on the fire, then this will stop boiling.	If the bone of the frog is placed in a cooking pot while this is boiling, then it will stop boiling.
108.11	*om.*	*om.*	If you want to suppress sexual desire in a woman, split a frog from its back to its mouth in the name of this woman and her mother, put the frog on the ground and order the woman to step over it and sleep supine, then run the frog over her back; from that moment, she will never desire sexual intercourses again.

108.12	زبل الضفدع يسحق ويداف بدهن ورد ويدهن به جسد المحموم فتزول عنه الحمى باذن الله	زبل الضفادع يسحق بدهن ورد ويدهن به من كانت به الحمى اللازمة التي لا تفارقها فيطرد الحمى	زبل الضفدع اذا اذيف بدهن ورد ودهن به اطراف المحموم تذهب حماه لوقته
108.13	اذا لسع الانسان ثعبان او اسود سالخ تأخذ ضفدعا فيشقه نصفين وتلصق الشقة الواحدة على اللسعة ساعتا جيدا وشيلها وألصق الشقة الاخرى وخليها ساعتا جيدا وشيلها فيسكن باذن الله	اذا أخذ ضغفدا عاطريا ووضعت على لسع الحيات والعقارب نفعت	اذا أخذ ضفدع وشق نصفين ولصقت الجميع علي لدغة الأفعى نفعت الملدوغ نفعا جيدا
108.14	اذا اردت أن تعرف الانثى من الذكر من الضفادع فخذ ضفدعا واغرز في ظهره ابرة فان خرج منها الدم فهو ذكر وان لم يخرج دم فهو انثى	*om.*	اذا اردت ان تفرق الذكر من الانثى في الضفادع اغرز ابرة في ظهر اي ضفدعة شيت فالذي يخرج من ظهر منه الدم ذكر والذي لم يخرج من ظهر انثى
108.15	يؤخذ ضفدع يحرق ويسحق ويؤخذ رماده فيبجّ في الانف يقطع الرعاف باذن الله تعالى	الضفادع اذا احرقت وأخذ رمادها فيسحق وينفخ في الانف قطع الرعاف وحبس الدم	اذا احرق الذكر وسحق ونقع ونفخ من رماده في انف صاحب الرعاف ينقطع لوقته
108.16	رماد الضفدع اذا عجن بالزيت وطلى به على مواضع داء الثعلب انبت الشعر باذن الله تعالى	رماده اذا عجن بزيت وطلى موضع داء الثعلب ينبت فيه الشعر	رماد الضفدع اذا عجن بالزيت وطلى به داء الثعلب انبت شعره
108.17	*om.*	تأخذ ضفدعا طويلة الرجلين فاسلخ جلدها واجعل فيه لسان هدهد وقلبه وعلقه عليك فلا يستطيع عدوك يكلمك	*om.*
108.18	*om.*	دم الضفدع الصغير اذا طلى على اصول الشعر الذي قد نتف لم يعد نباته	دم الضفدع الصغير اذا طلى به اصول الشعر التي لم تنبت منها [فانها تنبت منها]

108.12	Frog droppings: if they are ground, diluted with rose oil, and rubbed on the body of a feverish man, then the fever will leave him, with the permission of God, may He be exalted.	Frog droppings: if they are ground with rose oil, and this is used to anoint the one affected by the compelling fever that does not stop, then this will chase the fever away.	Frog droppings: if they are diluted with rose oil and rubbed on the extremities of a feverish man, then the fever will instantly cease.
108.13	If a snake or a black snake bites a man, take a frog and split it in two, apply promptly one half on the bite and then remove it; then, apply the other half, drain it at the right moment, then remove it, and the bite will heal, with the permission of God.	If a sweet-smelling frog is taken and applied on the bite of snakes and scorpions, this will be useful for it.	If a frog is taken, split it in two and the whole of it is applied on the bite of the viper, then this will be very beneficial to the man who has been bitten.
108.14	If you want to recognize the female frog from the male one, take a frog and pierce its back with a needle: if the back bleeds, then it is male, if, instead, it does not bleed, then it is female.	*om.*	If you want to distinguish the female frog from the male one, pierce the back of any frog with a needle; the one whose back bleeds is a male, whereas the one whose back does not bleed is a female.
108.15	If a frog is taken, burnt, ground, and its ash applied into the nose, then this will stop the bleeding, with the permission of God, may He be exalted.	If the frogs are burnt, their ash taken, ground, and blown inside the nose, then this will stop the nose bleeding and staunch the blood.	If a male frog is burnt, ground, and moistened, then the bleeding nose is filled with its ash, the bleeding will instantly stop.
108.16	Frog ash: if it is kneaded with oil and rubbed on the areas affected by alopecia, then this will make the hair grow again, with the permission of God, may He be exalted.	Its ash: if it is kneaded with oil and rubbed on the area of the alopecia, then the hair will grow there again.	Frog ash: if it is kneaded with oil and rubbed on the alopecia, then this will make the hair grow again.
108.17	*om.*	Take a frog with long legs, skin it, put the tongue of a hoopoe and its heart inside the skin, hang it on your person, and then your enemy will be unable to talk to you.	*om.*
108.18	*om.*	Blood of a small frog: if it is rubbed on the roots of the hair when it has been pulled out, then it will not grow again.	Blood of a small frog: if it is rubbed on the roots of the hair that does not grow, then will grow again.

١٠٩. السمك الطري

	a	b	c
	—	السمك الطري	—
109.1	—	تأخذ مرارة شبوط ومرارة ذئب فصيرهما في صوفة لون وتحتملها المرأة حين تطهر قبل ان يأتيها الرجل فاذا جامعها حبلت	—
109.2	—	مرارة السمك المان ما هيج يسعط به الدابة التي بها جنون فيذهب عنها الجنون	—
109.2	—	تأخذ مرارة سمكة فتطلي بها ما شئتَ من عود او غير ذلك اجتمع عليه الذباب	—

109. Freshwater Fish

	a	b	c
	–	**The freshwater fish**	–
109.1	–	Carp bile and wolf bile: if they are put inside a coloured woollen cloth, and a woman carries it when she is not menstruating and before that the man visits her, then, if they copulate, she will get pregnant.	–
109.2	–	Gall of the fish *al-mān* that acts against excitement: if the animal that has been taken by madness sniffs it, then the madness will leave it.	–
109.3	–	If some fish gall is taken, and you rub it on whatever branch you want—or on something else—then the flies will gather there.	–

١١٠. السمك المالح

	a	b	c
	—	السمك المالح	باب منافع السمك المالح
110.1	—	السمك المالح اذا [طلى] عضة الكلب نفعه	السمك المالح اذا طلى به عضة الكلب الكلب ابرأته
110.2	—	*om.*	اذا اردت ان لا تسكر في المقام خذ شيئا من سمك مالح وشمها فانك لا تسكر
110.3	—	اذا رأيت ان السكر لا يعقل فشممه ماء السمك المالح حين يشمه يرجع اليه عقله	فان رأيت سكر اناء قد غلب عليه فشمه رائحة السمك المالح فانه يصحوا ويرجع الى عقله
110.4	—	عين السمك المالح تسحق ويتخذ منه فتيلة قطن ينفع من القولنج ويحل الطبيعة	اذا أخذ السمك المالح وسحق وعجن وعمل فتيلة وحمله من يشتكي القولنج انحل طبيعه وزال المه
110.5	—	لوجع الاذن يقطر في الاذن ماء السمك فانه يسكن الضربان باذن الله تعالى	اذا قطرت في الاذن من ماء السمك المالح سكن ضربانها والمها ودويها باذن الله تعالى
110.6	—	غرا السمك يطلي على بياض الاظفار يزيد لونه	*om.*
110.7	—	وينفع من عضة الكلب الكلب ومن حرق النار مع ادويته	*om.*
110.8	—	بيض السمك اذا أكل هيج القيء واحدث الهيضة	*om.*

110. Saltwater Fish

	a	b	c
	—	**The saltwater fish**	**Chapter on the useful properties of the saltwater fish**
110.1	—	If the saltwater fish is rubbed on the bite of the dog, then it will be useful for it.	If the saltwater fish is rubbed on the bite of the rabid dog, then this will cure it.
110.2	—	*om.*	If you do not want to get drunk, take some saltwater fish and smell it, then you will not get drunk.
110.3	—	If you see that a drunk person is not in his mind, then let him smell the water of the saltwater fish; and when he smells it, he will regain his sense.	If you see that a drunk man has already been overwhelmed by the pitch, then let him smell the scent of saltwater fish, and he will be better and regain his sense.
110.4	—	Saltwater fish eye: if it is ground, put in a cotton compress, this will be useful against the colic, and will have a purgative effect.	Saltwater fish: if it is taken, ground, kneaded, made into a compress, and the man suffering from a colic carries it, then he will be purged, and its pain will cease.
110.5	—	Against the pain in the ear: if the water of the fish is applied in drops inside the ear, then the pangs will cease, with the permission of God, may He be exalted.	If some water of [saltwater] fish is applied in drops inside the hear, then its pangs and its pain will cease, and it will heal, with the permission of God, may He be exalted.
110.6	—	Fish glue: if it is rubbed on the white spot on the nails, then this will improve its colour.	*om.*
110.7	—	It is useful also against the bite of the rabid dog, and against the burnings of the fire, this will cure them.	*om.*
110.8	—	Fish eggs: if they are eaten, this will provoke the vomit, and will provoke diarrhoea with vomit as well.	*om.*

110.9	—	الطريح اذا سلخ ووضع على النشر ازاله قناطير الدهن المستخرج من عينها ينفع من تلين الصلابات	om.
110.10	—	مرارته تنفع لصبغ الصوف الابيض	om.
110.11	—	وان طلى بها مع خل وخردل على البرص صبغه	om.
110.12	—	السمك المعروف بأرفا اذا دق ووضع على الصداع الشديد ازاله	om.
110.13	—	الذكون سمكة اذا أخذ شحمه وشرب نفع من الماء ويدر البول ويغزره	om.
110.14	—	وان غمس فيه فتيلة واسرجت واطفئت وشممتها امرأة بها خنق	om.
110.15	—	والسمكة بالشبهة بالتمسا اذا أكلها الملدوغ بالافعى نفعه ومن العقارب وسائر السموم	om.
110.16	—	وان سحقت بخل ووضعت على عضد الارنب نفعه	om.
110.17	—	اذا أخذ كبده ومرارته يحلقا الشعر وتفعل كبده ذلك وحدها	om.
110.18	—	اذا شويت الوف لحمه يزيد في الباه	om.
110.19	—	واذا طبخ سكباج نفع صاحب الاستسقاء والجذام	om.

110.9	–	*Al-ṭarīḥ* fish [?]: if it is skinned, chopped up, covered with several measures (*qanāṭīr*) of the oil extracted from its eye, then this will be useful to soften different kinds of callousness.	*om.*
110.10	–	Its gall is useful to dye white wool.	*om.*
110.11	–	If this—mixed with vinegar and mustard seeds—is rubbed on the leprosy, thin this will dye it.	*om.*
110.12	–	If the fish known as *arfā* [?] is ground and applied on the intense headache, then this will make it cease.	*om.*
110.13	–	The *dakūn* [?] is a fish, if its fat is taken and drunk, this will be useful to the water, will make the urine flow, and make it abundant.	*om.*
110.14	–	If a wick is soaked in it and a woman lights a lantern, extinguishes it, and smells it, then she will suffocate.	*om.*
110.15	–	The fish that resembles the *tamsā* [?]: if the man who has been bitten by a viper, or stung by scorpions, or by another poisonous animal eats it, then this will be useful to him.	*om.*
110.16	–	If it is ground with vinegar, and applied on the arm of the hare [kind of bandage?], this will be useful to it.	*om.*
110.17	–	If its liver and its gall are taken, then these will shave the hair, and its liver does this alone as well.	*om.*
110.18	–	If the *al-waff* fish [?] is roasted, then its flesh will increase the sexual desire.	*om.*
110.19	–	If it is prepared as *sikbāǧ* [mashed meat cooked in vinegar], then it will be useful to the man affected by dropsy and leprosy.	*om.*

110.20	—	ويأمن أكله من الرياح السوء ومن السحر	*om.*
110.21	—	كبده اذا اكل نفع من وجع الكبد	*om.*
110.22	—	دم الوق اذا اكتحل به احد عمى	*om.*
110.23	—	وينفع من اليرقان والصفار من الوجع	*om.*
110.24	—	وان طلى به البهق غيّر لونه	*om.*
110.25	—	مرارته اذا اكتحل بها انسان نفعت من الغشاوة	*om.*

110.20	—	Eating it saves from the evil spirits, and from magic.	*om.*
110.21	—	Its liver: if it is eaten, this will be useful against the liver complaint.	*om.*
110.22	—	*Al-daqq* fish [?] blood: if is is applied on the eyes of somebody, then he will become blind.	*om.*
110.23	—	It is useful against the jaundice and the yellow complexion [that derives] from the pain.	*om.*
110.24	—	If it is rubbed on the vitiligo, then this will change its colour.	*om.*
110.25	—	Its gall: if it is applied on the eyes of a man, then this will be useful against the cataract.	*om.*

Appendix

Synoptic table of the manuscript tradition

	(a)		(b)			(c)		
	B Berlin Pet. II 244	S Istanbul, Sehid Ali Pasha 2096	G Gotha 67/2	T Istanbul, Saray Ah-met III 2055	W Wien 1481/2	L Leipzig 770	C Cairo, *Dār al-Kutub*, ṬT 305	
1. Man	ذكر منافع اعضاء ابن ادم [2]	ذكر منافع اعضاء ابن ادم [151r]	الانسان [33r]	منافع الانسان [3v]	انسان [135v]	باب منافع الانسان [2v]	منافع الانسان [2]	**١. الانسان**
Woman	–	–	المراة [33r]	–	المراة [136v]	–	–	
Child	–	–	الصبي [33r]	–	–	–	–	
	–	–	–	باب السباع [9v]	السباع [137r]	–	–	
2. Lion	ذكر منافع الاعضاء الاسد [8]	ذكر منافع اعضاء الاسد [156r]	الاسد [34v]	الاسد [9v]	الاسد [137r]	باب منافع الاسد [5v]	باب منافع الاسد [5]	**٢. الاسد**
3. Wolf	ذكر منافع اعضاء الذئب [12]	ذكر منافع اعضاء الذئب [160r]	الذئب [35v]	–	الذئب [138r]	باب منافع الذئب [6v]	باب منافع الذئب [5]	**٣. الذئب**
	ذكر منافع اعضاء الثعلب [16]	ذكر منافع اعضاء الثعلب [164r]	See No.13	–	See No.13	See No.13	See No.13	
4. Hyena	ذكر منافع اعضاء الضبع [18]	ذكر منافع اعضاء الضبع [167r]	الضبع [36v]	–	الضبع [138v]	باب منافع الضبع [8r]	باب منافع الضبع [7]	**٤. الضبع**
5. Bear	ذكر منافع اعضاء الدب [21]	ذكر منافع اعضاء الدب [169r]	الدب [37v]	الدب [10v]	الدب [139v]	باب منافع الدب [9r]	باب منافع الدب [8]	**٥. الدب**
6. Jerboa	ذكر منافع اعضاء اليربوع [23]	ذكر منافع اليربوع [172r]	–	اليربوع [11r]	اليربوع [139v]	–	–	**٦. اليربوع**
	–	–	الخنزير واليربوع [38r]	–	–	–	–	
7. Pig	ذكر منافع اعضاء الخنزير [24]	ذكر منافع اعضاء الخنزير [173r]	–	الخنزير [11r]	الخنزير [140r]	باب منافع الخنزير [9v]	باب منافع الخنزير [9]	**٧. الخنزير**
8. Dog	ذكر منافع اعضاء الكلب [26]	ذكر منافع اعضاء الكلب [148v]	الكلب [38v]	الكلب [11v]	الكلب [140r]	باب منافع الكلب [10r]	باب منافع الكلب [9]	**٨. الكلب**

	(a)		(b)			(c)		
	B Berlin Pet. II 244	**S** Istanbul, Sehid Ali Pasha 2096	**G** Gotha 67/2	**T** Istanbul, Saray Ahmet III 2055	**W** Wien 1481/2	**L** Leipzig 770	**C** Cairo, *Dār al-Kutub*, ṬT 305	
9. Hare	ذكر منافع اعضاء الارنب [32]	ذكر منافع اعضاء الارنب [42r]	الارنب [40r]	الارنب [13r]	الارنب [141r]	باب منافع الارنب [11v]	باب منافع الارنب [12]	**٩. الارنب**
10. Gazelle	ذكر منافع اعضاء الغزال [35]	ذكر منافع اعضاء الغزالة [146r]	الغزال [40v]	الغزال [15r]	الغزال [141v]	باب منافع الغزال [12v]	باب منافع الغزال [13]	**١٠. الغزال**
11. Mountain Goat	ذكر منافع اعضاء الوعل [38]	ذكر منافع اعضاء الوعل [49r]	الوعل [41r]	–	الوعل [142v]	باب منافع الوعل [13v]	باب منافع الوعل [14]	**١١. الوعل**
12. Deer	ذكر منافع اعضاء الايل [39]	ذكر منافع اعضاء الأيّل [50r]	الايل [41v]	الايل [15v]	الاريل [142v]	باب منافع الايل [14r]	باب منافع الاريل [14]	**١٢. الايل**
13. Fox	See after No. 3	ذكر منافع اعضاء الثعلب [53]	الثعلب [42r]	الثعلب [16r]	الثعلب [143r]	باب منافع الثعلب [14v]	باب منافع الثعلب [15]	**١٣. الثعلب**
14. Crocodile	ذكر منافع اعضاء التمساح [41]	ذكر منافع اعضاء التمساح [54v]	التمساح [42v]	التمساح [17r]	التمساح [143r]	باب منافع التمساح [15v]	باب منافع التمساح والسرطان [16]	**١٤. التمساح**
15. Cow	ذكر منافع اعضاء البقر [42]	ذكر منافع اعضاء البقر [55v]	البقر [43r]	البقرة [17v]	البقرة [143v]	باب منافع البقر [15v]	باب منافع البقر [17]	**١٥. البقر**
16. Horse	–	ذكر منافع اعضاء الفرس [59r]	الخيل [45r]	الفرس [20r]	الفرس [145v]	باب منافع الفرس [18r]	باب منافع الفرس [20]	**١٦. الفرس**
					End of W			
17. Mule	–	ذكر منفع اعضاء البغل [64r]	البغال [46r]	البغل [22r]		باب منافع البغل [19r]	باب منافع البغل [22]	**١٧. البغال**
18. Donkey	See after No. 23	ذكر منافع اعضاء الحمار [64v]	الحمير [46v]	الحمار الاهلي [22v]		باب منافع الحمار [19r]	باب منافع الحمار [22]	**١٨. الحمار**
19. Wild Donkey	See after No. 23	ذكر منافع اعضاء حمار الوحش [67v]	–	الحمار الوحشي [67v]		باب منافع حمار الوحش [20r]	باب منافع حمار الوحش [23]	**١٩. حمار الوحش**

	(a)		(b)			(c)		
	B Berlin Pet. II 244	S Istanbul, Sehid Ali Pasha 2096	G Gotha 67/2	T Istanbul, Saray Ah- met III 2055	W Wien 1481/2	L Leipzig 770	C Cairo, *Dār al-Kutub*, ṬT 305	
20. Camel	ذكر منافع اعضاء الجمل [48]	ذكر منافع اعضاء الجمل [70r]	الجمل [48r]	الجمل [24v]		باب منافع الجمل [20v]	باب منافع الجمل [24]	**٢٠. الجمل**
21. Sheep	ذكر منافع اعضاء الخروف [50]	ذكر منافع اعضاء الخروف [6r]	الضان [49r]	الضان [25v]		باب منافع الضان [22v]	باب منافع الضان [26]	**٢١. الضأن**
	–	–	–	الايل [26r]II	–	–	–	
	–	–	–	الفرس [26v]II	–	–	–	
22. Goat	ذكر منافع اعضاء الماعز [54]	ذكر منافع اعضاء الماعز [38r]	الماعز [50v]	الماعز [28v]		باب منافع المعز [23r]	باب منافع المعز [27]	**٢٢. الماعز**
23. Wild Cow	–	باب منافع اعضاء بقر الوحش [11r]	بقر الوحش [52r]	بقر الوحش [31r]		باب منافع بقر الوحش [24r]	باب منافع بقر الوحش [29]	**٢٣. بقر الوحش**
	ذكر منافع اعضاء الحمار [58]	See No.18	See No.18	See No.18		See No.18	See No. 18	
	ذكر منافع اعضاء حمار الوحش [60]	See No.19	See No.19	See No.19		See No.19	See No.19	
	ذكر منافع اعضاء الخفاش [61]	See No.53	See No.53	See No.53		See No.53	See No.53	
	ذكر منافع اعضاء ابو تمر [65]	See No.54	–	–		–	–	
	ذكر منافع اعضاء الحمام [65]	See No.55	See No.55	See No.55		See No.55	See No.55	
	ذكر منافع اعضاء النمس [68]	See No. 27	See No. 27	–		See No. 27	See No. 27	

	(a)		(b)			(c)		
	B Berlin Pet. II 244	S Istanbul, Sehid Ali Pasha 2096	G Gotha 67/2	T Istanbul, Saray Ah-met III 2055	W Wien 1481/2	L Leipzig 770	C Cairo, *Dār al-Kutub*, ṬṬ 305	
24. Roe Deer	ذكر منافع اعضاء اليحمور [68]	ذكر منافع اعضاء اليحمور [72r]	اليحمور [52v]	اليحمور [31r]		باب منافع اليحمور [24r]	–	**٢٤. اليحمور**
	See No. 27	ذكر منافع اعضاء النمس [73v]	See No. 27	–		See No. 27	See No. 27	
25. Cheetah	ذكر منافع اعضاء النمر [70]	ذكر منافع اعضاء النمر [74v]	النمر [52v]	النمر [31v]		باب منافع النمر [24v]	باب منافع النمر [30]	**٢٥. النمر**
26. Elephant	ذكر منافع اعضاء الفيل [70]	ذكر منافع اعضاء الفيل [75r]	الفيل [53r]	الفيل [32r]		باب منافع الفيل [24v]	باب منافع الفيل [31]	**٢٦. الفيل**
27. Ichneumon	See before No. 24	See after No. 24	النمس [53v]	–		باب منافع النمس [25r]	باب منافع النمس [31]	**٢٧. النمس**
28. Stellion	[ذكر منافع اعضا الضب] [71]	ذكر منافع اعضاء الضب [76r]	الضب [53v]	–		باب منافع الضب [25r]	باب منافع الضب [31]	**٢٨. الضب**
29. Buffalo	–	ذكر منافع اعضاء الجاموس [11]	–	–		باب منافع الجاموس [25v]	باب منافع الجاموس [32]	**٢٩. الجاموس**
30. Cat	[السنور] [72]	ذكر منافع اعضاء السنور [12r]	السنور [53v]	–		باب منافع السنور [25v]	باب منافع السنور [32]	**٣٠. السنور**
31. Lynx	[ذكر منافع اعضا الفهد] [72]	ذكر منافع اعضاء الفهد [14v]	الفهد [55r]	–		باب منافع الفهد [26v]	باب منافع الفهد [33]	**٣١. الفهد**
32. Badger	[ذكر منافع اعضا الغرير] [72]	ذكر منافع اعضاء الغريري [91r]	–	–		–	–	**٣٢. الغرير**
33. Weasel	ذكر منافع ابن العرس [73]	ذكر منافع اعضاء العرس [91r]	ابن عرس [55r]	–		باب منافع بنات عرس [26v]	باب منافع بنات عرس [34]	**٣٣. ابن عرس**
34. Jackal and Chamois	–	–	–	–		باب منافع ابن اوي [27r]	باب منافع واوي [34]	**٣٤. ابن اوي والاروى**

	(a)		(b)			(c)		
	B Berlin Pet. II 244	S Istanbul, Sehid Ali Pasha 2096	G Gotha 67/2	T Istanbul, Saray Ah- met III 2055	W Wien 1481/2	L Leipzig 770	C Cairo, *Dār al-Kutub*, ṬT 305	
	ذكر منافع اعضاء بن اوي [73]	ذكر منافع اعضاء ابن اوي [92r]	الاروي [55r]	–		باب منافع الازوي [27r]	باب منافع الازدي [34]	
35. Monkey	ذكر منافع القرد [74]	ذكر منافع اعضاء القرد [92v]	القرد [55v]	–		باب منافع القرد [27r]	باب منافع القرد [34]	٣٥. القرد
36. Hyrax	–	ذكر منافع اعضاء الوبر [93]	الوبر [55v]	–		–	–	٣٦. الوبر
37. Beaver	[جراد كبير] [74]	ذكر منافع اعضاء القسطبون [15r]	See No. 36	–		–	–	٣٧. القسطوريون
38. Hedgehog	ذكر منافع اعضا القنفد [75]	ذكر منافع اعضاء القنفد [15v]	القنفد [55v]	–		باب منافع القنفد [27r]	باب منافع القنفد [35]	٣٨. القنفد
39. Indian Hedgehog	–	ذكر منافع اعضاء القنفد الهندي [18v]	...	–		باب منافع القنفد الهندي [28r]	–	٣٩. القنفد الهندي
40. *Kāša*	–	ذكر اعضاء الكاشة [20r]	...	–		–	–	٤٠. الكاشة
41. Salamander	[السمندل] [77]	ذكر منافع اعضاء السمندل [20v]	...	–		باب منافع السمندل [28v]	–	٤١. السمندل
42. Rhinoceros	[كركدن] [78]	ذكر منافع اعضاء كرك [21r]	...	–		باب منافع الكركند [28v]	–	٤٢. كركدن
	See No. 79	See No. 79	See No. 79	See No. 79		باب منافع الافعاء [29r]	See No. 79	
43. Mouse	ذكر منافع اعضاء الفار [79]	ذكر منافع اعضاء الفار [22r]	...	–		باب منافع الفار [29r]	باب منافع الفار [36]	٤٣. الفار

	(a)		(b)			(c)		
	B Berlin Pet. II 244	S Istanbul, Sehid Ali Pasha 2096	G Gotha 67/2	T Istanbul, Saray Ah- met III 2055	W Wien 1481/2	L Leipzig 770	C Cairo, *Dār al-Kutub*, ṬT 305	
44. Mole	ذكر منافع الخلد [80]	ذكر منافع اعضاء الخُلد [24v]	…	–		باب منافع الخلد [29v]	باب منافع الخلد [37]	٤٤. الخلد
45. Sandgrouse	ذكر منافع الحجل [82]	ذكر منافع اعضاء الحجل [27r]	…	–		باب منافع الحجل [30v]	باب منافع الحجل [38]	٤٥. الحجل
46. Vulture	[ذكر منافع النسر] [84]	ذكر منافع اعضاء النسر [29r]	…	–		باب منافع الدراج والنسر [31r]	باب منافع الداراج والنسر [38–39]	٤٦. النسر
47. Collared Pigeon	[ذكر منافع الفاختة] [85]	ذك منافع اعضاء الفواخت [31r]	…	–		باب منافع الفواخت [31v]	–	٤٧. الفواخت
48. Wood Pigeon	[ذكر منافع الورشان] [86]	ذكر منافع اعضاء الورشان [32r]	…	–		–	–	٤٨. الورشان
49. Hoopoe	[ذكر منافع الهدهد] [86]	ذكر منافع اعضاء الهدهد [32r]	…	–		باب منافع الهدهد [31v]	–	٤٩. الهدهد
50. Swallow	ذكر منافع اعضاء الواق [90]	ذكر منافع اعضاء الواق [36r]	…	الخطاف [32r]		باب منافع التوفر [32v]	–	٥٠. الخطاف
	End of B							
51. Quail		ذكر منافع اعضاء السلوي [37v]	…	السلوي [32v]		باب منافع السلوي [33r]	باب منافع السلوا [39]	١٥. السلوى
52. Sparrow		ذكر منافع اعضاء العصفور [78r]	…	العصفور [33r]		باب منافع العصفور [33v]	باب منافع العصفور [40]	٥٢. العصفور
53. Bat		ذكر منافع اعضاء الخفاش [80r]	…	الخفاش [34r]		باب منافع الخفاش [34r]	باب منافع الخفاش [40]	٥٣. الخفاش
54. *Abū Tamra* bird		ذكر منافع ابو تمرة [85v]	…	–		–	–	٤٥. ابو تمرة

	(a)		(b)			(c)		
	B Berlin Pet. II 244	S Istanbul, Sehid Ali Pasha 2096	G Gotha 67/2	T Istanbul, Saray Ah-met III 2055	W Wien 1481/2	L Leipzig 770	C Cairo, *Dār al-Kutub*, ṬT 305	
55. Pigeon		ذكر منافع اعضاء الحمام [86r]	…	الحمام [35v]		باب منافع الحمام [35v]	باب منافع الحمام [42]	٥٥. الحمام
56. Egyptian Vulture		ذكر منافع اعضاء الرخمة [88v]	…	الرخمة [37r]		باب منافع الرخم [36v]	–	٥٦. الرخم
57. Starling		–	…	الزرازير [37v]		–	–	٥٧. الزرزور
58. Kite		ذكر منافع اعضاء الحداة [90v]	…	الحداة [37v]		باب منافع الحداة [37r]	باب منافع الحداة [43]	٥٨. الحدأة
59. Crow		ذكر منافع الغراب [94v]	…	الغراب [38r]		باب منافع الغراب [37v]	باب منافع الغراب [43]	٥٩. الغراب
60. Owl		ذكر منافع اعضاء البومة [98v]	…	البومة [39v]		باب منافع البوم [38v]	باب منافع البوم [45]	٦٠. البوم
61. Rooster		ذكر منافع اعضاء الديك [101r]	…	الديك [40v]		–	–	٦١. الديك
62. Hen		ذكر منافع اعضاء الدجاجة [103v]	…	[الدجاجة] [41r]		–	–	٦٢. الدجاجة
63. Ostrich		ذكر منافع اعضاء النعامة [105v]	…	النعامة [42r]		–	–	٦٣. النعامة
64. Duck and Goose		ذكر منافع اعضاء البطة [106v]	الاوز والبط[56r]	الاوز [56r]		–	–	٦٤. الاوز والبط
65. Crane		ذكر منافع اعضاء الكركي [109r]	الكركي [56v]	الكركي [43r]		–	–	٦٥. الكركى
66. Bustard		ذكر منافع اعضاء الحباري [110v]	الحباري [56v]	الحباري [v43]		–	باب منافع الحباري [45]	٦٦. الحبارى
67. Saker		–	–	–		–	فصل [46]	٦٧. الصقر

	(a)		(b)			(c)		
	B Berlin Pet. II 244	S Istanbul, Sehid Ali Pasha 2096	G Gotha 67/2	T Istanbul, Saray Ahmet III 2055	W Wien 1481/2	L Leipzig 770	C Cairo, *Dār al-Kutub*, ṬT 305	
68. Peacock		In margine [111r]	الطاووس [57r]	الطاووس [43v]		باب منافع الطاوس [38v]	باب منافع الطاووس [46]	٦٨. الطاؤوس
69. Curlew		ذكر منافع اعضاء الكروان [111v]	الكروان [57r]	الكروان [43v]		باب منافع الكيروان [39r]	باب منافع الكيروان [46]	٦٩. الكروان
70. Eagle		ذكر منافع اعضاء عقرب الماء [111v]	العقاب [57r]	العقاب [44r]		باب منافع العقرب [39r]	باب منافع العقرب (عقاب) [46]	٧٠. العقاب
71. *Zummağ* falcon		–	–	الزمخ [44r]				٧١. الزمج
72. Sparrow Hawk		[...]	الباشق [57r]	الباشق والزمح واليؤيؤ [44r]		–	–	٧٢. الباشق
73. Merlin		[...]	اليؤيؤ [58v]	طير البوبو [44r]		–	–	٧٣. اليؤيؤ
74. Hawk		[...]	البازي [57v]	البازي [44r]		–	–	٧٤. الباز
75. Green Woodpecker		–	–	الشقراق [44v]		–	–	٧٥. الشقراق
76. Guinea Fowl		–	–	دجاجة الحبش [44v]		–	–	٧٦. دجاج الحبش
77. Turtle Dove		[...]	الشفانين [57v]	الشفانين [44v]		–	–	٧٧. الشفانين
78. Wild Pigeon		[...]	اليمامة [58r]	حمامة البحر [45r]	–	باب منافع اليمام [39v]	باب منافع اليمام [47]	٧٨. اليمام
				خشاش الارض [45r]				
79. Snake		ذكر منافع اعضاء الحية البرصاء [113v]	الحية [58r]	الحية [58r]	See after No. 42	باب منافع الحية [39v]	باب منافع الحية [47]	٧٩. الحية
80. Scorpion		ذكر منافع العقرب البري [118r]	العقارب [58v]	العقارب [46v]		باب منافع العقرب ايضا [40v]	باب منافع العقرب [48]	٨٠. العقرب
81. Ladybird		–	بقر بني اسرايل [59r]	ام قيس [47r]		–	–	٨١. بقر بني اسرائل

	(a)		(b)			(c)		
	B Berlin Pet. II 244	S Istanbul, Sehid Ali Pasha 2096	G Gotha 67/2	T Istanbul, Saray Ahmet III 2055	W Wien 1481/2	L Leipzig 770	C Cairo, *Dār al-Kutub*, ṬT 305	
82. Lizard		ذكر منافع الجراذون السماني [120v]	الجراذين [59r]	الجردون [47v]		باب منافع الحردون [41v]	باب منافع الجردون [49]	٨٢. الحرذون
83. Dung Beetle		–	الجعل الكبير [60r]	العجل [48r]		–	–	٨٣. الجعل
84. Chameleon		ذكر منافع العضاية وهي الحرباء [122v]	العضاية [60r]	العضابة [48r]		باب منافع العظايا [41v]	باب منافع العظاية [50]	٨٤. العضاية
85. Blister Beetle		–	الذراريح [60r]	الذراريح [48v]		–	–	٨٥. الذراريح
86. White Worm		–	–	شحمة الارض [48v]		–	–	٨٦. شحمة الارض
87. Gecko		ذكر منافع سام أبرص وهو الوزعة [124r]	سامّ ابرص [60v]	سامّ أبرص [48v]		باب منافع الوزغ [42r]	باب منافع الوزغ وهو السآم ابرص [51]	٨٧. سامّ أبرص
88. Fly		[124v]	الذباب [60v]	الذباب [49r]		باب منافع الذباب [42v]	باب منافع الذباب [51]	٨٨. الذباب
89. Spanish Fly		–	–	–		باب منافع الذباب الاخضر See after No.110	–	٨٩. الذباب الاخضر
90. Hornet		الزنبور [125r]	الزنبور [60v]	–		–	–	٩٠. الزنبور
91. Mantis		–	جمل اليهود [60v]	–		–	–	٩١. جمل اليهود
92. Ant		ذكر منافع النمل [126r]	النمل [61r]	–		–	–	٩٢. النمل
93. Scarab		الخنفساة [126v]	الخنفساة [61v]	الخنفساء [49r]		–	–	٩٣. الخنفساء
94. Bedbug		–	–	الفسافس See after No. 110	–	–	–	٩٤. الفسافس
95. Lice		–	القمل [61v]	القمل [45v] Only chapter title		–	–	٩٥. القمل

	(a)		(b)			(c)		
	B Berlin Pet. II 244	**S** Istanbul, Sehid Ali Pasha 2096	**G** Gotha 67/2	**T** Istanbul, Saray Ahmet III 2055	**W** Wien 1481/2	**L** Leipzig 770	**C** Cairo, *Dār al-Kutub*, ṬṬ 305	
			End of G					
96. Flea		ذكر منافع الحلم وهي دودة [127r]		See after No.110		–	–	٩٦. الحلم
97. Spider		منافع العنكبوت [128v]		العنكبوت [49v]		–	–	٩٦. الحلم
		–		السمك الطري [49v] See No. 109		–	–	
		See No. 101		السرطان النهري [49v]		–	–	
		See No. 102		السرطان البحري [50r]		–	–	
98. *Kanǧ*		ذكر منافع الكنج وهي دابة تشبه الحرباء [128v]		See after No. 110		–	–	٩٨. الكنج
99. Earthworm		الخراطيم [130r]		See after No. 110		–	–	٩٩. الخراطين
100. Sperm Whale		ذكر منافع حوت الماء [131v]		–		–	–	١٠٠. حوت الماء
101. River Crab		ذكر منافع السرطان النهري [132r]		See after No. 100		–	–	١٠١. السرطان النهري
102. Sea Crab		–		See after No. 100		–	–	١٠٢. السرطان البحري
103. Whale		ذكر منافع الحوت [134r]		–		–	–	١٠٣. الحوت

	(a)		(b)			(c)		
	B Berlin Pet. II 244	S Istanbul, Sehid Ali Pasha 2096	G Gotha 67/2	T Istanbul, Saray Ah- met III 2055	W Wien 1481/2	L Leipzig 770	C Cairo, *Dār* *al-Kutub*, ṬT 305	
104. Turtle		ذكر منافع الساحفاة [135r]		–		باب منافع السلحفاة See after No. 106	باب منافع السلحفاة See after No. 106	**١٠٤. السلحفاة**
105. River Snail		ذكر منافع الحلزون الذي يكون على الانهار [136v]		–		–	–	**١٠٥. الحلزون الانهار**
106. Pearl Oyster		ذكر منافع الصدف [137r]		See after No. 110		باب منافع الصدف [42v]	باب منافع الصدف [51]	**١٠٦. الصدف**
		See No. 104		See No. 104		باب منافع السلحفاة [43r]	باب منافع السلحفاة [52]	
107. Leech		منافع العلق [140]		See after No. 110		باب منافع العلق [43v]	باب منافع العلق [53]	**١٠٧. العلق**
108. Frog		[الضفدع] [140r]		الضفادع [50r]		باب منافع الضفدع [44r]	باب منافع الضفدع [53]	**١٠٨. الضفدع**
							End of C	
109. Freshwater Fish		–		السمك الطري [49v]		–		**١٠٩. السمك الطري**
110. Saltwater Fish		–		السمك المالح [50v]		باب منافع السمك المالح [45r]		**١١٠. السمك المالح**
		See No. 106		الصدف [51v]		See No. 106	See No. 106	
		See No. 98		الكنج [52r]		See No. 100	See No. 100	
		–		See No. 90 الفسافس [52r]		–	–	
		See No. 96		الحلم [52v]		See No. 96	See No. 96	
		See No. 99		الحراطير [52v]		See No. 99	See No. 99	

	(a)		(b)			(c)		
	B Berlin Pet. II 244	**S** Istanbul, Sehid Ali Pasha 2096	**G** Gotha 67/2	**T** Istanbul, Saray Ah-met III 2055	**W** Wien 1481/2	**L** Leipzig 770	**C** Cairo, *Dār al-Kutub*, ṬT 305	
		See No. 107		[53r] العلق		See No. 107	See No 107	
		See No. 104		السلحفاة [53v]		See No. 104	See No. 104	
				End of T				
						باب منافع الذباب الاخضر [45r] See No. 89		

Thematic Index

Diseases of body, body parts and organs

Sex and love

Reproduction and Birth

Sleep and Insomnia

Cosmetics

Nature, husbandry, agriculture and hunting

Vermin and obnoxious animals

Crafts

Tricks

At court

Evil eye and magic

Poisons and antidotes

Arabic-English Glossary

1 Animal parts and substances

Armpit	إبط
Outer opening of the urethra	إحْليل
Bowels	أحْشاء
Duodenum	اعفاج
Intestine	أمعاء
Rennet	إنْفحة
See also منفحة	
Body	بَدَن
Extremity of the ribs	بستامزك
Saliva	بُصاق
Roe	بطارخ
Abdomen, belly	بَطْن
Droppings	بَعْرة
Phlegm	بَلْغَم
Urine	بَوْل
Breast	ثَدي
Forehead	جَبْهَة
Forehead, temples	جَبين
Eyelid	جَفْن
Skull	جُمْجُمة
Abdomen	جَوْف
Chest	جَيْب
Eyebrow	حاجب
Groin	حقو
Throat (back of the)	حَلْق
Gullet	حُلقوم
Breast	حِلمة
Palate	حَنَك
Craw of a bird	حَوصلة
Menstrual blood	حَيْضة
Hip, waist	خاصِرة
Menstruation	حَيْض
Excrement	خُرْء
Vertebra	خَرَزة
Testicle	خُصيَة
Hoof	خُفّ
Back	دُبْر
Grease	دَسَم
Forearm	ذراع
Droppings (of bird)	ذَرق
Penis	ذَكَر
Tail	ذَنَب
Foot, paw	رِجْل
Excrement	رَجيع
Uterus	رَحم
Nape	رَقَبة
Knee	ركبة
Excrement	رَوْث
Lung	رِئة
Saliva	ريق
Dung	زَبْل
Fuzz	زَغب
Appendance of the liver	زيادة الكبد
Umbilicus	سُرة
Legs (lower part)	سِفْلة
Slough	سَلْخ
Hump	سَنام
Fat	شَحْم
Lip	شَفة

Spine	صُلْب
Molar	ضِرْس
Spleen	طِحال
Hoof 0loven	ظِلْف
Ivory	عاج
Nerves	عَصَب
Juice	عُصارة
Arm	عَضُد
Bone	عِظْم
Neck	عُنْق
Epiglottis	غَلْصَمَة
Milk of a pregnant woman	غيل
Leg	فَخْذ
Anus	فم الصفرة
Temple	فود
Gizzard	قانِصة
Leg	قائمة
Skull	قِحْف
Penis	قَضيب
Foreskin	قُلفة
Liver	كَبِد
Shoulder, shoulder blade	كَتِف
Tibia, shinbone	كُراع
Anklebone	كَعْب
Claw	كَفّ
Kidney	كُلْوة \ كُلْية \ كُلى
Milk	لَبَن
Milk (sour)	لبن حامض
Milk (cow)	لَبَن حَليب
Gum	لِثة
Jawbone	لُحي
Tongue	لسان
Saliva	لُعاب
Uvula, throat	لِهاية/لهاة
Bladder	مَثانة
Marrow	مُخّ
Claws	مَخالب
Gall	مرارة
Placenta	مَشيمة
Entrails	مُصران
Liver	معاليق
Stomach	مَعِدة
Joints	مفاصل
Buttocks	مَقْعَدة
Nostril	مَنْخَرة
Rennet	منفحة

See also إِنْفَحة

Beak	مِنْقار
Sperm	مَنى
Wax	مُوم
Erection	نعظ
Nipples	نهود
Fur	وَبَر
Fat	وَدَك
Hip, thigh	ورك
Dirt	وَسَخ
Hand	يَد

2 Other simples

Antimony	إِثْمَد
Calendula	أَذَرْيون
Arak	اراك
Rice	أَرُز
Myrtle	آس

Aster	واسطراطيقوس
Gum ammoniac	اشْق \ وَشْق
Clover dodder	افْتيمون
Absinth	افْسَنْتين
Camomile	أقحوان
Indian gooseberry	أمْلَج
Anise	أنيسون
Myrobalan	أهليلج
Aubergine	باذِنْجان
Broad bean	باقِلى
Ben tree	بان
Seed	بِزْر
Dark psyllium	بِزْر قَطوناء
Onion	بَصَل
Sea onion	بصل الفأر
Legumes	بَقْل
Purslane	بَقْلة حمقاء
Cashew	بَلاذِر
Balsam of Mecca	بَلْسان
Beleric (bastard myrobalan)	بَليلج
White henbane	بَنْج
Sweet Violet	بَنَفْسَج
Borax	بَوْرَق
Armenian borax	بورق ارمني
Dates	تَمْر
Tin	تِنْكار
Bisabol myrrh	جاوشير
Rocket	جَرْجير
Julep, rose water	جُلّاب
Castoreum	جَنْدُ بادَسْتِر
Nut	جَوْز
Orpine	جوز بري
Blue morning-glory	حَب النيل
African bowstring hemp	حَرَق
African lycium	حَضَض
Fenugreek	حُلبة
Asafoetida	حِلتيت
Beach grass	حَلْفاء
Henna	حناء
White henna	حناء ابيض
Chick-pea	حِمّص
Wheat	حِنْطة
Colocynth	حَنْظَل
Chalk	حُوّاري
Mustard	خَرْدَل
Lettuce	خَسّ
Marshmallow	خِطْمي
Lemon grass	خلال المامون
Vinegar	خَلّ
Wine	خَمْر
Galangal	خَولَنجان
Cucumbers	خيار
Spiny broom	دار شَيشعان
Cinnamon	دار صيني
Long pepper	دار فِلْفِل
Leopard’s bane	دَرونَج
[Essential] oil	دُهْن
Fennel	رازَيانج
Ragweed	زُرْبيح
Jelly	رُبّ
Dates (fresh)	رُطب
Pomegranates	رُمّان
Basil	رَيْحان
Yellow vitriol	زاج اصفر

Meerschaum	زُبْد البَحْر
Pharaonic glass	زُجاج فِرْعَوْني
Long aristolochia	زَراوَنْد طويل
Realgar (red arsenic)	زَرْنيخ احمر
Saffron	زَعْفران
Pitch	زِفْت
Lily	زَنْبَق
Ginger	زَنْجَبيل
Cinnabar	زُنْجُفْر
Rue	سَذاب
Sedge	سُعْد
Galingale	سُعْد هندي
Quince	سَفَرْجَل
Persian giant fennel	سَكبِينَج
White sugar	سُكَّر أبيض
Sugar candy, rock candy	سكَّر نبات
Rock sugar	طَبَرْزَد سُكَّر
Oxymel	سَكَنْجَبِين
Turnip	سلجم
Beet	سَلْق
Cassia	سَليخة
Sumach	سُمّاق
Sesame	سُمْسُم
Semolina	سميد
Hyacinth	سُنْبُل
Nardus	سنبل الطيب
Sandarac	سِنْدَرُوس
Liquorice	سُوس
Iris	سوسَن
Fumitory	شاهْتَرج
Alum	شَبّ
Yemeni alum	شبّ يماني
Dill	شِبِث
Wine	شُراب
Barley	شَعير
Red anemones	شَقائق النُعْمان
Wax	شَمع
Indian hemp	شَهْدانَج
Fennel flower	شُونيز
Sesame oil	شِيرَج
Pepperwort	شيطْرَج
Aloe	صَبِر
Vermillion	صَبْغة
Thyme	صَعْتَر
Wild thyme	صَعْتَر جبلي
Pine resin	صَمْغ الصَنَوْبَر
Lotus	ضال
Gypsum	طَباشير
Pitch (liquid)	طِلاء
Root/roots	عِرق/عُروق
Tutsan	عَرينَة
Honey	عَسَل
Gall nut	عَفْص
Black berry	عُلَّيْق
Grapes	عِنَب
Ambergris	عَنْبَر
Sarcocolla	عَنْزَروت
Red squill	عُنْصُل
Sneezewort	عَواطيس
Laurel	غار
Rowan	غُبَيْراء
Cyclamen	غرطنياثا
Saffron	غُمْرة

Radish	فُجل
Bdellium	فَرْك
Black pepper	فِلفِل
White pepper	فِلفِل ابيض
Pennyroyal	فُوذَنْج
Origanum	فُوذَنْج جبلي
Dyer's madder	فوّة
Tuber	قاقس
Capers	قُبّار
Squirting cucumber	قِثّاء الحمار
Alfalfa	قُرْط
Cinnamon	قِرْفة
Clover	قَرَنْفيل/قَرَنْفِل
Sugar cane	قَصَب
Cotton	قُطن
Tar	قَطران
Wheat	قَمْح
Cauliflower	قُنّبيط
Galbanum	قِنّة
Pandang oil plant	كادي
Mediterranean moon carrot	كاشِم
Camphor	كافور
Red brine (vinegar sauce)	كامَخ احمر
Mustard	كَبَر
Sulphur	كِبْريت
Yellow sulfur	كِبْريت اصفر
Linen	كَتّان
Goat's thorn	كَثيراء
Astragale	كَثيراء بيضاء
Leek	كُرّاث
Wild leek	كُرّاث نبطي
Caraway	كَراوْيا

Vetches	كَرْسَنة
Celery	كَرَفْس\ كرفس نبطي
Coriander	كُزْبَرة \ كسبرة
Fumitory	كُشْفَرة
Clover dodder	كُشوث/كُشُت
Lime	كِلْس
Cumin	كَمّون كِرماني
Incense	كُنْدُر
Hellebors	كُنْدُس
Laudanum	لاذن
Frankincense	لُبان
Myrrh	مُرّ
Silver foam	مرتج
	مرتك
Marjoram	مَرْزَنْجوش
Vinegar sauce	مُرّي
Ointment	مَرْهَم
Musk	مِسْك
Iraqi Musk	مسك عراقي
Apricot	مِشْمِش
Mastic	مُصْطَكي
Blue bdellium	مُقْل (ازرق)
Bdellium of the Jews	مقل اليهود
Salt	مِلْح
Bitter salt	ملح مُر
Rock salt	مِلْح اندراني
Storax	ميعة
Wine	نَبيذ
Dog's tooth grass	نجيل\نُجل
Starch	نُشاء
Soda	نَطْرون
Ammonia	نَوشاذر

White acacia	هَراس
Asparagus	هَليون
Rose	وَرْد
Curcuma	وَرْس
Gum ammoniac	وَشْق \ اشْق
Mandrake	يَبْروح

3 Diseases

Retention	احتباس
Urine retention	احتباس البول
Menstrual retention	احتباس الحيض
Convulsions, spasm	اختلاج
Tremor	ارتعاش
Flaccidity	استرخاء
Dropsy	استسقاء
Bowel movement	استطلاق
Diarrhea	اسهال
Inflammation	انتفاخ
Gangrene	آكِلة
Sty	برة
Pustules	بَثْر
Pleurisy	بِرْسام
Spots	بُروشة
Leprosy	بَرَص
Phlegm	بَلْغَم
Breathlessness, breath difficulties	بُهْر
Vitiligo	بَهَق
Haemorrhoids	بَواسير
Glaucoma	بَياض
Chilblains	تثلج
Indigestion	تُخْمة
Dripping	تقطير
Warts	ثُؤْلول/ثآليل
Smallpox	جُدَري
Elephantiasis	جُذام
Scabies	جَرَب
Wound	جُرْح
Pleurisy	جَنْب
Nyctalopia	جُهْر
Pustules	حَبّ
Impetigo	حَزازة
Stones	حَصاة
Dry scabies	حَصَف
Itch	حكة
Erysipelas	حُمْر\حمرة
Hectic fever	حُمّي الدق
Quartan fever	حُمّي رُبع
Intermittent fever	حمي الغِبّ
Tertian fever	حمي مثلثة
Fever with shivers	حُمّي نافض
Palpitations	خَفَقان
Scrofula	خَنازير
Suffocation	خوانيق
Alopecia	داء الثَعْلَب
Bubo	دبول
Ulcer	دُبَيْلة
Lachrymation	دَمْعة
Varicose veins	دوالي
Worms	دُود
Buzz	دَوِي
Asthma	رَبْو
Convulsions	رَجفان
Convulsions	رَجيف
Proplapse, flaccidity	رخاء

Moistness	رطوبة
Nose bleed	رُعاف
Tremor	رعشة
Inflammation of the eye	رَمَد
Winds	ريح
Dysentery	زَحير
Magic	سِحْر
Obstruction	سَدَد
Cancer	سَرطان
Cough	سُعال
Chronic cough	سعال قديم
Apnoea	سقوط النفس
Incontinence	سَلَس
Sore	سَلْعة
Consumption	سِلّ
Poison	سَمّ
Stoutness	سُمْن
Insomnia	سَهَر
Skin eruption with itch	شَرى
Laceration	شَقّ
Migraine	شَقيقة
White hair	شَيب
Scabies	شَرْي
Headache	صُداع
Epilepsy	صَرْع
Yellow bile	صفار
Yellow colour, paleness	صفرة
Deafness	صَمَم
Deafness	طراش
Pang, sharp pain	ضَرْب
Obscuration of the eyesight	ظُلْمة
Ulcer (animals)	عَرَن
Difficult breath	عُسْر النفس
Bite	عِضّة
Sterility	عُقْر
Cataract	غَشاوة
Rheum	عُمْش
Indisposition	غشي
Paralysis	فالِج
Night terror	فَزَع
Winds	فساء
Lesion of the first vertebra of the neck	فهاق
Irregular breath	فواق
Particles in the eye	قذاة
Ulcer	قَرْح
Ringworm	قَرَع
Colic	قَولَنج
Tetter	قُوبة
Catarrh	قَيح
Stiffness	كُزاز
Fracture	كَسْر
Freckles	كَلَف
Bite, sting	لَدْغ
Sting	لَسْعَة
Facial paralysis	لَقوة
Effeminate man	مُخنّث
Excrescence on the leg of working beasts	مَشَش
Gripes	مَغْص
Feverish heat	مَليلة
Odour	نَتِن
Loss of blood	نَزْف
Catarrh	نَزْلة
Fistula	ناصور/ناسور
Forgetfulness	نسيان

Evil eye	نَظْرة	Contusion	وُثْي
Gout	نِقْرِس	Swelling	وَرامة
Freckles, discolored spots	نَمَش	Swelling, intumescence	وَرَم
Small swollen pustules	نَمْل	Obsession	وَسواس
Tingle	نملة	Leprosy	وَضَح
Emaciation	هزال	Delivery	وِلادة
Excitement	هَيْج	Jaundice	يَرَقان

English-Arabic Glossary

1 Animal parts and substances

Abdomen, belly	بَطْن
Abdomen	جَوْف
Anklebone	كَعْب
Anus	فم الصفرة
Appendance of the liver	زيادة الكبد
Arm	عَضُد
Armpit	إبط
Back	دُبْر
Beak	مِنْقار
Bladder	مَثانة
Body	بَدَن
Bone	عِظْم
Bowels	أحْشاء
Breast	ثَدي
Breast	حِلمة
Buttocks	مَقْعَدة
Chest	جَيْب
Claw	كَفّ
Claws	مَخالب
Craw of a bird	حَوصلة
Dirt	وَسَخ
Droppings	بَعْرة
Droppings (of bird)	ذَرْق
Dung	زَبْل
Duodenum	اعفاج
Entrails	مُصران
Epiglottis	غَلْصَمَة
Erection	نعظ
Excrement	خُرْء
Excrement	رَجيع
Excrement	رَوْث
Extremity of the ribs	بستامزك
Eyelid	جَفْن
Eyebrow	حاجب
Fat	شَحْم
Fat	وَدَك
Fingers	إصْباع
Foot	رِجْل
Forearm	ذراع
Forehead	جَبْهَة
Forehead, temples	جَبين
Foreskin	قُلفة
Fur	وَبَر
Fuzz	زَغب
Gall	مرارة
Gizzard	قانصة
Grease	دَسَم
Groin	حقو
Gullet	حُلقوم
Gum	لِثة
Hand, paw	يَد
Hip, waist	خاصِرة
Hip, thigh	ورك
Hoof	خُفّ
Hoof (cloven)	ظِلْف
Hump	سَنام
Intestine	أمعاء
Ivory	عاج
Jawbone	لُحي

Joints مفاصل

Juice عُصارة

Kidney كُلْوة \ كُلْية \ كُلى

Knee ركبة

Leg فَخْذ

Leg قائمة

Legs (lower part) سِفْلة

Lip شَفة

Liver كَبِد

Liver معاليق

Lung رِيّة

Marrow مُخّ

Menstrual blood حَيْضة

Menstruation حَيْض

Milk لَبَن

Milk (cow) لَبَن حَليب

Milk (sour) لبن حامض

Milk of a pregnant woman غيل

Molar ضِرْس

Nape رَقَبة

Neck عُنُق

Nerve عَصَب

Nipples نهود

Nostril مَنْخَرة

Outer opening of the urethra إحْليل

Palate حَنَك

Penis ذَكَر

Penis قضيب

Phlegm بَلْغَم

Placenta مَشيمة

Rennet إنْفَحة

See also منفحة

Rennet منفحة

See also إنْفَحة

Roe بطارخ

Saliva بُصاق

Saliva ريق

Saliva لُعاب

Shoulder, shoulder blade كَتِف

Skull جُمْجُمة

Skull قِحْف

Slough سَلْخ

Sperm مَنى

Spine صُلْب

Spleen طِحال

Stomach مَعِدة

Tail ذَنَب

Temple فود

Testicle خُصيَة

Throat (back of the) حَلْق

Tibia, shinbone كُراع

Tongue لسان

Umbilicus سُرة

Urine بَوْل

Uterus رَحم

Uvula, throat لِهاية/لهاة

Vertebra خَرَزة

Wax مُوم

2 Other simples

Absinth افْسَنْتين

African bowstring hemp حَرَق

African lycium حَضَض

Alfalfa قُرْط

Aloe	صَبِر
Alum	شَبّ
Ambergris	عَنْبَر
Ammonia	نَوشاذر
Anise	أنيسون
Antimony	إثْمَد
Apricot	مِشْمِش
Armenian borax	بورق ارمني
Arak	اراك
Asafoetida	حِلتيت
Asparagus	هَليون
Aster	واسطراطيقوس
Astragale	كَثيراء بيضاء
Aubergine	باذِنْجان
Balsam of Mecca	بَلْسان
Barley	شَعير
Basil	رَيْحان
Bdellium	فَرْك
Bdellium of the Jews	مقل اليهود
Beach grass	حَلْفاء
Beet	سَلْق
Beleric	بَليلج
Ben tree	بان
Bisabol myrrh	جاوشير
Bitter salt	ملح مُر
Black berry	عُلَّيق
Black pepper	فِلفِل
Blue bdellium	مُقْل (ازرق)
Blue morning-glory	حَب النيل
Borax	بَوْرَق
Broad bean	باقِلى
Calendula	أذَرْيون

Camomile	أقحوان
Camphor	كافور
Capers	قُبّار
Caraway	كَراوْيا
Cashew	بَلاذِر
Cassia	سَليخة
Castoreum	جَنْدُ بادَسْتِر
Cauliflower	قُنَّبيط
Celery	كَرَفْس\ كرفس نبطي
Chick-pea	حِمّص
Cinnabar	زُنْجُفْر
Cinnamon	دار صيني
Cinnamon	قِرْفة
Clover	قَرَنْفيل/قَرَنْفِل
Clover dodder	افتيمون
Clover dodder	كُشوث/كُشُت
Colocynth	حَنْظَل
Coriander	كُزْبَرة \ كسبرة
Cyclamen	غرطنياثا
Wheat	قَمْح
Cotton	قُطُن
Cucumber	خيار
Cumin	كَمّون كِرماني
Curcuma	وَرْس
Dark psyllium	بِزْر قَطوناء
Dates	تَمْر
Dates (fresh)	رُطب
Dill	شِبِث
Dog's tooth grass	نجيل\نُجل
Dyer's madder	فوّة
[Essential] oil	دُهْن
Fennel	رازِيانج

Fennel flower	شُونيز
Fenugreek	حُلبة
Frankincense	لُبان
Fumitory	شاهْتَرج
Fumitory	كُسْفَرة
Galangal	خَولَنجان
Galbanum	قِنّة
Galingale	سُعْد هندي
Gall nut	عَفْص
Ginger	زَنْجَبيل
Goat's thorn	كَثيراء
Grapes	عِنَب
Gum ammoniac	اشق \ وَشق
Gypsum	حُوّاري
Gypsum	طَباشير
Hellebors	كُنْدُس
Henna	حناء
Honey	عَسَل
Hyacinth	سُنْبُل
Incense	كُنْدُر
Indian gooseberry	أمْلَج
Indian hemp	شَهْدانَج
Iraqi musk	مسك عراقي
Iris	سوسَن
Jelly	رُبّ
Julep	جُلّاب
Laudanum	لاذُن
Laurel	غار
Leek	كُرّاث
Legumes	بَقْل
Lemon grass	خلال المامون
Leopard's bane	دَرونَج
Lettuce	خَسّ
Lily	زَنْبَق
Lime	كِلْس
Linen	كَتّان
Liquorice	سُوس
Long aristolochia	زَراوَنْد طويل
Long pepper	دار فِلْفِل
Lotus	ضال
Mandrake	يَبْروح
Marjoram	مَرْزَنْجوش
Marshmallow	خِطْمي
Mastic	مُصْطَكي
Mediterranean moon carrot	كاشِم
Meerschaum	زُبْد البَحْر
Musk	مِسْك
Mustard	خَرْدَل
Mustard	كَبَر
Myrobalan	أهليلج
Myrrh	مُرّ
Myrtle	آس
Nardus	سنبل الطيب
Nut	جَوْز
Ointment	مَرْهَم
Onion	بَصَل
Origanum	فُوذَنْج جبلي
Orpine	جوز بري
Oxymel	سَكَنْجَبين
Pandang oil plant	كادي
Pennyroyal	فُوذَنْج
Pepperwort	شيطَرَج
Persian giant fennel	سَكبينَج
Pharaonic glass	زُجاج فِرْعَوْني

Pine resin	صَمْغ الصَنَوْبَر
Pitch	زِفْت
Pitch (liquid)	طِلاء
Pomegranates	رُمّان
Purslane	بَقْلة حمقاء
Quince	سَفَرْجَل
Radish	فُجْل
Ragweed	زُرْبيح
Realgar (red arsenic)	زَرْنيخ احمر
Red anemones	شَقائق النُعْمان
Red brine (vinegar sauce)	كامَخ احمر
Red squill	عُنْصُل
Rice	أرُزّ
Rock salt	مِلْح اندراني
Rock sugar	طَبَرْزَد سُكّر
Rocket	جَرْجير
Root/roots	عِرق/عُروق
Rose	وَرْد
Rowan	غُبَيْراء
Rue	سَذاب
Saffron	زَعْفَران
Saffron	عُمْرة
Salt	مِلْح
Sandarac	سِنْدَرُوس
Sarcocolla	عَنْزَروت
Sea onion	بصل الفأر
Sedge	سُعْد
Seed	بِزْر
Semolina	سميد
Sesame	سُمْسُم
Sesame oil	شِيرَج
Silver foam	مرتج
	مرتك
Sneezewort	عَواطيس
Soda	نَطْرون
Spiny broom	دار شَيشعان
Squirting cucumber	قِثّاء الحمار
Starch	نُشاء
Storax	ميعة
Sugar candy	سكّر نبات
Sugar cane	قَصَب
Sulphur	كِبْريت
Sumach	سُمّاق
Sweet Violet	بَنَفْسَج
Tar	قَطران
Thyme	صَعْتَر
Tin	تِنْكار
Tuber	قاقس
Turnip	سلجم
Tutsan	عَرِينَة
Vermillion	صَبْغة
Vetches	كَرْسَنَة
Vinegar	خَلّ
Vinegar sauce	مُرّي
Wax	شَمع
Wheat	حِنْطة
White acacia	هَراس
White henbane	بَنْج
White henna	حناء ابيض
White pepper	فِلفِل ابيض
White sugar	سُكّر أبيض
Wild leek	كُرّاث نبطي
Wild thyme	صَعْتَر جبلي
Wine	خَمْر

Wine	شُراب
Wine	نَبيذ
Yellow vitriol	زاج اصفر
Yellow sulfur	كِبْريت اصفر
Yemeni alum	شبّ يماني

3 Diseases

Alopecia	داء الثَّعْلَب
Asthma	رَبْو
Bite	عِضّة
Bite, sting	لَدْغ
Bowel movement	استطلاق
Breathlessness, breath difficulties	بُهْر
Bubo	دبول
Buzz	دَوِي
Cancer	سَرطان
Cataract	غشاوة
Catarrh	قَيْح
Catarrh	نَزلة
Chilblains	تثلج
Chronic cough	سعال قديم
Colic	قولَنج
Consumption	سِلّ
Contusion	وُثي
Convulsions, spasm	اختلاج
Convulsions	رَجفان
Convulsions	رَجيف
Cough	سُعال
Deafness	صَمَم
Deafness	طراش
Delivery	وِلادة
Difficult breath	عُسْر النفس
Diarrhea	اسهال
Dripping	تقطير
Dropsy	استسقاء
Dry scabies	حَصَف
Dysentery	زَحير
Effeminate man	مُخنّث
Elephantiasis	جُذام
Emaciation	هزال
Epilepsy	صَرْع
Erysipelas	حُمْرا حمرة
Evil eye	نَظْرة
Excitement	هَيْج
Excrescence on the leg of working beasts	مَشَش
Facial paralysis	لَقوة
Fever	حُمّى
Fever with shivers	حُمّى نافض
Feverish heat	مَليلة
Fistula	ناصور/ناسور
Flaccidity	استرخاء
Forgetfulness	نسيان
Fracture	كَسْر
Freckles	كَلَف
Freckles, discolored spots	نَمَش
Gangrene	آكِلة
Glaucoma	بَياض
Gout	نِقْرِس
Gripes	مَغْص
Haemorrhoids	بَواسير
Headache	صُداع
Hectic fever	حُمّى الدق
Impetigo	حَزازة
Incontinence	سَلَس

Indigestion	تُخْمة
Indisposition	غشى
Inflammation	انتفاخ
Inflammation of the eye	رَمَد
Insomnia	سَهَر
Intermittent fever	حُمّى الغِبّ
Irregular breath	فواق
Itch	حكة
Jaundice	يَرَقان
Laceration	شَقّ
Lachrymation	دَمْعة
Leprosy	بَرَص
Leprosy	وَضَح
Lesion of the first vertebra of the neck	فهاق
Loss of blood	نَزْف
Magic	سِحْر
Menstrual retention	احتباس الحيض
Migraine	شَقيقة
Moistness	رطوبة
Night terror	فَزَع
Nose bleed	رِعاف
Nyctalopia	جُهْر
Obscuration of the eyesight	ظُلْمة
Obsession	وَسواس
Obstruction	سَدَد
Odour	نَتِن
Palpitations	خَفَقان
Paralysis	فالِج
Pang, sharp pain	ضَرْب
Particles in the eye	قذاة
Phlegm	بَلْغم
Pleurisy	بِرْسام
Pleurisy	جَنْب
Poison	سَمّ
Proplapse, flaccidity	رخاء
Pustules	بَثْر
Pustules	حَبّ
Quartan fever	حُمّي رُبع
Retention	احتباس
Rheum	عُمْش
Ringworm	قَرَع
Scabies	جَرَب
Scabies	شَرْي
Scrofula	خَنازير
Skin eruption with itch	شَرى
Small swollen pustules	نَمْل
Smallpox	جُدَري
Sore	سَلْعة
Spots	بُروشة
Sterility	عُقْر
Stiffness	كُزاز
Sting	لَسْعَة
Stones	حَصاة
Stoutness	سُمْن
Sty	برة
Suffocation	خوانيق
Swelling	وَرامة
Swelling, intumescence	وَرَم
Tertian fever	حُمّى مثلثة
Tetter	قُوَبة
Tingle	نملة
Tremor	ارتعاش
Tremor	رعشة
Ulcer	دُبَيْلة

Ulcer	قَرْح
Ulcer (animals)	عَرَن
Urine retention	احتباس البول
Varicose veins	دوالي
Vitiligo	بَهَق
Warts	ثُؤْلول/ثآليل
White hair	شَيب
Wind	ريح / رِياح
Winds	فساء
Worms	دُود
Wound	جُرْح
Yellow bile	صفار
Yellow colour, paleness	صفرة